Recent Results in Cancer Research 53

Fortschritte der Krebsforschung
Progrès dans les recherches sur le cancer

A. Clarysse   Y. Kenis   G. Mathé

Cancer Chemotherapy

Its Role in the Treatment Strategy of
Hematologic Malignancies and Solid Tumors

With 154 Figures

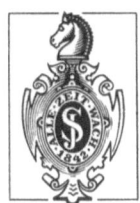

Springer-Verlag
Berlin   Heidelberg   New York 1976

Revised and enlarged edition of:
MATHÉ et KENIS: La Chimiothérapie des Cancers, 3e édition
Copyright © 1973, 1975 by
Expansion Scientifique Française, Paris

ALBERT CLARYSSE, MD, FACP, Chief, Division of Cancer
Chemotherapy, Sint Janshospitaal, Bruges, Belgium,
and Former Assistant Professor of Medicine, University
of Utah School of Medicine, Salt Lake City, U.S.A.

YVON KENIS, MD, Division of Cancer Chemotherapy,
Institut Jules Bordet, Brussels, Belgium

GEORGES MATHÉ, MD, Professor of Oncology, University
of Paris Sud; Institut de Cancérologie et d'Immunogénétique,
Hopital Paul Brousse; Division of Hematology,
Institut Gustave Roussy, Villejuif, France

Sponsored by the Swiss League against Cancer

ISBN 978-3-540-07055-9   ISBN 978-3-642-81010-7 (eBook)
DOI 10.1007/978-3-642-81010-7

Library of Congress Cataloging in Publication Data. Clarysse, A. 1936— Cancer
chemotherapy. (Recent results in cancer research; v. 53.) Rev. and enl. translation of the 3d ed. of La chimiothérapie des cancers; by G. Mathé and Y. Kenis.
Includes bibliographical references and index. 1. Cancer — Chemotherapy.
2. Antineoplastic agents. I. Kenis, Yvon, joint author. II. Mathé, Georges, 1922—
joint author. III. Mathé, Georges, 1922— La chimiothérapie des cancers. IV. Title.
V. Series. [DNLM: 1. Antineoplastic agents — Therapeutic use. 2. Neoplasms —
Drug therapy. Wl RE106P v. 53/QZ267 C614c.] RC261.R35 vol. 53 [RC271.C5]
616.9'94'008s [616.9'94'061] 75-43554.

Introduction

This book is addressed primarily to the practicing oncologist
and hematologist and to others who may not be able personally
to scan the plethora of papers discussing the use of cytotoxic
agents in the treatment of cancer. In addition, anyone in any
way concerned with the problem of cancer or its treatment
— be he internist, surgeon, radiotherapist, family physician,
basic researcher, or pharmacologist — will find some useful
information here. We especially wish physicians who may see
cancer patients in their practice to be informed about the
progress being made in the management of advanced cancer,
particularly the indications for therapy and the results. Our
greatest concern is that every patient should receive the best
therapy currently available.

This text is the first English edition of *La chimiothérapie des
cancers* by G. Mathé. The two earlier editions have been completely revised, enlarged, and updated. Some of the authors
have worked on both sides of the Atlantic, so that European
and American points of view have been integrated, hopefully
to advantage.

The first part outlines the basic principles of cancer chemotherapy. Certain aspects of cellular and molecular biology, and
of tumor cell characteristics and kinetics are reviewed because
they are necessary to an understanding of the mechanisms of
action of cytotoxic drugs. The reader is given the experimental
data on which current chemotherapy protocols are based and
shown how they are applied to the clinical situation. In view
of the importance of organized cooperative trials, several
chapters describe the different phases of preclinical and clinical
trials and the practical aspects of treatment with cytotoxic
agents.

A considerable portion of this review has been devoted to a
discussion of general principles because they constitute the
rationale upon which current and future chemotherapeutic
protocols are based. As our understanding of these principles
increases, it is no longer enough to hand out cookbook-type
recipes for cancer chemotherapy.

On several occasions we have, for sake of clarity, made state-
ments on issues that are still under debate; for example, the
classification of cytotoxic agents according to their effect on
the cell cycle.

The second part of the book deals with the treatment of various hematologic malignancies and solid tumors. All through this textbook, we discuss chemotherapy in the context of the overall treatment strategy, the aim of which is to cure the patient. A cure requires that all cancer cells be killed. The strategy includes four treatment modalities, each of which may play a specific rote in the achievement of a cure, according to the stage of the disease at which the patient presents for treatment.

For each disease entity we have reviewed the effectiveness of the various conventional and experimental cytotoxic agents, used singly and in various combinations. The reader will appreciate that such information can only be relative. Most of it is based on data obtained by a number of authors, using different schedules and different criteria to evaluate response, and treating different patient populations, often in trials that are not comparable. When a particular regimen is clearly superior, we have indicated this. The authors do not claim to be without some personal bias, but every effort has been made to consider different opinions. Special recommendations are based on treatment schedules for which adequate data have been published. At the Institut de Cancérologie et d'Immunogénétique and at the Institut Gustave Roussy we are investigating protocols that exploit the phenomena of cell synchronization, recruitment, and potentiation. We hope by these means to improve existing regimens, but we must wait until we have sufficient data to justify their use.

The reader may sometimes have the impression that not much in the way of conclusions can be drawn from the results listed in various tables. Unfortunately, this is all too true. This vagueness serves to stress the necessity for controlled trials and organized studies to obtain answers to specific questions.

The need for more uniformity in terminology, staging classifications and procedures, criteria for evaluating responses, and methods for reporting results is also repeatedly emphasized. Without uniformity in such matters, the institutions and treatment groups cannot be compared.

We constantly stress the need for a concerted effort in the management of cancer patients: at the time of diagnosis and at various stages in the course of the illness, a case should be discussed by a surgeon, a radiotherapist, a chemotherapist and nowadays an immunotherapist. We anticipate that in the years to come a significant effort will be made to employ systematic chemotherapy and immunotherapy to supplement surgery or radiotherapy in apparently localized disease. If the results of treating residual disease by systematic chemotherapy have so far been of questionable value, this may be because it was carried out under suboptimal conditions. The next decade should confirm whether adjuvant therapy of good quality is capable of improving the overall cure rate of one in three cancer patients. The cooperative approach is usually practicable only in centers or clinics that specialize in the treatment of cancer, but it in no way excludes the participation of the

family doctor. On the contrary, he becomes an integral part
of a team that takes care of his patient from diagnosis until
death, if not cure.
This work is based on the observations of many dedicated and
competent researchers and clinicians. Some important contributions may well have escaped our attention and hence fail to
appear in this text. We also realize the temporary value of a
work of this nature. Chemotherapy is a rapidly changing discipline and many recommendations made today may no longer
be valid a couple of years from now.
We have tried to keep the contents updated as much as
possible during the time-consuming process of publication.
Complementary data can be found in G. Mathé:
Cancer Active Immunotherapy, Immunoprophylaxis and Immunorestoration. Springer-Verlag, 1976. Readers are urgent
to check the original articles for the correctness of dosage
schedules, modes of administration, toxicity and special
precautions.

Acknowledgements

We wish to thank JENNIFER TOVEY, MARIE-ANNE BONNAMY
and NICOLE VRIZ for secreterial assistance. The reading of the
manuscript by Dr. LOUIS BALIZET enabled us to cut out some
of the errors in the English language. We are also indebted to
the contributors to former French editions of this text and to
the publishers, Springer-Verlag.

A. CLARYSSE, Y. KENIS, G. MATHÉ

Contents

Chapter 1
The History of Cancer Chemotherapy

Surgery, the first form of treatment for cancer, was already known to the Egyptians but cures were limited to localized disease. At the turn of the present century it was realized that radiotherapy could accomplish the same effect in certain localized radiosensitive tumors. Chemotherapy did not establish itself as a mode of therapy until World War II. Nevertheless, caustic applications were used as long ago as 500 BC, and at various times in the past 1500 years concentrated acids or alkalis and various metals or metalloids, such as arsenic, mercury, zinc chloride, copper salts, silver nitrates and salts of antimony, have been advocated for the local treatment of cancer. EISENMANN treated skin papillomas with podophyllotoxin preparations (1860) (1). The systemic administration of chemicals was introduced by LISSAUER (1865), who reported marked symptomatic improvement following the use of potassium arsenite (Fowler's solution) in leukemia (2). However, the early results of chemotherapy were unimpressive. Several breakthroughs occurred in the late 1930's and resulted in the first effective chemotherapy. Among these were the observation that colchicine acts as a mitotic poison (DUSTIN, LITS, 1934) (3,4), the introduction of estrogens for prostatic cancer (HUGGINS and HODGES, 1941) (5), androgens for breast cancer (LOESER, 1939) (6), actinomycin (WAKSMAN and WOODRUFF, 1940) (7), nitrogen mustard (GILMAN et al., 1942) (8), and the discovery of the lymphopenic effect of corticosteroids (DOUGHERTY and WHITE, 1944) (9). FARBER obtained the first remissions in childhood acute leukemia with aminopterin in 1948 (10) and demonstrated the clinical value of actinomycin D (11), thereby generating interest in substances produced by micro-organisms. Although the antimitotic action of podophyllotoxin and colchicine had been known for some time, mitotic poisons had no great importance until the discovery of the leukopenic effect of the Vinca alkaloids by BEER (1955) (12).

In spite of initial enthusiasm, cancer chemotherapists soon learned that remissions are almost always temporary and that emergence of resistance is the rule rather than the exception. Furthermore, the realization that cytotoxic drugs never kill 100 percent of the tumor cells but only a constant fraction, irrespective of the number present (13), may have supplied another argument for those who wanted to abandon this approach to the cancer problem. However, subsequent progress has confirmed the value of this discipline, both as a form of therapy in clinical oncology, and as an investigational tool in cell biology. A large number of agents has become available. We have learned to administer them in more effective schedules and combinations and in association with radiotherapy or surgery. The value of cytotoxic drugs has been confirmed by the cures obtained in choriocarcinoma and in Burkitt's lymphoma (14, 15, 16), two tumors in which immune mechanisms are important, and by the long-term survival rates in certain acute leukemias and hematosarcomas. The results for solid tumors are admittedly less dramatic. Additionally, the introduction of chemotherapeutic agents into molecular biology has permitted the study of cellular mechanisms, especially the role of nucleic acids in protein synthesis.

About the same time that it was learned that chemotherapy rarely kills the last cell, immunotherapy appeared on the scene. This treatment is based on the premise that tumor cells possess specific antigens that can elicit both a humoral and a cellular response from the host. Immunotherapy follows "zero-order kinetics", that is a specific number of immunocompetent cells or antibodies is required for the lysis of each tumor cell. The advantage of this method is that all tumor cells, including the last one, can be destroyed. Both experimental and clinical trials indicate that immune mechanisms can destroy only a small number of cells, not more than 10^5. Therefore, immunotherapy has been utilized to eliminate residual disease after the bulk of the tumor population has been reduced by other treatment modalities (17).

Thus we now have four treatment modalities available to treat malignant disease: surgery, radiotherapy, chemotherapy, and immunotherapy (still largely experimental). Each of these modes of therapy has its proper indications, and several or all of them may be called upon at some stage or another in the general strategy aimed at the total destruction of the tumor cell population (18). It is within the perspective of this overall cancer strategy that we discuss the role of chemotherapy.

In recent years it has been realized that chemotherapy is most effective against a small number of tumor cells. This has led to the use of chemotherapy early in the disease or as an adjuvant immediately after primary treatment with surgery or radiotherapy has reduced the bulk tumor mass. This approach has already yielded encouraging results in the treatment of Wilms' tumor, osteogenic sarcoma, Ewing's sarcoma, Hodgkin's disease and breast cancer. It is anticipated that adjuvant chemotherapy will play an important role in the treatment of cancer in the years to come.

REFERENCES

1. EISENMANN,   : Über die locale Wirkung der Sabina. Virchows. Arch. 18, 171 (1860).
2. LISSAUER,   : In Bendorf: Zwei Fälle von Leukämie. Berl. klin. Wschr. 40, 403 (1865).
3. DUSTIN, A.P.: Contribution à l'étude de l'action des poisons caryoclasiques sur les tumeurs animales. Action de la colchicine sur le sarcome greffé, type Crocker, de la souris. Bull. Acad. roy. Méd. Belg. 14, 487 (1934).
4. LITS, F.: Contribution à l'étude des réactions cellulaires provoquées par la colchicine. C.R. Soc. Biol. (Paris) 115, 1421 (1934).
5. HUGGINS, C., HODGES, C.V.: Studies on prostatic cancer. I. The effect of castration, of estrogen and of androgen injection on serum phosphatases in metastatic carcinoma of the prostate. Cancer Res. 1, 293 (1941).
6. LOESER, A.A.: Male hormone in the treatment of cancer of the breast. Acta U.I.C.C. 4, 375 (1939).
7. WAKSMAN, S.A., WOODRUFF, H.B.: Bacteriostatic and bactericidal substances produced by a soil actinomyces. Proc. Soc. exp. Biol. (N.Y.) 45, 609 (1940).
8. GILMAN, A.: The initial clinical trial of nitrogen mustard. Amer. J. Surg. 105, 574 (1963).

9. DOUGHERTY, T.F., WHITE, A.: Influence of hormones on lymphoid tissue structure and function. Role of pituitary adrenotrophic hormone in regulation of lymphocytes and other cellular elements of blood. Endocrinology 35, 1 (1943).
10. FARBER, S., DIAMOND, L.K., MERCER, R.D., SYLVESTER, R.F., WOLFF, J.A.: Temporary remissions in acute leukemia in children produced by folic acid antagonist, 4-aminopteroyl-glutamic acid. New Engl. J. Med. 238, 787 (1948).
11. FARBER, MADDOCK, C., SWAFFIELD, M.: Studies on the carcinolytic and other biological activity of actinomycin D. Proc. amer. Ass. Cancer Res. 2, 104 (1956).
12. BEER, C.T.: The leucopenic action of extracts of Vinca rosea. British Empire Cancer Campaign, 33rd Annual Report 487 (1955).
13. SKIPPER, H.E., SCHABEL, Jr., F.M., WILCOX, W.S.: Experimental evaluation of potential anticancer agents. XIII. On the criteria and kinetics associated with "curability" of experimental leukemia. Cancer Chemother. Rep. 35, 1 (1964).
14. LI, M.C., HERTZ, R., SPENCER, D.B.: Effect of methotrexate therapy upon choriocarcinoma and chorioadenoma. Proc. Soc. exp. Biol. Med. 93, 361 (1956).
15. BURKITT, D., HUTT, M.S.R., WRIGHT, D.H.: The African lymphoma. Preliminary observations on response to therapy. Cancer 18, 399 (1965).
16. NGU, V.A.: The African lymphoma (Burkitt tumor): survivals exceeding two years. Brit. J. Cancer 19, 101 (1965).
17. MATHE, G.: Active immunotherapy. Advanc. Cancer Res. 14,1 (1971).
18. MATHE, G.: La dernière cellule. Presse méd. 75, 2591 (1967).

Chapter 2
Basic Cell Biology

Tremendous progress has been made in the past two decades in our knowledge of the structure and function of cells. In order to understand
carcinogenesis and cancer chemotherapy, one must be familiar with the
basic biology of both the normal and the cancer cell. Chemotherapy attempts to destroy tumor cells through interference with essential molecular processes. The ideal cancer drug would be one that kills tumor
cells without damaging the normal cells of the host. Unfortunately the
cause of cancer remains obscure and it is impossible to pin down definite differences between normal and cancer cells. Cancer chemotherapy is
therefore largely empirical and nonspecific; it damages normal cells
too, especially rapidly proliferating ones, though hopefully to a
lesser extent than malignant cells.

A. THE NORMAL CELL

1. The Cell Structure

The cell is the smallest complete structural and functional unit in
the body (1-3). In unicellular organisms all vital processes take place
in a single cell. Higher organisms, including man, originate their development in a single fertilized germ cell. Even in multicellular organisms the cell is still the primary unit of all functions that maintain life.

Traditionally, the cell is described as a mass of cytoplasm containing a
nucleus with its nucleoli (Fig. 2-1). Various organelles can be distinguished with the electron microscope. The cell, nucleus and organelles
are all lined by membranes, called "unit membranes." The presumed general structure of these membranes is that of a double layer of polar lipid
molecules; embedded in this lipid matrix are proteins that make up the
membrane's active sites. Unit membrane is semipermeable, allowing metabolic exchange with the surrounding environment (4).

The nucleus is the most important component of the cell. It is made up
largely of chromosomes; these are the cellular location of genes, and
they control and regulate the hereditary characteristics, function, and
reproduction of the cell. Each chromosome consists of a giant molecule
of DNA plus supporting protein. Each gene is a portion of the DNA molecule. Chromosomes are visible as such only during mitosis; between cell
divisions they are contained in the irregular clumps of chromatin.

The nucleus also contains one or more nucleoli, which are rich in RNA
and probably involved in the synthesis of ribosomal RNA. Chromatin and
nucleoli are bathed in the nuclear juice or nucleoplasm. The nucleus

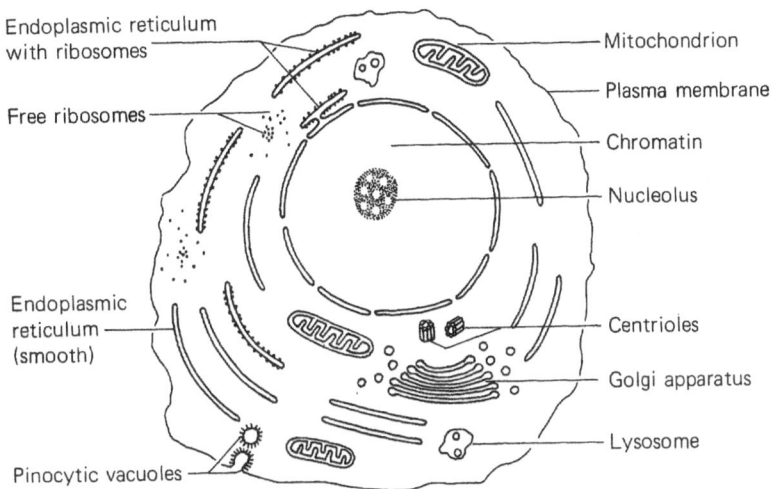

Fig. 2-1. Schematic view of the ultrastructure of the cell in interphase

has a double-layered <u>membrane</u> and the spaces between the two layers
are referred to as <u>perinuclear cisterns</u>. The nuclear membrane has pores
that are closed by a thin, homogeneous membrane. Molecules as large as
RNA can pass from the nucleus into the cytoplasm, thus indicating that
the nuclear membrane is quite permeable.

Extending throughout most of the cytoplasm is the <u>endoplasmic reticulum</u>,
a complex system of tubules of unit membrane usually arranged in paral-
lel rows (<u>5, 6</u>). The endoplasmic reticulum is contiguous with the nuclear membrane and may be either smooth (agranular) or rough (granular).
<u>Agranular</u> endoplasmic reticulum may, depending on the cell type, be
the site of steroid synthesis, detoxification processes, or glycogen
storage. <u>Granular</u> endoplasmic reticulum owes its roughness to the presence on its surface of ribosomes that take part in protein synthesis.
<u>Ribosomes</u> can also be found freely dispersed in the cytoplasm. They are
small organelles composed of roughly equal parts of protein and RNA
(ribosomal RNA) and are structured in two subunits, one large and one
small.

The <u>Golgi apparatus</u> is a system of sacs, vesicles, and vacuoles of
unit membrane, usually located near the nucleus (<u>7</u>). It is particularly
prominent in secreting cells, where it is found between the nucleus and
the secretory pole of the cell. The role of the Golgi apparatus appears
to be concerned with the packaging of the proteins, hormones, and enzymes secreted by the cell into membrane-lined secretory granules that
then find their way to the surface of the cell.

The cytoplasm also contains <u>mitochondria</u>, generally elongated bodies,
the size, shape, number, and distribution of which varies with the function of the cell. They are made up of two unit membranes surrounding
an inner lumen that contains a protein and lipid matrix. Mitochondria
are the power generators of the cell. Products of the catabolic breakdown of carbohydrates, lipids and proteins are supplied to the mitochondria and are oxidized by the enzymes of the citric-acid cycle (Krebs
cycle), which are contained in the outer membrane. The inner membrane
contains the enzymes of the electron-transport chain and provides a
means for trapping the energy derived from the oxidative reactions in

the form of the high-energy phosphate bond of ATP (oxidative phosphory-lation). This energy then becomes available to the cell for energy-re-quiring processes (8). Mitochondria also contain some DNA and are ca-pable of synthesizing some of the mitochondrial proteins. The mitochon-drial DNA appears to represent a genetic system that is separate from but not independent of nuclear inheritance.

Lysosomes also form a heterogeneous group of cytoplasmic organelles; they are sacs of unit membrane filled with hydrolytic enzymes primarily concerned with the digestive and lytic processes of the cell: elimina-tion of undesirable exogenous substances and autolysis of nonviable portions of the cell. (9, 10, 11). They vary in size, number, and en-zyme content with the type of cell and its physiologic status. The en-tire scope of their physiologic and pathologic significance has not yet been elucidated.

The structure and function of the centrioles, two short cylinders lo-cated near the nucleus, is described below under cell division.

2. Molecular Biology

The advances made in unravelling the structure of the cellular compo-nents have been equalled by those achieved in understanding their func-tion at the molecular level.

The importance of the nucleus as the director of cellular function is thought to be due to the nucleoproteins in its chromatin. They deter-mine the genetic characteristics of the cell and are involved in pro-tein synthesis (12, 13). The synthesis of proteins is extremely impor-tant in cell function, since all the enzymes that catalyze chemical re-actions and most of the important structures of the cell are basically composed of proteins.

(i) Structure of Nucleic Acids
Nucleoproteins are conjugated proteins that consist of nucleic acid as the prosthetic group plus a protein, generally histone or protamine. The exact function of histones is not clearly known, but they are thought to exert an inhibitory function (14, 15). Genes that are not functioning tend to combine with histones (Fig. 2-2). There are two types of nucleic acid: deoxyribonucleic acid (DNA) and ribonucleic acid (RNA) (12, 13). Most of the DNA is found in the nucleus, with a small amount in the mitochondria. Genes are portions of the DNA mole-cule. Three types of RNA can be distinguished: messenger RNA (mRNA), ribosomal RNA (rRNA), and transfer RNA (tRNA). All three diffuse from the nucleus through the nuclear membrane into the cytoplasm, where they play a major role in protein synthesis.

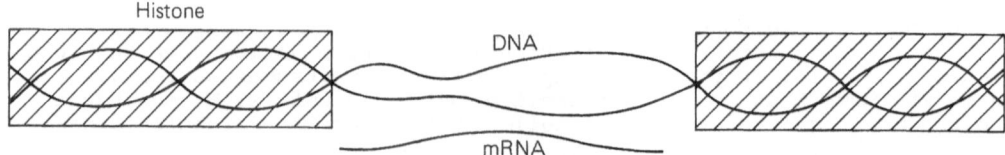

Fig. 2-2. Inhibitory role of histones in transcription

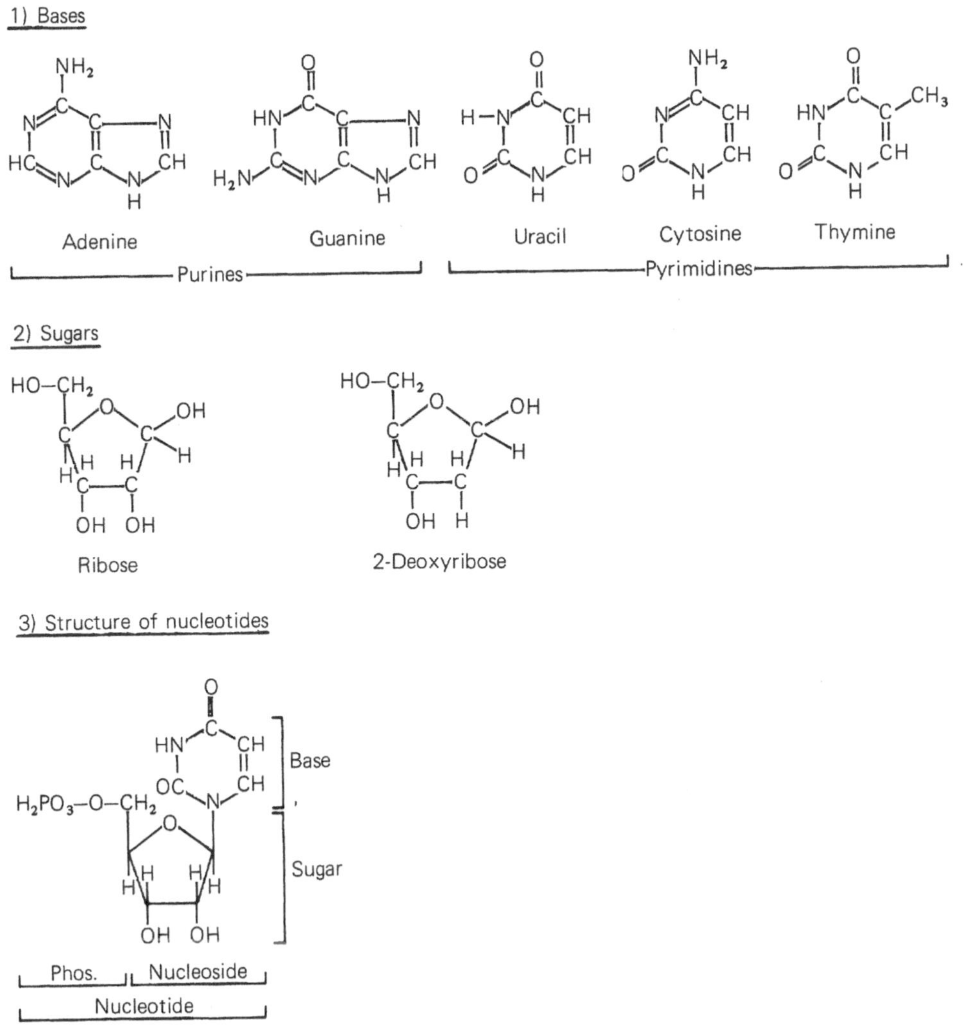

1) Bases

| Adenine | Guanine | Uracil | Cytosine | Thymine |

Purines — Adenine, Guanine

Pyrimidines — Uracil, Cytosine, Thymine

2) Sugars

Ribose   2-Deoxyribose

3) Structure of nucleotides

Phos. | Nucleoside

Nucleotide

Fig. 2-3. The composition of nucleotides, the structural units of nucleic acids

Nucleic acids are polynucleotides (12, 13, 16). A nucleotide consists of a purine or pyrimidine base, a pentose sugar (deoxyribose in DNA and ribose in RNA), and phosphate group (Fig. 2-3; Table 2-1). The pyrimidines are cytosine, present in all nucleic acids, thymine, found mainly in DNA, and uracil found in RNA. The purines, adenine and guanine, occur in both DNA and RNA. The nitrogenous base is attached to the 1' carbon of the pentose. Nucleotides are linked to form nucleic acids by phosphodiester linkage between the 3' carbon of one sugar and the 5' carbon of the neighboring sugar.

DNA is made up of two polynucleotide chains, coiled together in the form of a helix (Fig. 2-4) (17). The backbone of the helix consists of the sugar molecules joined by the 3'5' phosphodiester linkages, which run in opposite directions in the two chains. The bases are located on

Table 2-1. Nomenclature of purine and pyrimidine nucleotides

Base	Nucleoside	Nucleotide monophosphate	Nucleotide diphosphate	Nucleotide triphosphate
Adenine	Adenosine (A)	Adenine ribonucleotide Adenosine monophosphate (AMP) Adenylic acid	Adenosine diphosphate (ADP)	Adenosine triphosphate (ATP)
Guanine	Guanosine (G)	Guanine ribonucleotide Guanosine monophosphate (GMP) Guanylic acid	Guanosine diphosphate (GDP)	Guanosine triphosphate (GTP)
Cytosine	Cytidine (C)	Cytosine ribonucleotide Cytidine monophosphate (CMP) Cytidylic acid	Cytidine diphosphate (CDP)	Cytidine triphosphate CTP)
Uracil	Uridine (U)	Uracil ribonucleotide Uridine monophosphate (UMP) Uridylic acid	Uridine diphosphate (UDP)	Uridine triphosphate (UTP)
Thymine	Thymidine (dT) (thymine deoxy- riboside)	Thymine deoxyribonucleotide Thymidine monophosphate (dTMP) Thymidylic acid	Thymidine diphosphate (dTDP)	Thymidine triphosphate (dTTP)

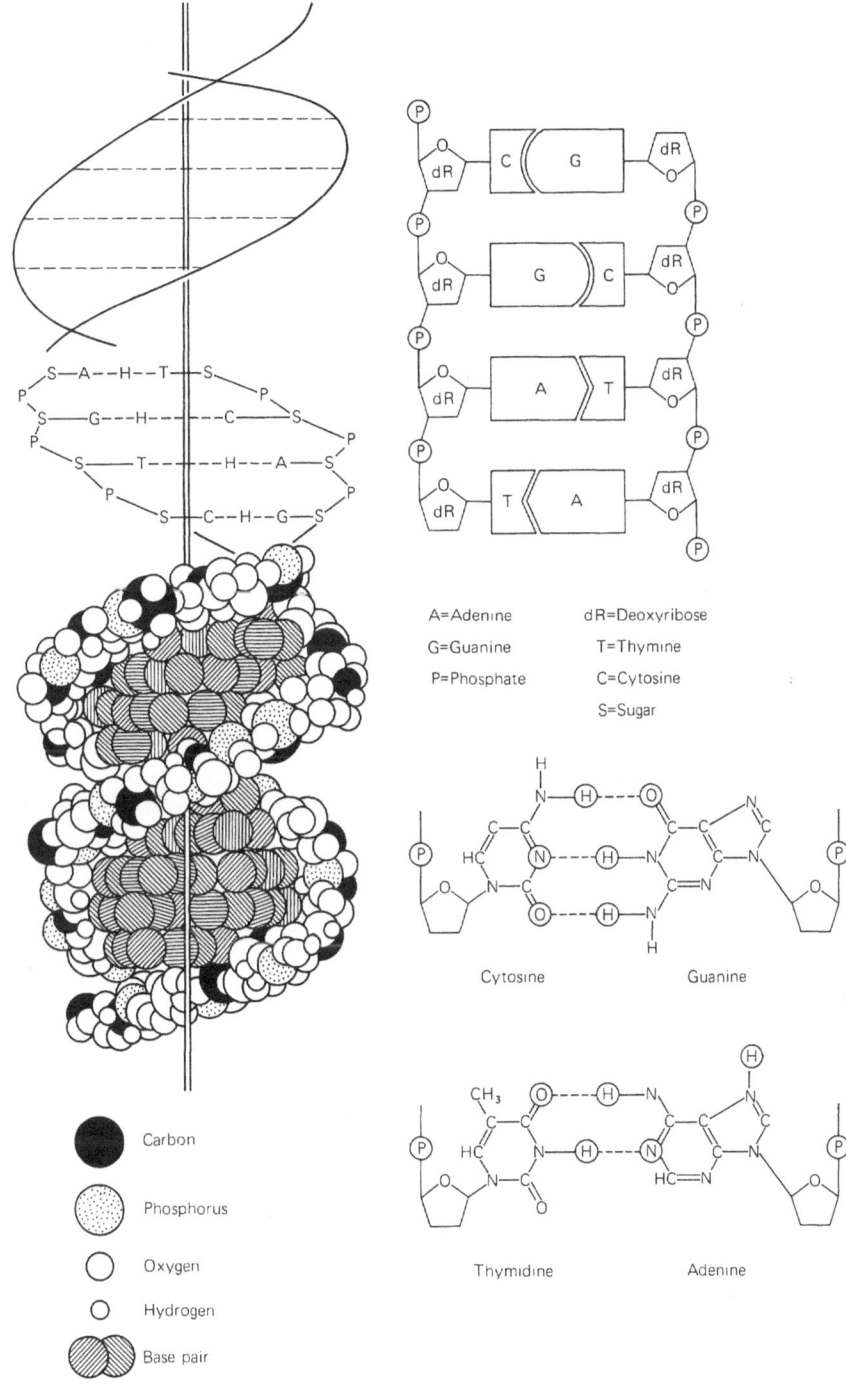

A=Adenine dR=Deoxyribose
G=Guanine T=Thymine
P=Phosphate C=Cytosine
S=Sugar

Cytosine   Guanine

Thymidine   Adenine

Carbon

Phosphorus

Oxygen

Hydrogen

Base pair

Fig. 2-4. Double helical structure of DNA and hydrogen bonding between the bases of the two nucleotide chains

9

the inside of the helix, the phosphates on the outside. The two chains
are held together by hydrogen bonds involving the keto and the amino
groups of opposing bases. Guanine is always linked to cytosine by three
hydrogen bonds and adenine to thymine by two hydrogen bonds (18). The
sequence of bases in one chain automatically determines that of its
partner. It is the specificity of the base pairing that ensures the
faithful replication of the nucleic-acid chains.

The structure of RNA is very similar to that of DNA (Fig. 2-5). It is
also a polymer of the four main nucleotides, but it forms a single
chain instead of the double stranded helix, the sugar residue is ribose
instead of deoxyribose, and it contains uracil instead of thymine. Its
structure is such that it is complementary to DNA chains.

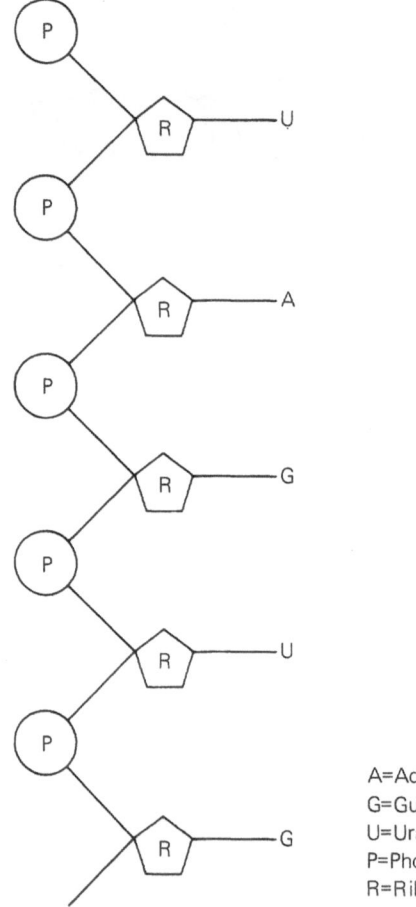

A=Adenine
G=Guanine
U=Uracil
P=Phosphate
R=Ribose

Fig. 2-5. The structure of RNA

(ii) Function of Nucleic Acids
DNA has two major functions: It serves both as a template for its own
replication and as a template for RNA synthesis. The former process is
responsible for the transmission of genetic characteristics and the
latter regulates protein synthesis, which is the means by which genes
carry out their function (12, 13, 19).

At cell division the two strands of the DNA helix, while progressively separating, act as templates for the formation of their complementary strands (Fig. 2-6). The enzyme DNA polymerase is necessary to link the nucleotides by 3'5' phosphodiester bonds. Thus, each daughter cell receives a genetic make-up identical to that of the parental cell.

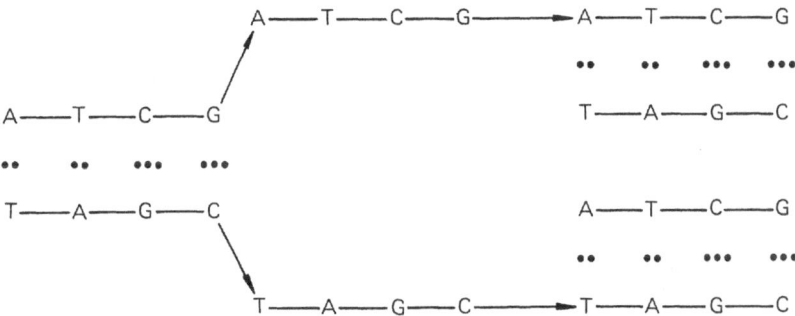

Fig. 2-6. The replication of DNA

The genetic information is conveyed by the sequence of the nucleotide bases in the DNA molecule (the genetic code) (20). Each sequence of three bases, called a triplet or codon, determines the type of amino acid that will be inserted in the protein-peptide chain. Genes control the structure and the function of the cell through the synthesis of structural proteins and protein enzymes.

All three types of RNA are involved in the important process of protein synthesis (Fig. 2-7) (12, 13, 19). Messenger RNA, by way of its nucleotide sequence, transfers the genetic information encoded by the triplets of the nuclear DNA to the ribosomes in the cytoplasm. This process is referred to as transcription (Fig. 2-8). The synthesis of mRNA upon a DNA template proceeds in a similar way to DNA replication, and the enzyme RNA polymerase is necessary to link the nucleotide precursors. The length of the mRNA molecule depends on the size of the protein to be synthesized. Accurate transmission of the message is assured by the base-pairing rule (A=U; G≡C). Actual protein synthesis takes place in the ribosomes in the cytoplasm.

Each of the 20 different amino acids is brought into the ribosome by a specific RNA molecule, transfer RNA, for insertion into the peptide chain. (Fig. 2-9). The polynucleotide chain of tRNA is thought to have a secondary structure in the shape of a clover leaf. The specificity for a given amino acid resides in the sequence of three bases (the anticodon), which is complementary to the three bases on the mRNA (the codon) that code for the particular amino acid carried. Before they can take part in the protein synthesis amino acids must be activated by reaction with an energy source, ATP. This reaction requires amino-acyl RNA synthetase, an enzyme specific for each amino acid. The activated amino acid is then transferred to its specific tRNA and the activated amino acid-RNA complex is ready to participate in protein synthesis in the ribosomes.

The ribosomes are spherical particles consisting of subunits, one large and one small, made up of ribosomal RNA and protein. Ribosomal RNA is probably synthesized in the nucleolus as a single chain (21). This chain is cleaved into several smaller subunits which migrate into the cytoplasm. Little is known about the internal structure and function of rRNA.

11

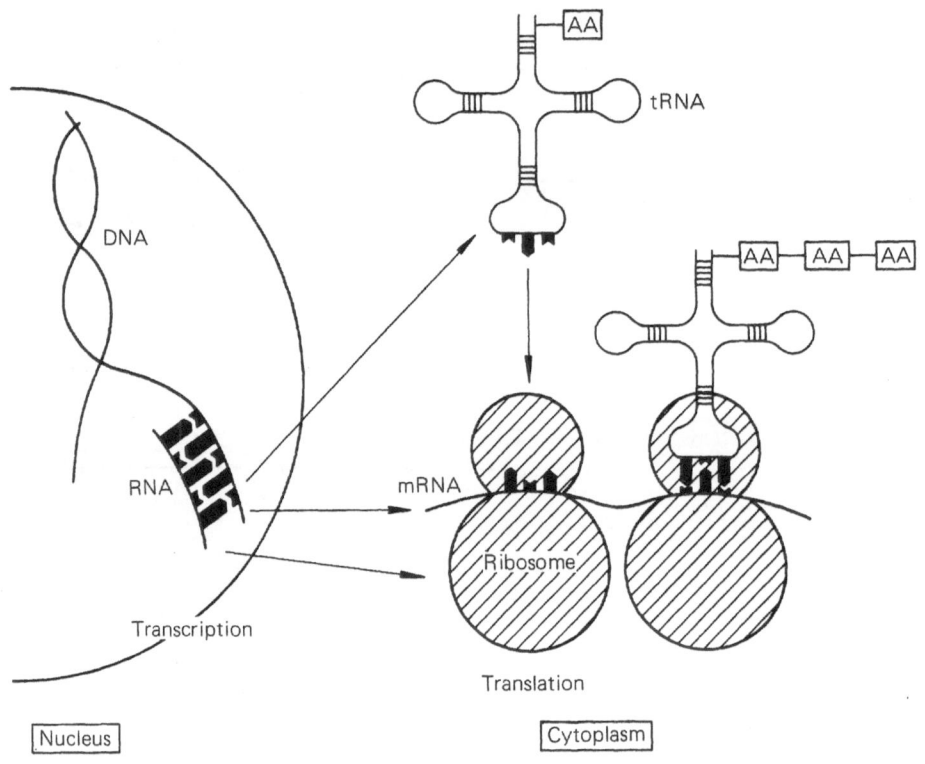

Fig. 2-7. Diagrammatic outline of protein synthesis: transcription and translation

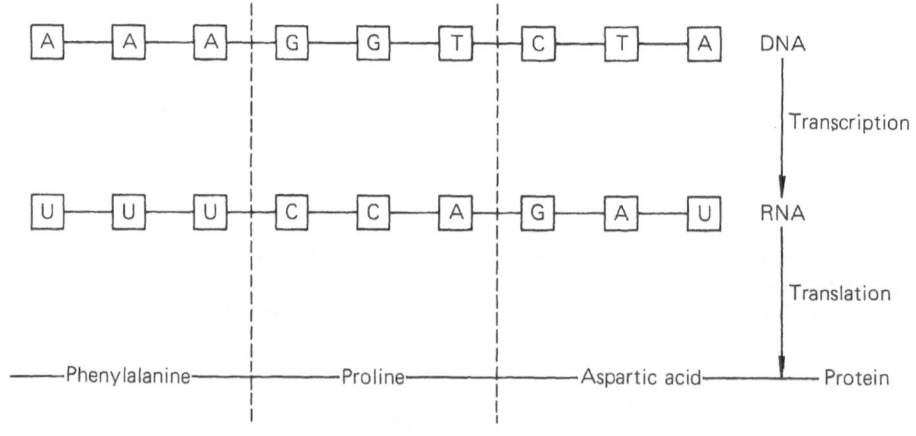

Fig. 2-8. An example of transcription and translation

Messenger RNA attaches to ribosomes and moves across them bringing successive triplets into position to select the appropriate amino acid-tRNA complexes. This process is known as <u>translation</u>. The peptide chain assembly begins at the amino-terminal end and continues by the addition

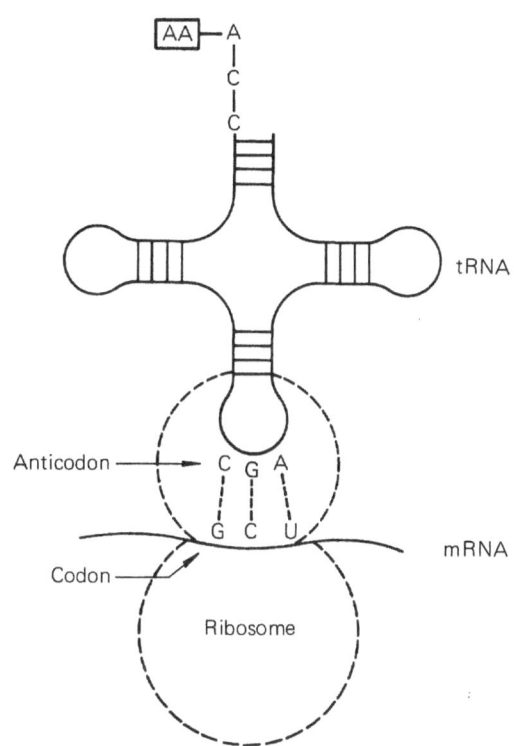

Fig. 2-9. Diagram of an amino-acyl tRNA molecule showing the clover leaf shape. The anticodon of the tRNA is complementary to a sequence of 3 bases (the codon of the mRNA)

of amino acids, enzymatically linked by the formation of peptide bonds, in a particular sequence dictated by the RNA template. Once the poly-peptide is completed, it is released from the ribosome.

Cells possess control mechanisms to make sure that proteins are syn-thesized in the required amounts at the appropriate times. JACOB and MONOD postulated that chromosomes carry several types of genes (22, 23). Adjacent to one or more structural genes that code for structural pro-teins or enzymes is an operator gene (Fig. 2-10), which controls the structural genes. One or more structural genes together with their ope-rator gene form a unit called an operon. The operator gene itself is controlled by a third factor, the regulator gene. The operator gene can be turned off by attachment of a repressor molecule produced by the regulator gene.

(iii) Synthesis of Nucleic Acids
Nucleic acids are obviously some of the most important components of the cell. An adequate supply of purine and pyrimidine nucleotides to serve as building blocks for DNA and RNA is essential to the function and survival of the cell. Nucleotides can come from one or two sources: the salvage pathway, or de novo synthesis (Fig. 2-11) (13). The salvage pathway reuses bases obtained by catabolism of cells or ingested bases, but de novo synthesis in the cell is the major source of nucleotides. Figure 2-12 illustrates the series of reactions leading to a purine nucleotide. The synthesis of the purine ring begins on the 1 carbon

13

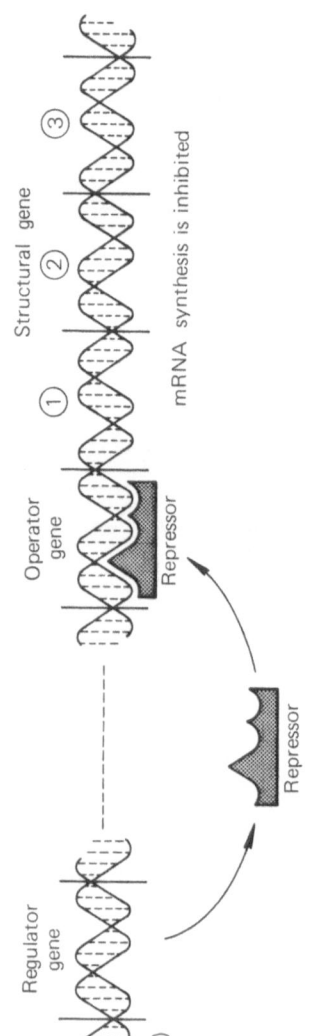

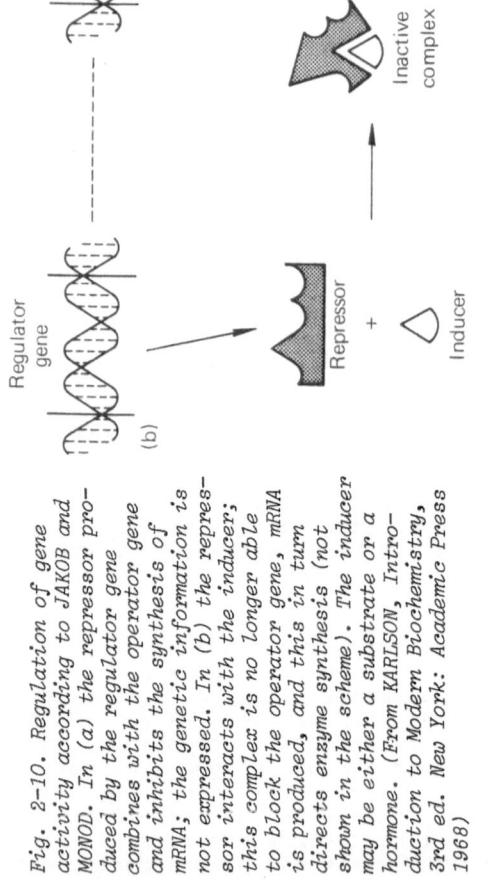

Structural gene

① ② ③

Operator gene

Regulator gene

Repressor

Repressor

(a) mRNA synthesis is inhibited

Operator gene

Regulator gene

Repressor + Inducer

Inactive complex

mRNA is produced

(b)

Fig. 2-10. Regulation of gene activity according to JAKOB and MONOD. In (a) the repressor pro- duced by the regulator gene combines with the operator gene and inhibits the synthesis of mRNA; the genetic information is not expressed. In (b) the repres- sor interacts with the inducer; this complex is no longer able to block the operator gene, mRNA is produced, and this in turn directs enzyme synthesis (not shown in the scheme). The inducer may be either a substrate or a hormone. (From KARLSON, Intro- duction to Modern Biochemistry, 3rd ed. New York: Academic Press 1968)

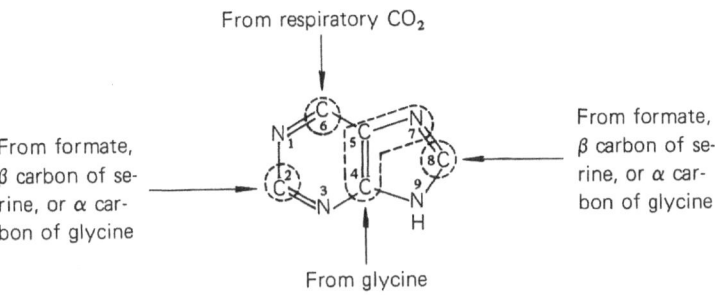

From respiratory CO_2

From formate, β carbon of serine, or α carbon of glycine

From formate, β carbon of serine, or α carbon of glycine

From glycine

N in 1 from amino N of aspartic acid.
N in 3 and 9 from amide N of glutamine.

Fig. 2-11. Sources of carbon and nitrogen in the purine nucleus (From HARPER (13))

of a sugar phosphate, 5-phosphoribosyl-1-pyrophosphate (PRPP), which is provided by the hexose monophosphate shunt. All subsequent compounds leading to the formation of purine are therefore formed as ribonucleotides. The first purine nucleotide synthesized is inosine monophosphate (IMP). IMP serves as a precursor for adenosine monophosphate (AMP) and guanosine monophosphate (GMP). Purine nucleotides can also be formed directly from free purines or purine nucleosides but these pathways are of secondary importance.

Pyrimidine biosynthesis begins with the formation of carbamyl aspartic acid (ureidosuccinic acid) (Fig. 2-13). Orotic acid, the first pyrimidine ring to be synthesized, reacts with PRPP and is decarboxylated to uracil monophosphate (UMP). UMP is the precursor of cytosine monophosphate (CMP) and thymidylic acid (TMP). TMP is an essential compound for DNA synthesis, which is selectively inhibited in its absence.

Several feedback mechanisms regulate the biosynthesis of purine and pyrimidines. IMP and UMP can be transformed into a number of different nucleotides by alterations of functional groups, by coupling of additional phosphate residues, or by reduction of ribose to deoxyribose nucleotides at the disphosphate level. Ribo- and deoxyribonucleotides are phosphorylated to the triphosphate level prior to incorporation into nucleic acids (Fig. 2-14).

Folic acid is an essential vitamin in nucleic-acid synthesis. It is either furnished to the cell from dietary sources or is synthesized by the cell (Fig. 2-15). It is converted by a series of enzymatic reactions to tetrahydrofolic acid (THFA); derivatives of THFA are important as one-carbon fragment donors in the synthesis of purine and pyrimidine bases (Fig. 2-16).

3. Cell Division

Cell division or mitosis ensures growth and repair of tissues and organs by providing daughter cells more or less identical to the parent cell (24-28). The process proceeds in several phases (Fig. 2-17). Following mitosis, the cell enters the interphase, during which the chromosomes are invisibly embedded in the nuclear chromatin. The interphase itself is subdivided into three phases: G_1, S, and G_2. G_1 is also called the first gap period in DNA synthesis, but this phase is anything but a rest period as far as RNA and protein synthesis is concerned. G_1 is the

15

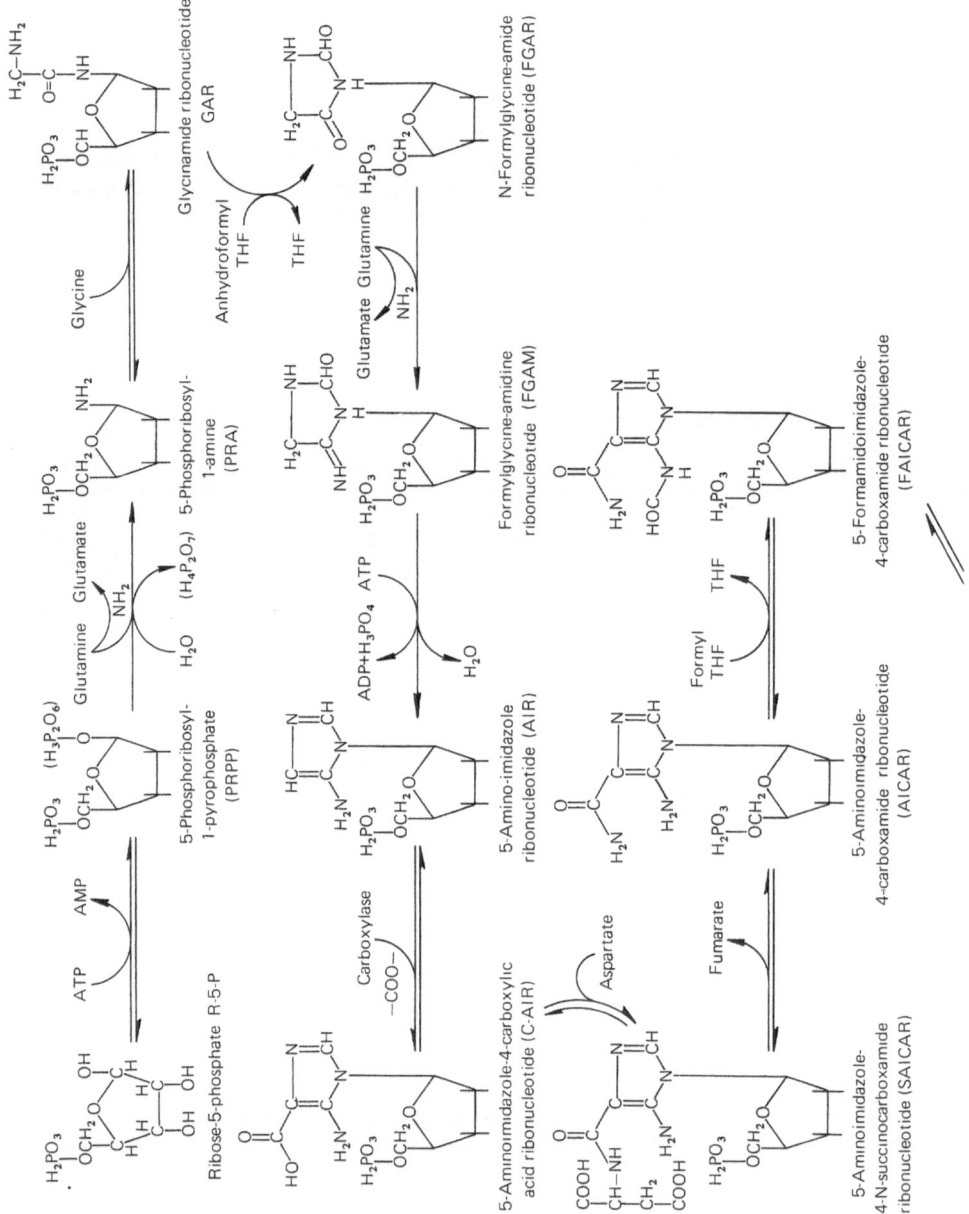

Fig. 2-12. Purine nucleotide synthesis

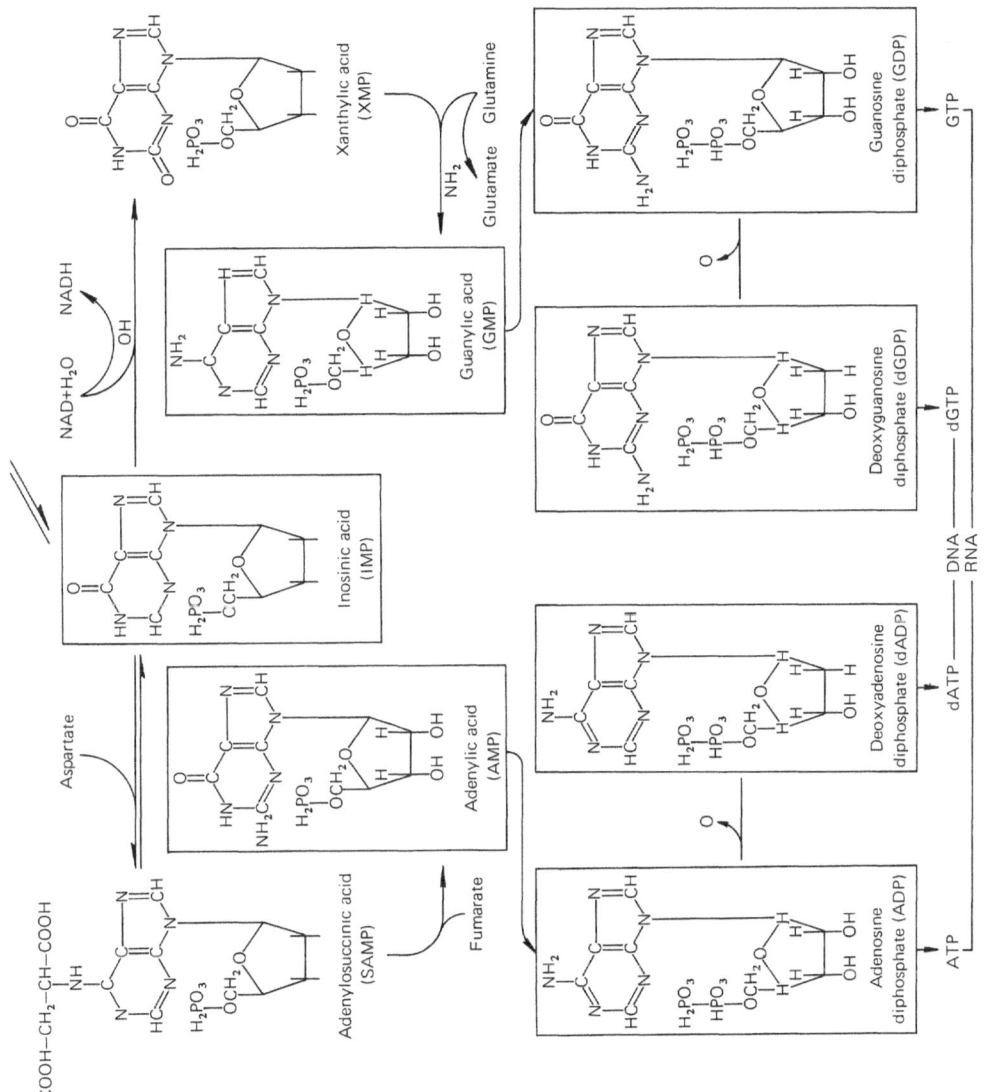

Fig. 2-12. *Purine nucleotide synthesis*

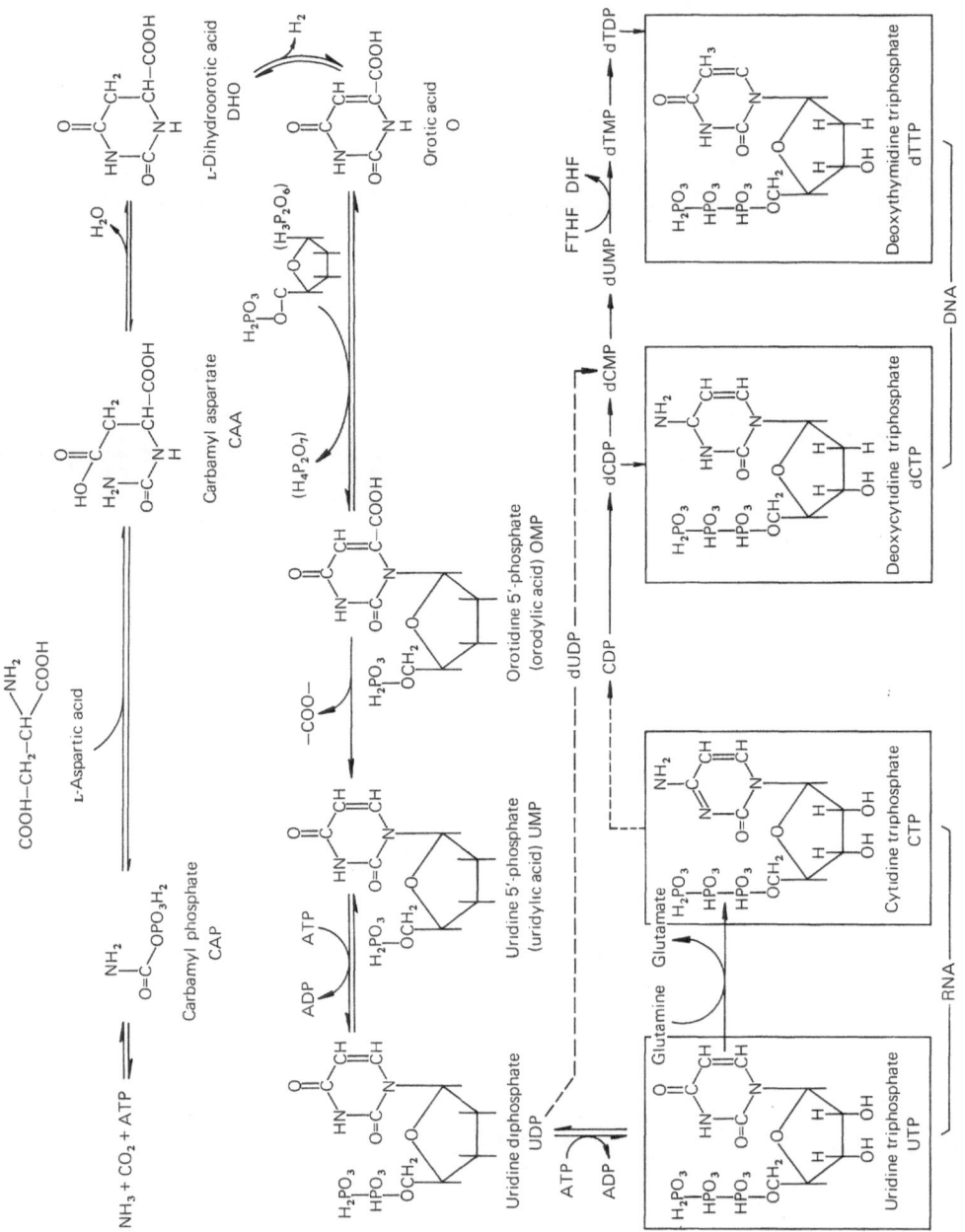

Fig. 2-13. Pyrimidine nucleotide synthesis

18

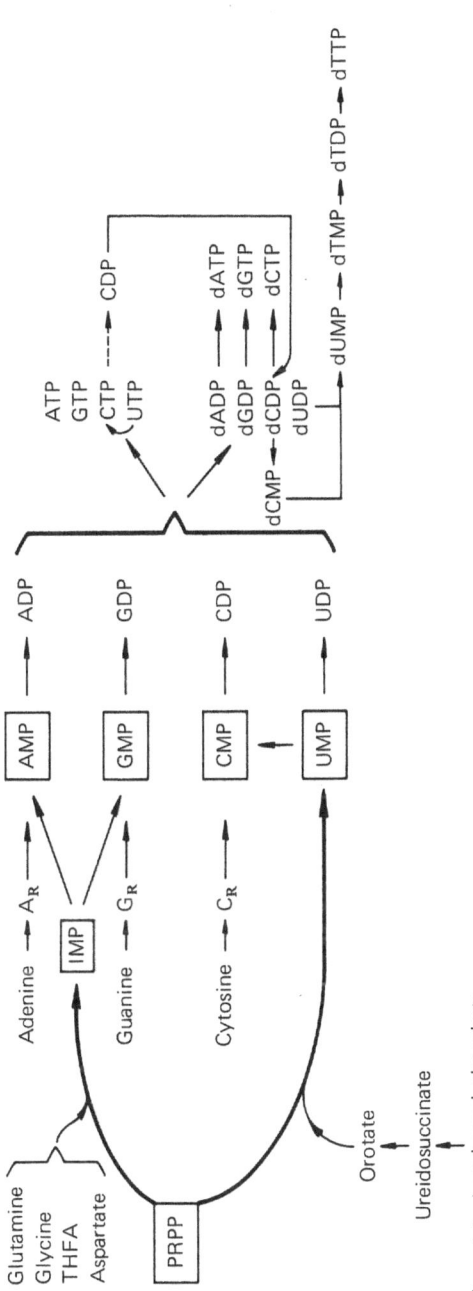

Fig. 2-14. Schematic representation of purine and pyrimidine biosynthesis and interconversions. (See Table 2-1 and Figs. 2-12 and 2-13 for abbreviations)

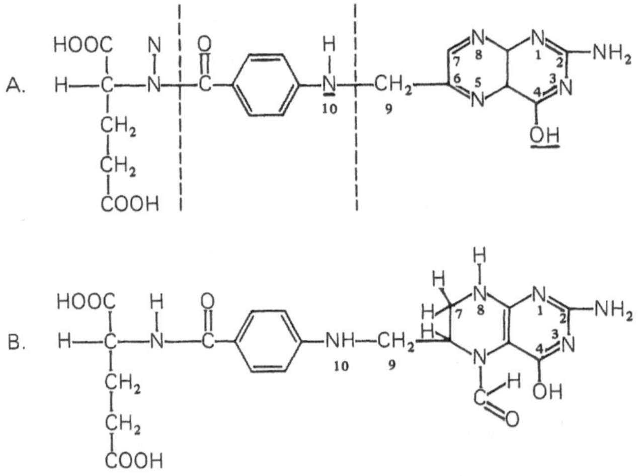

Fig. 2-15. A. Folic acid (pteroylglutamic acid), B. Folinic acid or citrovorum factor (N^5-formyltetrahydrofolic acid)

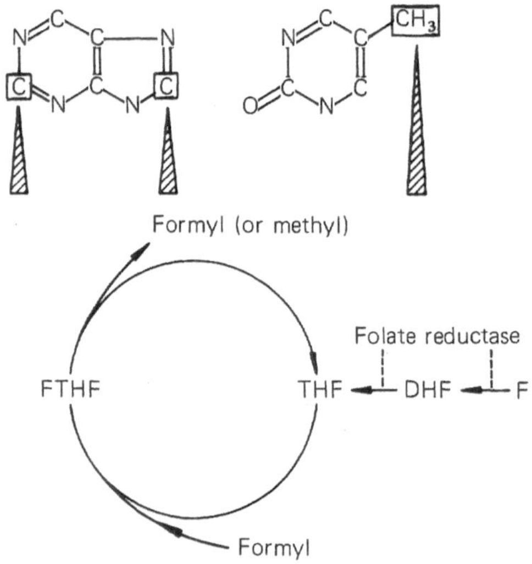

Fig. 2-16. Tetrahydrofolic acid derivatives, acting as formyl carriers, are required for the incorporation of one-carbon units into positions 2 and 8 of the purine nucleus and for the methylation of deoxyuridine monophosphate (dUMP) to thymidine monophosphate (dTMP). DHF = dihydrofolic acid, THF = tetrahydrofolic acid, FTHF = formyltetrahydrofolic acid

phase of the cell cycle. It is followed by the S phase, during which DNA is synthesized and the chromosome complement is duplicated (Fig. 2-18). DNA synthesis can be demonstrated by measuring the uptake of radioactive tritiated thymidine into the nascent DNA (29, 30). Between the S phase and the mitotic phase is a short second gap, G2; the appearance of fine filaments around the centrioles suggests that protein

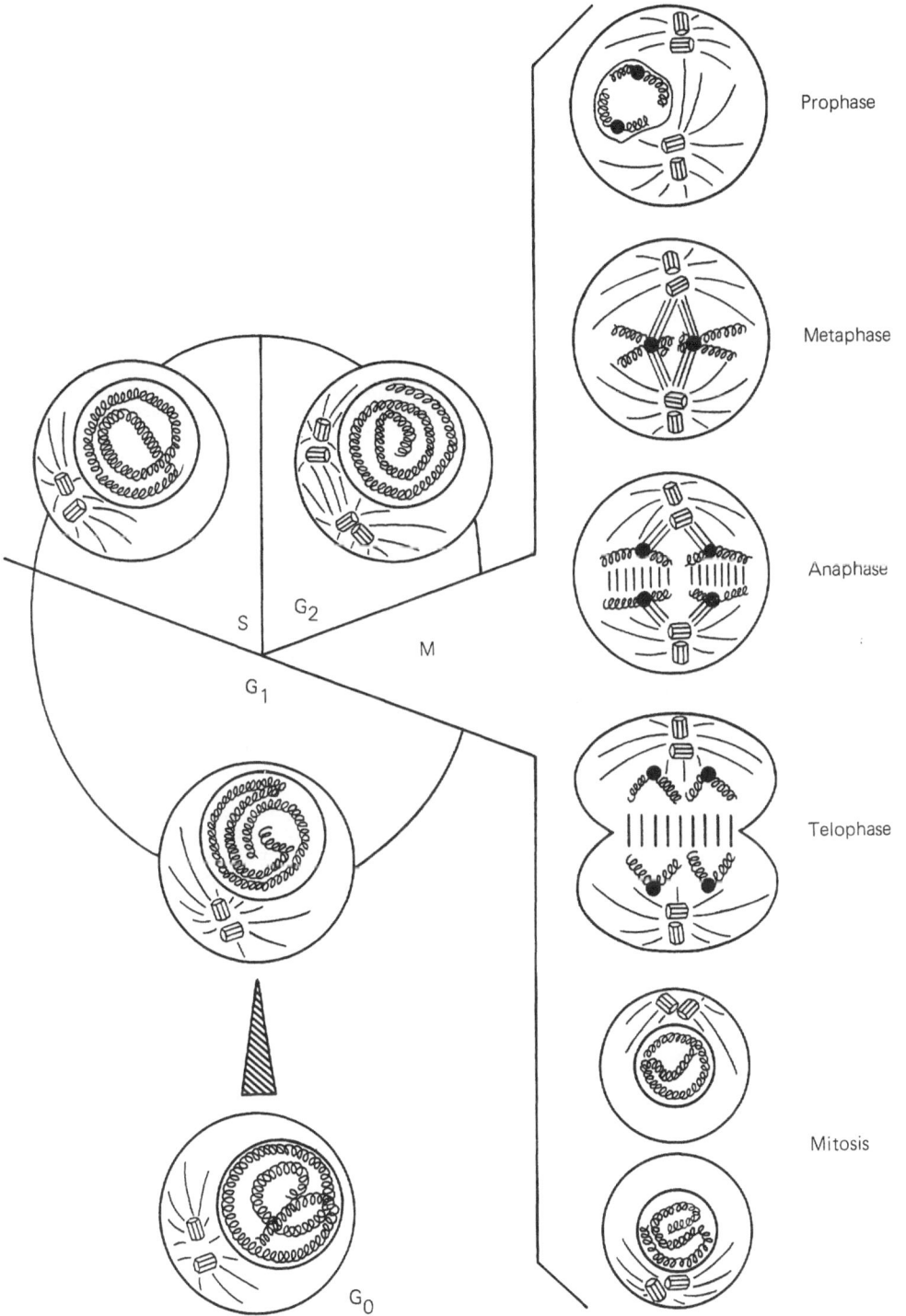

Prophase

Metaphase

Anaphase

Telophase

Mitosis

S

G_2

M

G_1

G_0

Fig. 2-17. The different phases of the cell cycle. G_1 postmitotic phase (first gap period), S phase of DNA synthesis, G_2 premitotic phase (second gap period), M mitosis, G_0 resting phase

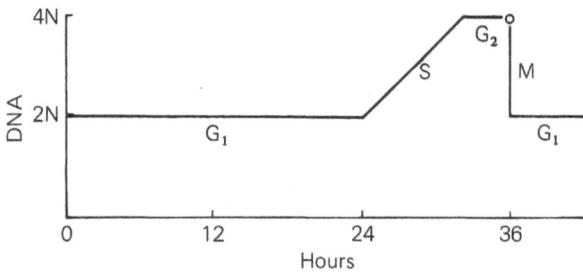

Fig. 2-18. The synthesis of DNA during the cell cycle. ((from LATJA) (24)). 2N diploid quantity of DNA, 4N tetraploid quantity of DNA

synthesis for the mitotic spindle is taking place (31). The mitotic phase (M) is subdivided into prophase, metaphase, anaphase, and telo-phase. During prophase the chromosomes condense into more compact bodies and divide into 2 chromatids held together by a centromere. The DNA he-lix of each chromatid receives one strand from the newly synthesized DNA and one strand from the template DNA. RNA synthesis stops early in prophase and the nucleoli and membranes begin to dissolve. The cen-trioles move to opposite poles and the spindle begins to form. The chro-mosomes line up along the equatorial plane of the spindle, each pair of chromatids being fixed by the centromere on a different fiber of the mitotic spindle. This gives the characteristic appearance of the cell in metaphase. Blocking cells in metaphase with mitotic poisons allows the chromosomes to be counted and their morphology studied. Their number (2N) varies with the species, but is constant in normal cells of a par-ticular species. Human cells contain 46 chromosomes, 22 pairs of auto-somes, and one pair of sex chromosomes (XX in female cells, XY in male cells). Late in metaphase the centromere of each chromosome divides, and the number of chromosomes is doubled (4N). Immediately the daughter chromosomes begin to move away from each other to opposite poles, assis-ted by the fibers of the mitotic spindle, which seem to contain contrac-tile proteins similar to those in muscles. This separation of the chro-mosomes is the crucial event in anaphase. Vesicular elements, probably originating in the endoplasmic reticulum, settle on the surface of the chromosomes, fuse, and form a double membrane around each chromosome. During telophase, when the chromosomes reach the two poles, these mem-branes coalesce to form the nuclear membrane. The chromosomes then take on the appearance characteristic of interphase, nucleoli reappear and the spindle disappears. Division of the cytoplasm is associated with the nuclear division, but the underlying mechanism is not understood (32).

Chap. 3 describes how chemotherapeutic agents act by interfering with either the synthesis or the function of nucleotides, nucleic acids, proteins, or the mitotic spindle.

B. THE CANCER CELL

For decades scientists of various disciplines have searched for differ-ences between the cancer cell and the normal cell, in the hope of under-standing the process of carcinogenesis and of developing specific rather than empirical chemotherapy. Differences have been noted in the bioche-mical reactions, surface properties, chromosome constitution, and kine-tics of malignant cells. However, none of these changes is unique for or common to all malignancies. Furthermore, it is impossible to tell whether the alterations noted in cancer cells are an essential part of carcinogenesis or just secondary changes.

1. Biochemical Characteristics

Almost 50 years ago WARBURG observed that increased glycolysis is a characteristic pattern of energy metabolism in malignant tissues (33-35). He proposed that the basic abnormality in cancer cells was an injury to the respiratory mechanisms, resulting in continued production of lactic acid from glucose. However, increased glycolysis, though common, is neither a unique nor a constant feature of malignant tissues. Moreover, it has never been unequivocally established whether the increased lactic acid results from augmented production (an abnormality in the glycolytic pathway) or decreased breakdown (an abnormality in the oxidative phosphorylation). The activity of Krebs cycle in tumors has been reported to be either normal or decreased. Abnormalities in the rate of ATP hydrolysis, of glucose or phosphate entry into malignant cells, of the glycolytic enzymes, or of the reoxidation of $NADH_2$ have all been put forward as explanations for the increased glycolysis in malignant tissues (36, 37).

WEBER, studying a spectrum of Morris hepatomas with different growth rates noted a progressive decrease in the synthetic pathway and an increase in the catabolic pathway of the carbohydrate metabolism with increasing growth rate (38). In lipid metabolism both are decreased. In contrast, in protein and nucleic-acid metabolism the anabolic pathways become progressively dominant and the catabolic pathways decline with increasing tumor growth. This metabolic pattern is not simply a reflection of rapid growth, since it differs from that of regenerating liver.

Tumors also display altered isozyme patterns (39-41). In hepatomas isozymes that are responsive to hormones or regulatory metabolites may disappear to be replaced by isozymes that are normally low or absent in the fully differentiated hepatocyte. Some of these may be characteristic of fetal or neonatal livers, or of other organs. Such changes would be expected to influence the metabolic pattern and growth rate of hepatomas.

Tumor cells contain less cyclic AMP than normal cells; this is a significant observation, since cAMP may control cell proliferation and differentiation (42). Contact between cells normally leads to an increase in cAMP, culminating in inhibition of initiation of DNA synthesis, thereby inhibiting cell growth. A defect in this response to contact may result in uncontrolled growth of tumor cells.

Biochemical differences have thus far rarely been the basis of specific cancer chemotherapy, with the exception of L-asparaginase (43). Certain tumors lose the capacity to synthesize asparagine, an amino acid that is not essential for normal tissues. Tumors that have become dependent on an exogenous supply are nonviable if asparagine in the extracellular space is destroyed by asparaginase.

The sensitivity of mammary tumors to hormones is determined by the presence or absence in the cytoplasm of a specific protein that binds estrogen and then transports it to the nucleus, where the estrogen exerts its effect by binding to the chromatin (44).

2. Surface Properties

The membranes of malignant cells exhibit distinct changes as against
normal cells (42, 45). This is seen in vitro from the loss of contact
inhibition or the selective agglutination of tumor cells by wheat-germ
agglutinin, soybean agglutinin, and Concanavalin A. Immunologic techniques reveal the presence of tumor-specific or fetal antigens and a
lowered concentration of the normal antigens. Membrane lipids, glyco-
protein, and glycosphingolipids are altered, and tumor cells are often
surrounded by a thicker layer of mucopolysaccharides than are normal
cells (46).

3. Chromosome Constitution

Abnormalities in the number and the morphology of chromosomes are frequent in cancer cells (47). However, with the exception of the Philadelphia chromosome, these changes are quite inconstant and variable (48).
It is possible that newer techniques, for example fluorescent staining,
may reveal specific marker chromosomes in other malignancies (Burkitt's
tumor) (49). It has been one of the major contributions of cytogenetic
studies to reveal that tumor populations are heterogeneous, being composed of competing clones of cells with different and continuously
changing genotypes that allow the tumor population to adapt to a changing environment. The inconstancy of the chromosomal alterations makes
it difficult to evaluate their significance in relation to the origin,
development, and behavior of malignancies. It has been found that cells
with chromosomal instability or abnormalities are susceptible to malignant transformation (50). Unrestrained growth, the essential characteristic of tumor cells, is passed on from parent cells to progeny. This
suggests that cancer is due to an alteration at the chromosomal level;
this may be an accumulation of somatic mutations or the insertion of
viral genome into the host chromosome. Alternatively, cancer could be
an example of irreversible differentiation.

4. Tumor-Cell Kinetics

We next consider the cellular composition and the growth pattern of
malignant tissues. It is often believed that rapid proliferation is a
fundamental characteristic of malignant cells as compared to their normal counterparts. However, BRESCIANI has shown that cancer cells do not
necessarily replicate at the full speed characteristic of the cell line
(51). The cell-cycle time (Tc) of an experimental mammary mouse tumor,
though shorter than that of the normal mammary cells, was not as short
as that of mammary gland under hormone stimulation. Normal tissues, such
as bone marrow and the bowel epithelium, can divide more rapidly than
malignant cells. Cancer should be regarded, not as abnormal growth -
malignant cells grow and divide by the same mechanisms as normal cells -
but rather as an abnormality of the regulation of growth. Intimately
associated with this feature is a deficiency in differentiation and a
loss of repression of cell migration (52).

Cells are not always in reproductive cycle. Some cells are said to be
in a "resting" phase or G$_0$ (53, 54). Hepatocytes provide an example:
normally they do not divide in the adult but they can be triggered into
cell cycle by partial hepatectomy. When regeneration is completed they
return to the G$_0$ phase. That tumor cells can be in a resting state has
been inferred from the slow growth rate of certain tumors and the appearance of metastases many years after effective control of the primary tumor (55). Special techniques, such as continuous labeling with
tritiated thymidine to saturate the population, confirm the existence

of resting tumor cells. Cells in G_0 do not contribute any cell input into the cell population. Their DNA content is postmitotic (G_1), and nothing is known about the possible biochemical differences between cells in G_0 and G_1 or the control and the extent of their conversion from the nonproliferative state (G_0) to the proliferative state. It is debatable whether they in fact represent a specific class of cells or just cells with a very long G_1 (Fig. 2-19). However since such cells are not sensitive to cell-cycle-dependent drugs, they may be the source of late relapses and are therefore of real concern to the chemotherapist.

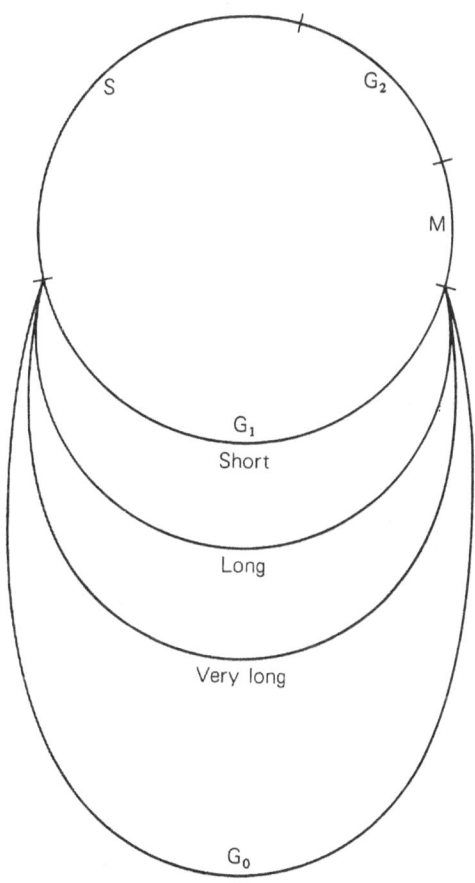

Fig. 2-19. The concept of resting cells: prolonged G_1 or G_0

A tumor can be thought of as consisting of four types of cells (Fig. 2-20) (56, 57).
A. Dividing tumor cells ("cells in cycle"). This is the only compartment that adds cells to the population and it is the most sensitive to cytotoxic agents.
B. Resting, temporarily nondividing cells ("cells in G_0"). We have already referred to their refractoriness to cycle-dependent agents.
C. Differentiated, permanently nondividing cells. Since these are destined to die, they are of little concern to the chemotherapist.
D. Dying cells.

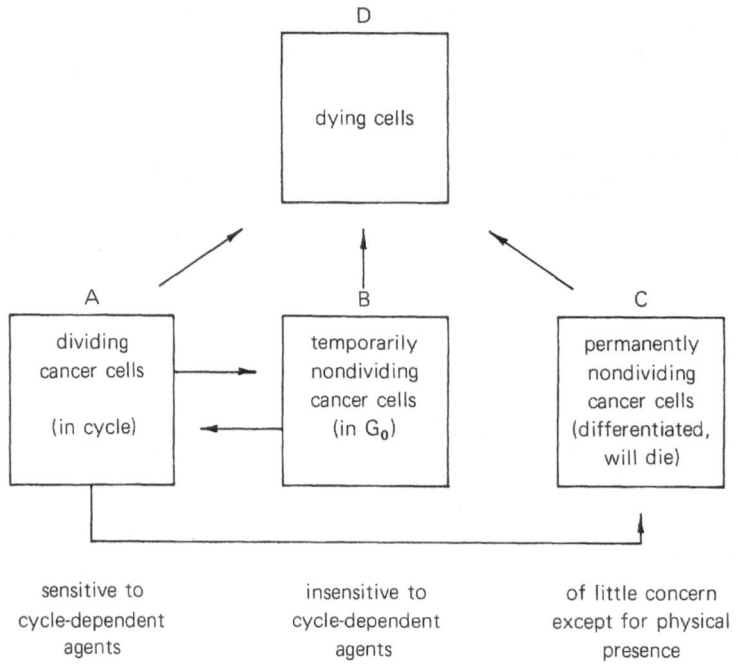

Fig. 2-20. *Cell types in an individual tumor mass*

Tumor growth patterns were first studied by measuring tumor masses on serial chest roentgenograms (58, 59). The doubling time (DT), that is the time interval required for the tumor mass to double, can thereby be determined (Table 2-2) (60).

Table 2-2. Growth rates of different human tumors (From CHARBIT et al. (60))

Pathology	Geometric mean of the DTs (days)	Median DTs
1. Lung metastasis of embryonal tumors	27.0	25
2. Lymphomas	28.9	32
3. Malignant mesenchymal tumors	41.4	37
4. Lung metastasis of squamous cell carcinomas	58.0	56
5. Primary squamous cell carcinoma	81.8	80
6. Lung metastasis of adenocarcinoma	82.7	89
7. Primary adenocarcinoma	166.3	207

Tumor growth, like growth of normal tissues (e.g. human fetus) follows a Gompertz curve, that is an exponentially decreasing exponential function (Figs. 2-21 and 2-22) (61). Early growth is exponential; during this logarithmic phase the growth fraction is high, the volume doubling time is short, and large numbers of cells are sensitive to cell-cycle-dependent drugs. As the tumor mass enlarges, the growth rate becomes progressively slower and the growth curve may reach a plateau, that is

26

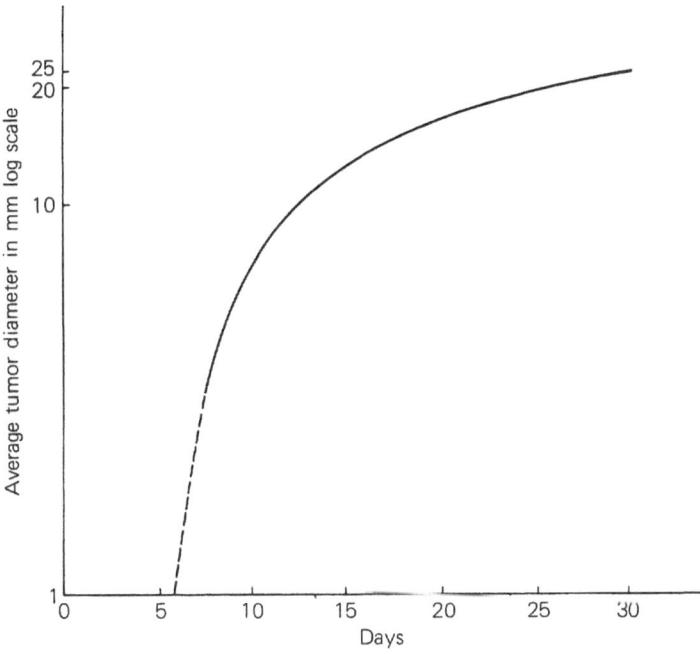

Fig. 2-21. Tumor growth following s.c. injection of 10⁴ L1210 leukemia
cells in mice. Growth follows a Gompertz curve

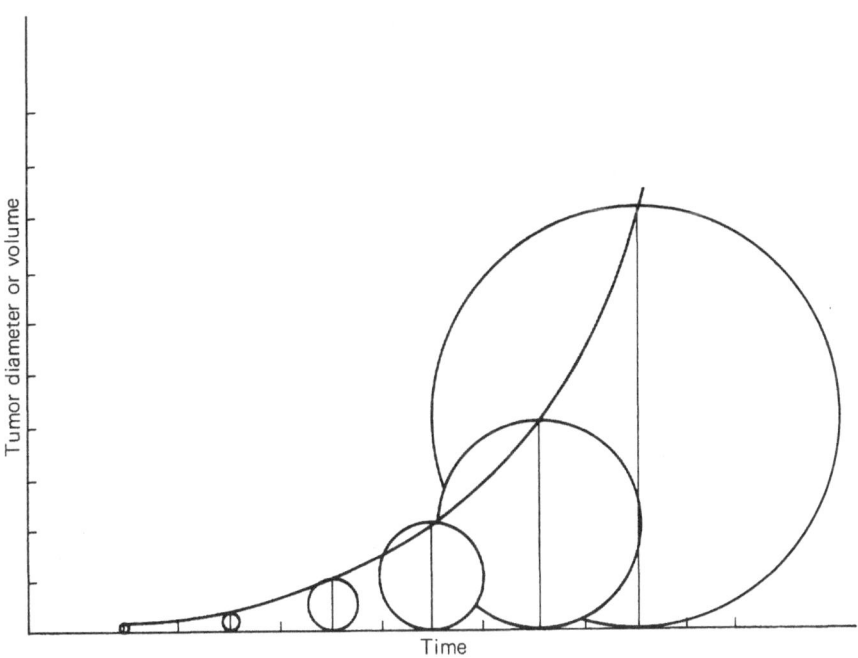

Fig. 2-22. Exponential tumor growth. The doubling time of the tumor volume is one third of the doubling time of the diameter since the volume
of the sphere is proportional to the diameter to the power of three

cell input equals cell loss. This stationary phase is characterized by a low growth fraction, and a long doubling time, and the sensitivity of the total population to cell-cycle-dependent agents decreases as an increasing number of cells remain for prolonged periods in G_1 or enter G_0. In some tumors the cell-cycle time may become longer as the tumor grows, while in others it remains fairly constant. A stationary-phase growth pattern is likely to have been reached in most human tumors by the time a diagnosis is made. It should be pointed out that the so-called "accelerated phase" of a tumor in fact resulted from an error of recording. A tumor with a constant doubling time, when plotted on an arithmetical scale, will appear to be growing slowly at first, then faster, while a logarithmic scale reveals that growth is constant (Fig. 2-23).

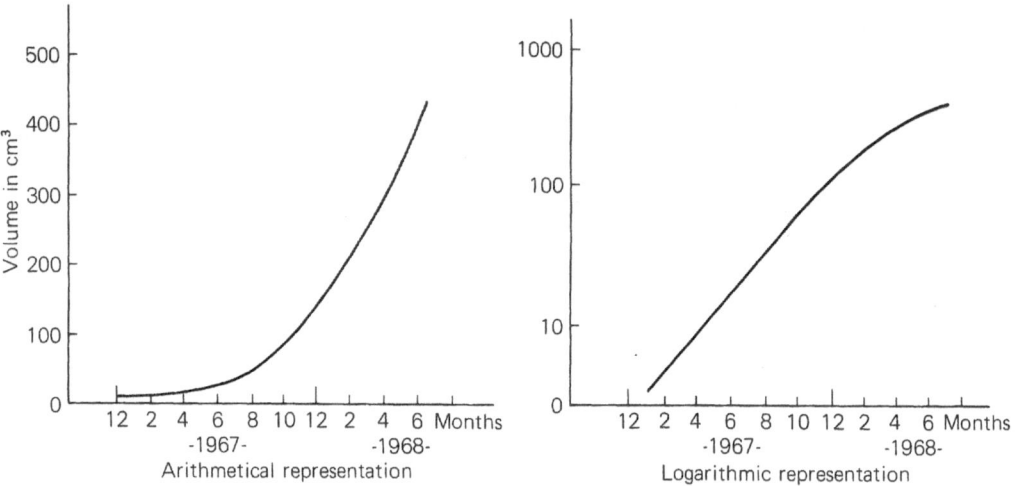

Fig. 2-23. Growth of a pulmonary metastasis of a squamous epithelial carcinoma originating in the head and neck area. (From SAEGESSER and PETTAVEL, Oncologie chirurgicale, Vol. 1, Paris: Masson 1971)

Various techniques have been developed for the study of the characteristics of the cell cycle in experimental tumors and in a few human tumors (62). The labeled mitosis technique consists in labeling with tritiated thymidine a cohort of cells engaged in DNA synthesis (Fig. 2-24). Tumor biopsies are taken at regular intervals following the injection and autoradiographs made. The number of labeled mitoses per 100 mitoses is plotted against time following the pulse label, which allows the labeled cohort to be followed through successive mitoses. If all the cells in the population under study had the same cell-cycle time (Tc), a series of trapezoid-shaped waves would be obtained, generated by each passage of the cohort through mitosis, from which the duration of G_2, M, S, G_1 and hence Tc could be calculated (Fig. 2-24). An actual curve, however, shows considerable damping of the trapezoids due to the variation in the Tc's of the individual cells making up the population. The degree of damping is a measure of the spread in the distribution of the cell-cycle times. Many tumors have such a wide spread of Tc's that the Tc distribution is more representative than a mean or median value. If the spread is extensive, a second wave may not appear in the curve, indicating that the labeled cells had lost their synchrony before the second mitosis. Tc, GF, and cell loss are the three most important parameters in cell kinetics; of these, cell loss is the most difficult to measure accurately.

Cell loss can be estimated by measuring the birth rate of cells within a tumor (the potential doubling time, PDT, or the doubling time of the population in the absence of cell loss) and comparing this with its actual volume growth rate (the observed doubling time, DT) (63, 64). The rate of the cell loss φ = 1- PDT : DT. Such calculations indicate that the cell loss is very considerable in most tumors (Table 2-3). Cell loss occurs through exfoliation from the skin or pleura, migration via lymphatic and vascular channels, and cell death. Tumor cells die either like differentiated end-cells in normal tissues, or as a result of a cellular defect (e.g. ineffective mitosis), changes in their environment (lack of nutrients or accumulation of toxic catabolites), or immunologic attack by the host. The extent of cell loss can cause considerable divergence in the actual growth curves of tumors that have identical potential doubling times. The tumor mass may grow, remain stable, or regress, depending on whether cell loss is smaller, equal to, or larger than the cell input from the dividing compartment. Thus, the clinical evaluation of tumor masses may not accurately reflect either the proliferative activity of a given tumor or the effect of a given treatment. Furthermore, the growth fraction in various parts of a particular tumor mass may be different, depending on local factors such as vascularization (Fig. 2-25) (65).

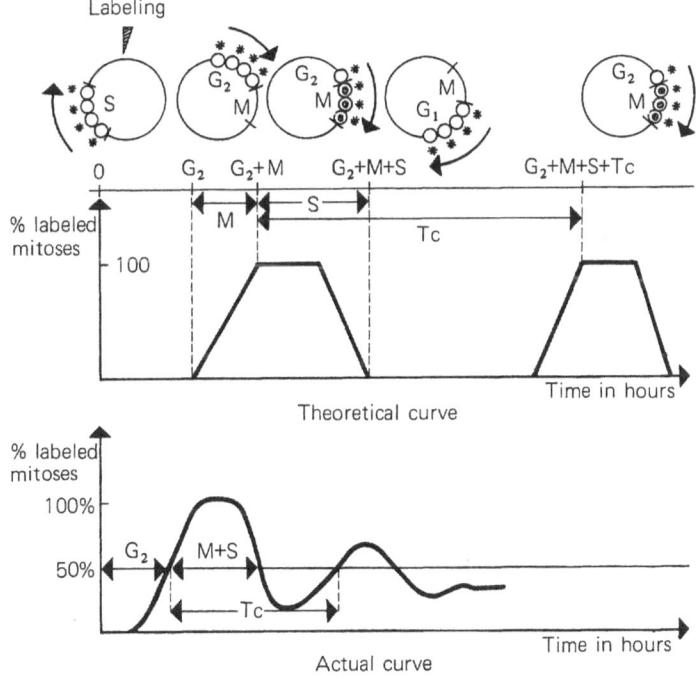

Fig. 2-24. Calculation of the average duration of the cell cycle (Tc), G2, M, and S using the method of labeled mitoses. A theoretical and an actual curve are represented

The study of tumor growth patterns and kinetics has been of great value
to the oncologist (66,67). Cytotoxic agents have been classified according to their effect on the cell cycle (see Ch. 5). Since most antitumor
drugs interfere with active cellular processes, it is not surprising
that the majority of drugs affect cells in the proliferative cycle. Drugs
that affect cells as long as they are in cycle are referred to as cell-
cycle-dependent. If their effect is limited to cells in a particular
phase of the cycle, for exemple S or M, they are classified as cell-
phase-dependent agents. The cytocidal action of irradiation is independent of the cell cycle; thus it is equally toxic to proliferating and
resting cells.

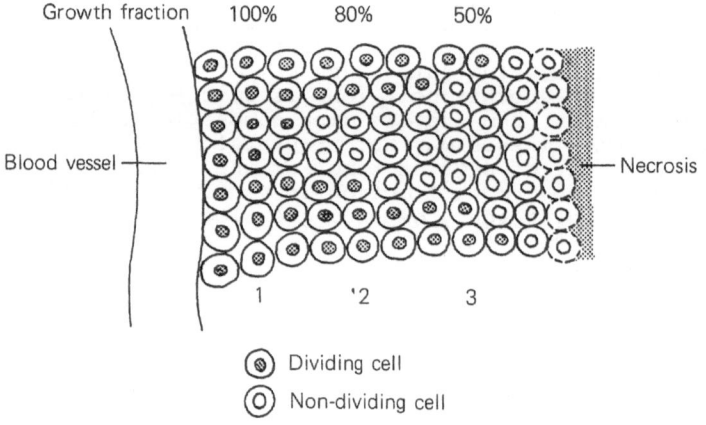

*Fig. 2-25. Growth fractions in three zones located (1) near the blood
vessel, (2) midway between the blood vessel and the necrotic area and
(3) near the necrotic area*

Table 2-3. The labeling indices of human tumors. (From LAMERTON and
STEEL (64))

Site of tumor	Median labeling index %	Potential doubling time (days)	Principal authors
Breast	1.1	43	WOLBERG and BROWN
Central nervous system	2	23.4	KURY and CARTER
Melanoma	3.3	14.2	–
Colon	4.5	10.4	WOLBERG
Uterus, Cervix	4.8	9.8	TITUS and SHORTER
Stomach	6.9	6.8	LIEB and LISCO
Tongue	7.2	6.5	TITUS and SHORTER
Lung, Larynx	15	3.1	–
Lymphosarcoma, Burkitt's tumor	32	1.5	COOPER

The type of growth exponential versus stationary must be taken into consideration in planning the treatment of a malignancy. Solid tumors are generally in the stationary phase at the time of diagnosis. It is therefore not surprising that they respond less well to chemotherapy than acute leukemias or Burkitt's tumor, where most of the cells are in cycle (68). The sensitivity of solid tumors to chemotherapy might improve if we could develop drugs active against resting cells or devise methods to bring resting cells into cycle. This "recruitment" can be effected, as has been shown in experimental systems, by reducing the number of cells in the population, thereby bringing the remaining cells into the exponential part of the growth curve. This is the rationale for recommending surgical reduction of tumor masses that cannot be completely resected (see p. 235). The same rationale applies to chemotherapy programs that use cell-cycle-dependent drugs followed in sequence by cell-phase-dependent agents (69). Another theoretical approach to solid tumors would be to convert cells with proliferative integrity (compartments A + B, Fig. 2-20) by some biochemical manipulation into compartment C cells that would be eliminated by natural cell death.

A special class of tumor cells not previously mentioned are those in the so called "tumor sanctuaries". Cells in areas such as the central nervous system pose a special problem to the oncologist because the concentrations of cytotoxic drugs that can reach them are inadequate.

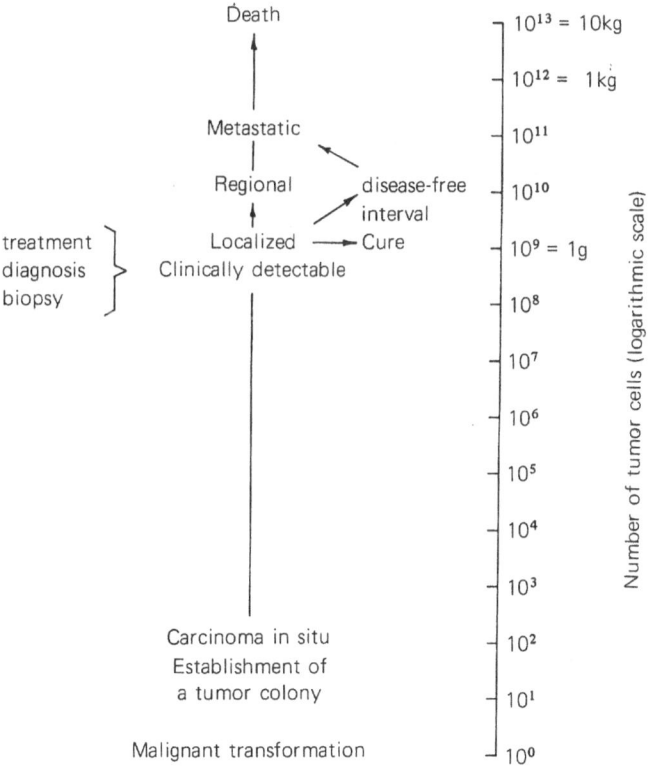

Fig. 2-26. The natural history of a malignancy and the correlation of the clinical course with the number of tumor cells

It is true that the clinical response of malignancies does not always fit the predictions of kinetic studies (70). However, rather than invalidating the usefulness of kinetic considerations, this should stimulate us to pursue such studies to remedy our inadequate understanding.

In summary, it can be stated that cancer cells are distinguished by their capacity to multiply and invade in situations where normal cells are restricted. This abnormal behavior in the result of a heritable alteration in the mechanisms that control the initiation of DNA replication. The exact nature of the defect and the control mechanism have not yet been elucidated. Some alterations have been observed in the biochemical reactions, surface properties, and chromosome constitution of malignant cells, but it is very likely that these are secondary to the primary defect. The only difference between the proliferation of cancer cells and normal cells is that cancer cells have lost the capacity to regulate cell reproduction. Cell reduction in normal tissues (e.g., liver, bone marrow) will stimulate a compensatory production until the number is restored; this process is controlled by growth stimulators and inhibitors, such as hormones and chalones (71). Tumor cells may not respond, or only partially, to these growth-regulating factors.

In medical practice, cancer comprises some 100 clinically distinct illnesses characterized by the property that the cells multiply and invade where normal cells do not. It is generally believed that malignant transformation starts in a single cell. The derangement of the normal mechanisms controlling the growth, division, and movement of the cells may result in the establishment of a clone of malignant cells (Fig. 2-26). The earliest clinical stage is carcinoma in situ. Once the number of cells has reached 10^9, or 1 g in weight, the tumor may become clinically detectable. If diagnosed and treated at this stage, the patient has a good chance of cure; if untreated, malignant cells will eventually find their way into regional lymph nodes or disseminate via the blood stream. By the time a patient dies of a widespread malignancy or leukemia, he may harbor up to 10^{12} to 10^{13} tumor cells (1 to 10 Kg). This is the magnitude of the tumor population that must be destroyed to cure a patient at this stage.

REFERENCES

1. LOEVY, A.G., SIEKEVITZ, P.: Cell Structure and Function, Vol. 1, New York: Rinehart and Wiston 1963.
2. SWANSON, C.P.: The cell, Vol. 1, 2 ed. New York: Prentice Hall 1964.
3. ROSS, L.M.: The Cell. Clinical Symposia Ciba 25, 4 (1973).
4. BENNET, H.S.: The concept of membrane flow and membrane vesiculation as mechanisms for active transport and ion pumping. J. biophys. biochem. Cytol., suppl. 2, 99 (1956).
5. PORTER, K.R.: The submicroscopic morphology of protoplasm. Harvey Lect. 51, 175 (1956).
6. PALADE, G.E.: Studies on the endoplasmic reticulum. II. Simple dispositions in cells in situ. J. biophys. biochem. Cytol. 1, 567 (1955).
7. WHALEY, G., DAUWALDER, M., KEPHART, J.E.: Golgi apparatus: influence on cell surface. Science 175, 596 (1972).
8. LEHNINGER, A.L.: Oxidative phosphorylation. Harvey Lect. 44, 176 (1953).
9. deDUVE, C.: Lysosomes: a new group of cytoplasmic particles. In: Subcellular Particles, Vol. 1, p. 128 (ed. T. Havashi). New York: Ronald Press 1959.

10. BEAUFAY, H., VAN CAMPENHOUT, E., deDUVE, C.: Tissue fractionation studies. II. Influence of various hepatotoxic treatments on the state of some bound enzymes in rat liver. Biochem. J. 73, 617 (1959).

11. VERITY, M.A., ANDIMAN, R., MUNSAT, T.L., SMITH, R.E., SZEGO, C.M.: The lysosome: a role in disease. Ann. intern. Med. 78, 725 (1973).

12. WATSON, J.D.: Molecular Biology of the Gene. Menlo Park: W.A. Benjamin 1970.

13. HARPER, H.A.: Review of physiological chemistry. Los Altos: Lange Medical Publications 1975.

14. HUANG, R.C., BONNER, J.: Histone, a suppressor of chromosomal RNA synthesis. Proc. nat. Acad. Sci. 48, 1216 (1962).

15. BUTLER, J.A.V.: Role of histones and other proteins in gene control. Nature 207, 1041 (1965).

16. CRICK, F.H.C.: Structure of nucleic acids and their role in protein synthesis, Vol. 1, Cambridge, Cambridge Univ. Press Mass.: 1957.

17. WATSON, J.D., CRICK, F.H.C.: Molecular structure of nucleic acids: a structure for deoxyribose nucleic acid. Nature 171, 737 (1953).

18. SHAPIRO, H.S., CHARGAFF, E.: Studies on the nucleotide arrangement in desoxyribonucleic acids. IV. Pattern of nucleotide sequence in the desoxyribonucleic acid on rye germ and its fraction. Biochim. biophys. Acta 39, 68 (1960).

19. COHEN, G.N., GROS, F.: Protein biosynthesis. Annu. Rev. Biochem. 29, 525 (1960).

20. YCAS, M.: The coding hypothesis. Int. Rev. Cyto. 13, 1 (1962).

21. RHO, J.H., BONNER, J.: The site of ribonucleic acid synthesis in the isolated nucleus. Proc. nat. Acad. Sci. 47, 1611 (1961).

22. JACOB, F. MONOD, J.: Genetic regulatory mechanisms in the synthesis of proteins. J. molec. Biol. 3, 318 (1961).

23. JACOB, F., MONOD, J.: On the regulation of gene activity. Cold Spr. Harb. Symp. quant. Biol. 26, 193 (1961).

24. LAJTHA, L.G.: On DNA labeling in the study of the dynamics of bone marrow cell populations. In: The Kinetics of Cellular Proliferation, (ed. F. Stohlman) Vol. 1, p. 173. New York: Grune and Stratton 1959.

25. MAZIA, D.: Mitosis and the physiology of cell division. In: The Cell (eds. J. Brachet, A.E. Mirsky) Vol. 3, p. 77. New York: Academic Press 1961.

26. LAURENCE, L.: The Cell in Mitosis. Vol. 1, New York: Academic Press 1963.

27. BASERGA, R.: Biochemistry of the cell cycle: a review. Cell Tissue Kinet. 1, 167 (1968).

28. BASERGA, R.: Biochemical events in the cell cycle. In: Human Tumor Cell Kinetics Monograph 30, p. 1. National Cancer Institute 1969.

29. TAYLOR, J.H., WOODS, P.S. HUGHES, W.L.: The organization of chromosomes as revealed by autoradiografic studies using tritium-labeled thymidine. Proc. nat. Acad. Sci. (Wash.) 43, 122 (1957).

30. TAYLOR, J.H.: Autoradiography with tritium-labeled substances. Advanc. biol. med. Phys. 7, 107 (1960).

31. RUTHMANN, A.: The fine structure of the meiotic spindle of crayfish. J. biophys. biochem. Cytol. 5, 177 (1959).

32. BRACHET, J.: Biochemical cytology, Vol. 1. New York: Academic Press 1957.

33. WARBURG, O.: Stoffwechsel der Tumoren. Vol. 1. Berlin: Springer 1926.

34. GREENSTEIN. J.P.: Biochemistry of cancer, 2 ed., Vol. 1. New York: Academic Press 1954.

35. PITOT, M.C.: Some biochemical aspects of malignancies. Annu. Rev. Biochem. 35, 335 (1966).

36. NORDMANN, R.: Les altérations du metabolisme énergétique dans les tissus cancéreaux Rev. franc. Etudes clin. biol. 10, 607 (1965).

37. RACKER, E.: Bioenergetics and the problem of tumor growth. Amer. Scientist. $\underline{60}$, 56 (1972).
38. WEBER, G.: Molecular correlation concept of neoplasia. Advanc. Enzyme Regulation. $\underline{4}$, 115 (1966).
39. WEINHOUSE, S.: Isozymes in cancer. Cancer Res. $\underline{31}$, 1166 (1971).
40. CRISS, W.E.: A review of isozymes in cancer. Cancer Res. $\underline{31}$, 1523 (1971).
41. WEBER, G., QUEENER, S.F., MORRIS, H.P.: Imbalance in ornithine metabolism in hepatomas of different growth rates as expressed in behavior of l-ornithine carbamyl transferase activity. Cancer Res. $\underline{32}$, 1933 (1972).
42. EMMELOT, P.: Biochemical properties of normal and neoplastic cell surfaces: A review. Europ. J. Cancer $\underline{9}$, 319 (1973).
43. OETTGEN, H.F., OLD, L.J., BOYSE, E.A., CAMPBELL, H.A., PHILIPS, F.S., CLARKSON, B.D., TALLAL, L., LEEPER, R.D., SCHWARTZ, M.K., HO KIM, J.: Inhibition of leukemias in man by l-asparaginase. Cancer Res. $\underline{27}$, 2619 (1967).
44. McGUIRE, W.L., HUFF, K., JENNINGS, A., CHAMNESS, G.C.: Mammary carcinoma: A specific biochemical defect in autonomous tumors. Science $\underline{175}$, 335 (1972).
45. BURGER, M.M.: Surface properties of neoplastic cells. Hosp. Practice, $\underline{55}$ (Jul. 1973).
46. PAINTRAND, M., ROSENFELD, C.: Etude ultrastructurale de la glyco-calix des leucocytes humains normaux et leucémiques en culture permanente. Comparaison entre deux lignées d'origine normale et deux lignées d'origine leucémique. C.R. Acad. Sci. $\underline{274}$, 415 (1972).
47. KOLLER, P.C.: The role of chromosomes in cancer biology. Recent Results in Cancer Research, Vol. 38. Berlin-Heidelberg-New York: Springer Verlag 1971.
48. NOWELL, P.C., HUNGERFORD, D.A.: Chromosome studies in human leukemia. II. Chronic granulocytic leukemia. J. Nat. Cancer Inst. $\underline{27}$, 1013 (1961).
49. MANOLOV, G., MANOLOVA, Y.: Marker band in one chromosome 14 from Burkitt lymphomas. Nature $\underline{237}$, 33 (1972).
50. GERMAN, J.: Oncogenic implications of chromosomal instability. Hosp. Practice $\underline{93}$ (Feb. 1973).
51. BRESCIANI, F.: Cell proliferation in cancer. Europ. J. Cancer $\underline{4}$, 343 (1968).
52. PRESCOTT, D.M.: Biology of cancer and the cancer cell: normal and abnormal regulation of cell reproduction. CA, $\underline{22}$, 262 (1972).
53. MENDELSOHN, M.L.: Autoradiographic analysis of cell proliferation in spontaneous breast cancer of C3H mouse. II. The growth fraction. J. Nat. Cancer Inst. $\underline{28}$, 1015 (1962).
54. DE VITA, V.T.: Cell kinetics and the chemotherapy of cancer. Cancer Chemother. Rep. Part 3, $\underline{2}$, 23 (1971).
55. SUGARBAKER, E.V., KETCHAM, A.S., COHEN, A.M.: Studies of dormant tumor cells. Cancer $\underline{28}$, 545 (1971).
56. LAJTHA, L.G., GILBERT, C.W.: Kinetics of cellular proliferation. Adv. biol. med. Phys. $\underline{11}$, 1 (1967).
57. SKIPPER, H.E., PERRY, S.: Kinetics of normal and leukemic leucocyte populations and relevance to chemotherapy. Cancer Res. $\underline{30}$, 1883 (1970).
58. COLLINS, V.P., LOEFFLER, R.K., TIVEY, H.: Observations on growth rates of human tumors. Am. J. Roentgenol. $\underline{76}$, 988 (1956).
59. MEYER, J.A.: The concept and significance of growth rates in human pulmonary tumors. Ann. thorac. Surg. $\underline{14}$, 309 (1972).
60. CHARBIT, A., MALAISE, E.P., TUBIANA, M.: Relation between the pathological nature and the growth rate of human tumors. Europ. J. Cancer $\underline{7}$, 307 (1971).
61. LAIRD, A.K.: Dynamics of tumor growth. Br. J. Cancer $\underline{18}$, 490 (1964).

62. TUBIANA, M.: The kinetics of tumor cell proliferation and radio-
    therapy. Brit. J. Radiol. 44, 325 (1971).
63. STEEL, G.G.: Cell loss as a factor in the growth rate of human
    tumours. Europ. J. Cancer 3, 381 (1967).
64. LAMERTON, L.F., STEEL, G.G.: Cell population kinetics in normal
    and malignant tissues. In: Progress in Biophysics and Molecular
    Biology, Vol. 18, p. 245. Oxford: Pergamon Press 1968.
65. TANNOCK, I.F.: Relation between cel proliferation and the vascular
    system in a transplanted mouse mammary tumour. Brit. J. Cancer 22,
    258 (1968).
66. COOPER, E.H.: Cell kinetics and the growth of solid tumours in man.
    In: The Design of Clinical Trials in Cancer Therapy, p. 156 (ed.
    M. Staquet) Brussels: Editions Scientifiques Européennes 1972.
67. STRYCKMANS, P.: Kinetic aspects of leukemia therapy. In: The Design
    of Clinical Trials in Cancer Therapy, p. 132 (ed. M. Staquet)
    Brussels: Edition Scientifiques Européennes 1972.
68. COOPER, E.H., FRANK, G.L., WRIGHT, D.H.: Cell proliferation in
    Burkitt tumours. Europ. J. Cancer 2, 377 (1966).
69. SCHABEL, Jr. F.M.: The use of tumor growth kinetics in planning
    "curative" chemotherapy of advanced solid tumors. Cancer Res. 29,
    2384 (1969).
70. HALL, T.C.: Limited role of cell kinetics in clinical cancer chemo-
    therapy. Nat. Cancer Inst. Monogr. 34, 15 (1971).
71. BULLOUGH, W.S., LAURENCE, E.B.: The lymphocytic chalone and its
    antimitotic action on a mouse lymphoma in vitro. Europ. J. Cancer
    6, 525 (1970).

Chapter 3

Classification of Chemotherapeutic Agents According to their Mechanisms of Action

This chapter deals mainly with the mechanisms of action of the various drugs used in cancer chemotherapy (1-12, 220). There are various ways of classifying these agents, the best known method being based on the broad mechanism of action or the source of the drug (Table 3-1). However,

Table 3-1. Conventional classification of cytotoxic drugs

---

1. Alkylating agents
2. Antimetabolites
       folate analogs
       purine analogs
       pyrimidine analogs
       amino-acid analogs
3. Antibiotics
4. Plant alkaloids
5. Enzymes
6. Miscellaneous drugs
7. Steroid hormones
8. Radioactive isotopes

---

we prefer to think of cytotoxic drugs in terms of site of action. This is especially important in view of the current trend in cancer chemotherapy to design protocols that use drugs with different mechanisms of action sequentially or in combination. We distinguish drugs that (1) interfere with the biosynthesis of nucleic acids and proteins, (2) interfere with duplication, transcription, and translation, (3) interfere with the mitotic spindle, and (4) drugs with a complex or poorly understood mechanism of action that cannot easily be assigned to any of the other three groups. In Chap. 5 we classify chemotherapeutic agents according to their effects on the cell cycle.

For convenience, data on the pharmacology, dose schedules, toxicity, and indications of the principal agents are summerized in Table 3-2 at the end of this chapter.

A. DRUGS INTERFERING WITH BIOSYNTHESIS OF DNA, RNA, and PROTEINS

Nucleic acids are built up from nucleotide units and proteins from amino-acids. The biosynthesis of purines and pyrimidines and the role

of folate in these processes is outlined in Chap. 2. Antitumor drugs
can interfere at a variety of sites in this scheme (Fig. 3-1). Most

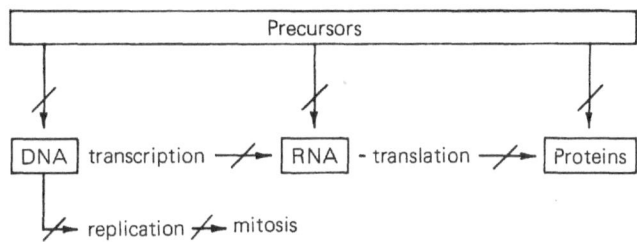

Fig. 3-1. Schematic representation of the potential sites of action of
cytotoxic agents. Different steps in DNA synthesis, DNA replication,
mitosis, translation and protein synthesis can be interrupted (indicated by a crossed bar)

agents in the class under discussion are referred to as analogs, antagonists, or antimetabolites. The compounds thus designated are structural analogs of normal metabolites or coenzymes, and they interfere
with normal cellular metabolism either by inhibiting specific enzymatic
steps or by fraudulent incorporation as a building unit. Four groups
are distinguished: folate, purine, pyrimidine, and amino-acid analogs
(13-15).

1. Folic Acid Analogs

Substitution of an amino group for the 4-hydroxy group of folic acid
produced a potent antagonist, aminopterin, that allowed FARBER to obtain the first remissions in acute childhood leukemia (16). Of the
many related compounds synthesized, 4-amino-N^{10}-methylpteroyl glutamic acid, or methotrexate (MTX), is the drug in most frequent clinical
use at the present time (Fig. 3-2) (17-23, 221, 235).

Folic acid coenzymes are involved in the transfer and utilization of
the single carbon (C1) moiety. Before it can function as a C1 carrier,
folic acid must be reduced to dihydrofolic acid and then to tetrahydrofolic acid (Fig. 2-16). These reactions are catalyzed by folate and
dihydrofolate reductase. Tetrahydrofolic acid accepts single carbon
fragments from various sources to generate the active folate coenzymes,
N^5 and N^{5-10} methylene tetrahydrofolate, that are utilized as carbon
donors in the synthesis of the methyl group of thymidylic acid, the
insertion of C2 and C8 in the purine ring, and the synthesis of the ß
carbon of serine (see Figs. 2-11, 2-12 and 2-13). Thymidylate synthesis requires substrate amounts of folate coenzymes, while purine synthesis appears to require only catalytic amounts. Methotrexate binds extremely tightly but reversibly to dihydrofolate reductase, thereby depleting the folate coenzymes. The resulting inhibition of thymidylate
synthesis and thus of DNA synthesis of cells in S phase seems to be the
key event leading to unbalanced growth and cell death (Fig. 3-3). Purine
synthesis, and hence RNA synthesis, are inhibited as well as serine and
methionine synthesis. The relative roles of the "thymidineless" and
the "purineless" state in causing cell death are not clear on the basis
of currently available experimental data (18, 23). Methotrexate not
only interferes with the function of dihydrofolate reductase, it also
inhibits thymidylate synthetase, thereby further interfering with the

37

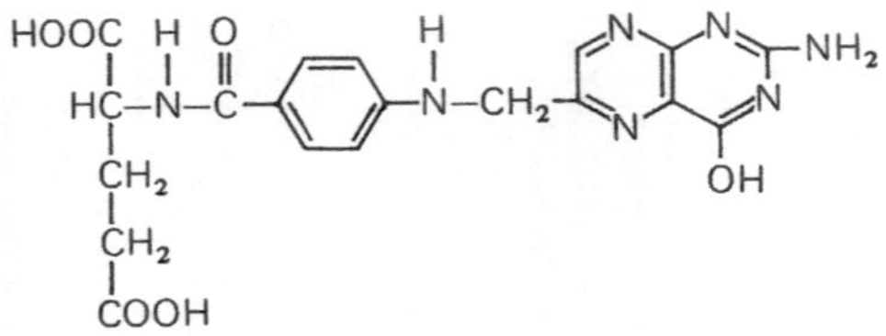

HOOC HO O
HC–N–C
|
CH₂
|
CH₂
|
COOH

N–CH₂

H

Pteroyl glutamic acid
Folic acid

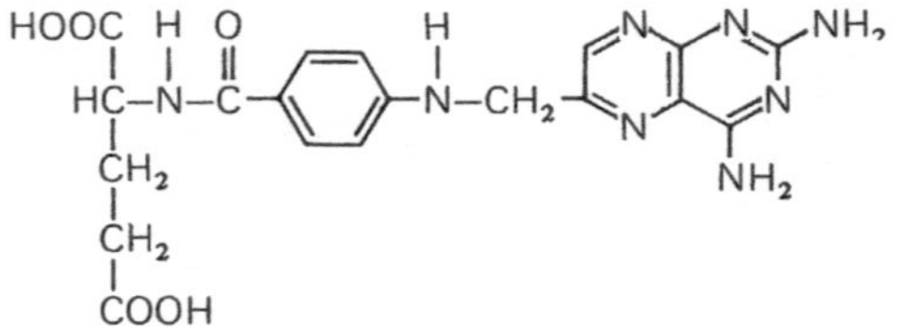

HOOC H O
HC–N–C
|
CH₂
|
CH₂
|
COOH

N–CH₂

H

4-Aminopteroyl glutamic acid
Aminopterin

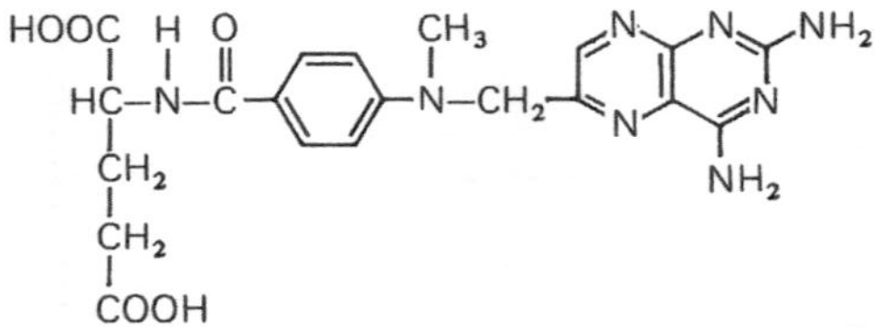

HOOC H O
HC–N–C
|
CH₂
|
CH₂
|
COOH

N–CH₂
|
CH₃

4-Amino-N¹⁰-methylpteroylglutamic acid
Methotrexate

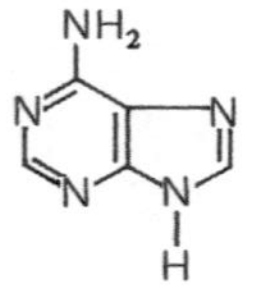

NH₂

Adenine

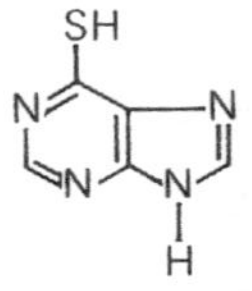

SH

6-Mercaptopurine

SCH₃

HOH₂C
HO OH

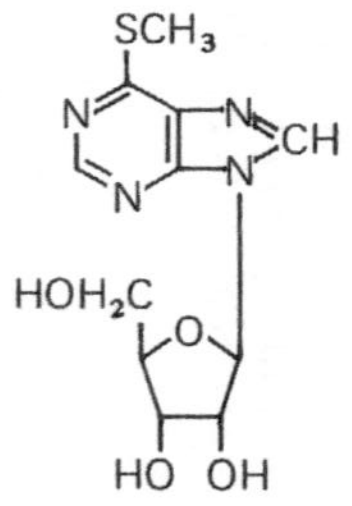

6-(Methylmercapto)purine ribonucleoside
6-MMPR

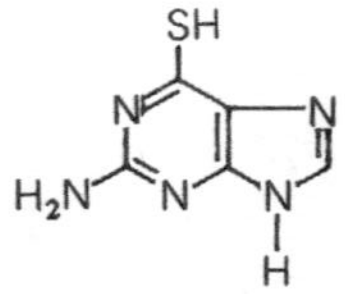

SH

H₂N

6-Thioguanine

H₂N–C
||
O

N

H

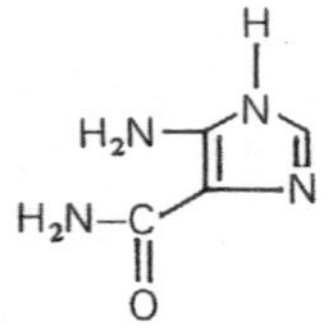

5-Amino-imidazole-4-carboxamide

CH₃
|
CH₃–N–N=N

H₂N–C
||
O

N

H

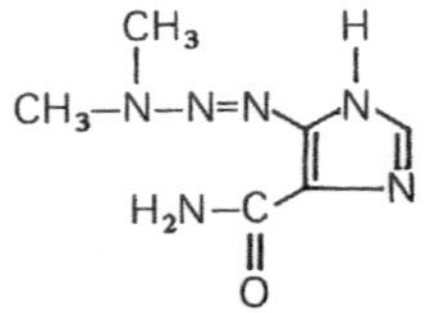

5(3,3-Dimethyl-1-triazeno)
imidazole-4-carboxamide (DIC)

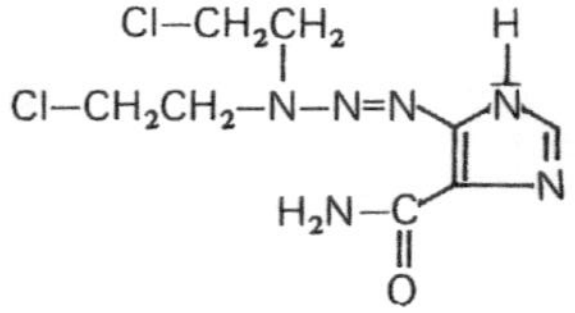

Cl–CH₂CH₂
|
Cl–CH₂CH₂–N–N=N

H₂N–C
||
O

N

H

5-[3,3-Bis(2-chloroethyl)-1-triazeno]
imidazole-4-carboxamide (TIC mustard)

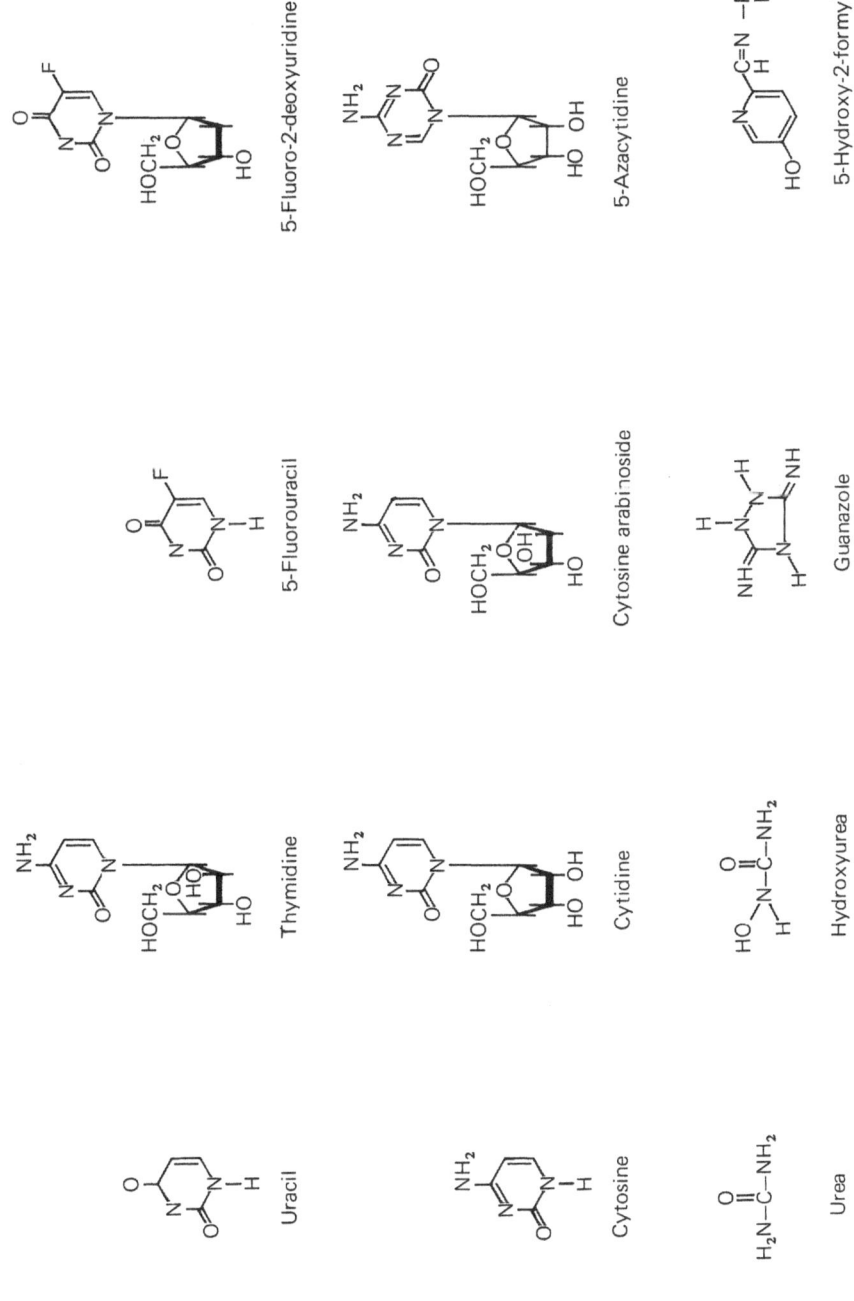

Fig. 3-2. Chemical structure of normal metabolites and of some of the antimetabolites used in cancer chemotherapy. Hydroxyurea, guanazole, and 5HP are not structural analogs of normal metabolites. They inhibit ribonucleotide reductase, the enzyme that supplies desoxyribonucleotides

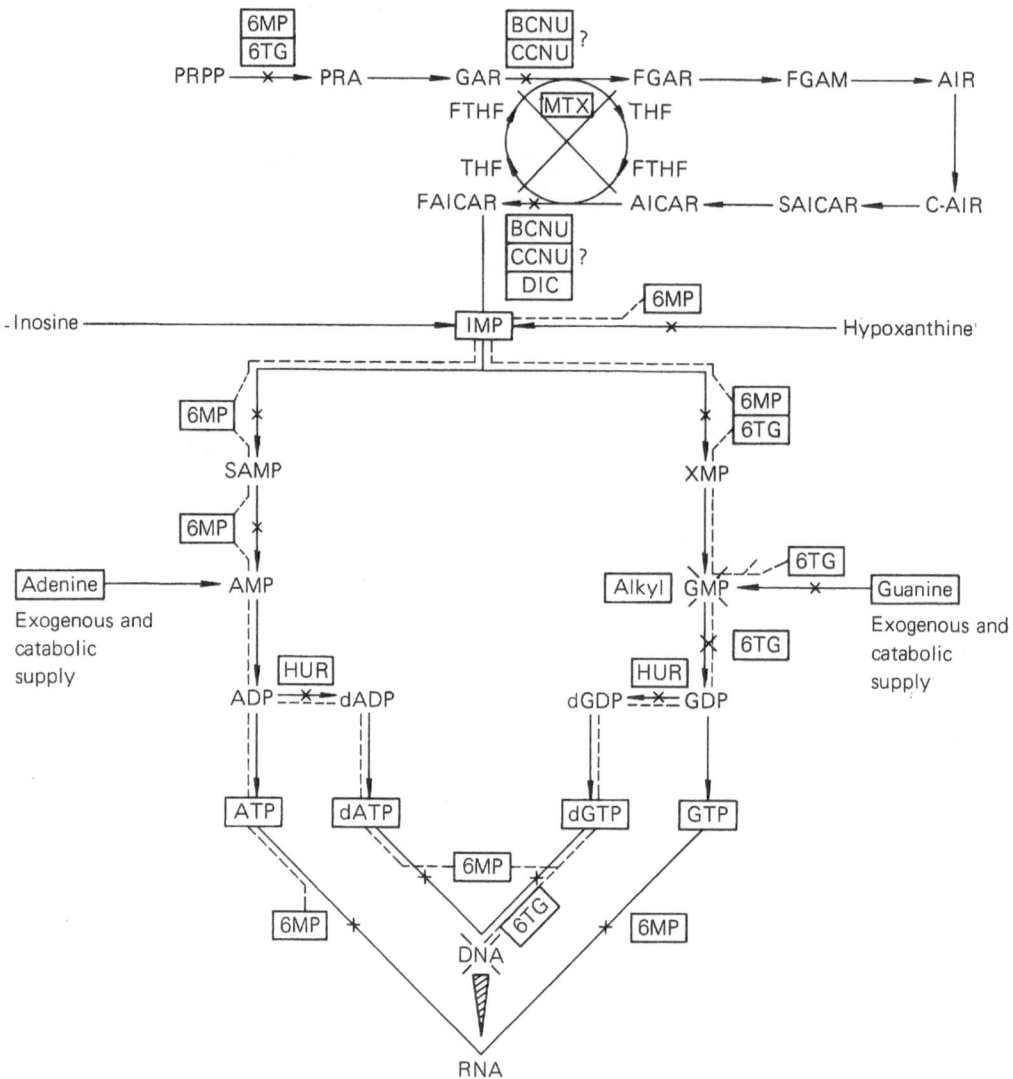

*Fig. 3-3. Sites of action of cytotoxic agents which interfere with pu-
rine biosynthesis (indicated by X); metabolic pathways in which cytotoxic drugs are incorporated (indicated by a dotted line). See Fig. 2-
12 for abbreviations*

synthesis of thymidylic acid. Folinic acid or citrovorum factor (N^5-
formyl tetrahydrofolate) (see Fig. 2-15) can circumvent the inhibition
of dihydrofolate reductase and prevent the toxic effects of MTX if administered before irreversible cell damage has occured, usually within
4 hours (<u>235</u>).

2. Purine Analogs

6-Mercaptopurine (6-MP), is a structural analog of adenine and hypoxanthine (24-28, 13) (see Fig. 3-2). To exert its biological effect it
must be converted to a 6-MP ribonucleotide(6-thioinosinate or T-IMP)
by hypoxanthine-guanine phosphoryl transferase, an enzyme for which it
competes with hypoxanthine. T-IMP acts as a pseudofeedback inhibitor
of amido transferase, the enzyme that catalyzes the initial reaction
in the de novo purine synthesis (conversion of PRPP to PRA) (see Fig.
3-3). T-IMP in addition blocks by competitive inhibition the two enzymes
in the conversion of IMP$\rightarrow\hspace{-0.3em}/\hspace{-0.3em}\rightarrow$SAMP$\rightarrow\hspace{-0.3em}/\hspace{-0.3em}\rightarrow$AMP and the enzyme of the conversion
of IMP$\rightarrow\hspace{-0.3em}/\hspace{-0.3em}\rightarrow$XMP, thereby reducing the supply of GMP. Thus, 6-MP inhibits
synthesis of both DNA and RNA by inhibition early in de novo synthesis
of purines and by interfering with purine nucleotide interconversion
steps. It also affects the utilization of exogenous purines. It is not
known whether some of the purine anabolites are incorporated into nucleic acids. Some of the metabolic alterations induced by 6-MP may be
due to the formation of 6-MMPR ribonucleotide (24).

6-(Methylmercapto)purine ribonucleoside (6-MMPR), an adenosine analog,
is converted by adenosine kinase to a 5-monophosphate ribonucleotide (6-
MMPR-P) (9, 29, 30) (see Fig. 3-2). Phosphorylation does not seem to
proceed beyond the monophosphate level therefore 6-MMPR is not incorporated into nucleic acids. 6-MMPR, like 6-MP, exerts a potent pseudofeedback inhibition on de novo purine synthesis by inhibiting amido
transferase. The combination of 6-MP with 6-MMPR has resulted in a
synergistic antitumor action in several in vivo and in vitro systems
(29).

6-Thioguanine (6-TG), a guanine analog, is metabolized to its nucleotide 6-thioguanosine-5-phosphate (6-thio GMP) (see Figs. 3-2 and 3-3)
(31-33). It can be further phosphorylated and incorporated into both
DNA and RNA. Thio-DNA cannot replicate and this is thought to be the
major cause of cell death. 6-Thio GMP in addition causes pseudofeedback
inhibition of amido transferase (PRPP$\rightarrow\hspace{-0.3em}/\hspace{-0.3em}\rightarrow$PRA), and inhibition of ino-
sinic dehydrogenase (IMP$\rightarrow\hspace{-0.3em}/\hspace{-0.3em}\rightarrow$XMP$\longrightarrow$GMP) and of guanylate kinase (GMP
$\rightarrow\hspace{-0.3em}/\hspace{-0.3em}\rightarrow$GDP). Such metabolic blockades should markedly limit the supply of
guanine nucleotide for nucleic acid and coenzyme synthesis.

The triazenoimidazole carboxamides, analogs of 5-aminoimidazole-4-car-
boxamide, a precursor in de novo purine synthesis, were initially developed as inhibitors of purine synthesis (see Figs. 3-2 and 3-3) (34-40).
Their action is not fully understood. They seem also to have an alkylating action, probably through one of their metabolites. 5-(3,3-Dime-
thyl-1-triazeno)imidazole-4-carboxamide (DIC) and 5-{3,3-bis(2-chlor-
ethyl)-1-triazeno}imidazole-4-carboxamide (TIC-mustard) are being evaluated in clinical trials (38-40).

3. Pyrimidine Analogs

A variety of analogs of the pyrimidine bases and nucleosides have been
obtained by substitution on the ring, modifications of the pyrimidine
ring structure, or changes in the sugar moiety of the nucleoside (14,
15). 5-Fluorouracil (5 FU) is the most frequently in clinical use (Fig.
3-2) (15, 41-43). It is converted first to the ribonucleoside, FUR, a
toxic compound with little selectivity for neoplastic cells, which is
then phosphorylated to the mono- (F-UMP), di- and triphosphoribonucleo-
tide. The consequences of such incorporation have been different in
the various systems tested, but translation errors can occur. F-UMP is
also reduced to the deoxynucleotide F-dUMP, which inhibits thymidylate
synthetase, the enzyme that catalyzes methylation of deoxyuridylate to

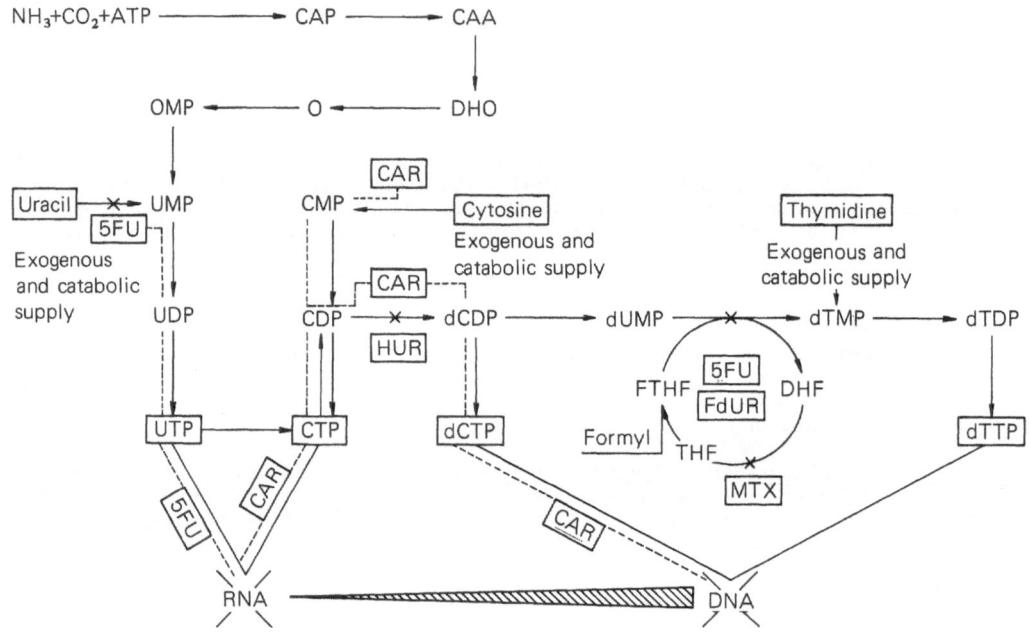

Fig. 3-4. Sites of action of cytotoxic agents which interfere with pyrimidine biosynthesis (indicated by X); metabolic pathways in which cytotoxic drugs are incorporated (indicated by a dotted line). See Fig. 2-13 for abbreviations

thymidylate (dUMP→dTMP) (Fig. 3-4). The "thymidineless" state leads to impaired DNA synthesis and cell death. There is no evidence that F-dUMP is further phosphorylated and incorporated into DNA. 5-Fluoro-2-deoxy-uridine (FUdR) (see Fig. 3-2) can be converted by intracellular deoxy-uridine kinase into F-dUMP and was introduced for more direct inhibition of thymidylate synthetase that can be obtained with 5 FU (Fig. 3-4) (44). However, FUdR is broken down to 5 FU with its attendant disadvantages (formation of FUR).

The substitution of iodine for the fluoride of FUdR yields 5-iodo-2'-deoxy-uridine (IUdR), a compound that can be incorporated into DNA in place of thymidylic acid. It has antiviral activity, especially against herpes virus, and possesses radiation-sensitizing properties.

Cytosine arabinoside (CAR) is an analog of 2-deoxycytidine that contains D-arabinose as the pentose moiety (see Fig. 3-2) (9, 45-53). It must be phosphorylated by deoxycytidine kinase to its active derivatives, ara-C-diphosphate (ara-CDP) and ara-C-triphosphate (ara-CTP). Phosphorylated derivatives of CAR inhibit the reductase responsible for the conversion of cytidine(5')diphosphate to (2')deoxy-cytidine (5')diphosphate (CDP→dCDP), and DNA polymerase. Both these reactions interfere with DNA synthesis (Fig. 3-4). Furthermore, small amounts of ara-CTP can be incorporated into DNA and RNA, thereby interfering with their function.

5-Azacytidine is an analog of cytidine in which N is substituted for the C in the position 5 of the pyrimidine ring (see Fig. 3-2) (54, 55). It seems to be incorporated into DNA and RNA and inhibits nucleic acid and protein synthesis. This agent is currently undergoing Phase I and II studies.

The triazene analog of uridine, 6-azauridine, after conversion to 6-aza-urydilate inhibits the enzymatic formation of uridylic acid from its carboxylated precusor, orotidylic acid, in de novo pyrimidine biosynthesis, thereby inhibiting nucleic acid synthesis (56). As expected, patients receiving this drug excrete large amounts of orotic acid and orotidine. This drug has been of limited value clinically.

4. Other Agents with Similar Action

Hydroxyurea (HUR), causes a specific inhibition of DNA synthesis of the cell in S phase without blocking the production of RNA or protein (Fig. 3-2) (9, 57-65). The impairment of DNA synthesis seems to be the result of an inhibition of ribonucleotide reductase, the enzyme that supplies deoxyribonucleotides (Fig. 3-4). There is some evidence that HUR may derange DNA structure and interfere with other metabolic processes, such as an early step in pyrimidine synthesis, but these sites of action are less well defined. HUR synchronizes cells (see p. 108) and hinders the repair process in cells that have been damaged but not destroyed by radiation. Hydroxyurea is thus being evaluated in conjunction with radiotherapy to augment the effects of radiation.

Two other compounds that act primarily by inhibiting the ribonucleotide diphosphate reductase system are guanazole (7, 66) and 5-hydroxy-2-formylpyridine thiosemicarbazone (5HP) (Fig. 3-2) (5, 9, 67, 222). Their clinical usefulness is under study.

Around 1960 the nitrosoureas were introduced as a new class of antitumor agents (7, 68-70). They have the basic nitrosourea configuration with the addition of chloroethyl and cyclohexyl groups. BCNU |1,3-bis (2-chloroethyl)-1-nitrosourea| (71), CCNU |1-(2-chloroethyl)-3-cyclohexyl-1-nitrosourea| (72-76, 223), and MeCCNU |1-(2-chloroethyl)-3-(4-methylcyclohexyl)-1-nitrosourea| (77, 78, 224) are already in clinical use (Fig. 3-5). Their high lipid solubility facilitates rapid transport into the cell and across the blood-brain barrier; the latter characteristic has prompted their use in the brain tumors and CNS leukemia. Inhibition of DNA and RNA synthesis accounts for their oncolytic effect.

BCNU: 1,3-bis(2-chloroethyl)-1-nitrosourea

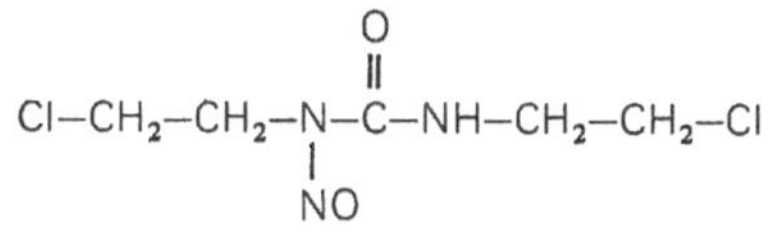

(Carmustine)

CCNU: 1-(2-chloroethyl)-3-cyclohexyl-1-nitrosourea (Lomustine)

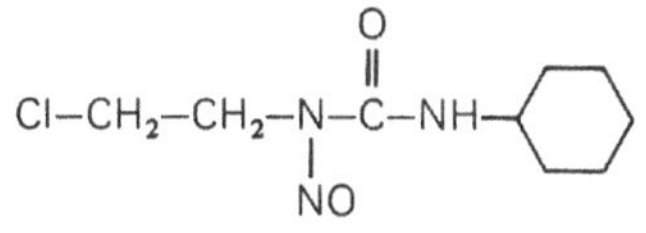

MeCCNU: 1-(2-chloroethyl)-3-(4-methyl cyclohexyl)-1-nitrosourea

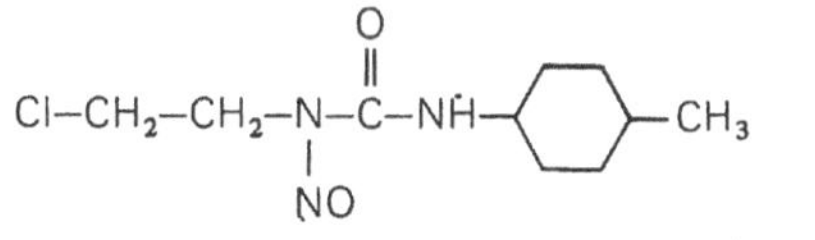

Fig. 3-5. Chemical structure of the nitrosoureas

They are rapidly broken down and the active compounds seem to be degradation products rather than the intact molecule. Although they have an
alkylating effect, they differ from conventional alkylating agents.
CCNU and MeCCNU, having only one alkylating side-chain, are incapable
of cross-linking DNA. Nitrosoureas act at different phases of the cell
cycle from known alkylating agents, and some tumors resistant to the
latter may respond to nitrosoureas. Their alkylating effect may be due
to the formation of diazohydroxide and/or 2-chloroethylamine. CCNU is
cleaved into a highly reactive cyclohexyl isocyanate intermediate that
binds extensively to the amino acid residues of proteins, and the un-
stable ethylene diazohydroxide that binds both to base residues of nucleic acids and to proteins (Fig. 3-6). In addition to this structural
modification of nucleic acids and proteins, nitrosoureas also inhibit
several enzymatic steps in nucleic acid synthesis. These include inhibition of nucleotidyl transferase, inhibition of ribonucleotide conversion to DNA and to a lesser extent to RNA, and interference with
the utilization of histidine in 1-carbon metabolism through inhibition
of forminotransferase, the enzyme that transfers the formino group
from FIGLU to FH4. MeCCNU is uniquely effective against advanced Lewis
lung tumor in mice, a slow-growing tumor with low growth fraction and
long doubling time. It was hoped from the superiority of MeCCNU in
this system that is would be equally active in human tumors that have
similar growth characteristics.

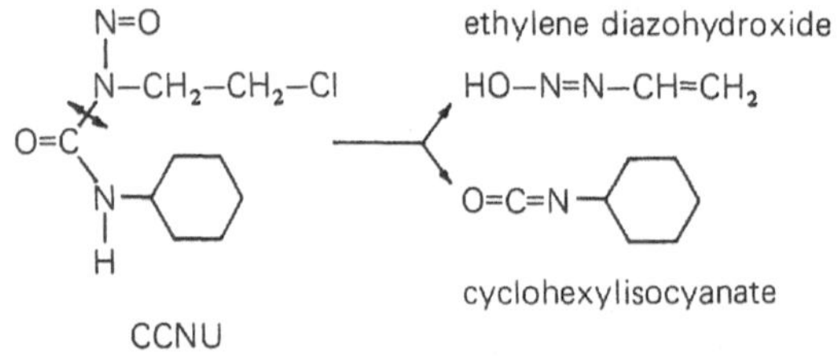

Fig. 3-6. Cleavage of CCNU

Streptozotocin (STZ) a 1-methyl,nitrosourea-glucosamine obtained from
Streptomyces achromogenes, is an antibiotic structurally related to
the nitrosoureas (Fig. 3-7) (79-82). It inhibits DNA synthesis and to
a lesser extent RNA and protein synthesis. The glucosamine carrier
may account for its specificity for the ß cells of the pancreas and
its activity in insulinomas.

Although the mechanism of the action of methylglyoxal-bis-guanylhydrazone (methylGAG, MGGH) is not fully understood, there is evidence that
it binds to DNA and thereby inhibits the synthesis of both DNA and RNA
(Fig. 3-8) (83-86). It also behaves as a mitochondrial poison. This

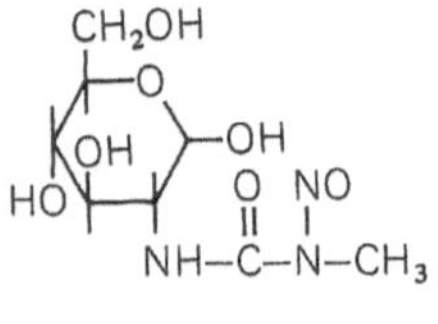

Fig. 3-7. Streptozotozin

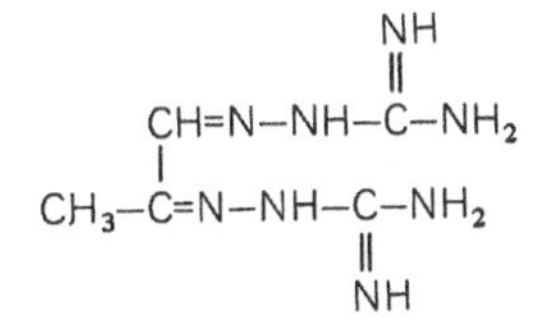

$$\begin{array}{c} \quad\quad\quad\quad NH \\ \quad\quad\quad\quad \| \\ CH{=}N{-}NH{-}C{-}NH_2 \\ | \\ CH_3{-}C{=}N{-}NH{-}C{-}NH_2 \\ \quad\quad\quad\quad \| \\ \quad\quad\quad\quad NH \end{array}$$

Fig. 3-8. Methylglyoxal-bis-guanylhydrazone

compound has shown activity against acute myeloblastic leukemias, but its toxicity and narrow therapeutic index have restricted its use and it has been rarely used in chemotherapy of solid tumors (226).

Procarbazine (PCZ) 1-methyl-2para(isopropylcarbamoyl)benzyl-hydrazine HCl is the most active of a series of derivatives of methylhydrazine that possess antitumor activity (Fig. 3-9) (9, 87-90). It causes suppression of DNA, RNA, and protein at several sites of action. Hydrogen peroxide, formed through auto-oxidation of the drug, can degrade DNA. High concentrations of hydrogen peroxide, formaldehyde, and other potential metabolites, such as N-hydroxymethyl derivatives and formylhydrazine, inhibit DNA and RNA polymerase. The N-methyl group of PCZ can con-

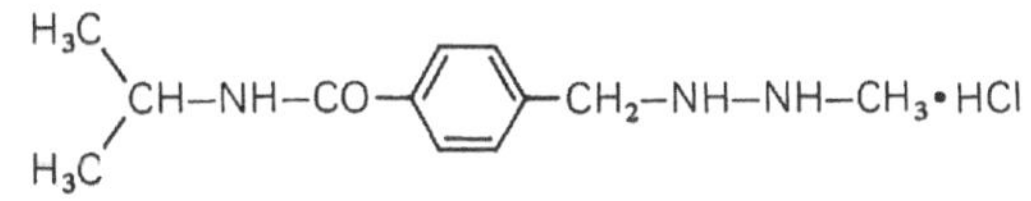

$$\begin{array}{c} H_3C \\ \quad\quad\diagdown \\ \quad\quad\quad CH{-}NH{-}CO{-}\!\!\!\bigcirc\!\!\!{-}CH_2{-}NH{-}NH{-}CH_3 \cdot HCl \\ \quad\quad\diagup \\ H_3C \end{array}$$

Fig. 3-9. 1-Methyl-2 para(isopropylcarbamoyl)benzyl-hydrazine HCl, pro-
carbazine

tribute to the formate pool (1-carbon pool) or be used for methylation of RNA (and DNA). Selective methylation of position 7 of guanine has been reported, especially in RNA (53). Interference with the normally occurring methylation of RNA (and DNA) by PCZ would contribute to its oncolytic effect. The importance of the N-methyl group is stressed by the fact that only methyl-substituted hydrazines have antitumor activity. When prescribing this drug, it should be remembered that it is a monoamine oxidase inhibitor.

B. INHIBITORS OF PROTEIN SYNTHESIS

L-Asparaginase, an enzyme extracted from E. coli and some other organisms, for example Erwinia carotovora, catalizes the hydrolysis of L-asparagine into aspartic acid and ammonium, so depleting the circulating pool of L-asparagine (Fig. 3-10) (9, 91-98). Normal cells synthesize this amino acid from glutamine and aspartic acid. Some malignant cells, mostly of lymphoid origin, lack asparagine synthetase and become dependent on a supply of asparagine in the extracellular space for their protein synthesis. ROBERTS et al. have shown that another enzyme, glutaminase, alone or in combination with L-asparaginase, has tumor activity in asparaginase-resistant Ehrlich carcinomas (99). The same combination of enzymes has potent selective cytocidal activity for human leukemic leukocytes. Glutamine antagonists, such as azaserine, diazo-oxo-norleucine, and azotomycin, which interfere with the synthesis of asparagine or the metabolism of glutamine, would also be expected to augment the tumor activity of L-asparaginase.

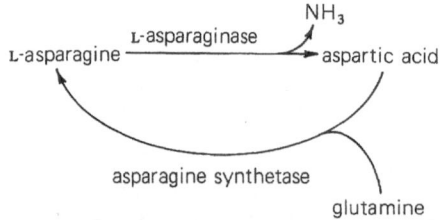

Fig. 3-10. Mechanism of action of L-asparaginase. Certain malignant cells, especially some of lymphoid origin, lack asparagine synthetase, the enzyme that catalyzes the synthesis of asparagine from glutamine and aspartic acid

C. DRUGS INTERFERING WITH REPLICATION, TRANSCRIPTION, AND TRANSLATION

The drugs discussed under this heading, rather that interfering with the synthesis of nucleotides, affect the nucleic acids directly or interrupt the processes of replication, transcription, and translation.

1. Alkylating Agents

Alkylating agents contain highly reactive, electrophilic alkyl groups that readily form covalent linkages with nucleophilic (electron-rich) substances (100-104). Thus, negatively charged groups, for example phosphate, amino, sulfhydryl, hydroxyl, carboxyl, and imidazole groups, are especially susceptible to alkylation. A portion of the alkylating agent is added to the nucleophilic site by substitution of a hydrogen atom in the receptor molecule.

The activity of a number of cellular constituents can thus be altered. The effects on nucleic acids and DNA synthesis are the most important in the context of this discussion. The phosphate groups and several portions of the nucleotide bases can be alkylated. The 7 position of guanine is most frequently involved. This can lead to mispairing of the substituted base (G=T instead of G=C) in nucleic acid replication or transcription. Alternatively, the purine ring may be opened or the guanine residue excised (depurination), either of which can result in serious damage to the DNA molecule, including chain rupture. Cells in late G_1 or early S phase are particularly sensitive to alkylation. Polyfunctional alkylating agents, containing 2 or more alkyl groups, are much more effective than monofunctional alkylators and can form bridges within a single molecule (intrastrand) or between two strands (interstrand). Cross-linking of the two strands of DNA, so preventing separation and replication, is thought to be a major mode of action of alkylating agents (Fig. 3-11). Other cellular functions, including glycolysis, respiration, protein synthesis, and various enzyme activities, may also be disturbed. Very high doses cause interphase death due to generalized cell damage; but with moderate doses cell death is delayed until the cell attempts division. Intracellular repair enzymes may restore the damaged DNA to a certain extent by excising affected parts.

Nitrogen mustard (HN2), methyl-bis(β-chloroethyl)amine hydrochloride, is the prototype of this class of agents (Fig. 3-12). Mustards owe their physiological activity to an intramolecular cyclization of one of the 2-chloroethyl side-chains whereby an ethylene-imonium inter-

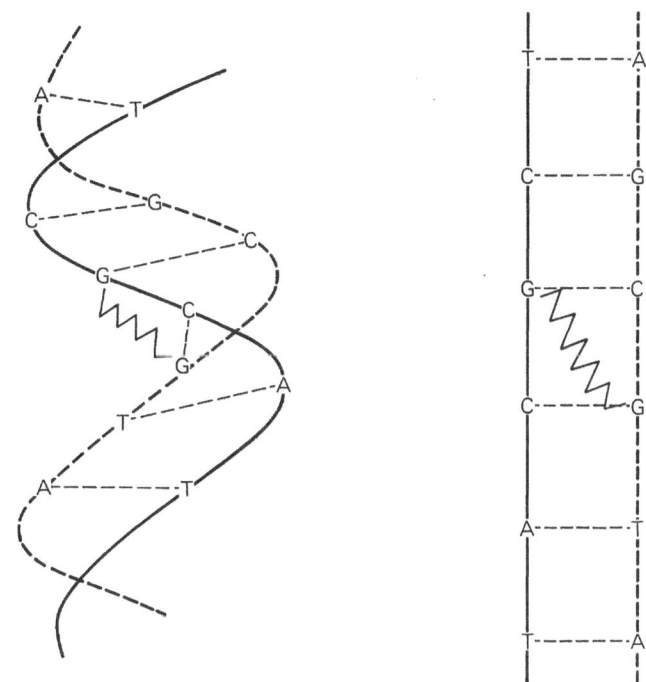

Fig. 3-11. Bridge formation between the two strands (interstrand) of DNA by alkylating agents

mediate is formed. In this process the tertiary amine is converted to a quaternary ammonium compound, which in turn forms a carbonium ion that avidly reacts with a number of cellular constituents (Fig. 3-13). The second chloroethyl moiety then cyclizes, which allows it to react with another site of the same or another molecule. The driving force for initial cyclization is the displacement of electrons away from the nitrogen atom. This reaction is therefore facilitated by the presence at R of electron-repelling substituents such as a methyl group. Nitrogen mustard cyclizes within minutes, whereas mustards with less effective repelling substituents at R, for example phenylbutyric acid or phenylalanine, cyclize at a much slower rate and can therefore be used orally.

Several classes of alkylating agents are available for clinical use:
1. bischloroethylamines
2. ethylene-imines
3. sulfonic esters
4. (epoxides)

(i) Bischloroethylamines

A large number of alkylating agents have been synthesized by altering the third substituent on the trivalent nitrogen, the two 2-chloroethyl groups being responsible for the alkylating activity (Fig. 3-12B). Among the aliphatic derivatives are nitrogen mustard (HN2) and the less commonly used mannomustine (Fig. 3-14). Several aromatic derivatives are effective tumor agents. Chlorambucil (CLB), a phenylbutyric

47

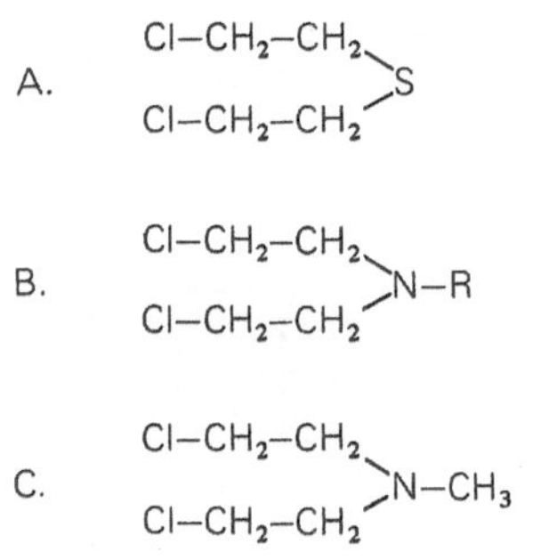

A. Cl–CH₂–CH₂
    Cl–CH₂–CH₂ 〉S

B. Cl–CH₂–CH₂
    Cl–CH₂–CH₂ 〉N–R

C. Cl–CH₂–CH₂
    Cl–CH₂–CH₂ 〉N–CH₃

*Fig. 3-12. A. Mustard gas, B. structural formula of bischloroethylamines,
C. nitrogen mustard*

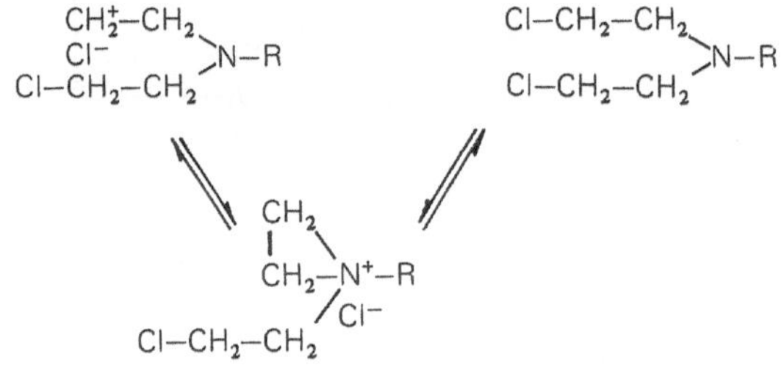

CH₂⁺–CH₂
Cl⁻   〉N–R
Cl–CH₂–CH₂

Cl–CH₂–CH₂
        〉N–R
Cl–CH₂–CH₂

CH₂
CH₂–N⁺–R
      Cl⁻
Cl–CH₂–CH₂

*Fig. 3-13. Biological activity of bischloroethylamines: intramolecular
cyclization of one of the two chloroethyl side chains yields an ethylene-imonium intermediate. This quaternary ammonium compound in turn
forms a carbonium ion that avidly reacts with a number of cellular
constituents*

acid substituted mustard, has been very useful in the control of chronic lymphoid leukemia (Fig. 3-15) (105). The synthesis of cyclophosphamide (CPM), a cyclic phosphamide ester of nitrogen mustard, was the result of an attempt to produce an agent with greater tumor selectivity
(Fig. 3-15) (106-109,227). The drug inactive in vitro, must be cleaved
at the nitrogen-phosphorus linkage before the bis(chloroethyl) portion
can be ionized. Since some tumor tissues have high phosphatase or phosphamidase activity, it was hoped that enzymatic activation in tumor
sites would result in the desired effect. However, we now know that the
hepatic microsomal mixed-function oxidase system activates the drug. Several metabolites have been proposed as the active compounds. Iphosfa-

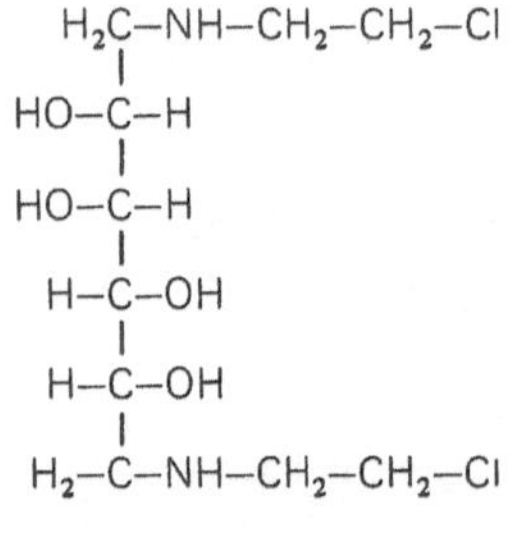

H₂C–NH–CH₂–CH₂–Cl
|
HO–C–H
|
HO–C–H
|
H–C–OH
|
H–C–OH
|
H₂–C–NH–CH₂–CH₂–Cl   *Fig. 3-14. Mannomustine*

48

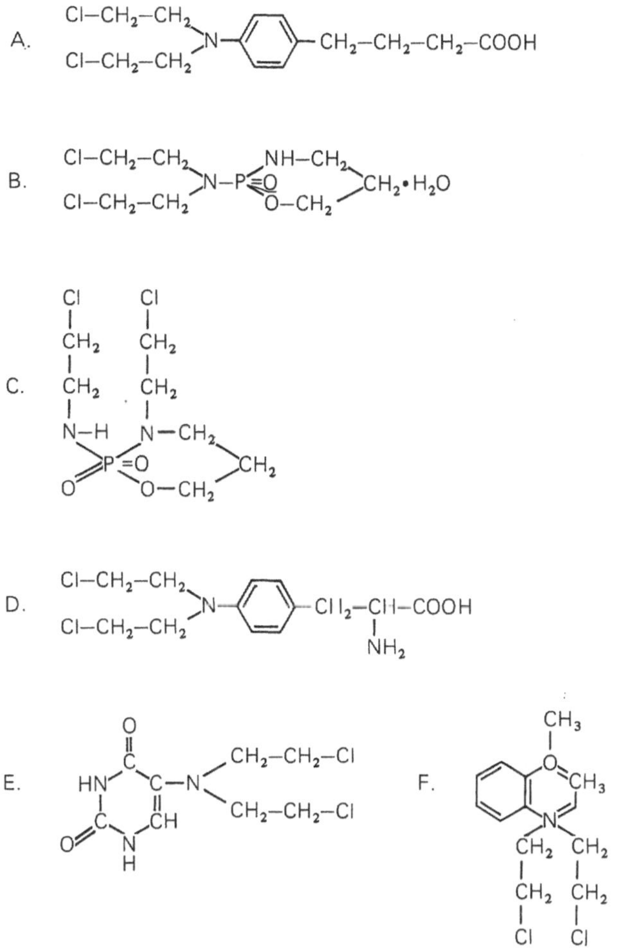

A.

$$Cl-CH_2-CH_2$$
$$Cl-CH_2-CH_2$$ N—⟨benzene⟩—$CH_2-CH_2-CH_2-COOH$

B.

$$Cl-CH_2-CH_2$$
$$Cl-CH_2-CH_2$$ $N-P{\equiv}O$ with $NH-CH_2$ and $O-CH_2$ forming $CH_2 \bullet H_2O$

C.

```
      Cl      Cl
      |       |
      CH₂     CH₂
      |       |
      CH₂     CH₂
      |       |
      N–H    N–CH₂
        \P=O       CH₂
       /    \O–CH₂
      O
```

$$Cl \quad Cl$$
$$CH_2 \quad CH_2$$
$$CH_2 \quad CH_2$$
$$N{-}H \quad N{-}CH_2$$
P=O, O, O{-}CH_2, CH_2

D.

$$Cl-CH_2-CH_2$$
$$Cl-CH_2-CH_2$$ N—⟨benzene⟩—$CH_2-CH-COOH$ with NH_2

E.

Uracil mustard structure:
HN–C(=O)–C–N with CH_2-CH_2-Cl and CH_2-CH_2-Cl; ring with O=C–N–H, CH

F.

Mitoclomine structure with CH_3, O, CH_3, N, CH_2 CH_2, CH_2 CH_2, Cl Cl

Fig. 3-15. Aromatic mustards: A. chlorambucil, B. cyclophosphamide, C. iphosfamide, D. melphalan, E. uracil mustard, F. mitoclomine

mide, an analog of cyclophosphamide, is under clinical investigation because of its superior cytotoxic activity in L1210 leukemia (7, 110, 111). Melphalan (MPH) was synthesized on the assumption that an amino acid on the nitrogen might allow it to be incorporated into intracellular pathways of protein synthesis, thus transporting the alkylating moiety into the cell (Fig. 3-15). Since phenylalanine is a precusor in melamin synthesis, some selective effect was anticipated in malignant melanoma. Instead, the drug proved to be most useful in myeloma. The mustard radical has also been attached to a pyrimidine precursor as uracil mustard (Fig. 3-15) (112, 113).

Mitoclomine is an experimental compound in which a bischloroethyl group is carried by a modified vitamin K5 molecule; it has been shown that synthetic vitamin K is concentrated by some tumor systems and it possesses radiosensitizing properties (Fig. 3-15). It has a selective effect on lymphocytes (114).

(ii) Ethylene-Imines

Since the mustards exert their effect via ethylene-immonium, a highly
reactive cyclical intermediate, it seemed logical to search for active
ethylene-imine derivatives (Fig. 3-16). A large number of compounds
have been synthesized, but only those used in clinical oncology are
described here. Triethylene melamine (TEM) contains three ethylene-
imino groups attached to a triazine moiety (Fig. 3-16). We also mention
hexamethylmelamine (HMM), which structurally resembles TEM but has two
methyl groups in place of each of the TEM-ethylene groups. (Fig. 3-16)
(116-119). However, it has been suggested that hexamethylmelamine may
not function as an alkylating agent but rather as a pyrimidine antimetabolite. Indeed, its metabolism differs significantly from that of TEM.
The clinical value of this drug is under investigation. Triethylene-
thiophosphoramide (thioTEPA) (Fig. 3-16) (120) is the most used among
the phosphoramides and trenimon (triethyleneimino 2,3,5-benzoquinone)
among ethyleneiminobenzoquinones (Fig. 3-16).

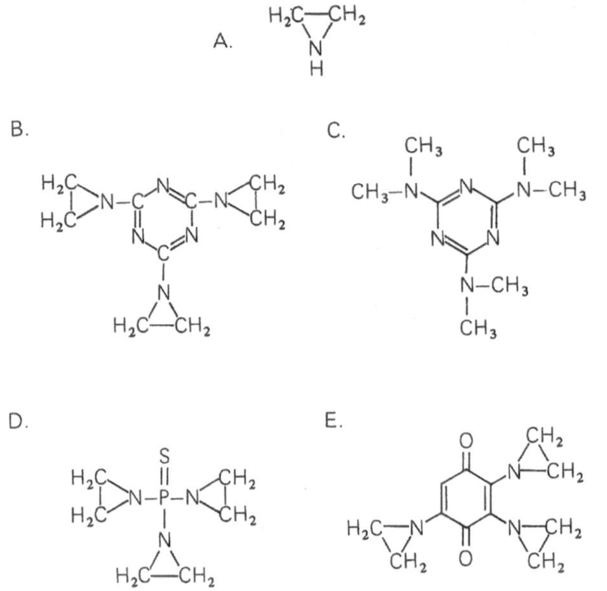

Fig. 3-16. Ethylene-imines: A. ethylene-imine, B. triethylenemelamine
(TEM), C. hexamethylmelamine (HMM) (not an ethylene-imine), D. triethylene thiophosphoramide (thio-TEPA), E. triethylene-imino 2,3,5-benzo-
quinone (trenimon)

(iii) Sulfonic Esters

Sulfonic esters are a different class of alkylating agents. In a series
in which two sulfonyl groups ($-O-SO_2-CH_3$) were joined together by a
chain of CH_2 groups to form bifunctional alkylating agents, busulfan
(BSF) (dimethyl-sulfonyl-oxy 1,4 butane) showed selective toxicity for
the myeloid series and remains the drug of choice for the treatment
of chronic myeloid leukemia (Fig. 3-17) (121). 1-Propanol, 3-3'-imino-
di-dimethanesulfonate (ester) hydrochloride (Yoshi 864) is a sulfonic
acid ester of aminoglycol. It has alkylating groups similar to busulfan
and may be an alkyl agent active against chronic myeloid leukemia and
possibly other tumors (228, 229).

50

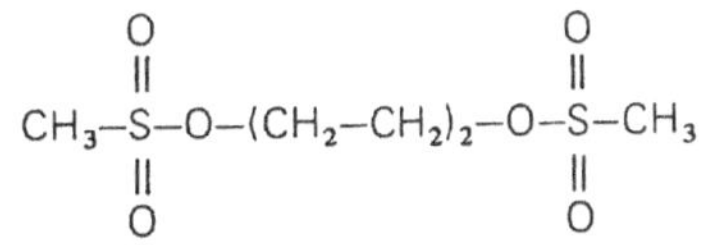

$$CH_3-S-O-(CH_2-CH_2)_2-O-S-CH_3$$

(with O above and O below each S, double bonds)

Fig. 3—17. Busulfan

(iv) Other Agents with Alkylating Action

The cytotoxic effect of two derivatives of piperazine, pipobroman (1,4-bis(3-bromopropionyl)piperazine) (Fig. 3-18 A) (122, 123) and piposulfan (N,N'-bis(3methane-sulfonoxypropanoyl)piperazine) (Fig. 3-18 B) (124) is usually thought to be due to alkylation. Both agents have some activity in chronic myeloid leukemia and polycythemia.

A.
$$Br-CH_2CH_2-C-N \quad N'-C-CH_2CH_2-Br$$

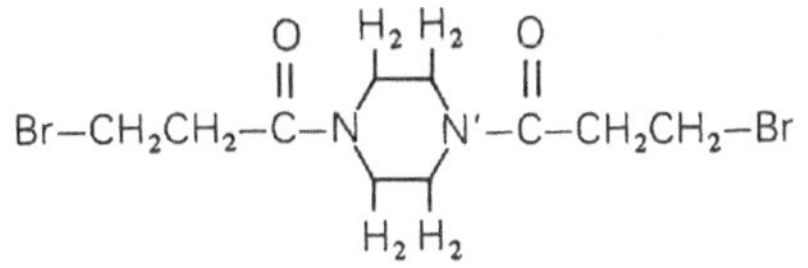

B.
$$CH_3-SO_2O-CH_2-CH_2-C-N \quad N-C-CH_2-CH_2-OSO_2-CH_3$$

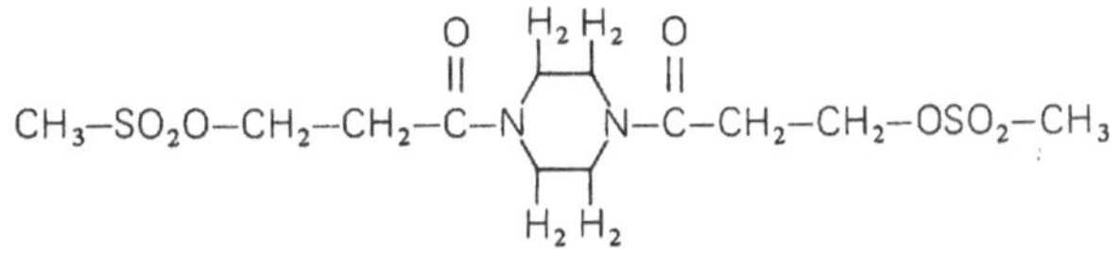

Fig. 3-18. A. 1,4-bis(3-bromopropionyl)piperazine, pipobroman, B. N,N'-bis(3-methane-sulfonoxypropanoyl)piperazine, piposulfan

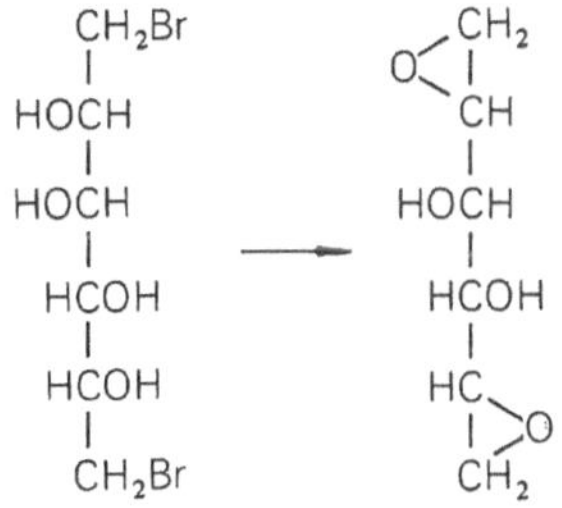

$$
\begin{array}{ccc}
CH_2Br & & CH_2 \\
| & & O< | \\
HOCH & & CH \\
| & & | \\
HOCH & & HOCH \\
| & \longrightarrow & | \\
HCOH & & HCOH \\
| & & | \\
HCOH & & HC \\
| & & |>O \\
CH_2Br & & CH_2 \\
\end{array}
$$

Fig. 3-19. Conversion of dibromomannitol into 1,2:5,6-dianhydro-D-mannitol, a diepoxide with alkylating activity

Dibromomannitol also seems to act as an alkylating agent (Fig. 3-19) (125). Its pharmacologic action is partly mediated through its conversion in vivo into 1,2:5,6-dianhydro-D-mannitol, a diepoxide with alkylating activity. Dibromomannitol has been most effective in the treatment of chronic myeloid leukemia (126), though it is not superior to myeleran (127). The value of dibromodulcitol (Fig. 3-20) is still under investigation (128-132, 230).

Inorganic platinum compounds, a new class of antitumor agents, form bridges between the two strands of DNA (133-135). DNA synthesis is inhibited while RNA and protein synthesis are less affected. Phase I and II studies of diamminodichloroplatinum (DDP) (Fig. 3-21) are in progress (136, 231).

51

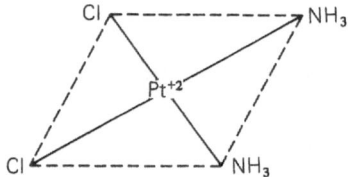

```
        CH₂—Br
         |
    H—C—OH
         |
   HO—C—H
         |
   HO—C—H
         |
    H—C—OH
         |
        CH₂—Br
```

Fig. 3-20. Dibromodulcitol

```
    Cl ╱------------→ NH₃
      ╱ ╱            ╱ ╱
     ╱ ╱   Pt⁺²     ╱ ╱
    ╱ ╱            ╱ ╱
   Cl ←----------╱→ NH₃
```

Fig. 3-21. Cis-platinum diamminodichloride (PDD)

Finally, we mention some agents that have several mechanisms of action, alkylation among them. Mitomycin C (MTC) (isolated from <u>Streptomyces</u> <u>caespitosus</u>) is a complex structure with several potentially active groupings such as the aziridine ring and the aminoquinone and methylure-thane moieties (Fig. 3-22) (<u>137-139</u>). After activation in vitro it acts like a bifunctional alkylating agent: cross-links form between the two strands of DNA and inhibit its replication. However, unlike the other alkylating agents, MTC does not alkylate the N-7 position of the guanine residues in DNA (<u>138</u>). RNA and protein synthesis are suppressed at high doses. <u>Porfiromycin</u> (Fig. 3-22 B), a methyl deriva-tive of MTC obtained from <u>Streptomyces</u> ardus and Streptomyces verti-<u>cellatus</u>, is undergoing clinical investigation (<u>140</u>). Several drugs discussed earlier under compounds interfering with nucleotide biosyn-thesis have, in addition, an alkylating effect. We refer to imidazole carboxamide (DIC) and the nitrosourea derivatives (BCNU, CCNU, and MeCCNU).

<u>ICRF-159</u> [1,2-bis(3,5-dioxopiperazine-1-yl)propane] (Fig. 3-23), a bio-dioxopiperazine originally designed as a potential intracellularly

```
                    O              O
                    ‖              ‖                 ┌─────────────┐
  H₂N                       CH₂OCNH₂                │ Aziridine ring │
  H₃C                       OCH₃                    │      \  /      │
                    N        N—R                     │       C        │
                    ‖                                │       |  N—H   │
                    O                                │       C        │
                                                     │      /  \      │
                                                     └─────────────┘
```

A.   —R=H
B.   —R=CH₃

Fig. 3-22. A. Mitomycin C, B. porfiromycin

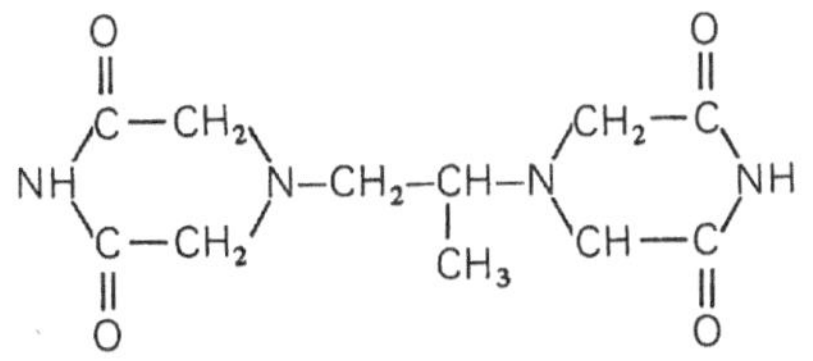

Fig. 3-23. 1,2-bis(3,5-dioxopiperazine-1-yl)propane, ICRF-159

activated chelating agent, is a potent inhibitor of DNA synthesis, while having relatively little effect on RNA and protein synthesis (141-145). In view of its structure, it is possible that it may exert a radiomimetic effect by acting as a mono- or bifunctional alkylating agent. Its chelating effect may be responsible for its protective action against daunorubicin toxicity (146-147).

2. Agents Interfering with Transcription

A series of compounds, often referred to as antibiotics because they are extracted from microorganisms, share a common mechanism of action (5, 53, 148). They bind to DNA, thereby inhibiting transcription or the synthesis of DNA-dependent RNA.

Actinomycin D (ACD) (or dactinomycin) was isolated from Streptomyces present in soil (Fig. 3-24) (149). On a molar basis, it is the most potent antineoplastic agent available. The actinomycins consist of a chromophore moiety, actinocin, which is responsible for the yellow color and the complexing with DNA, coupled to two cyclic oligopeptides (Fig. 3-25). For stable complex formation, DNA must be helical and possess guanine residues, preferably in the minor groove of the DNA helix (Fig. 3-26). ACD does not bind to RNA. It inhibits RNA synthesis preferentially, especially that of ribosomal RNA, since the DNA coding for it is rich in guanine. At higher concentrations, synthesis of all species of RNA is inhibited, and high levels (not attainable in vivo) inhibit DNA synthesis directly.

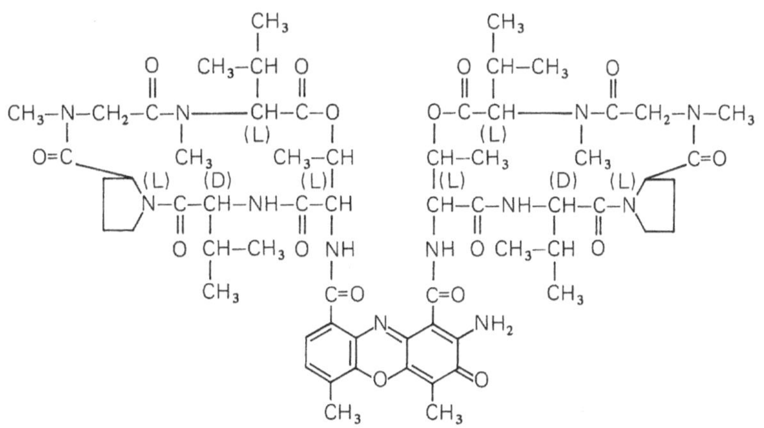

Fig. 3-24. Actinomycin D

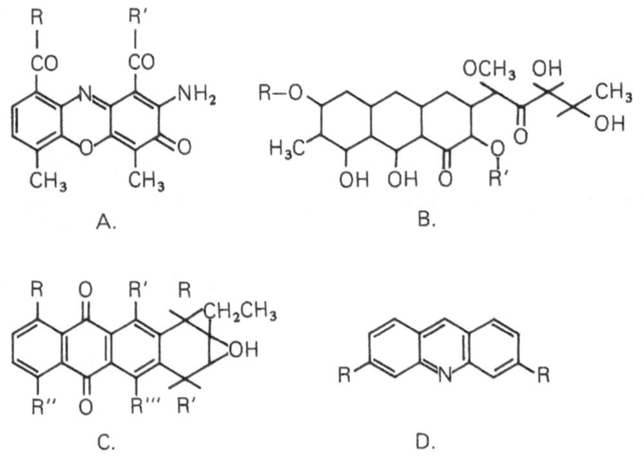

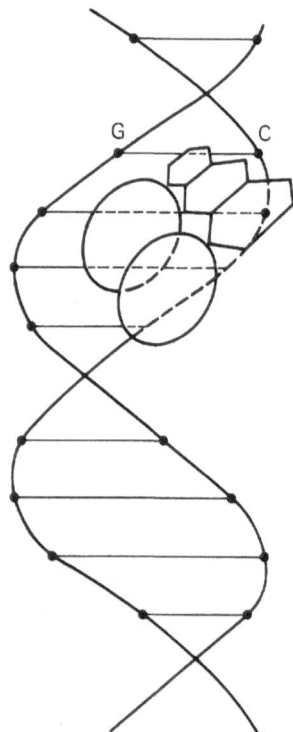

Fig. 3-25. *Structure of the chromophore moiety of: A. actinomycins, B. chromomycins, C. anthracyclines, D. acridines*

Fig. 3-26. *Schematic view of the binding between the chromophore moiety of actino-mycin D and a guanine of DNA (from Waring, M.J., Nature 219, 1320 (1968))*

The binding of <u>mithramycin</u> (MTM) (Fig. 3-27), a chromomycin extracted from <u>Streptomyces plicatus</u>, like that of actinomycin D, requires guanine and the helical structure (<u>150–152</u>). RNA synthesis is inhibited, but it has little effect on DNA synthesis. Its clinical use is limited to to embryonal carcinomas of the testes (<u>152</u>).

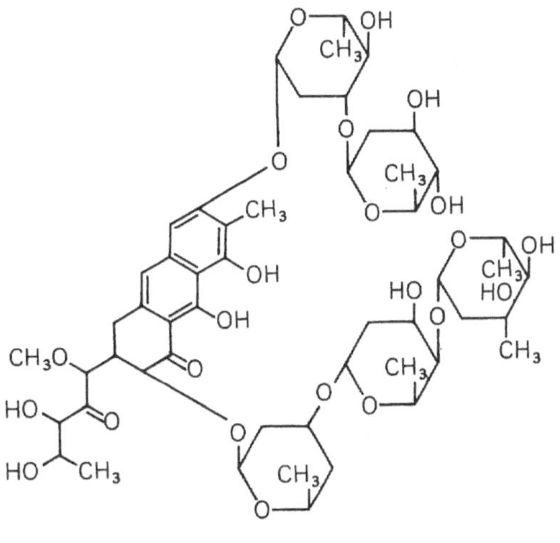

Fig. 3-27. Mithramycin

Daunorubicin (DRB) (Fig. 3-28 A) (153-156) (extracted from Streptomyces peucetius or ceruleorubidus) and adriamycin (ADM) (Fig. 3-28 B) (157-162, 236) (extracted from Streptomyces peucetius var. caesius) belong to the anthracycline group of antibiotics. They are identical in structure, a pigmented aglycone (see Fig. 3-25) in glycoside linkage with a amino sugar, except that the hydrogen atom in the acetyl radical of daunorubicin is replaced by a hydroxyl group in adriamycin. They bind to DNA, intercalating between adjacent base pairs, and inhibit both DNA and RNA synthesis. Although anthracycline antibiotics can bind to RNA, this binding is rather weak. Carminomycin differs from daunorubicin by the absence of a methoxyl group at C4, which is substituted by a hydroxyl group (232).

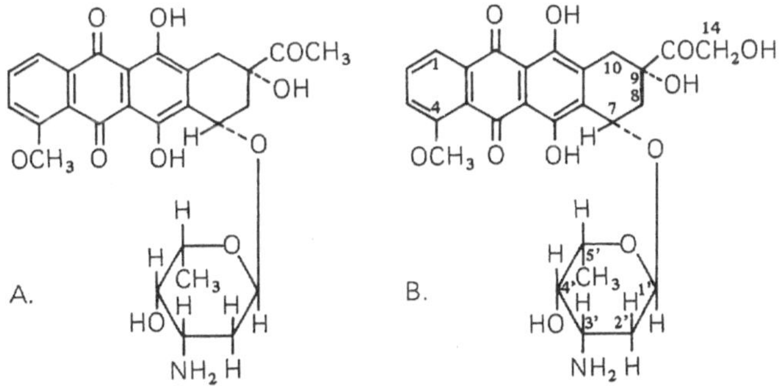

Fig. 3-28. A. Daunorubicin, B. adriamycin

The interaction of antibiotics with DNA has been compared to the interaction of acridines with DNA. It may therefore be appropriate to discuss at this point quinacrine (3-chloro-7-methoxy-9-(1-methyl-4-diethyl-aminobutylamino)-acridine) (Fig. 3-29), a synthetic agent that is useful in the treatment of malignant effusions because it has a cytocidal action on neoplastic cells and causes chemical inflammation of the serous membranes (163). Quinacrine is a relatively nonspecific enzyme inhibitor that acts by binding with proteins in general. There is also evidence that it binds to DNA and RNA. We also mention here 9-methoxy-ellipticine, an alkaloid extracted from leaves of Ochrosia borbonica (Fig. 3-30) (197, 198).

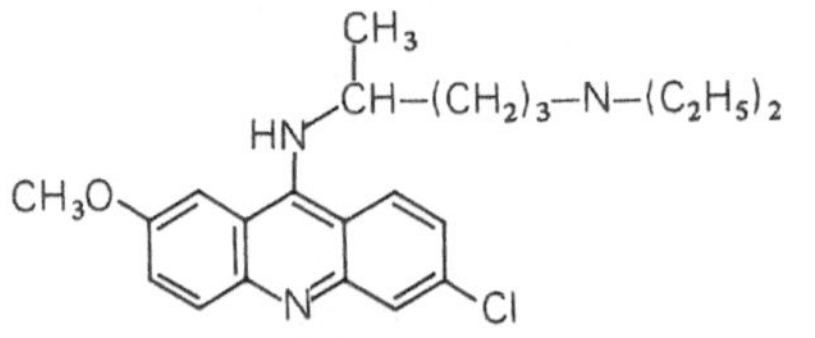

Fig. 3-29. Quinacrine

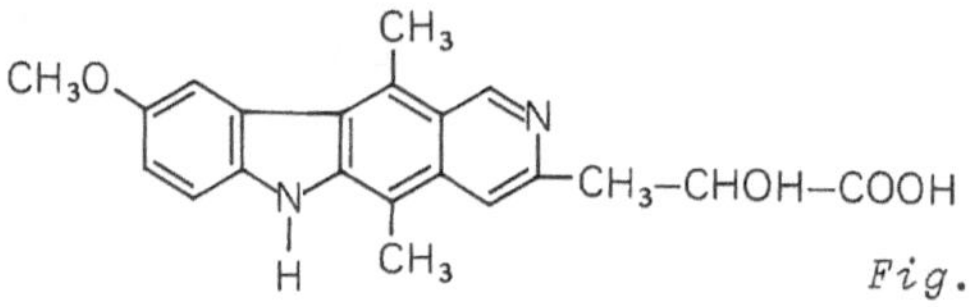

Fig. 3-30. 9-Methoxy-ellipticine

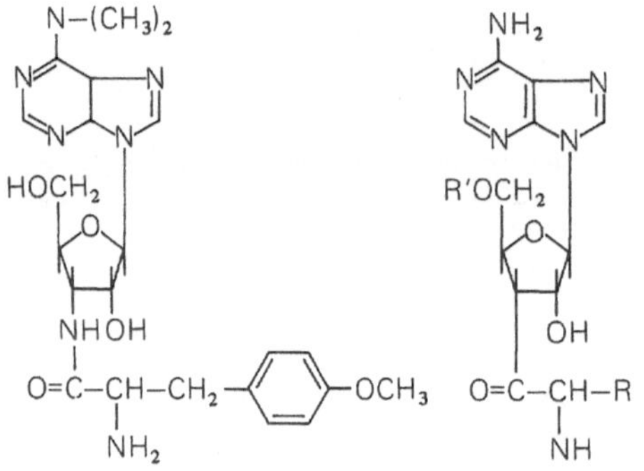

Fig. 3-31. The structure of puro-mycin (A) compared with that of an amino-acyl tRNA molecule (B)

3. Agents Interfering with Translation

Puromycin (Fig. 3-31), extracted from Streptomyces alboniger, inhibits
the formation of polypeptides or the synthesis of protein by interfering with the insertion into the growing peptide chain of the activated
amino acid-tRNA, which is released before its synthesis is completed
(164). Note the similarity between the structure of this antibiotic
and that of tRNA.

We have already mentioned the action of procarbazine at the level of
transfer RNA, selective methylation of position 7 of guanine, which
may contribute to its carcinostatic activity (53).

D. AGENTS WITH RADIOMIMETIC EFFECT

Bleomycin (BLM), a glycopeptide antibiotic isolated from fermentation
products of Streptomyces verticillus, can be separated by chromatography
into 13 peptides (7 in group A and 6 in group B) (165-175). The fraction
A_2 is the major component of the mixture and accounts for more than
50 percent of the clinical preparation. Further analysis by hydrolysis
yields 7 components. By binding to DNA, bleomycin inhibits DNA synthesis, while synthesis of RNA and protein is apparently unimpaired. It
also causes DNA strand breaks, hence its classification as a radiomimetic agent. Progression into mitosis is blocked, with cells accumulating into G_2, by concentrations that have no effect on the biosynthesis
of nucleic acids. The drug is concentrated by squamous epithelium, particularly by tissues that produce keratin (165, 175).

Streptonigrin (Fig. 3-32) (176), extracted from Streptomyces flocculus, also damages DNA. It has been postulated that H_2O_2, a product of the intracellular anaerobic oxidation of streptonigrin, is the lethal agent which interacts with DNA to produce single-strand breaks with single-hit kinetics analogous to X-irradiation. RNA, protein synthesis, and anaerobic glycolysis are inhibited, and cellular ATP levels are markedly reduced. Streptonigrin is closely related to, if not identical, with rufochromomycin, extracted from Streptomyces rufochromogenes. The antitumor activity of neocarzinostatin, a single-chain molecule composed of 10 g amino-acid residues, isolated from Streptomyces carzinostaticus, is probably based on radiomimetic characteristics (233).

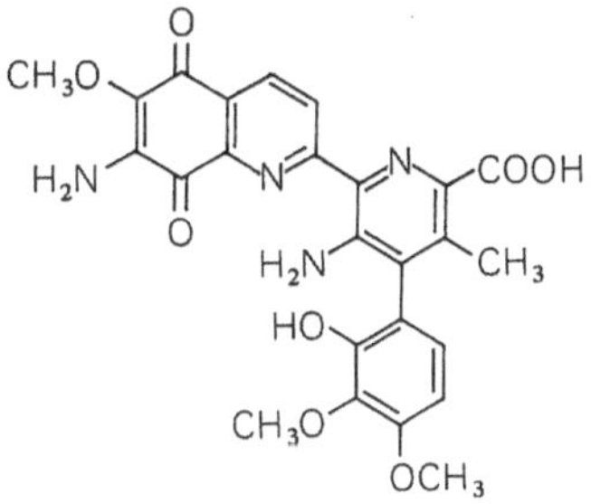

Fig. 3-32. Streptonigrin

E. AGENTS INTERFERING WITH THE MITOTIC SPINDLE

A series of plant alkaloids or their derivatives arrest cell division in metaphase. They are known as "mitotic or spindle inhibitors, arresters, or poisons" (9).

Colchicine is often used in experimental medicine but no longer as a clinical antineoplastic agent. The use of demecolcine in the treatment of chronic myeloid leukemia has been superseded by busulfan. By far the most widely used drugs in this class are the alkaloids vincristine (VCR) and vinblastine (VLB), isolated from the periwinkle Catharanthus roseus (177-190). Their structure is complex (Fig. 3-33); they are identical, except that vincristine has an aldehyde group where vinblastine has a methyl group; yet their tumor spectrum and toxicity are quite different. Cells are arrested in metaphase since Vinca alkaloids disrupt the formation of the mitotic spindle by binding to a cytoplasmic precusor protein of the spindle. This binding may occur during S phase, which is when cells are most sensitive to Vinca alkaloids, but the consequences do not become apparent until the next mitosis is attempted. The protein affected by Vinca alkaloids is a constituent of all cell structures containing microtubular elements, so that other cellular functions such as motility and phagocytosis may be affected. While a decrease in the biosynthesis of DNA, RNA, and protein has been reported, the results of various studies, using different test systems and drug concentrations (some of them not attainable in humans) are not in agreement. CREASEY reported preferential inhibition of the synthesis of tRNA (in Ehrlich ascitis cells) (178) but this was not confirmed by WAGNER, who found preferential inhibition of rRNA (in human epidermoid cells) (184). CREASEY more recently reported inhibition of RNA synthesis through effects on DNA-dependent RNA polymerase (181).

Two semisynthetic derivatives of podophyllotoxin, VM 26 (4'-demethyl-epipodophyllotoxin-β-D-thenylidine) (EPT) (Fig. 3-34 A) (191-194, 234), and VP 16231 (4'-demethylepipodophyllotoxin-ethylene-glycoside) (Fig.

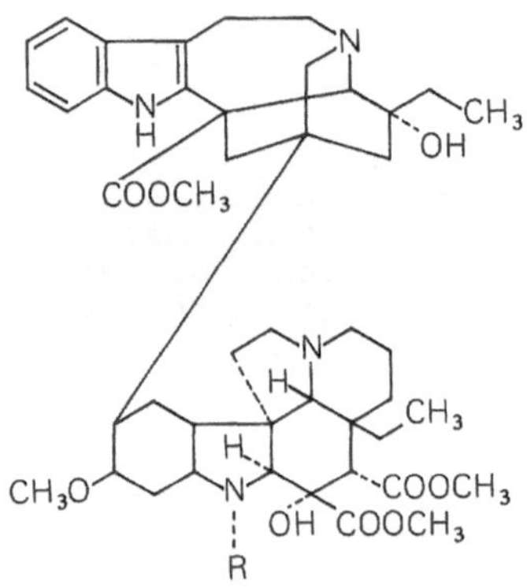

Vincristine: R=O=C—H
Vinblastine: R=CH₃

Fig. 3-33. The Vinca alkaloids

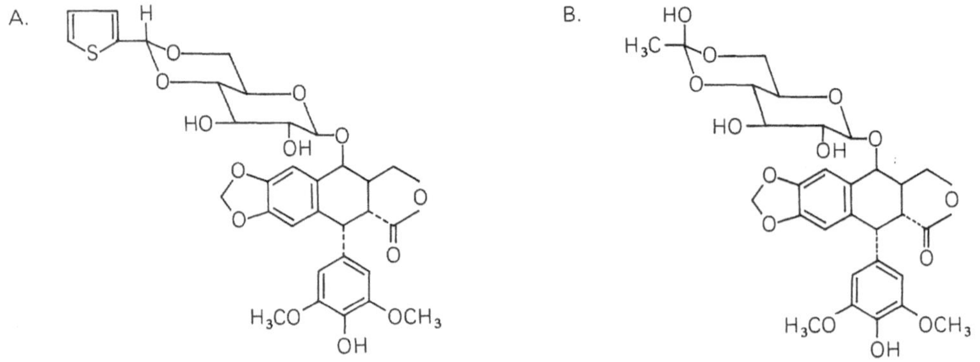

Fig. 3-34. A. 4'-demethyl-epipodophyllotoxin-β-D-thenylidine, EPT, VM 26, B. 4'-demethyl-epipodophyllotoxin-ethylidene-glycoside, EPE, VP 16213

3-34 B) (EPE) (192, 195, 196, 234) have recently been introduced for testing in human tumors. Like other mitotic poisons, they arrest cells in mitosis but they also prevent cells from entering prophase. The synchronizing effect of mitotic poisons is discussed on p. 144.

F. OTHER CYTOTOXIC AGENTS

Several drugs, most of them still undergoing investigation, cannot be classified in any of the preceding categories.

6- Aminochrysene (Chrysenex) (Fig. 3-35), a polycyclic amine, produces regressions of spontaneous mammary tumors in mice and blocks the carcinogenic action of methylcholanthrene (199, 200). Since some responses have been noted in chronic myeloid leukemia and breast cancer, other derivatives are being synthesized and screened (199).

Poly-IC (polyinosinic-polycytidylic acid) (201-206) is a synthetic, double-stranded RNA polymer that is capable of inducing interferon production in various animal species and in man (204). Growth of seve-

58

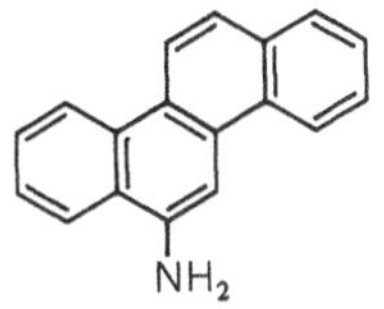

Fig. 3-35. 6-Aminochrysene

ral experimental tumors, both virus- and non-virus induced, has been
inhibited (201). However, it is not clear whether this is due to the
induction of interferon, to direct cytotoxic action (202), or to a form
of immune stimulation (203). Clinical experience in man is still limited (206-208).

Tilorone, another inducer of interferon, has inhibitory activity against
both DNA and RNA viruses and Walker 256 carcinosarcoma (209). Phase I
and II studies are in progress (210). This tumor is also inhibited by
rifampicin, an inhibitor of RNA-dependent DNA polymerase (reverse transcriptase) (209).

To conclude this section, we mention some experimental studies that
may open up new approaches to the medical treatment of cancer.

Chalones are tissue- but not species-specific mitotic inhibitors, produced by the tissues to control the rate of cell proliferation. At
least four different tumor types are inhibited (211-213). Several substances under study are capable of inhibiting cancer dissemination and
metastasis formation. Triton WR 1339, a non-ionic detergent, is thought
to inhibit tumor dissemination by enhancing the activity of the reticulo-endothelial system or by affecting the adhesiveness and movement
of cancer cells (214-216).

Tumor spread is also limited by ICRF 159, presumably through its effect
on the development of blood vessels in the invading margins of primary
tumors (144). The antitumor activity of vitamin A has been related to
its labilizing effect on lysosomes (217, 218).

Agents capable of stimulating the immune defenses are currently undergoing intensive investigation since the importance of immune mechanisms
in the control of cancer has been appreciated (219).

Fig. 3-36 summarizes the principal mechanisms of action of the more
important chemotherapeutic agents.

59

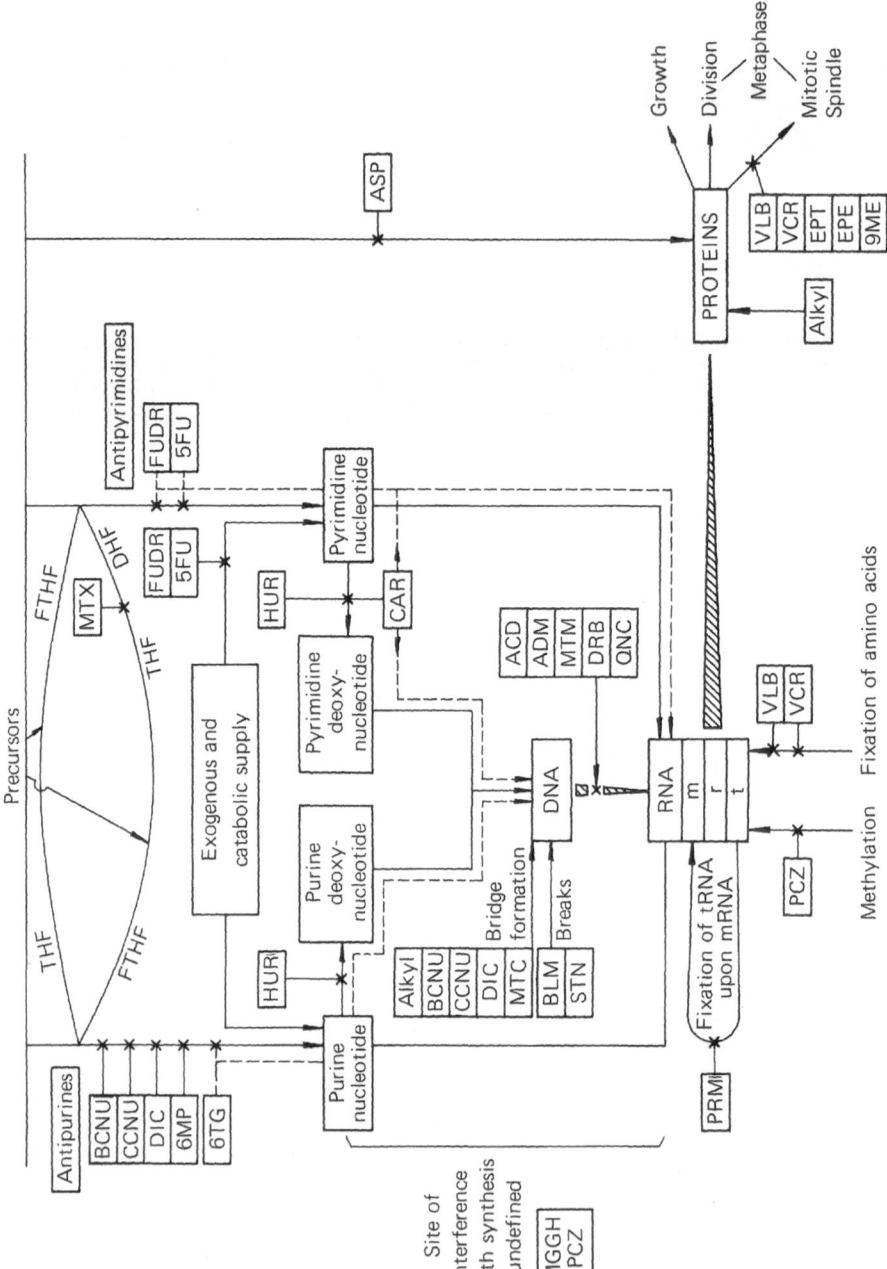

Fig. 3-36. Biochemical mechanisms of action of the more important drugs used in cancer che-motherapy

ACD	actinomycin D	HUR	hydroxyurea
ADM	adriamycin	9-ME	9-methoxy-ellipticine
Alkyl	alkylating agents	6-MP	6-mercaptopurine
ASP	L-asparaginase	MGGH	methyl-GAG
BCNU	bis-chloroethyl nitrosurea	MTC	mitomycin C
BLM	bleomycin	MTM	mithramycin
CAR	cytosine arabinoside	MTX	methotrexate
CCNU	chloroethyl-cyclohexyl nitrosurea	PCZ	procarbazine
DIC	imidazole carboxamide	PRM	puromycin
DRB	daunorubicin	QNC	quinacrine
EPT	epipodophyllotoxin-thenylidene	STN	streptonigrin
EPE	epipodophyllotoxin-ethylidene	6-TG	6-thioguanine
5-FU	5-fluoro-uracil	VCR	vincristine
FUdR	5-fluoro-deoxyuridine	VLB	vinblastine

Table 3-2. Principal chemotherapeutic agents

Drugs	How supplied	1. Mechanism of action 2. Plasma half-life 3. Metabolism 4. Excretion 5. Condition calling for dose reduction	Dosage	Side-effects	Indications (± in order of decreasing activity)
1. FOLIC ACID ANALOGS					
Methotrexate Amethopterin Methotrexate ® MTX	2.5-mg tabs 5- and 50 mg vials	1. Folic-acid antagonist 2. Triphasic plasma disappearance with T½ of 0.8, 3.5, and 27 h. Extensive enterohepatic circulation 3. Remains for weeks in body, bound to DHF reductase 4. 90% excreted unchanged in urine in 48 h 5. Impairment of renal or hepatic function Aspirin and sulfonamide displace albumin-bound MTX and increase toxicity	15-30 mg/m² p.o., i.v., i.m., every 4 days 60 mg/m², i.m., i.v., weekly 12-18 mg/m² p.o., i.m., i.v., daily for 5 days every 2-3 weeks 75 mg/m² a), i.v., q. 8 h x 6 with folinic acid 25 mg/m², i.m., q. 6 h x 12, starting 8 h after last dose of MTX Intrathecal: 5-10 mg/m², 1 to 3 days per week	BM depression, reversible; WBC nadir: ± day 7 GI: stomatitis, diarrhea, vomiting Hepatic: fibrosis, cirrhosis Renal Pulmonary: infiltrates Skin: pigmentation, alopecia Mucus membranes: conjunctivitis, vulvitis, vaginitis, proctitis Osteoporosis Paraplegia, leucoencephalopathy (following intrathecal MTX)	Acute lymphoid leukemia Gestational choriocarcinoma Burkitt's tumor Acute myeloid leukemia Most solid tumors, especially: H + N, breast, osteogenic sarcoma, testis, ovary, lung, cervix
2. PURINE ANALOGS					
6-Mercaptopurine Purinethol ® 6-MP	50-mg tabs	1. Purine analog 2. T½ = 1.5 h 3. Rapidly oxidized to thiouric acid 4. Renal excretion: parent compound and metabolites, 50% in 24 h 5. Allopurinol delays metabolism of 6-MP, increases its potency 2 to 4 times Impairment of renal or hepatic function	80-100 mg/m² p.o., 2.5 mg/kg daily	BM depression Stomatitis Cholestatic icterus	Acute lymphoid leukemia Acute myeloid leukemia Chronic myeloid leukemia Choriocarcinoma
6-Thioguanine Thioguanine ®	40-mg tabs	1. Purine analog 2. Rapidly converted to 2-ami-	80-120 mg/m² p.o., 2.5-3.0 mg/kg daily	BM depression Icterus	Acute myeloid leukemia (6-TG + CAR)

Table 3-2. (continued)

Drug	Pharmacology / Metabolism	Dosage	Toxicity	Indications
6-TG	no-6-methylmercaptopurine 3. Renal excretion: partly as thiouric acid 4. Impairment of renal or hepatic function. Allopurinol does not delay metabolism of 6-TG; no dose reduction required			Chronic myeloid leukemia (blastic crisis)
Imidazolcarboxamide Dacarbazine® DIC 100- and 200-mg vials	1. Purine analog and alkylating action 2. T$\frac{1}{2}$ = 30–45 min 3. Demethylation by liver microsomal enzymes to 5-amino-4-imidazole carboxamide (AIC) 4. Renal excretion: 45% within 6 h (50% as DIC, 50% as AIC) 5. Phenobarbital and dilantin may enhance the metabolism of DIC	250 mg/m², i.v., daily for 5 days; repeat every 21–28 days	GI: anorexia, nausea, vomiting, rarely diarrhea BM depression, delayed; WBC nadir: ± day 25 Transient flu-like illness local cellulitis	Melanoma Soft-tissue sarcomas
3. PYRIMIDINE ANALOGS				
5-Fluorouracil Fluorouracil® 5-FU 500-mg vials	1. Pyrimidine analog 2. T$\frac{1}{2}$ = 15–20 min 3. Primarily in liver 4. Renal excretion: 10–30% Expired as CO_2: 60–80% 5. Impaired liver function	400–500 mg/m² | Max. 12 mg/kg | 800 mg, i.v., daily for 4 days, followed by: 200–250 mg/m² or 6 mg/kg | every other day x 4; repeat after 4-week interval Loading dose as above, followed after recovery by: 500–600 mg/m² | i.v., 15 mg/kg | weekly 500–600 mg | i.v., 15 mg/kg | weekly, without loading dose	GI: nausea, vomiting, diarrhea, enteritis, stomatitis BM depression Alopecia Hyperpigmentation Cerebellar ataxia	Breast cancer Gastrointestinal adenocarcinomas Hepatoma Ovarian carcinoma Skin (topical application)
Cytosine arabinoside Cytosar® 100- and 500-mg vials	1. Pyrimidine analog 2. Biphasic plasma disappearance with T$\frac{1}{2}$ = 3–15 min	100–200 mg/m², daily, 1.5–3 mg/kg infusion (divided into 2 doses	GI: nausea, vomiting, stomatitis, diarrhea BM depression, megalo-	Acute myeloid leukemia Acute lymphoid

Table 3-2. (continued)

CAR		and 111-157 min 3. Rapidly deaminated to arabinofuranosyl uracil (Ara-U), mainly by liver 4. 90% excreted in 24 h by liver and kidneys 5. Impaired liver function	12 h apart), for 5-10 days, until toxicity or BM hypoplasia Intrathecal: 5-10 mg/m² 3 days per week	blastoid changes Fever, flu-like illness Hepatic (rare) Neck stiffness, convuls-ions (intrathecal)	leukemia (CNS intrathecally) Chronic myeloid leukemia (blastic crisis) Burkitt's tumor

4. OTHER INHIBITORS OF NUCLEIC ACID SYNTHESIS

Hydroxyurea Hydrea ® HUR	500-mg capsules	1. DNA inhibitor 2. $T_{\frac{1}{2}}$ = 1.5 to 5 h 3. Metabolized to urea by liver and kidneys 4. Renal excretion: 50-80%	1000-2000 mg/m² p.o., daily 20-50 mg/kg (in 2 divided doses) 2000-3000 mg/m² p.o., every 60-80 mg/kg 3 days	GI: nausea, vomiting, stomatitis BM depression, megaloblastoid changes Alopecia Skin rash	Chronic myeloid leukemia (resistant to BSF) Melanoma Hypernephroma
BCNU 1,3-bis(2-chloroethyl)-1-nitrosourea Carmustine	100-mg vials	1. Inhibition of DNA and RNA synthesis 2. $T_{\frac{1}{2}}$ = 1.5 h 3. Degradation products are probably the active compounds 4. Primarily excreted by kidneys as degradation products	100 mg/m², i.v., daily for 2 days 200 mg/m², i.v., single injection; repeat at 6- to 8-week intervals	GI: nausea, vomiting BM depression, delayed (4-6 weeks) Hepatic Renal	Brain (primary tumors and metastases) Acute lymphoid leukemia (CNS involvement) Hodgkin's disease, Non-Hodgkin's lymphomas, mycosis fungoides Myeloma, melanoma Lung, breast cancer
CCNU 1-(2-chloroethyl)-3-cyclohexyl-1-nitrosourea Lomustine	40- and 100-mg capsules	1. Inhibition of DNA and RNA synthesis 2. No intact drug detectable in plasma; $T_{\frac{1}{2}}$ of chloroethyl moiety = 72 h of cyclohexyl, carbonyl = 5 h 3. Degradation products are probably the active compounds 4. 60% excreted in urine in	130 mg/m², p.o.; repeat at 6- to 8-week intervals	GI: nausea, vomiting BM depression, delayed (4-6 weeks)	Gastrointestinal adenocarcinomas Brain tumors Hodgkin's disease Non-Hodgkin's lymphomas Lung cancer

Table 3-2. (continued)

Drug	Supply	Mode of action/pharmacology	Dosage	Toxicity	Indications
MeCCNU 1-(2-chloroethyl)-3-(4-methyl cyclohexyl-1-nitrosourea	20-, 50-, and 100-mg caps	48 h as metabolites; no intact drug 1. Inhibition of DNA and RNA synthesis 2. No intact drug detectable in plasma 3. Degradation products are active compounds 4. 60% excreted in urine in 48 h as metabolites; no intact drug	150-200 mg/m², p.o.; repeat at 6- to 8-week intervals	GI: nausea, vomiting BM depression, delayed (4-6 weeks)	Brain tumors Hodgkin's disease Non-Hodgkin's lymphomas Colorectal carcinomas Lung cancer
Streptozotocin STZ	2000-mg vials	1. Antibiotic structurally related to the nitrosoureas. Inhibits primarily DNA synthesis 4. 10-20% recovered in urine 5. Pre-existing renal disease	1 gm/m², i.v., weekly (monitor urinalysis, BUN, plasma creatinine and creatinine clearance)	GI: nausea, vomiting Renal: proteinurea, Fanconi's syndrome, uremia, anuria Hepatic: abnormal function studies Hypoglycemia BM depression: rare	Functional and non-functional pancreatic islet-cell carcinoma Pancreatic adenocarcinoma carcinoid tumors
Methyl-GAG Methylglyoxal-bisguanylhydrazone MGGH	1000-mg vials	1. Inhibition of DNA and RNA synthesis by linking to DNA 2. Rapidly cleared from blood 3. Metabolism not well understood 4. 25% excreted in urine during first 24 h, the rest slowly over 3 weeks 5. INHIBITORS OF PROTEIN SYNTHESIS	150-200 mg/m², infusion every 2 days	GI: nausea, vomiting, stomatitis, diarrhea BM depression Hypoglycemia	Acute myeloid leukemia
N-Methylhydrazine Procarbazine Matulane ® PCZ	50-mg caps	1. Inhibitor of DNA, RNA, and protein synthesis 2. T½ = 8 min 3. Formation of several metabolites 4. Major portion excreted in urine; 25% in first 24 h 5. INHIBITORS OF PROTEIN SYNTHESIS	100-200 mg/m², p.o., daily	GI: nausea, vomiting BM depression Psychic alterations: depression, aggravated by phenothiazine Mild MAO inhibitor: flushing after alkohol	Hodgkin's disease Non-Hodgkin's lymphomas Myeloma Melanoma Lung cancer
L-Asparaginase Crastinin ®	10,000-U vials	1. Inhibition of protein synthesis 2. T½ = 8-30 h; cumulative	10,000-15,000 U/m², i.v. per day; 3-7 days per week for 10-28 days	GI: nausea, vomiting, anorexia, weight loss Fever, hypersensitivity	Acute lymphoid leukemia Acute myeloid leu-

65

Table 3-2. (continued)

Drug	Supply	Pharmacology	Dose	Reactions	Indications
ASP		increase in plasma level with repetitive administration		reactions / Hepatic: abnormal function studies, fatty metamorphosis; hyperproteinemia, including albumin and fibrinogen; hyperlipidemia / Pancreatitis (rare); hyperglycemia / Coagulation defects / Somnolence, lethargy, confusion / BM: granulocytopenia, lymphopenia, thrombocytopenia (mild, transient)	kemia / Lymphosarcoma

6. ALKYLATING AGENTS

Drug	Supply	Pharmacology	Dose	Reactions	Indications
Mechlorethamine / Nitrogen mustard / Mustargen ® / HN2	10-mg vials	1. Alkylating agent / 2. 90% cleared from blood in 0.5 to 1 min / 3. Undergoes rapid chemical transformation and combination with either H_2O or reactive compounds in the cell / 4. 50% excreted in urine in first 24 h in detoxified form	15 mg/m² / 0.4 mg/kg — i.v., single dose, or in divided doses over 2-4 consecutive days; repeat at 3- to 6-week intervals	GI: nausea, vomiting, local vesicant / BM depression; nadir at 6-21 days	Hodgkin's disease / Non-Hodgkin's lymphomas / Lung cancer / Intra-arterial, intrapleural injections / Mycosis fungoides (topical)
Chlorambucil / Leukeran ® / CLB	2-mg tabs	1. Alkylating agent / 2. / 3. no information / 4.	4-8 mg/m² / 0.1-0.2 mg/kg — p.o., daily initially; maintenance adjusted to hematologic tolerance / 10-15 mg/m², p.o., daily for 1 week every other week	BM depression	Chronic lymphoid leukemia / Hodgkin's disease / Non-Hodgkin's lymphomas / Macroglobulinemia / Cancer of the testis, ovary, breast / Choriocarcinoma
Cyclophosphamide / Cytoxan ®	50-mg tabs / 100-,	1. Alkylating agent / 2. $T\frac{1}{2}$ = 4-6.5 h / 3. Must be metabolized, main-	1000 mg/m² / 30-40 mg/kg — i.v., single dose, or in divided do-	BM depression; WBC nadir: day 8-10, restoration by day 15-	Hodgkin's disease / Non-Hodgkin's lymphomas

Table 3-2. (continued)

Drug	Preparation	Pharmacology	Dose	Toxicity	Indications
CPM	200- and 500-mg vials	...ly in the liver, before becoming active 4. Renal excretion: 50-70% in 48 h (68% as metabolite, 32% as active drug) 5. Impaired hepatic or renal function. Several drugs (barbiturates, corticosteroids, phenothiazides, allopurinol and others) may change CPM metabolism, activity, and toxicity	...ses over 2-4 days; repeat at 2-3 week interval (intermittent therapy) 100 mg/m² | p.o., 2.0-2.5 mg/kg | daily (continuous therapy)	21; less thrombocytopenia GI: anorexia, nausea, vomiting Alopecia Hemorrhagic cystitis Cardiac toxicity (after very large doses)	Burkitt's tumor Mycosis fungoides Acute lymphoid leukemia Chronic lymphoid leukemia Myeloma Wilms' tumor Ewing's sarcoma Neuroblastoma Cancer of the ovary, breast, and lung
Melphalan L-Phenylalanine mustard Alkeran ® MPH	2-mg tabs	1. Alkylating agent 2. In active form in blood for 1-6 h 4. Metabolites excreted in urine	10 mg/m² | p.o., daily 0.25 mg/kg | for 4 days; repeat at 6-week intervals (intermittent therapy)	BM depression, delayed GI: nausea, vomiting	Myeloma Macroglobulinemia Cancer of the ovary and breast
Busulfan Myleran® BSF	2-mg tabs	1. Alkylating agent 2. Over 90% of drug cleared from blood in 2-3 min 4. 10-50% excreted in urine as metabolic products, chiefly methane sulfonic acid	4 mg/m², p.o., daily, until WBC 10-15,000; maintenance adjusted to hematologic tolerance (continuous therapy) 4 mg/m², p.o., daily until WBC 10-15,000; no therapy until WBC > 50,000 (intermittent therapy)	BM depression, mainly leukopenia Amenorrhea Hyperpigmentation Pulmonary fibrosis Wasting syndrome, with features of Addison's disease Cellular dysplasia Testicular atrophy	Chronic myeloid leukemia Polycythemia vera Myelofibrosis
Mitoclomin MCM	100-mg caps	1. Alkylating agent	100 mg, p.o., daily or 3 days per week	BM depression GI: nausea, diarrhea	Chronic lymphoid leukemia
Triethylene thiophosphoramide ThioTEPA ®	15-mg vials	1. Alkylating agent 2. Most of the drug is cleared from the plasma within a few minutes 3. Excreted in urine, most in 24-48 h	6 mg/m² | i.m., i.v., 0.2 mg/kg | daily for 4 days; repeat at 4-week intervals 6 mg/m² | i.m., i.v., 0.2 mg/kg | weekly	BM depression	Cancer of the ovary and breast Intracavitary injection for malignant effusions Local instillation for bladder cancer

Table 3-2. (continued)

Pipobroman Vercyte® PPB	10- and 25-mg tabs	1. Alkylating agent	1-1.5 mg/kg, p.o., initially; 0.1-0.2 mg/kg for maintenance	BM depression GI: nausea, vomiting, diarrhea	Chronic myeloid leukemia Polycythemia vera
Dibromomanitol DBM	100-mg tabs	1. Alkylating agent 4. 70% excreted as metabolites after 24 h, 24% unchanged	100-250 mg/m², p.o., daily; 400 mg/m², p.o., once weekly; 150-500 mg/m², p.o., daily for 7 days alternating with 7 days therapy	BM depression	Chronic myeloid leukemia Polycythemia vera
Mitomycin C Mutamycin® MTC	5-mg vials	1. Alkylating agent 2. Disappears rapidly from blood 3. Metabolism in vivo is unknown 4. 35% of intact drug recovered in urine within a few hours	1.0-1.5 mg/m², i.v., daily until toxicity; total dose should not exceed 50 mg/m² 20-25 mg/m², i.v., single dose; repeat at 3-week intervals	BM depression, delayed; especially thrombocytopenia Local cellulitis GI: anorexia, nausea, vomiting, stomatitis, diarrhea Alopecia	Cancer of the ovary, breast, H + N, lung, cervix, and gastrointestinal tract Chronic myeloid leukemia Lymphomas Melanoma

7. AGENTS INTERFERING WITH TRANSCRIPTION

Actinomycin D Dactinomycin Cosmegen® ACD	0.5-mg vials	1. Antibiotic; inhibits RNA synthesis 2. 85% cleared from blood in 2 min 4. Urinary excretion 12-20% Biliary excretion 50-90% in 24 h	0.3-0.5 mg/m², i.v., daily for 5 days; repeat at 2-4 week intervals 0,5 mg/m², i.v., once weekly	GI: anorexia, nausea, vomiting, stomatitis, diarrhea Local cellulitis BM depression Fever Alopecia; dermatitis (especially in previously irradiated areas)	Wilms' tumor Choriocarcinoma Testicular tumors Neuroblastoma, Ewing's sarcoma, soft-tissue sarcomas, rhabdomyosarcoma Carcinoid tumor Melanoma
Mithramycin Mithracin® MTM	2.5-mg vials	1. Antibiotic; inhibits RNA synthesis 2. 3. Insufficient data 4.	1.0-1.5 mg/m² 50 µg/kg infusion every other day until toxicity; repeat courses 4 weeks after beginning of previous one, but mini-	Malaise, fever, nausea, vomiting; Bleeding diathesis Abnormalities of hepatic and renal function Skin rash, facial flush	Embryonal carcinoma of testis Hypercalcemia associated with malignancies

68

Table 3-2. (continued)

Agent/Supply	Pharmacology	Dose	Toxicity	Indications
		mum 2 weeks after last dose For hypercalcemia: 0.025 mg/kg, infusion; repeat if no decline in serum Ca in 24-48 h, or if Ca returns to hypercalcemic levels	CNS reactions: headache, irritability, lethargy BM depression: leukopenia thrombocytopenia Hypocalcemia	
Daunorubicin DRB 20-mg vials	1. Antibiotic; inhibits DNA and RNA synthesis 2. $T\frac{1}{2}$ = 30-50 h 3. DRB is converted to daunorubicinol 4. Total DRB urinary excretion = 25%, daunorubicinol is a major component; also significant biliary excretion 5. Impaired hepatic function	40 mg/m², i.v., daily for 3-5 days; repeat at 3- to 4-week intervals 10-30 mg/m², i.v., twice weekly Maximum total dose: 600 mg/m²	BM depression Cardiac toxicity: acute: ECG changes, arrhythmias chronic: CHF (cumulative, dose-dependent) Alopecia Stomatitis Cellulitis, phlebitis	Acute lymphoid leukemia Acute myeloid leukemia Chronic myeloid leukemia, blastic crisis
Adriamycin ® Adriablastina ® ADM 10- and 50-mg vials	1. Antibiotic; inhibits DNA and RNA synthesis 2. Biphasic plasma disappearance with $T\frac{1}{2}$ = 1.1 h and 16.7 h 3. ADM is extensively metabolized in man 4. Total urinary excretion: 5% of administered dose (ADM plus metabolites); significant biliary excretion (± half of the parent compound and an additional 30% as conjugates) 5. ADM toxicity aggravated by hepatic dysfunction	60-75 mg/m², i.v., repeat at 3-week intervals (most commonly used schedule) 30 mg/m², i.v., daily for 3 days; repeat at 4-week intervals 10 mg/m², i.v., daily for 4 days, off therapy for 3 days; repeat cycle Maximum total dose: 550 mg/m²	BM depression (especially leukopenia) Cardiac toxicity: 1. transient ECG changes 2. myocardiopathy ("pump" failure) dose-dependent Stomatitis Nausea, vomiting Fever Alopecia	Acute lymphoid leukemia Acute myeloid leukemia Hodgkin's disease, non-Hodgkin lymphomas, soft-tissue sarcomas, osteogenic sarcoma Wilms' tumor, neuroblastoma, Ewing's sarcoma Cancer of breast, ovary, lung, bladder, and thyroid

8. AGENTS WITH RADIOMIMETIC EFFECT

Agent/Supply	Pharmacology	Dose	Toxicity	Indications
Bleomycin ® Blenoxane ® BLM 15-mg vials	1. Antibiotic; radiomimetic effect 2. $T\frac{1}{2}$ = 1.5 h 3. Relative high concentration	10 mg/m², i.m., or i.v., twice weekly until total dose of 300 mg	Fever, chills Rash, hyperpigmentation, hyperkeratosis, dyskeratosis, alopecia	Hodgkin's disease Non-Hodgkin lymphoma Squamous-cell car-

Table 3-2. (continued)

			Anorexia, nausea, stomatitis	cinomas: skin, vulva, H + N, penis, esophagus, and cervix
		4. 25-50% of administered dose excreted in urine in 24 h (as active BLM 20-40%)	Pulmonary, toxicity: pneumonitis, fibrosis Hypersensitivity reactions	Mycosis fungoides Testicular tumors

9. AGENTS INTERFERING WITH THE MITOTIC SPINDLE

Drug	Supply	Pharmacology	Toxicity	Indications
Vincristine Oncovin® VCR	1- and 5-mg vials	1. Plant alkaloid; mitotic poison 2. Cleared from blood within 30 sec 3. Metabolized in liver 4. Excreted by liver into the bile 5. Impaired hepatic function or biliary obstruction 1.0-2.0 mg/m², i.v., weekly (toxicity can be delayed by not exceeding a total dose of 2 mg per week in adults)	Neurotoxicity: peripheral neuropathy (areflexia, paresthesias, jaw pains), muscle weakness, paralytic ileus Alopecia Local cellulitis Little BM depression at dosages used	Acute lymphoid leukemia Acute myeloid leukemia Chronic myeloid leukemia (blastic crisis) Hodgkin's disease Non-Hodgkin lymphomas **Wilms' tumor** **Rhabdomyosarcoma** **Ewing's sarcoma** Neuroblastoma Retinoblastoma Soft-tissue sarcomas Melanoma Cancer of breast, testis, brain, ovary, and cervix
Vinblastine Velban® VLB	10-mg vials	1. Plant alkaloid; mitotic poison 2. Cleared from blood within 30 sec; 60% binds to platelets 3. Metabolized in liver 4. Excreted by liver into bile 5.0-6.0 mg/m², i.v., weekly	BM depression: leukopenia (nadir, day 5-10) less thrombocytopenia Local cellulitis Anorexia, nausea, vomiting Less neurotoxicity than VCR Alopecia	Hodgkin's disease, non-Hodgkin lymphomas Cancer of breast and testis (teratocarcinoma) Choriocarcinoma (resistant to MTX, ACD) Histiocytosis X

Table 3-2. (continued)

4'-Dimethyl-epipodophyl-lotoxin-β-D-thenylidene glucoside VM26 EPT	50-mg amps	1. Semisynthetic derivative of podophyllotoxin; mitotic poison 2. $T_{1/2}$ = 10 h 3. Urinary and biliary excretion	30 mg/m^2, infusion (30-60 min), daily for 5 days; repeat at 10- to 21-day intervals 70 mg/m^2, infusion, once weekly 40-115 mg/m^2 infusion, twice weekly	BM depression: leukopenia, less thrombocytopenia, nausea, vomiting, diarrhea Hypotension following i.v. push injection Alopecia Anaphylaxis (rare)	Non-Hodgkin lymphomas, Hodgkin's disease Cancer of bladder and brain
4'-Dimethyl-epipodophyl-lotoxin-β-D-ethylidene glucoside VP 16-213 EPE	100-mg vials 100-mg caps	1. Semisynthetic derivative of podophyllotoxin; mitotic poison 2. $T_{1/2}$ = 10 h 4. Urinary excretion: 85% in 24 h	50-60 mg/m^2, infusion, daily for 5 days, or 100-120 mg/m^2, p.o., daily for 5 days; repeat at intervals of 5 to 25 days 120 mg/m^2 p.o. or i.v., weekly	BM depression (in 30%) Anorexia, nausea, vomiting Alopecia	Acute monocytoid leukemia Acute myelomonocytoid leukemia Reticulosarcoma Cancer of breast, bladder, kidney, and thyoid

a. Consult reference 235 for additional high-dose methotrexate regimens.

REFERENCES

1. DOWLING, Jr., M.D., KRAKOFF, I.H., KARNOFSKY, D.A.: Mechanism of action of anticancer drugs. In: Chemotherapy of Cancer, p. 1 (ed. W. H. Cole), Philadelphia: Pa.: Lea and Febiger 1970
2. GOODMAN, L.S., GILMAN, A.: The pharmacological basis of therapeutics, 4 ed., Vol. 1, New York: MacMillan 1975
3. LIVINGSTON, R., CARTER, S.: Single agents in cancer chemotherapy. New York: IFI/Plenum 1970
4. CLINE, M.J.: Cancer chemotherapy. Philadelphia-London-Toronto: W.B. Saunders (1971)
5. YOUNG, C.W., BURCHENAL, J.H.: Cancer chemotherapy. Annu. Rev. Pharmacol. 11, 369 (1971)
6. BERGEVIN, P.R., TORMEY, D.C., BLOM, J.: Guide to the use of cancer chemotherapeutic agents. Modern Treatment, 9, 185 (1972)
7. CARTER, S.K.: Current status of new agents. Cancer Chemoter. Rep. 3, 33 (1972)
8. BURCHENAL, J.H., CARTER, S.K.: New cancer chemotherapeutic agents. Cancer 30, 1639 (1972)
9. SARTORELLI, A.C., CREASEY, W.A.: Cancer chemotherapy. Annu. Rev. Pharmacol. 9, 51 (1969).
10. OLIVERIO, V.T., ZUBROD, C.G.: Clinical pharmacology of the effective antitumor drugs. Annu. Rev. Pharmacol. 5, 335 (1965).
11. ADAMSON, R.H.: Metabolism of anticancer agents in man. Ann. N.Y. Acad. Sci. 179, 432 (1971).
12. HARRAP, K.R.: Pharmacologic disposition of anticancer agents. In: The Design of Clinical Trials in Cancer Therapy, p. 292 (ed. M. Staquet). Brussels: Editions Scientifiques Européennes 1972.
13. ELION, G.B.: The comparative metabolism of "Imuran" and 6-mercaptopurine (6-MP) in man. Proc. amer. Ass. Cancer Res. 10, 21 (1969).
14. ROY-BURMAN, P.: Analogues of nucleic acid components. Mechanisms of action. In: Recent Results in Cancer Research 25. Berlin-Heidelberg: Springer 1970.
15. HITCHINGS, H., ELION, G.B.: Mechanisms of action of purine and pyrimidine analogues. In: Cancer Chemotherapy II, p. 23 (eds. I. Brodsky, S.B. Kahn, J.H. Moyer). New York: Gune and Stratton 1972.
16. FARBER, S., DIAMOND, L.K., MERCER, R.D., SYLVESTER, R.F., WOLFF, J.A.: Temporary remissions in acute leukemia in children produced by folic acid antagonist, 4 aminopteroyl-glutamic acid. New Engl. J. Med., 238, 787 (1948).
17. ANDERSON, L.L., COLLINS, G.J., OJIMA, Y., SULLIVAN, R.D.: A study of the distribution of methotrexate in human tissues and tumors. Cancer Res. 30, 1344 (1970).
18. BORSA, J., WHITMORE, G.F.: Cell killing studies on the mode of action of methotrexate on L-cells in vitro. Cancer Res. 29, 737 (1969).
19. HARRAP, K.R., HILL, B.T., FURNESS, M.E., HART, L.I.: Sites of action of methotrexate: intrinsic and acquired drug resistance. Ann. N.Y. Açad. Sci. 186, 312 (1970).
20. HENDERSON, E.S., ADAMSON, R.H., OLIVERIO, V.T.: The metabolic fate of tritiated methotrexate. II. Absorption and excretion in man. Cancer Res. 25, 1018 (1965).
21. WERKHEISER, W.C.: Specific binding of 4-amino folic acid analogues by folic acid reductase. J. Biol. Chem. 236, 888 (1963).
22. BERTINO, J.R., JOHNS, D.G.: Folate antagonists. In: Cancer Chemotherapy II, p. 9 (eds. I. Brodsky, S.B. Kahn, J.H. Moyer). New York: Grune and Stratton 1972.
23. HRYNIUK, W.M.: Purineless death as a link between growth rate and cytotoxicity by methotrexate. Cancer Res. 32, 1506 (1972).
24. BENNETT, Jr., L.L., ALLAN, P.W.: Formation and significance of 6-methylthiopurine ribonucleotide as a metabolite of 6-mercaptopurine. Cancer Res. 31, 152 (1971).

25. BROCKMAN, R.W., CHUMLEY, S.: Inhibition of formylglycinamide ribonucleotide synthesis in neoplastic cells by purines and analogs. Biochim. Biophys. Acta 95, 365 (1965).
26. ELION, G.B.: Biochemistry and pharmacology of purine analogues. Fed. Proc. 26, 898 (1967).
27. HITCHINGS, G.H.: Chemotherapy and comparative biochemistry: G.H. A. Clowes Memorial Lecture, Cancer Res. 29, 1895 (1969).
28. MOORE, G.E., BROSS, I.D.J., AUSMAN, R., NADLER, S., JONES, Jr., R., SLACK, N., RIMM, A.A.: Effects of 6-mercaptopurine (NSC-755) in 290 patients with advanced cancer. Eastern clinical drug evaluation program. Cancer Chemother. Rep. 52, 655 (1968).
29. WANG, M.C., SIMPSON, A.I., PATERSON, A.R.P.: Combinations of 6-mercaptopurine (NCS-755) and 6-(methylmercapto)purine ribonucleoside (NSC-40774) in therapy of Ehrlich ascites carcinoma. Cancer Chemother. Rep. 51, 101 (1967).
30. HO, H.W., FREI, III E.: Pharmacological studies of the antitumor agent 6-methylthiopurine ribonucleoside. Cancer Res. 30, 2852 (1970).
31. LEPAGE, G.A.: Incorporation of 6-thioguanine into nucleic acids. Cancer Res. 20, 403 (1960).
32. LEPAGE, G.A., JONES, M.: Further studies on the mechanism of action of 6-thioguanine. Cancer Res. 21, 1590 (1961).
33. LEPAGE, G.A., WHITECAR, Jr., J.P.: Pharmacology of 6-thioguanine in man. Cancer Res. 31, 1627 (1971).
34. SAUNDERS, P.P.: Studies of the mechanism of action of the antitumor agent 5(4)-(3,3-dimethyl-1-triazeno)-imidazole-4(5)-carboxamide in Bacillus subtilis. Biochem. Pharmacol. 19, 911 (1970).
35. SKIBBA, J.L., ERTÜRK, E., JOHNSON, R.O., BRYAN, G.T.: Inhibition 14C-thymidine uptake in proliferating rat tissues by 4(5)-(3,3-dimethyl-1-triazeno)-imidazole-5 (4)-carboxamide (NSC 45388, DIC). Proc. amer. Ass. Cancer Res. 7, 2 (1971).
36. SKIBBA, J.L., RAMIREZ, G., BEAL, D.D., BRYAN, G.T.: Metabolism of 4(5)-(3,3-dimethyl-1-triazeno)-imidazole-5(4)-carboxamide to 4(5)-amino-imidazole-5(4)-carboxamide in man. Biochem. Pharmacol. 19, 2043 (1970).
37. MIZUNO, N.S., HUMPHREY, E.W.: Metabolism of 5-(3,3-dimethyl-1-triazeno)-imidazole-4-carboxamide (NSC-45388) in human and animal tumor tissue, Cancer Chemother. Rep. 56, 465 (1972).
38. CARTER, S.K., FRIEDMAN, M.A.: 5-(3,3-dimethyl-1-triazeno)-imidazole-4-carboxamide (DTIC, DIC, NSC-45388), a new antitumor agent with activity against malignant melanoma. Europ. J. Cancer 8, 85 (1972).
39. VOGEL, C.L., DeVITA, V.T., DENHAM, C., FOLEY, H.T., FIELD, R.B.: Preliminary clinical trials and clinical pharmacologic studies with 5-(3,3-bis(2-chloroethyl)-triazeno)-imidazole-carboxamide (NSC-82196) given orally. Cancer Chemother. Rep. 55, 159 (1971).
40. BAGLEY, Jr., C.M., CANELLOS, G.P., YOUNG, R.C., GALLELLI, J.F., DE VITA, Jr., T.: Clinical trials with 5-(3,3-bis(2-chloroethyl-1-triazeno)imidazole-4-carboxamide (NSC-82196) given intravenously. Cancer Chemother. Rep. 56, 387 (1972).
41. MUKHERJEE, K.L., BOOHAR, J., WENTLAND, D., ANSFIELD, F.J., HEIDELBERGER, C.: Studies on fluorinated pyrimidines. XVI. Metabolism of 5-fluorouracil-2'-C14 and 5-fluoro-2'-deoxyuridine-2-C14 in cancer patients. Cancer Res. 23, 49 (1963).
42. MUKHERJEE, K.L., CURRERI, A.R., JAVID, M., HEIDELBERGER, C.: Studies of fluorinated pyrimidines. XVII. Tissue distribution of 5-fluorouracil2-C14 and 5-fluoro-2'-deoxyuridine in cancer patients. Cancer Res. 23, 67 (1963).
43. HEIDELBERGER, C.: Fluorinated pyrimidines. In: Progress in Nucleic Acid Research and Molecular Biology, 4, p. 1 (eds. J.N. Davidson, W.E. Cohn). New York: Academic Press 1965.
44. ANSFIELD, F.J., CURRERI, A.R.: Further clinical comparison between 5-fluorouracil (5-FU) and 5-fluoro-2'-deoxyuridine. Cancer Chemother. Rep. 32, 101 (1963).

45. CHU, M.Y., FISHER, G.A.: A proposed mechanism of action of 1-β-D-arabinofuranosyl-cytosine as an inhibitor of the growth of leukemic cells. Biochem. Pharmacol. 11, 423 (1962).
46. CHU, M.Y., FISHER, G.A.: Effect of cytosine arabinoside on the cell viability and uptake of deoxypyrimidine nucleosides in L 5178Y cells. Biochem. Pharmacol. 17, 741 (1968).
47. FURTH, J.J., COHEN, S.S.: Inhibition of mammalian DNA polymerase by the 5'-tri-phosphate of 9-β-D-arabinofuranosyladenine. Cancer Res. 27, 1528 (1967).
48. FURTH, J.J., COHEN, S.S.: Effect of the 5' triphosphate of 1-β-D-arabinofuranosyladenine on the enzymatic synthesis of nucleic acid in mammalian tissues. Proc. amer. Ass. Cancer Res. 9, 23 (1968).
49. FINKELSTEIN, J.Z., SCHER, J., KARON, M.: Pharmacologic studies of tritiated cytosine arabinoside (NSC-63878) in children. Cancer Chemother. Rep. 54, 35 (1970).
50. BAGULEY, B.C., FALKENHANG, E.M.: Plasma half-life of cytosine arabinoside (NSC-63878) in patients treated for acute myeloblastic leukemia. Cancer Chemother. Rep. 55, 291 (1971).
51. FREI, III E., BICKERS, J.N., HEWLETT, J.S., LANE, M., LEARY, W.V., TALLEY, R.W.: Dose schedule and antitumor studies of arabinosyl cytosine (NSC 63878). Cancer Res. 29, 1325 (1969).
52. BURKE, P.J., OWENS, Jr., A.H., COLSKY, J., SHNIDER, B.I., EDMONSON, J.H., SCHILLING, A., BRODOVSKY, H.S., WALLACE, Jr., H.J., HALL, T.C.: A clinical evaluation of a prolonged schedule of cytosine arabinoside. Cancer Res. 30, 1512 (1970).
53. BURCHENAL, J.H., KREIS, W.: Antibiotics, L-asparaginase and new agents. In: Cancer Chemotherapy II, p. 41 (eds. I. Brodsky, S.B. Kahn, J.H. Moyer) New York: Grune and Stratton 1972.
54. WEISS, A.J., STRAMBAUGH, J.E., MASTRANGELO, M.J., LAUCIUS, J.F., BELLET, R.E.: Phase I study of 5-azacytidine (NSC-102816). Cancer Chemother. Rep. 56, 413 (1972).
55. VOGLER, W.R., ARKUM, S.N.: Phase I study of 5-azacytidine. Proc. amer. Ass. Cancer Res. 14, 59 (1973).
56. HANDSCHUMACHER, R.E., CALABRESI, P., WELCH, A.D., BONO, V., FALLEN, H., FREI, E.: Summary of current information on 6-azauridine. Cancer Chemother. Rep. 21, 1 (1962).
57. PFEIFFER, S., TOLMACH, L.J.: Inhibition of DNA synthesis in HeLa cells by hydroxyurea. Cancer Res. 27, 124 (1967).
58. KRAKOFF, I.H., BROWN, N.C., REICHARD, P.: Inhibition of ribonucleoside diphosphate reductase by hydroxyurea. Cancer Res. 28, 1559 (1968).
59. ROSENKRANZ, H.S., JACOBS, S.J., CARR, H.S.: Studies on hydroxyurea VIII. The deoxyribonucleic acid of hydroxyurea-treated cells. Biochim. Biophys. Acta, 161 428 (1968).
60. BECKLOFF, G.L.: Pharmacological, metabolic and clinical experience with hydroxyurea. Clin. Trials J. 4, 873 (1967).
61. ROSNER, F., RUBIN, H., PARISE, F.: Studies on the absorption, distribution, and excretion of hydroxyurea (NSC-32065). Cancer Chemother. Rep. 55, 167 (1971).
62. FABRICIUS, E., RAJEWSKU, M.F.: Determination of hydroxyurea in mammalian tissues and blood. Rev. Europ. clin. biol. 16, 679 (1971).
63. KENNEDY, B.J., YARBRO, J.W.: Metabolic and therapeutic effects of hydroxyurea in chronic myeloid leukemia. J. amer. med. Ass. 195, 1038 (1966).
64. ARIEL, I.M.: Therapeutic effects of hydroxyurea. Cancer 25, 705 (1970).
65. VERLY, W.G., LEDRU, E.: Action of hydroxyurea on survival of EMS-treated or UV-irradiated HeLa cells. Rev. Europ. Etudes clin. et biol. 16, 788 (1971).
66. YABAR, D., HOLLAND, J.F., ELLISON, R.R., FREEMAN, A.: Clinical pharmacological trial of guanazole. Cancer Res. 33, 972 (1973).

67. DECONTI, R.C., TOFTNESS, B.R., AGRAWAL, K.C., TOMCHICK, R., MEAD, J.A.R., BERTINO, J.R., SARTORELLI, A.C., CREASEY, W.A.: Clinical and pharmacological studies with 5-hydroxy-2-formylpyridine thiosemicarbazone. Cancer Res. 32, 1455 (1972).

68. SYMPOSIUM ON THE NITROSOUREA. Cancer Chemother. Rep. Part 3, Vol. 4, No 3, 1-46 (1973).

69. CARTER, S.K., SCHABEL, F.M., BRODER, L.E., et al.: 1,3-bis(2-chloroethyl)-1-nitrosourea (BCNU) and other nitrosoureas in cancer treatment. Adv. Cancer Res. 16, 273 (1972).

70. OLIVERIO, V.T.: Toxicology and pharmacology of the nitrosoureas. Cancer Chemother. Rep. Part 3, Vol. 4, No 3, 13 (1973).

71. GROTH, D.P., D'ANGELO, J.M., VOGLER, W.R., MINGIOLI, E.S., BETZ, B.: Selective metabolic effects of 1,3-bis(2-chloroethyl)-1-nitrosourea upon de novo purine biosynthesis. Cancer Res. 31, 332 (1971).

72. WASSERMAN, T.H., SLAVIK, M., CARTER, S.K.: Clinical comparison of the nitrosoureas. Cancer 36, 1258 (1975).

73. CHUN HUI, CHENG, FUJIMURA S., GRUNBERGER, D., WEINSTEIN, I.B.: Interaction of 1-(2-chloroethyl)-3-cyclohexyl-1-nitrosourea (NSC 79037) with nucleic acids and proteins in vivo and in vitro. Cancer Res. 32, 22 (1972).

74. OLIVERIO, V.T., VIETZKE, W.M., WILLIMANS, M.K., ADAMSON, R.H.: The absorption, distribution, excretion, and biotransformation of the carcinostatic 1-(2-chloroethyl)-3-cyclohexyl-1-nitrosourea in animals. Cancer Res. 30, 1330 (1970).

75. HANSEN, H.H., SELAWRY, F.M., WALKER, M.D.: Clinical studies with 1-(2-chloroethyl)-3-cyclohexyl-1-nitrosourea (NSC-79037). Cancer Res. 31. 223 (1971).

76. BRODER, L.E., HANSEN, H.H.: 1-(2-chloroethyl)-3-cyclohexyl-1-nitrosourea (CCNU, NSC-79037): a comparison of drug administration at four-week and six-week intervals. Europ. J. Cancer 9, 147 (1973).

77. GOTTLIEB, J.A., McCREDIE, K.B., HERSH, E.M., FREI III, E.: Initial clinical studies with 1-2(chloro-ethyl)-3-(4-methylcyclohexyl)-1-nitrosourea (methyl'CCNU). Proc. amer. Ass. Cancer Res. 13, 79 (1972).

78. MAYO, J.G., LASTER, Jr., W.R., ANDREWS, C.M., SCHABEL. Jr., F.M.: Success and failure in the treatment of solid tumors. III. "Cure" of metastatic Lewis lung carcinoma with methyl-CCNU (NSC-95441) and surgery-chemotherapy. Cancer Chemother. Rep. 56, 183 (1972).

79. CARTER, S.K., BRODER, L., FRIEDMAN, M.: Streptozotocin and metastatic insulinoma. Ann. intern. Med. 74, 445 (1971).

80. DU PRIEST, Jr., R.W., MASSEY, W.H., FLETCHER, W.S.: Search for new cancer drugs: streptozotocin. Amer. Surg. 38, 514 (1972).

81. STOLINSKY, D.C., SADOFF, L., BRAUNWALD, J., BATERMAN, J.R.: Streptozotocin in the treatment of cancer: phase II study. Cancer 30, 61 (1972).

82. BRODER, L.E., CARTER, S.K.: Results of therapy with streptozotocin in the treatment of cancer: phase II study. Cancer 30, 61 (1972).

83. KOLMEIER, K.H., SILVERSTEIN, M.N., FLEISHER, G.A.: Anaerobic glycolysis in normal and leukemic bone-marrow leukocytes. Effect of methyl-glyoxal-bis guanylhydrazone dihydrochloride. Cancer 19, 1199 (1966).

84. SARTORELLI, A.C., IANNOTTI, A.T., BOOTH, B.A., SCHNEIDER, F.H., BERTINO, J.R., JOHNS, D.G.: Complex formation with DNA and inhibition of nucleic acid synthesis by methylglyoxal-bis(guanylhydrazone). Biochim. Biophys. Acta 103, 174 (1965).

85. FREIREICH, E.J., FREI, E., KARON, M.: Methylglyoxal-bis(guanylhydrazone): a new agent active against myelocytic leukemia. Cancer Chemother. Rep. 16, 183 (1962).

86. REGELSON, W., HOLLAND, J.F.: Clinical experience with methylglyoxal bis(guanylhydrazone) dihydrochloride: a new agent with clinical activity in acute myelocytic leukemia and the lymphomas. Cancer Chemother. Rep. 27, 15 (1963).

87. BROOKES, P., LAWLEY, P.D.: Mechanism of action of 1-methyl-2-p-(isopropylcarbamoyl)-benzylhydrazine hydrochloride (RO4-6467). In: 42nd Annual Report of the British Empire Cancer Campaign for Research, part II, p. 77 (1964).

88. KREIS, W., BURCHEMAL, J.H., HUTCHINSON, D.J.: Influence of a methyl-hydrazine derivative on the in vivo transmethyllation of the S-methy group of methionine onto purine and pyrimidine bases of RNA. Proc. amer. Ass. Cancer Res. 149, 38 (1968).

89. KREIS, W.: Metabolism of an antineoplastic methylhydrazine deriva-tive in a P 815 mouse neoplasm. Cancer Res. 30, 82 (1970).

90. OLIVERIO, V.T.: Pharmacologic disposition of procarbazine. In: Proceedings of the Chemotherapy Conference on Procarbazine (Ma-tulane: NSC-77213): development and application. (ed. S.K. Carter) Cancer Therapy Evaluation Branch. Bethesda, Md.: National Cancer Institute 1970.

91. SCHREK, R., DOLOWA, W.C., AMMERAAL, R.N.: L-asparaginase: toxici-ty to normal and leukemic human lymphocytes. Science 155, 329 (1967).

92. BROOME, J.D.: Studies on the mechanism of tumor inhibition by L-asparaginase. Effects of the enzyme on asparaginase levels in the blood, normal tissues and 6 C3HED lymphomas of mice; differ-ences in asparaginase formation and utilization in asparaginase-sensitive and -resistant lymphoma cells. J. exp. Med. 127, 1055 (1968).

93. TOMAO, F.A., SCHWARTZ, M.K., LASH, E., OETTGEN, H., KRAKOFF, I.H.: Blood levels and distribution of L-asparaginase in man. Proc. amer. Ass. Cancer Res. 10, 94 (1969).

94. OHNUMA, T., HOLLAND, J.F., FREEMAN, A., SINKS, L.F.: Biochemical and pharmocological studies with asparaginase in man. Cancer Res. 30, 2297 (1970).

95. GRUNDMANN, E., OETTGEN, H.F.: Experimental and clinical effects of L-asparaginase. In: Recent Results in Cancer Research, Berlin-Heidelberg: Springer-Verlag 1970.

96. CAPIZZI, R.L., BERTINO, J.R., SKEEL, R.T., CREASEY, W.A., ZANES, R., OLAYON, PERTERSON, R.G., HANDSCHUMAKER, R.E.: L-asparaginase - clinical, biochemical, pharmacological and immunological studies. Ann. intern. Med. 7, 893 (1971).

97. HASKELL, C.M., CANELLOS, G.P., LEVENTHAL, B.G., CARBONE, P.P., BLOCK, J.B., SERPICK, A.A., SELAWRY, O.S.: L-asparaginase. Therapeutic and toxic effects in patients with neoplastic disease. New Engl. J. Med. 281, 1028 (1969).

98. OHNUMA, T., HOLLAND, J.F., MEYER, P.A.: Therapy with Erwinia caro-tovora asparaginase after anaphylaxis to asparaginase from E. coli. Proc. amer. Cancer Res. 13, 117 (1972).

99. ROBERTS, J., HOLCENBERG, J.S., DOLOWY, W.C.: Antineoplastic acti-vity of highly purified bacterial glutaminase. Nature 227, 1136 (1970).

100. KARNOFSKY, D.A.: Comparative clinical and biological effects of alkylating agents. Ann. N.Y. Acad. Sci. 68, 657 (1958).

101. WHEELER, G.P.: Studies related to the mechanisms of action of cytotoxic alkylating agents: a review. Cancer Res. 22, 651 (1962).

102. VERLY, W.G., BRAKIER, L.: Mécanismes moléculaires de l'action toxique des agents alkylants. Rev. europ. Etudes clin. et biol. 15, 483 (1970).

103. LUDLUM, D.B.: Mechanism of action of chemotherapeutic drugs. Me-chanism of action of alkylating agents. In: Cancer Chemotherapy II, p. 1, (eds. I. Brodsky, S.B. Kahn, J.H. Moyer). New York: Grune and Stratton 1972.

104. ROBERTS, J.J., CRATHORN, A.R., BRENT, T.P.: Repair of alkylated DNA in mammalian cells. Nature 218, 970 (1968).
105. MOORE, G.E., BROSS, I.D.J., AUSMAN, R., NADLER, S., JONES, Jr., R., SLACK, N., RIMM, A.A.: Effects of chlorambucil (NSC-3088) in 374 patients with advanced cancer. Eastern clinical drug evaluation program. Cancer Chemother. Rep. 52, 661 (1968).
106. BROCK, N.: Pharmacologic characterization of cyclophosphamide (NSC-26271) and cyclophosphamide metabolites. Cancer Chemother. Rep. 51, 315 (1967).
107. BROCK, N., GROSS, R., HOHORST, H.J., KLEIN, H.O., SCHNEIDER, B.: Activation of cyclophosphamide in man and animals. Cancer 27, 1512 (1971).
108. SLADEK, N.E.: Evidence for an aldehyde possessing alkylating activity as the primary metabolite of cyclophosphamide. Cancer Res. 33, 651 (1973).
109. BAGLEY, Jr., C.M., BOSTICK, F.W., DEVITA, Jr., V.T.: Clinical pharmacology of cyclophosphamide. Cancer Res. 33, 226 (1973).
110. HILL, D.L., LASTER, Jr., W.R., KIRK, M.C., SALAH DAREER, STRUCK, R.F.: Metabolism of iphosphamide (2-(2-chloroethylamino)-3-(2-chloroethyl)tetrahydro-2H-1,3,2-oxazaphosphorine 2-oxide) and production of a toxic iphosphamide metabolite. Cancer Res. 33, 1016 (1973).
111. COHEN, M.H., MITTELMAN, A.: Initial clinical trials with isofosfamide. Proc. amer. Ass. Cancer Res. 14, 64 (1973).
112. SHANBROM, E., MILLER, S., HAAR, H., OPFELL, R.: Therapeutic spectrum of uracil-mustard, a new oral antitumor drug. J. amer. med. Ass. 174, 108 (1960).
113. KENNEDY, B.J., THEOLOGIDES, A.: Uracil mustard, a new alkylating agent for oral administration in the management of patients with leukemia and lymphoma. New Engl. J. Med. 264, 790 (1961).
114. FOX, M., REES, R.W.M., BENNETT, D.H.J., HENRY, L.: Investigations into the lymphopoenic and immuno-suppressive properties of the antitumor agent, mitoclomine. Lymphology 4, 35 (1971).
115. CALABRESI, P., WELCH, A.D.: Chemotherapy of neoplastic diseases. Annu. Rev. Med. 13, 147 (1962).
116. WAMPLER, G.L., MELLETTE, S.J., KUPERMINC, M., REGELSON, W.: Hexamethylmelamine (NSC-13875) in the treatment of advanced cancer. Cancer Chemother. Rep. 56, 505 (1972).
117. BERGEVIN, P.R., TORMEY, D.C., BLOM, J.: Clinical evaluation of hexamethylmelamine (NSC-13875). Cancer Chemother. Rep. 57, 51 (1973).
118. BLUM, R.H., LIVINGSTONE, R.B., CARTER, S.K.: Hexamethylmelamine. A new drug with activity in solid tumors. Europ. J. Cancer 9, 195 (1973).
119. WORZALLA, J.F., KAIMAN, B.D., JOHNSON, B.M., JOHNSON, R.O., BRYAN, G.T.: Metabolism of ring-^{14}C-hexamethylmelamine (NSC-13875, HMM) in rats. Proc. amer. Ass. Cancer Res. 14, 25 (1973).
120. ULTMAN, J.E., HYMANN, G.A., CRANDALL, C., NANJOKS, H., GELLHORN, A.: Triethylene thiophosphoramide (thio-tepa) in the treatment of neoplastic disease. Cancer 10, 902 (1957).
121. GALTON, D.A.G., TILL, M., WILTSHAW, E.: Busulfan (1,4-dimethanesulfonyloxy butane), myleran: summary of clinical results. Ann. N.Y. Acad. Sci. 68, 967 (1958).
122. Evaluation of two antineoplastic agents: pipobroman (Vercyte) and thioguanine. J. amer. Med. Ass. 200, 139 (1967).
123. MONTO, R.W., TEN PAS, A., BATTLE, Jr., J.D., ROHN, R.J., LOUIS, J., LOUIS, N.P.: A-8103 in polycythemia. J. amer. Med. Ass. 190, 97 (1964).
124. KENIS, Y.: Effect of piposulfan (NSC-47774) on maligant lymphomas and solid tumors. Cancer Chemother. Rep. 52, 433 (1968).

125. ELSON, L.A., JARMAN, M., ROSS, W.C.J.: Toxicity, hematological effects and antitumour activity of epoxides derived from disubstituted hexitols. Mode of action of mannitol myleran and dibromomannitol. Europ. J. Cancer 4, 617 (1968).

126. CASAZZA, A.R., CAHN, E.L., CARBONE, P.P.: Preliminary studies with dibromomannitol (NSC-94100) in patients with chronic myelogenous leukemia. Cancer Chemother. Rep. 51, 91 (1967).

127. CANELLOS, G.P., YOUNG, R.C., NIEMAN, P., DEVITA, V.T.: Dibromomannitol in the treatment of chronic granulocytic leukemia: a randomized comparison with busulfan. Amer. Soc. Clin. Oncol., Abstr. 31 (1973).

128. HORVATH, I.P., SELLEI, C., ECKHARDT, S., KRALOVANSKY, J.: Studies on the mechanism of action of dibromomannitol (DEM) and dibromodulcitol (DBD). Tenth International Cancer Congress (Houston). Abstract 672. 415 (1970).

129. SELLEI, C., ECKHARDT, S., HORVATH, I.P., KRALOVANSZKY, J., INSTITORIS, L.: Clinical and pharmacologic experience with dibromodulcitol (NSC-104800), a new antitumor agent. Cancer Chemother. Rep. 53, 377 (1969).

130. ANDREWS, N.C., WEISS, A.J., ANSFIELD, F.J., ROCHLIN, D.B., MASON, J.H.: Phase I study dibromodulcitol (NSC-104800). Cancer Chemother. Rep. 55, 61 (1971).

131. PHILIPS, R.W., BROOK, J.: Clinical experiences with dibromodulcitol (NSC-104800) in solid tumors. Cancer Chemother. Rep. 55, 567 (1971).

132. KEYES, Jr., J.W., SELAWRY, O.S., HANSEN, H.H.: Initial clinical trial of dibromodulcitol (NSC-104800) in patients with advanced cancer. Cancer Chemother. Rep. 55, 583 (1971).

133. ROSENBERG, B., VANCAMP, L., TROSKO, J.E., MANSOUR, V.H.: Platinum compounds: a new class of potent antitumor agents. Nature 222, 385 (1969).

134. KOCIBA, R.J., SLEIGHT, S.D.: Acute toxicologic and pathologic effects of cis-diamminedichloroplatinum (NSC-119875) in the male rat. Cancer Chemother. Rep. 55, 1 (1971).

135. DE CONTI, R.C., LANGE, R.C., HARDER, H.C., CREASEY, W.A.: Clinical and pharmacological studies with cis-diammine chloroplatinum (II) (cis-PT). Proc. amer. Ass. Cancer Res. 13, 96 (1972).

136. ROSSOF, A.H., SLAYTON, R.E., PERLIA, C.P.: Preliminary clinical experience with cis-diamminedichloroplatinum (II) (NSC 119875, CACP). Cancer 30, 1451 (1972).

137. IYER, V.N., SZYBALSKY, W.: A molecular mechanism of mitomycin action: linking of complementary DNA strands. Proc. nat. Acad.Sci. 50, 355 (1963).

138. TOMASZ, M.: Novel assay of 7-alkylation of guanine residues in DNA. Application to nitrogen mustard, triethylenemelamine and mitomycin C. Biochim. Biophys. Acta 213, 288 (1970).

139. MOORE, G.E., BROSS, I.D., AUSMAN, R., NADLER, S., JONES, R., SLACK, N., RIMM, A.A.: Effects of mitomycin C (NSC-26980) in 346 patients with advanced cancer. Cancer Chemother. Rep. 52, 675 (1968).

140. IZBICKI, R., AL-SARRAF, M., REED, M.L., VAUGHN, C.B., VAITKEVICIUS, V.K.: Further clinical trials with porfiromycin (NSC-56410) (large intermittent doses). Cancer Chemother. Rep. 56, 615 (1972).

141. HELLMANN, K., NEWTON, K.A., WHITMORE, D.N., HANHAM, I.W.F., BOND, J.V.: Preliminary clinical assessment of I.C.R.F. 159 in acute leukaemia and lymphosarcoma. Brit. Med. J. 1, 822 (1969).

142. CREIGHTON, A.M.: Bisdiketopiperazines: a new class of antitumor agents. Proc. 6th Intern. Congr. Chemother. 1, 167 (1970).

143. SHARPE, H.B.A., FIELD, E.O., HELLMANN, K.: Mode of action of the cytostatic agent "ICRF 159". Nature 226, 524 (1970).

144. SALSBURY, A.J., BURRAGE, K., HELLMANN, K.: Inhibition of metasta-
     tic spread by I.C.R.F. 159: selective deletion of a malignant
     characteristic. Brit. Med. J. 4, 344 (1970).
145. CREAVEN, P.J., COHEN, M.H., HANSEN, H.H., SELAWRY, O.S., TAYLOR,
     S.G.III: Phase I clinical trial of a single-dose and two weekly
     schedules of ICRF-159 (NSC-129943). Cancer Chemother. Rep. Part
     1, Vol. 58, 393 (1974).
146. WOODMAN, R.J., KLINE, I., VENDITTI, J.M.: Protection by (1,2-bis
     (3,5-dioxopiperazin-1-yl)propane) (ICRF-159) against daunomycin
     toxicity and enhanced antileukemic (L1210) efficacy of the com-
     bination. Proc. amer. Ass. Cancer- Res. 13, 31 (1972).
147. HERMAN, E.H., MHATRE, R.M., LEE, I.P., WARAVDEKAR, V.S.: Preven-
     tion of the cardiotoxic effects of adriamycin and daunomycin in
     the isolated dog heart (36432). Proc. Soc. Exp. Biol. Med. 140,
     234 (1972).
148. GOLDBERG, I.H., FRIEDMAN, P.A.: Antibiotics and nucleic acids.
     Annu. Rev. Biochem. 40, 775 (1971).
149. YOUNG, C.W.: Actinomycin and antitumor antibiotics. Amer. J.
     clin. Path. 52, 130 (1969).
150. YARBRO, J.W.: Mithramycin: mechanism of action. In: Proceedings
     of the Chemotherapy Conference on Mithramycin (Mithracin): Devel-
     opment and Application, (eds. S.K. Carter and M.A. Friedman).
     Cancer Therapy Evaluation Branch. Bethesda: National Cancer Insti-
     tute 1970.
151. KENNEDY, B.J.: Metabolic and toxic effects of mithramycin during
     tumor therapy. Am. J. Med. 49, 494 (1970).
152. KENNEDY, B.J.: Mithramycin therapy in advanced testicular neo-
     plasms. Cancer, 26, 755 (1970).
153. CALENDI, E., DI MARCO, A., REGGIANI, M., SCARPINATO, B., VALEN-
     TINI, L.: On physico-chemical interactions between daunomycin
     and nucleic acids. Biochem. Biophys. Acta 103, 25 (1965).
154. DI MARCO, A.: Daunomycin pharmacological activity at the cellular
     level. Path. et Biol. 15, 897 (1967).
155. ALBERTS, D.S., BACHUR, N.R., HOLTZMAN, J.L.: Distribution and
     excretion of daunomycin in man. Proc. Amer. Ass. Cancer Res. 10,
     3 (1969).
156. DI FRONZO, G., BONADONNA, G.: Distribution of tritiated daunomycin
     in man by a simplified method. Rev. Europ. Etud. clin. biol. 15,
     314 (1970).
157. DI FRONZO, G., GAMBETTA, R., BONADONNA, G.: Preliminary studies
     on the distribution and excretion of 3H-adriamycin in man. First
     Congress of the European Association for Cancer Research (abstr.),
     p. 25 (1970).
158. ROSSO, R., RAVAZZONI, C., ESPOSITO, M., SALA, R., SANTI, L.:
     Plasma and urinary levels of adriamycin in man. Europ. J. Cancer
     8, 455 (1972).
159. BENJAMIN, R.S.: Pharmacokinetics of adriamycin in patients with
     sarcomas. Cancer Chemother. Rep. Part 1, Vol. 58, 271 (1974).
160. INTERNATIONAL SYMPOSIUM ON ADRIAMYCIN, Vol. 1 (eds, S.K. Carter,
     A. DiMarco, M. Ghione, I.H. Krakoff, G. Mathê). Berlin-Heidelberg-
     New York: Springer-Verlag 1972.
161. EORTC INTERNATIONAL SYMPOSIUM: Adriamycin review, Vol. 1 (eds. M.
     Staquet, H. Tagnon, Y. Kenis et al.) Ghent: European Press Medi-
     kon 1975.
162. O'BRYAN, R.M., LUCE, J.K., TALLEY, R.W., GOTTLIEB, J.A., BAKER,
     L.H., BONADONNA, G.: Phase II evaluation of adriamycin in human
     neoplasia. Cancer 32, 1 (1973).
163. DOLLINGER, M.R., KRAKOFF, I.H., KARNOFSKY, D.A.: Quinacrine (ata-
     brine) in the treatment of neoplastic effucions. Ann. Intern. Med.
     68, 249 (1967).

164. MUELLER, G.C., KAJIWARA, K., STUBBLEFIELD, E., RUECKERT, R.R.: Molecular events in the reproduction of animal cells. I. The effect of puromycin on the duplication of DNA. Cancer Res. 22, 1084 (1962).

165. UMEZAWA, H., ISHIZUKA, M., MAEDA, K., TAKEUCHI, T.: Studies on bleomycin. Cancer 20, 891 (1967).

166. KUNIMOTO, T., HORI, M., UMEZAWA, H.: Modes of action of phleomycin, bleomycin and formycin on HeLa S3 cells in synchronized cultures. J. Antibiot. (Tokyo), Ser. A. 20, 277 (1967).

167. SUZUKI, H., NAGAI, K., YAMAKI, H., TANAKA, N., UMEZAWA, H.: On the mechanism of action of bleomycin: scission of DNA in vitro and in vivo. J. Antibiot. (Tokyo) 22, 446 (1969).

168. TANAKA, N.: Inhibition of transcription by pluramycin and bleomycin. J. Antibiot. (Tokyo) 23, 523 (1970).

169. FUJITA, H.: Studies in concentration of bleomycin.in blood, urine and tissues, Information provided by: Nippon Kayaku Co., Ltd. 1969.

170. OHNUMA, T., MARTIN, S.A., HOLLAND, J.F.: Bioassay of bleomycin. Proc. amer. Ass. Cancer Res. 12, 94 (1971).

171. OHNUMA, T., SELAWRY, O.S., HOLLAND, J.F., DEVITA, Jr., V.T., SHEDD, D.P., HANSEN, H.H., MUGGIA, F.M.: Clinical study with bleomycin: Tolerance to twice weekly dosage. Cancer 30, 914 (1972).

172. YAGODA, A., MUKHERJI, B., YOUNG, C., ETCUBANAS, E., LAMONTE, C., SMITH, J., TAN, C.T., KRAKOFF, I.H.: Bleomycin an antitumor antibiotic: Clinical experience in 274 patients. Ann. Intern. Med. 77, 861 (1972).

173. BLUM, R.H., CARTER, S.K., AGRE, K.: A clinical review of bleomycin. A new antineoplastic agent. Cancer 31, 903 (1973).

174. BARRANCO, S.C., LUCE, J.K., ROMSDAHL, M.M., HUMPHREY, R.M.: Bleomycin as a possible synchronizing agent for human tumor cells in vivo. Cancer Res. 33, 882 (1973).

175. DeLENA, M., GIZZON, A., MONFARDINI, S., BONADONNA, G.: Clinical, radiologic, and histopathologic studies on pulmohary toxicity induced by treatment with bleomycin. Cancer Chemother. Rep. 56, 343 (1972).

176. MILLER, D.S., LASZLO, J., McCARTY, K.S., GUILD, W.R., HOCHSTEIN, P.: Mechanism of action of streptonigrin in leukemic cells. Cancer Res. 27, 632 (1967).

177. MARSDEN, J.H.: Mechanism of action of the Vinca alkaloids. In Cancer Chemotherapy II, p. 33. (eds. I. Brodsky, S.B. Kahn, J.H. Moyer). New York: Grune and Stratton 1972.

178. CREASEY, W.A., MARKIW, M.E.: Biochemical effects of the Vinca alkaloids. I. Effects of vinblastine on nucleic acid synthesis in mouse tumor cells. Biochem. Pharmacol. 3, 135 (1964).

179. SAVEL, H.: The metaphase-arresting plant alkaloids and cancer chemotherapy. Progr. exp. Tumor Res. 8, 189 (1966).

180. CREASEY, W.A.: Modifications in biochemical pathways produced by the Vinca alkaloids. Cancer Chemother. Rep. 52, 501 (1968).

181. CREASEY, W.A.: Effect of the Vinca alkaloids on RNA synthesis in relation to mitotic arrest. Fed. Proc. 27, 760 (1968).

182. MALAWISTA, S.E., SATO, H., BENSCH, K.G.: Vinblastine and griseofulvin reversibly disrupt the living mitotic spindle. Science 160, 770 (1968).

183. KRISHAN, A.: Time-lapse and ultrastructure studies on the reversal of mitotic arrest induced by vinblastine sulfate in Earle's cells. J. nat. Cancer Inst. 41, 581 (1968).

184. WAGNER, E.K., ROIZMAN, B.: Effect of the Vinca alkaloids on RNA synthesis in human cells in vitro. Science 162, 569 (1968).

185. WILSON, L., BRYAN, J., RUBY, A., MAZIA, D.: Precipitation of proteins by vinblastine and calcium ions. Proc. nat. Acad. Sci. (Wash.) 66, 807 (1970).

186. WEISENBERG, R.C., TIMASHEFF, S.N.: Aggregation of microtubule subunit protein. Effects of divalent actions, colchicine and vinblastine. Biochemistry 9, 4110 (1970).

187. PLAGEMAN, P.G.W.: Vinblastine sulfate: Metaphase arrest, inhibition of RNA synthesis, and cytotoxicity in Novikoff rat hepatoma cells. J. nat. Cancer Inst. 45, 589 (1970).

188. HEBDEN, H.F., HADJFIELD, J.R., BEER, C.T.: The binding of vinblastine by platelets in the rat. Cancer Res. 30, 1417 (1970).

189. TAROCCO, R.P., BRUSA, L., PONZONE, A., PILERI, A.: Effects of vincristine on nucleic acid and protein metabolism in acute leukemia blast cells. Cancro 21, 25 (1968).

190. MORASCA, L., RAINISIO, C., MASERA, G.: Duration of cytotoxic activity of vincristine in the blood of leukemic children. Europ. J. Cancer 5, 79 (1969).

191. STÄHELIN, H.: 4'-Demethyl-epipodophyllotoxin thenyline glucoside (VM 26), a podophyllum compound with a new mechanism of action. Europ. J. Cancer 6, 303 (1970).

192. POUILLART, P.: Etude de la pharmacocinétique du VM26 et du VP 16213. Biomedicine (in prep.).

193. DOMBERNOWSKY, P., NISSEN, N., LARSEN, V.: Clinical investigation of a new podophyllum derivative, epipodophyllotoxin, 4[1]-demethyl-9-(4,6-O-2-thenylidene-β-D-glucopyranoside) (NSC 122819) in patients with malignant lymphomas and solid tumors. Cancer Chemother. Rep. 56, 71 (1972).

194. GOLDSMITH, M.A., CARTER, S.K.: 4'-demethyl-epipodophyllotoxin-B-D-thenylidene glucoside (VM-26). A brief review. Europ.J. Cancer 9, 477 (1973).

195. NISSEN, N.I., LARSEN, V., PEDERSEN, H., THOMSOM, K.: Phase I clinical trial of a new antitumor agent, 4'-demethylepipodophyllotoxin 9-(4,6-O-ethylidene-B-D-glucopyranoside) (NSC 141540; VP 16213). Cancer Chemother. Rep. 56, 769 (1972).

196. E.O.R.T.C.-Clinical Screening Group.: Epipodophyllotoxin VP 16213 in the treatment of acute leukaemias, haematosarcomas and solid tumours. Brit. Med. J. 3, 199 (1973).

197. LE MEN, J., HAYAT, M., MATHE, G., GUILLON, J.C., CHENU, E., HUMBLOT, M., MASSON, Y.: Méthoxy-9-ellipticine lactate. I. Experimental study (oncostatic and immunosuppressive actions; preclinical pharmacology). Rev. europ. Etudes clin. et biol. 15, 534 (1970).

198. GARCIA-GIRALT, E., MACIERA-COELHO, A.: Methoxy-9-ellipticine. II. Analysis in vitro of the mechanism of action. Rev. europ. Etudes clin. et biol. 15, 539 (1970).

199. TAGNON, H.J., COUNE, A., GARATTINI, S., ROSSO, R., LAMBELIN, G., GAUTIER, M., BUU-HOI, N.P.: The antitumoral activity of some derivatives of 6-aminochrysene. Europ. J. Cancer 6, 81 (1970).

200. GELZER, J., LOUSTALOT, P.: Chrysenex in experimental advanced mammary cancer. Eurp. J. Cancer 3, 79 (1967).

201. LEBY, H.B., LAW, L.W., RABSON, A.S.: Inhibition of tumor growth by polyinosinic-polycytidylic acid. Proc. nat. Acad. Sci., Wash. 62. 357 (1969).

202. FISHER, J.C., COOPERBAND, S.R., MANNICK, J.A.: Mechanism of tumor inhibition by poly I: C. Proc. amer. Ass. Cancer Res. 11, 26 (1970).

203. VANDEPUTTE, M., DATTA, S.K., BILLIAU, A., DE SOMER, P.: Inhibition of polyoma-virus oncogenesis in rats by polyriboinosinic-ribocytidylic acid. Europ. J. Cancer 6, 323 (1970).

204. FIELD, A.K., YOUNG, C.W., KRAKOFF, I.H., TYTELL, A.A., LAMPSON, G.P., NEMES, M.M., HILLEMAN, M.R.: Induction of interferon in human subjects by poly I-C. Proc. Soc. exp. Biol. (N.Y.) 136, 1180 (1971).

205. HOMAN, E.R., ZENDZIAN, R.P., ADAMSON, R.H.: Some aspects of the pharmacology and toxicology of polyinosinic: polycytidylic acid. Proc. amer. Ass. Cancer Res. 10, 40 (1969).
206. KRAKOFF, I.H., YOUNG, C.W., HILLEMAN, M.R.: Clinical pharmacology of poly I-C. A preliminary report. Proc. amer. Ass. Cancer Res. 11, 45 (1970).
207. MATHE, G., AMIEL, J.L., SCHWARZENBERG, L., SCHNEIDER, M., HAYAT, M., DE VASSAL, F., JASMIN, C., ROSENFELD, C., SAKOUHI, M., CHOAY, J.: Remission induction with poly I-C in patients with acute lymphoblastic leukaemia (preliminary results). Rev. europ. Etudes clin. et biol. 15, 671 (1970).
208. DEVITA, V.T., CANELLOS, C., CARBONE, P., BARON, S., LEVY, H., GRAINICK, H.: Clinical trials with the interferon inducer polyinosinic-cytidilic acid. Proc. amer. Ass. Cancer Res. 11, 21 (1970).
209. ADAMSON, R.H.: Antitumor activity of two antiviral drugs·- rifampicin and tilorone. Lancet 1, 398 (1971).
210. WAMPLER, G.L., KUPERMINC, M., REGELSON, W.: Tilorone (DEAE-fluorenone) HCl: clinical activity of the first of a new series of host defense stimulating agents. Amer. Soc. Clin. Oncol. Abstr. 80 (1973).
211. IVERSEN, O.H.: Some theoretical considerations on chalones and the treatment of cancer: a review. Cancer Res. 30, 1481 (1970).
212. BULLOUGH, W.S., LAURENCE, E.B.: The lymphocytic chalone and its antimitotic action on a mouse lymphoma in vitro. Europ. J. Cancer 6, 525 (1970).
213. MATHE: G.: Lymphocyte inhibitors fulfilling the definition of chalones and immunosuppression. Rev. europ. Etudes clin. et biol. 17, 548 (1972).
214. ROSSO, R., DONELLI, M.G., FRANCHI, G., GARATTINI, S.: Effect of Triton WR 1339 on cancer dissemination and metastases. Europ. J. Cancer 5, 77 (1969).
215. FRANCHI, G., MORASCA, L., REYERS-DEGLI-INNOCENTI, I., GARATTINI, S.: Triton WR 1339 (TWR), an inhibitor of cancer dissemination and metastases. Europ. J. Cancer 7, 533 (1971).
216. FRANCHI, G., REYERS DEGLI INNOCENTI, I., STANDEN, S., GARATTINI, S.: Triton WR 1339: effect on the reticulo-endothelial system (RES) activity in tumor-bearing mice. Europ. J. Cancer 9, 487 (1973).
217. BRANDES, D., ANTON, E., SCHOFIED, B., BARNARD, S.: Role of lysosomal labilizers in treatment of mammary gland carcinomas with cyclophosphamide (NSC-26271). Preliminary Chemother. Rep. 50, 47 (1966).
218. COHEN, M.H., CARBONE, P.P.: Enhancement of antitumor effect of alkylating agents by vitamin A. Proc. amer. Ass. Cancer Res. 10, 14 (1969).
219. MATHE, G.: Active immunotherapy. Advanc. Cancer Res. 14, 1 (1971).
220. CHABNER, B.A., MYERS, C.E., COLEMAN, N., JOHS, D.G.: Clinical pharmacology of antineoplastic agents. New Engl. J. Med. 292, 1107 and 1159 (1975).
221. FREI, E.III., JAFFE, N., TATTERSALL, M.H.N., PITMAN, S., PARKER, L.: New approaches to cancer chemotherapy with methotrexate. New Engl. J. Med. 292, 846 (1975).
222. KRAKOFF, I.H., ETCUBANAS, E., TAN, C., MAYER, K., BETHUNE, V., BURCHENAL, J.H.: Clinical trial of 5-hydroxypicolinaldehyde thiosemicarbazone (5-HP; NSC-107392), with special reference to its iron-chelating properties. Cancer Chemother. Rep. Part 1, Vol. 58, 207 (1974).
223. WASSERMAN, T.H., SLAVIK, M., CARTER, S.K.: Review of CCNU in clinical cancer therapy. Cancer Treat. Rev. 1, 131 (1974).
224. WASSERMAN, T.H., SLAVIK, M., CARTER, S.K.: Methyl-CCNU in clinical cancer therapy. Cancer Chemother. Rep. 1, 251 (1974).

225. SCHEIN, P.S., O'CONNELL, M.J., BLOM, J., HUBBARD, I.T. et al.: Clinical antitumor activity and toxicity of streptozotocin (NSC-85998). Cancer 34, 993 (1974).
226. SHNIDER, B.I., COLSKY, J., JONES, R., CARBONE, P.P.: Effectiveness of methyl-GAG (NSC-32946) administered intramuscularly. Cancer Chemother. Rep. Part 1, Vol. 58, 689 (1975).
227. GERSHWIN, M.E., GOETZI, E.J., STEINBERG, A.D.: Cyclophosphamide: use in practice. Ann. intern. Med. 80, 531 (1974).
228. HIRANO, M., MIURA, M., KAKIZAWA, H., et al.: Effect of two new sulfonic acid esters of aminoglycols on chronic myelogenous leukemia. Cancer Chemother. Rep. 56, 47 (1972).
229. ALTMAN, S.J., FLETCHER, W.S., ANDREWS, N.C., WILSON, W.L., PISCHER, T.: Yoshi 864 (NSC 102627) 1-propanol,3,3'-iminodi-dimethanesulfonate (ester) hydrochloride: a phase I study. Cancer 35, 1145 (1975).
230. ANDREWAS, N.C., WEISS, A.J., WILSON, T.: Phase II study of dibromodulcitol (NSC-104800). Cancer Chemother. Rep. Part 1, Vol. 58, 653 (1974).
231. HIGBY, D.J., WALLACE, H.J., ALBERT, D.J., HOLLAND, J.F.: Diamminodichloroplatinum: a phase I study showing responses in testicular and other tumors. Cancer 33, 1219 (1974).
232. CAUSE, G.F., BRASIINIKOVA, M.G., SHORIN, V.A.: A new antitumor antibiotic, carminomycin (NSC-180024). Cancer Chemother. Rep. Part 1, Vol. 58, 255 (1974).
233. SCHAEPPI, U., MENNINGER, F., FLEISCHMAN, R.W., BOGDEN, A.E., SCHEIN, P.S., COONEY, D.A.: Toxicity of neocarzinostatin (NSC-69856): an antitumor antibiotic with radiomimetic and antigenic characteristics. Cancer Chemother. Rep. Part 3, Vol. 5, 43 (1974).
234. MATHE, G., SCHWARZENBERG, L., POUILLART, P., OLDHAM, R., WEINER, R., et al.: Two epipodophyllotoxin derivatives VM 26 and VP 16213, in the treatment of leukemias hematosarcomas and lymphomas. Cancer 34, 985 (1974).
235. CHABNER, B.A., SLAVIK, M., editors: High-dose methotrexate therapy meeting, Bethesda, Maryland, December 19, 1974. Cancer Chemother. Rep. Part 3, Vol. 6, 1-82 (1975).
236. Proceedings of the Fifth New Drug Seminar on Adriamycin (Washington D.C., Dec. 16-17, 1974) and the Adriamycin New Drug Seminar (San Francisco, Jan. 15-16, 1975). Cancer Chemother. Rep. Part 3, 6, 83-397 (1975).

Chapter 4
Hormonal Agents Used in the Treatment of Cancer

The growth and function of many tissues are influenced by hormones.
Some of them, such as growth hormone, insulin, and thyroid hormone, act
on a great variety of tissues including some malignant ones but their
use in cancerology is limited. Insulin has a direct stimulating effect
on dimethylbenzanthracene-induced mammary carcinoma in rats (1); the
same tumor is also influenced by growth hormone and prolactin (2). Other
hormones, especially steroids, have a more restricted spectrum of target organs. They have been used for over 30 years in the palliation
of so-called "hormone-dependent" tumors. Cancers originating in organs
that are normally sensitive to either the maturing or the suppressant
action of hormones may maintain this sensitivity to a greater or lesser
extent (3). This explains the regression that can occur in breast cancer
in premenopausal women following oophorectomy or in prostate carcinomas
after orchiectomy. Similarly, androgens can have a beneficial effect
in carcinoma of the breast, and estrogens in prostate cancer.

By the same token, the administration of hormones, which under normal
physiologic conditions stimulate growth of certain organs, can result
in malignant transformation of these organs. This phenomenon has been
well documented in experimental animals (4); in humans the evidence
is more circumstantial. However, conditions associated with estrogen
overproduction tend to be more frequently associated with endometrial
carcinoma, and the sequence of events seems to be transition from hyperplasia to dysplasia, terminating in neoplasia. Tumors induced by hormone stimulation, at least in animals, are often hormone-dependent and
their growth ceases when the hormone is withdrawn. The effect of hormone
administration on a tumor is not necessarily direct; it may be the result of a secondary alteration in a complex interhormonal balance (Fig.
4-1). Therapy based on the dependence of malignant tissue on the hormones required for the development of its normal counterpart has the
advantage that it is organ-specific and involves less systemic toxicity
than most cytotoxic agents.

A. STEROID HORMONES

The different steroid hormones (corticosteroids, androgens, estrogens,
and progestins) all seem to interact with their respective target tissues in a similar manner (5-8). The hormone first binds to a specific
receptor protein in the cytoplasm of the target cell to form a relatively stable complex. This complex is then translocated into the nucleus where it is associated with a specific receptor site on the chromosomal DNA characteristic of the target tissue. The hormone-protein
complex induces synthesis of ribosomal and messenger RNA; mRNA determines the synthesis of specific proteins (enzymes) through which the

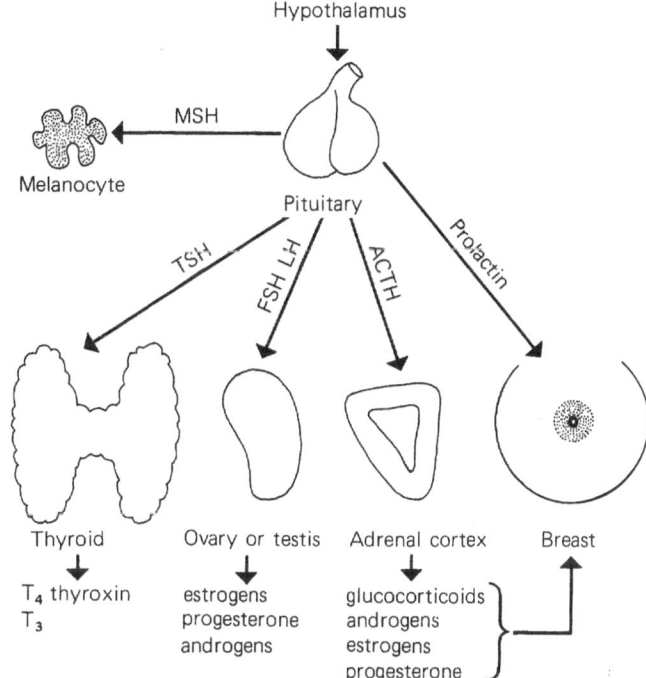

Fig. 4-1. Endocrine glands, hormones, and target organs

hormone exerts its action on the target tissue (9). The responsiveness of human breast carcinomas to estrogens has been correlated with the presence of an estrogen receptor (10).

The physiologic effects of the different classes of steroid hormones are quite variable, although they have a similar mechanism of action at the molecular level and a similar chemical structure.

Steroid hormones are derivatives of cholesterol and contain the cyclo-pentanoperhydrophenanthrene nucleus. (Fig. 4-2 A). The greek letter Δ indicates a double bond; groups that lie above the plane of each of the steroid rings are indicated by the greek letter β and a solid line (─OH), while those that lie below are indicated by α and a dotted line (─OH).

1. Corticosteroids

Corticosteroids are 21-C compounds with a double bond between C4 and C5, a keto group at C3, and an acetyl group at C17. Because they cause pyknosis and lysis of lymphocytes (11) and inhibit lymphocyte mitotic activity, they have been tried in acute and chronic lymphoid leukemia and lymphosarcomas, and as immunosuppressive agents (12). We are constantly reminded of their widespread influence on the intermediary metabolism and most organ systems by the multiplicity of the side-effects that accompany steroid therapy (see Table 4-1) (13). The exact mechanisms by which corticosteroids exert their wide range of influence are not known.

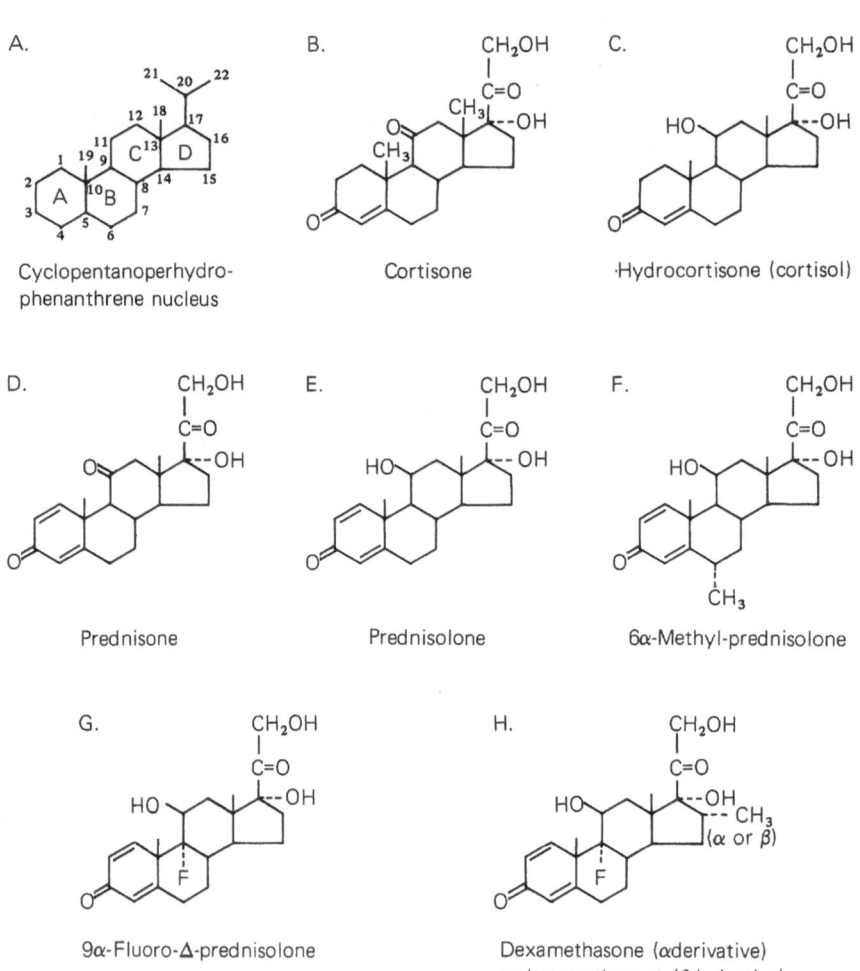

A. Cyclopentanoperhydro-phenanthrene nucleus

B. Cortisone

C. Hydrocortisone (cortisol)

D. Prednisone

E. Prednisolone

F. 6α-Methyl-prednisolone

G. 9α-Fluoro-Δ-prednisolone

H. Dexamethasone (αderivative) or betamethasone (βderivative)

Fig. 4-2. Structural formulas of corticosteroids commonly used in cancer chemotherapy

Corticosteroids are widely used in oncology either for a specific tumor effect or for various pharmacological effects useful in the palliation of complications. Antitumor effects are noted in leukemias, especially acute and chronic lymphoid leukemia, and lymphomas; they are seen less often in multiple myeloma and in selected cases of advanced breast and prostate carcinoma. The symptomatic use of steroids (often associated with other treatment modalities) has been reviewed in STOLL's textbook (3). Pressure symptoms of intracranial hypertension, spinal-cord compression, or superior vena cava obstruction may be relieved. The hypercalcemia associated with osteolytic metastases often responds promptly. Auto-immune hemolytic anemia also responds to steroid therapy, but thrombocytopenia rarely does. Nothing besides steroid therapy can be offered to a patient with radiation pneumonitis or myelitis. Painful liver metastases, obstructive and hepatocellular jaundice, and dyspnea caused by lymphangitic carcinomatosis may be alleviated. An improved appetite and a sense of wellbeing is often welcome in advanced cancer patients. However, the benefits of steroid therapy must always be weighed against its hazards. These include not only the well-known side-effects but also the possibility of tumor enhancement through its immunosuppressive effect (14) and facilitation of metastatic spread (15, 16).

Numerous steroid preparations are commercially available, but only those commonly used in the treatment of cancer are discussed here.

Cortisone and hydrocortisone (or cortisol, probably the physiologic glucocorticoid) are rarely used except in adrenal insufficiency or for replacement following adrenalectomy, because of their potent mineralocorticoid activity (see Fig. 4-2). Many modifications of these two older preparations have been made in attempts to decrease side-effects in proportion to therapeutic effect. Their sodium-retaining and potassium-losing effects have thus been reduced, but there is no convincing evidence of any significant qualitative difference in the so-called "anti-inflammatory" action of any of the commercially available corticosteroid preparations. There are, of course, significant differences in their potency and in the rate at which the body appears to metabolize different compounds.

Prednisone and prednisolone (Fig. 4-2), Δ-derivatives of cortisone and hydrocorticone, seem to be metabolized more slowly by the liver because of the additional double bond between C1 and C2, and a therapeutic effect can thus be obtained with a lower dose. 6α-methylprednisolone (Fig. 4-2) is about 15 to 25 percent more potent than prednisone. The introduction of a halogen in position 9α (9α-fluoro-hydrocortisone = fludrocortisone, and 9α-fluoro-Δ-prednisolone) (Fig. 4-2) increases the anti-inflammatory potency but also enhances the sodium-retaining effect. Fludrocortisone is used almost entirely in adrenal replacement therapy to supplement hydrocortisone and to insure adequate sodium retention.

Other synthetic steroids, such as triamcinolone (16α-hydroxy-9α-fluoro-prednisolone), dexamethasone (9α-fluoro-19α-methyl-hydrocortisone), betamethasone (9α-fluoro-16α-methyl-hydrocortisone), and paramethasone (6α-fluoro-16α-methyl-hydrocortisone), though more potent, offer no significant advantages over the more economical prednisone. Dexamethasone (Fig. 4-2) is customarily used in the treatment of intracranial hypertension (see p. 212).

Corticotropin or ACTH, which stimulates the adrenal cortex to release its own natural steroids, is no longer used in cancer chemotherapy.

In the treatment of malignant disease, steroids are often given initially in a fairly high dosage (40-100 mg prednisone) until the desired clinical response is achieved, whereupon the dosage is tapered to the minimal maintenance level or withdrawn altogether.

2. Androgens

Androgens stimulate the growth of several normal tissues (virilizing effect: development of secondary male sex characteristics, body hair, sebaceous glands, larynx, and increased erythropoiesis) and of certain malignant tissues (some cancers of the prostate and of the breast). On the other hand they also inhibit the development of certain normal tissues (breast, uterus, vaginal mucosa) and some malignancies.

Tumor responses are found in selected advanced cases of cancer of the breast (10-20%), prostate, and kidney. In addition, androgens are used to stimulate erythropoiesis (17) in myeloid metaplasia (18), chronic leukemia (19), and multiple myeloma, to improve hematopoietic tolerance to cytotoxic chemotherapy (20), and for their general anabolic effect in advanced cancers. There is no evidence that anabolic steroids can prevent the osteoporosis induced by corticosteroids.

While these beneficial effects are not commonly obtained, the side-effects almost always are (see Table 4-1). Virilization and increased
libido in women is especially distressing. The search continues for
androgenic compounds that maintain the antitumor or anabolic effects
without the virilizing properties.

Testosterone (Fig. 4-3) is a 19-C compound with a double bond between
C4 and C5, a keto group at C3, and hydroxyl group at C17. Several esters
have been prepared for i.m. injection, from which the drug is more
slowly absorbed (Fig. 4-3). Testosterone propionate is relatively short-
acting, while testosterone enanthate has a longer duration of action.
They are usually given 2 or 3 times per week. Methylation of testosterone at C17 decreases its inactivation in the liver, allowing oral administration. Methyltestosterone and halogenated derivative, 9α-fluoro-
11-hydroxy-17α-methyltestosterone, or fluoxymesterone, can thus be given orally (Fig. 4-3). They are short-acting and less potent than parenteral preparations. Oxymetholone (2-hydroxymethylene-17α-methyl-
17β-hydroxy-3-androstanone) is often used in aplastic anemia (21).

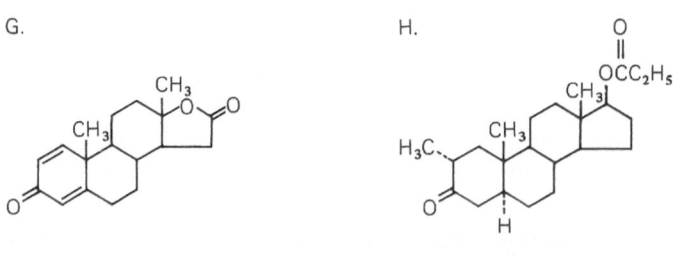

Fig. 4-3. Structural formulas of androgens commonly used in cancer chemotherapy

88

Liver functions must be watched since androgenic and anabolic steroids with alkyl groups substituted in the α position on C17 can produce liver dysfunction. A new oral preparation, 7β, 17α-dimethyltestosterone, or calusterone, was recently introduced for tumor treatment with a claim of potent antitumor efficacy with insignificant androgenicity (Fig. 4-3) (22). Unfortunately, initial response rates of over 50 percent were not confirmed in a study by the Cooperative Breast Cancer Group (23); however, the response rate of 28 percent (compared to 18 percent for testolactone) justifies further evaluation of this drug, especially in comparison with other oral preparations. Similar claims have been made for Δ1-testolactone and dromostanolone propionate or 2α-methyl-dihydrotestosterone propionate (Fig. 4-3) (24-26). While they are less virilizing, their response rates are no better than those of testosterone propionate.

In cancer therapy androgens are administered in much larger than physiologic doses and their effects may not be apparent for 6 to 12 weeks. Therapy is best started with a parenteral preparation, preferably a fast-acting one, so that its use can promptly be terminated if patients deteriorate or develop hypercalcemia shortly after initiation of androgen therapy. If the hormone is well tolerated, a switch can be made to the longer-acting parenteral esters. The older oral preparations (methyltestosterone, fluoxymesterone) may not be potent enough to induce a remission but can be used to maintain a remission induced by a parenteral agent. Calusterone will probably be more effective in the induction of remissions; studies are in progress (23).

Once androgen therapy has been started patients must be watched closely for tumor progression, hypercalcemia, and fluid retention. Liver function should be monitored with 17α-alkyl-substituted preparations. Androgen therapy can be continued once a remission is obtained as long as tumor regression persists. Occasionally a withdrawal response may be observed when the hormone is discontinued. Alternatively, androgens can be stopped once tumor regression is complete in observable lesions, to be reinstituted only when tumor progression is again noted. No data are available on the relative effectiveness of these two modes of administration.

3. Estrogens

Estrogens promote the growth and development of certain normal tissues (female reproductive organs and breasts) and some malignancies (breast cancer in premenopausal women) while they inhibit normal tissues (secondary male sex organs) and certain cancers. They are most useful for the treatment of advanced prostate cancers and of breast cancer in postmenopausal women (3).

The most potent natural estrogen, estradiol-17β, (Fig. 4-4) is an 18-C compound with a hydroxyl group at C3 and three double bonds in the A ring. It is inactivated in the liver, therefore it is ineffective when administered orally. Several esters of estradiol are marketed for i.m. injection (estradiol benzoate, cypionate, diprionate, and valerate). They have a duration of action ranging from 3 to 4 days to 3 to 4 weeks. Ethinyl estradiol (Fig. 4-4) is one of the most potent estrogens and is effective orally, since an alkyl group at C17 protects it from inactivation by the liver. By far the most popular estrogens for clinical use is the nonsteroid synthetic diethylstilbestrol (Fig. 4-4), which is potent, effective orally, and inexpensive. Other nonsteroid estrogens, such as benzestrol, dienestrol, and hexestrol offer no advantage over diethylstilbestrol and are more expensive. Chlorotrianisene (Fig. 4-4) has a long-acting effect claimed to be due to a higher level of storage in adipose tissue. It is presumed to be altered in the body

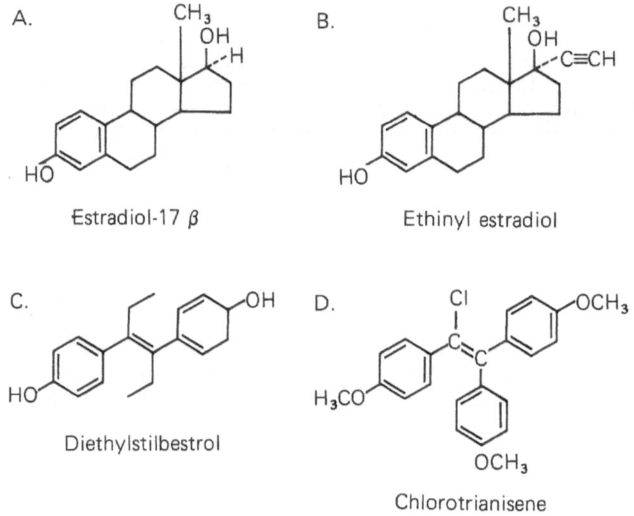

A.

CH₃

Estradiol-17 β

B.

CH₃

Ethinyl estradiol

C.

Diethylstilbestrol

D.

Chlorotrianisene

Fig. 4-4. Structural formulas of estrogens commonly used in cancer chemotherapy

before becoming effective and has been used most frequently for palliation of prostate cancer.

As a rule, there is no need to use parenteral estrogen preparations; diethylstilbestrol is the drug of choice. Estrogens, like androgens, can be used either continuously or intermittently (see p. 89). Anorexia, nausea, and vomiting are common early side-effects but can often be avoided by a gradual build-up from 5 mg to the full dose of 15 mg. Patients who cannot tolerate diethylstilbestrol may do better with ethinyl estradiol. Early in the course of treatment the patient must be closely observed for progression of disease, hypercalcemia, and fluid retention. Feminization in males and stress incontinence in females are unpleasant later manifestations. Patients should be warned about the possibility of uterine bleeding.

4. Progestational Agents

Progesterone is normally required for the maturation and secretion of the endometrium. This hormone was therefore tried in advanced endometrial carcinoma, with approximately one third of patients showing some responses (27). Selected breast cancer patients may also experience a beneficial effect but the use of progestins in renal carcinoma and malignant melanoma is still experimental.

Progesterone (Fig. 4-5), a 21-C steroid with an acetyl side chain at C17, methyl groups at C10 and C13, a keto group at C3, and a double bond between C4 and C5, is not used as such in oncology. Synthetic derivatives, referred to as progestins, are marketed that have a longer duration of action or an effect following oral administration. However, they do not mimic the physiological and pharmacological effects of progesterone. There are significant qualitative differences in their estrogenic, androgenic, anabolic, and antiestrogenic properties, which alter their side-effects and possibly their antitumor effect.

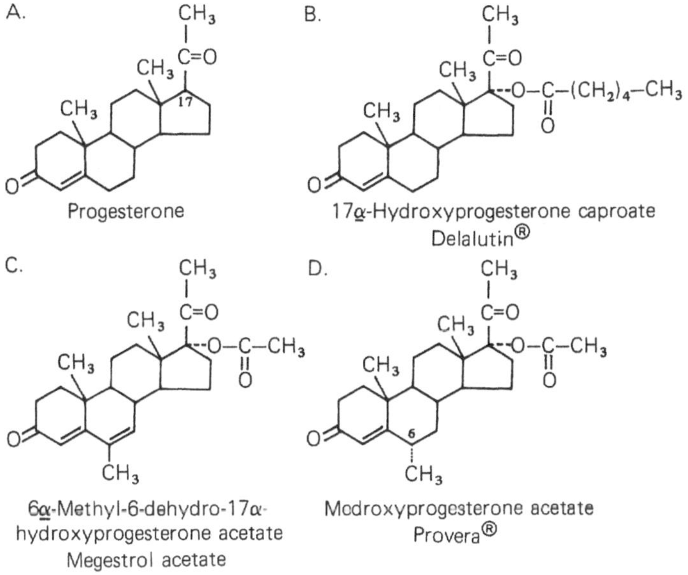

A. Progesterone

B. 17α-Hydroxyprogesterone caproate
Delalutin®

C. 6α-Methyl-6-dehydro-17α-
hydroxyprogesterone acetate
Megestrol acetate

D. Medroxyprogesterone acetate
Provera®

Fig. 4-5. *Structural formulas of progestational agents commonly used in cancer chemotherapy*

Progestins can be classified in 3 chemical groups. The derivatives of 17α-hydroxyprogesterone are most commonly used, especially 17α-hydroxyprogesterone caproate (Delalutin), an esterified derivative in oil solution for i.m. injection, and 17α-hydroxy-6α-methylprogesterone acetate and medroxyprogesterone acetate for i.m. and oral administration (Fig. 4-5). A new preparation, 6α-methyl-6-dehydro-17α-hydroxyprogesterone acetate (megestrol acetate) (Fig. 4-5), differs from medroxyprogesterone by the presence of a double bond between C6 and C7 and the position of the methyl group at C6. It is not inactivated by the liver and can be administered orally. Other synthetic progestins, derived either from testosterone or 19-nortestosterone, are used in contraceptive preparations. Progesterone therapy is relatively free from side-effects.

B. THYROID HORMONES

For completeness, we mention the use of thyroid hormones in certain thyroid cancers. Some of these regress when the output of the thyroid-stimulating hormone (TSH) of the pituitary is suppressed by thyroid administration. The active principles of the thyroid gland appear to be the iodine-containing amino acids, thyroxin (T_4) and triiodothyronine (T_3). L-triiodothyronine (sodium liothyronine, Cytomel) acts rapidly and can be taken orally (Fig. 4-6).

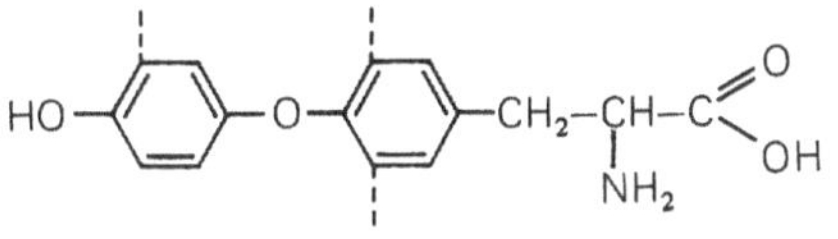

Fig. 4-6. *L-triiodothyronine*

C. OTHER SUBSTANCES WITH HORMONAL ACTIVITY

Several compounds that interfere with the production or the activity
of certain hormones have been under clinical and/or preclinical investigation. Mitotane (bis (chloro-4'-phenyl-chloro-1'-phenyl)-2,2'-dichloro-
1,1-ethane, or o,p'DDD) (Fig. 4-7) produces selective atrophy of the
zona fasciculata and zona reticularis of the adrenal cortex and interferes with the production of cortisol by several mechanisms (28, 29).
In the dog, o,p'-DDD inhibits adrenal G6PD, the enzyme responsible for
the regeneration of NADPH, an essential cofactor in hydroxylation reactions for steroid synthesis, such as the conversion of cholesterol
to Δ5-pregnenalone. This drug also alters the extraadrenal metabolism
of cortisol and inhibits growth of adrenal cortical carcinomas by a
poorly understood mechanism of action. Aminoglutethimide (Elipten)
(Fig. 4-8) also causes distinctive histologic changes in the adrenal
gland, inhibits the enzymatic conversion of cholesterol to Δ5-pregne-
nalone (hence steroid synthesis) and alters the extraadrenal metabolism
of cholesterol, not only in animals but also in patients with adrenal
cortical carcinomas.

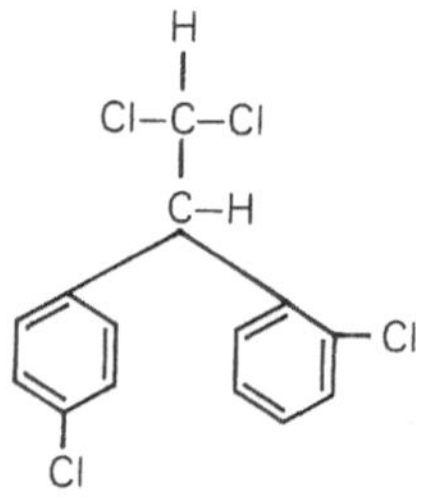

Fig. 4-7. Mitotane (o,p'DDD)

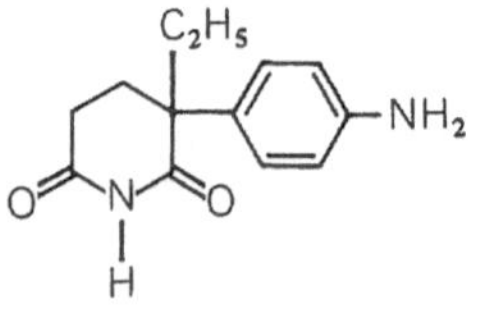

Fig. 4-8. Aminoglutethimide, Elipten

Antiestrogens such as nafoxidine (Fig. 4-9), transclomiphene, and tamoxifen (Fig. 4-10) exert their action by competing effectively with estradiol for its specific cytoplasmic receptor in the target tissue (30-32).
The same mechanism of action has been proposed for some of the compounds
discussed earlier, for example dromostanolone. The effectiveness of nafoxidine was confirmed by the EORTC BREAST CANCER GROUP (32).

The observation that prolactin plays a major part in the induction and
growth of mammary tumors led to the use of prolactin inhibitors; 1-
(morpholino-methyl)-4-phthalimido-piperidine dione-2,6, or CG 603, 2-
bromo-α-ergocryptine, and levodopa are therefore under study (33, 34).

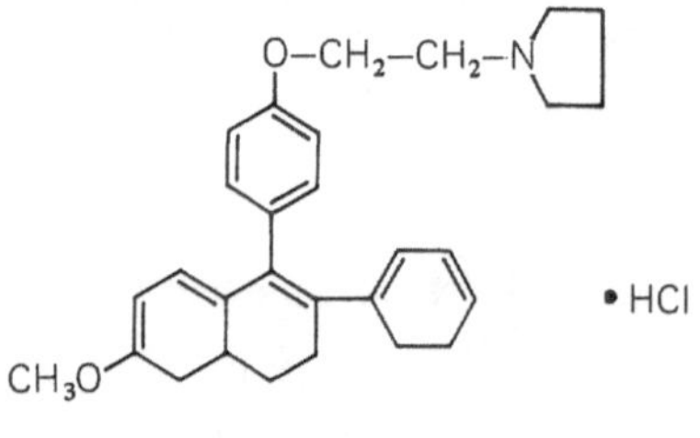

Fig. 4-9. Nafoxidine

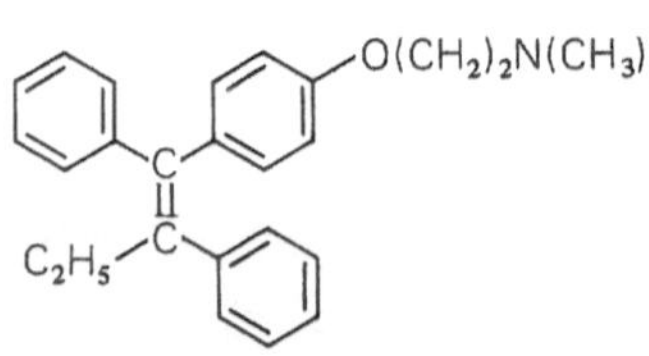

Fig. 4-10. Tamoxifen

Table 4-1. Prinicipal antitumor hormones

Compound	Preparations	Chemical characteristics	Dosage	Side-Effects	Indications
		1. CORTICOSTEROIDS			
Prednisone Meticorten® Deltasone®	1- and 5-mg tabs 2.5-, 5.0- and 50-mg tabs	Synthetic glucocorticoid, Δ_1-derivative of cortisone (double bond C_{1-2})	40-100 mg/m², daily initially. Taper dosage as desired effect is obtained and discontinue if possible; if not determine lowest dose to maintain the desired effect (possibly alternate day maintenance)	Fluid and electrolyte disturbances; Na and fluid retention CHF in susceptible patients K loss, hypokalemic alkalosis hypertension	Acute lymphoid leukemia Chronic lymphoid leukemia Hodgkin's disease Non-Hodgkin lymphomas Histiocytosis X Myeloma Macroglobulinemia Breast cancer Prostate cancer Intracranial hypertension Spinal cord compression Superior vena cava syndrome Hypercalcemia Autoimmune hemolytic anemia, thrombocytopenia Dyspnea due to pulmonary lymphangitic carcinomatosis
Prednisolone Delta-Cortef®	5-mg tabs	Synthetic glucocorticoid; Δ_1-derivative of hydrocortisone (double bond C_{1-2})		Gastrointestinal: Peptic ulcer GI bleeding	
9α-Fluoro-Δ-prednisolone Fluprednisolone Alphadrol®	0.75-and 1.5-mg tabs	Synthetic glucocorticoid; differs from prednisolone by presence of fluor at C_9		Endocrine-metabolic: negative N2 balance due to protein catabolism decreased CHO tolerance development of Cushingoid state secondary adrenocorticalpituitary unresponsiveness, especially in stress situations	
9α-Fluoro-16α-hydroxy-prednisolone Dexamethasone Decadron®	0.25-, 0.5-, 0.75-, and 1.5-mg tabs	9α-fluoro, 16-methyl-substituted steroid with a C_{1-2} double bond; enhanced glucocorticoid activity, reduced mineralocorticoid effect; used primarily for anti-inflammatory effect	For intracranial hypertension: 10 mg dexamethasone sodium phosphate injection initially, followed by 4 mg every 6 h, i.m. or p.o. Taper dosage and discontinue if possible. Some patients require	Musculoskeletal: myopathy: muscle weakness, atrophy Osteoporosis, compression fractures of vertebrae	

Table 4-1. (continued)

Compound	Preparations	Chemical characteristics	Dosage	Side-Effects	Indications
			low-dose maintenance: 2 mg b.i.d. or t.i.d.	aseptic necrosis of femoral and humoral heads	
9α-Fluorocortisol Fludrocortisone Florinef®	0.1-mg tabs	Halogenated derivative of hydrocortisone; possesses greatly enhanced mineralocorticoid activity; used primarily for replacement therapy in chronic adrenocortical insufficiency	For replacement therapy in chronic adrenal cortical insufficiency: 0.05 to 0.1 mg daily	Skin: thin, fragile skin, atrophy, petechiae, ecchymoses nodular panniculitis impaired wound healing	
				Ophthalmic: posterior subcapsular cataracts exophthalmus increased intraocular pressure	
				CNS effects: irritability, nervousness, excessive motor activity insomnia euphoria, depression, organic psychosis pseudotumor cerebri	
				Immunosuppression: increased susceptibility to infections	

2. ANDROGENS

Compound	Preparations	Chemical characteristics	Dosage	Side-Effects	Indications
Testosterone propionate		Short-acting testosterone salt; useful for initial	100 mg, i.m., 3 times per week	Fluid retention Masculinization:	Breast cancer Renal carcinoma

Table 4-1 (continued)

Compound	Preparations	Chemical characteristics	Dosage	Side-Effects	Indications
Oreton propionate®	100 mg/ml, 10 ml vials	parenteral therapy; not practical for long-term therapy		oily skin, acne, hirsutism hoarseness clitoral hypertrophy increased libido changes in psyche	Anemia associated with lymphomas, chronic lymphoid leukemia, myeloma myelofibrosis
				Nausea, vomiting	To improve tolerance to cytotoxic chemotherapy
Testosterone enanthate Delatestryl®	200 mg/ml 1- and 5-ml vials	Long-acting potent ester that produces a steady response; useful for long-term maintenance therapy	500-1200 mg, i.m. weekly	Cholestatic icterus: androgenic and anabolic steroids with alkyl groups substituted in the α position on C17	therapy General anabolic effect
c Testosterone cypionate Depot-testosterone cypionate®	50 mg/ml; 10 ml vials 100 and 200 mg/ml in 1- and 10 ml vials	Same as testosterone enanthate		Risk of aggravation of certain breast cancers	
Methyltestosterone Metandren® Oreton Methyl®	10- and 25-mg tabs 5- and 10- mg linguets 10- and 25-mg tabs 10 mg	Methylation of testosterone in C17; short-acting preparation for oral or buccal administration; less potent than long-acting esters of testosterone; not potent enough to be used initially but may be used for maintenance, once a remission has been induced	150-200 mg p.o., daily	Precipitation of hypercalcemia in breast cancer	
Fluoxymesterone Halotestin®	linguets 2-,5-, and 10 mg tabs	Halogenated derivative of methyl testosterone; short-acting, for oral administration; less potent	20-40 mg, p.o., daily		

Table 4-1 (continued)

Compound	Preparations	Chemical characteristics	Dosage	Side Effects	Indications
Ora-testryl® Ultandren®	5 mg tabs 5 mg tabs	than long-acting esters of testosterone			
7β, 17α-dimethyl-testosterone Caluste-rone Methosarb®	50 mg tabs	Minimized virilization	200-250 mg p.o., daily		
Δ1-Testo-lactone Teslac ®	100 mg/ml; and 5-mg vials; 50 mg tabs	Modified testosterone derivative containing a lactone group. Although chemically related to testosterone propionate, it is devoid of androgenic activity, yet capable of inducing tumor regressions	100 mg, i.m., 3 times per week 150-1000 mg, p.o., daily		
2α-methyl-dihydrotesto-sterone propionate Dromosta-nolone propionate Drolban®	50 mg/ml; 10-mg vials	Synthetic derivative of testosterone with decreased androgenic effect	100 mg, i.m., 3 times per week		

Table 4-1. (continued)

Compound	Preparations	Chemical characteristics	Dosage	Side Effects	Indications
		3. ESTROGENS			
Diethylstilbestrol DES Diethylstilbestrol ®	0.1-, 0.25-, 0.5-, 1.0-, 5-, and 25-mg tabs	Nonsteroidal estrogen	Breast cancer: 15 mg, p.o., daily (to avoid N + V: start with 5 mg daily and increase gradually, or give entire dose at bedtime with antiemetic) Prostate cancer: 1 mg, p.o., daily	Nausea, vomiting Stress incontinence Fluid and Na retention Feminization: gynecomastia, nipple and areolar pigmentation, testicular atrophy, impotence, altered hair distribution Uterine bleeding Aggravation of certain breast cancers Increased incidence of cardiovascular complications (dose-related)	Breast cancer (in postmenopausal women) Prostate cancer
Ethinyl estradiol Estinyl ®	0.5-mg tabs	Steroid related to estradiol (the principal ovarian estrogen)	Breast cancer: 3 mg, p.o., daily		
		4. PROGESTINS			
17α-Hydroxyprogesterone caproate Delalutin ®	125 mg/ml; 2- and 10-ml vials; 250 mg/ml, 1- and 5-ml vials	Esterified derivative of progesterone in oil solution for i.m. injection; has no estrogenic activity; seven times more potent than progesterone	1.000-1.500 mg, i.m., 2 or 3 times per week	Relatively free of side-effects Occasionally fluid retention Changes in epithelium of female genital tract and acinar cells of breast	Endometrial carcinoma Renal carcinoma Breast cancer

Table 4-1. (continued)

Compound	Preparations	Chemical characteristics	Dosage	Side Effects	Indications
17α-hydroxy 6α-methyl progesterone acetate Medroxy-progesterone acetate Depot Provera®	50 and 100 mg/ml; 1- and 5-ml vials; 400 mg/ml; 1-, 2.5-, and 10-ml vials	Derivative of progesterone for i.m. and p.o. administration; has no inherent estrogenic activity	500-1.000 mg, i.m., 2 to 5 times per week. (Minimum 3000 mg per week for first 5-6 weeks; maintenance: 400 mg/month)		
Provera®	2.5- and 10-mg tabs		200-400 mg, p.o., daily		
Farlutal® Farlutal-Depot®	100 mg tabs 150 mg (3ml) 500 mg (5ml)				
6α-methyl-6-dehydro-17α-hydroxyprogesterone acetate Megestrol acetate Megace®	20 mg tabs	Differs from medroxyprogesterone by presence of a double bond between C6-7 and by the position of the methyl group in C6; not inactivated by the liver, can be administered orally	40 mg, p.o., daily		

5. ANTIESTROGENS

Compound	Preparations	Chemical characteristics	Dosage	Side Effects	Indications
Tamoxifen Nolvadex			20-40 mg, p.o., daily	nausea, vomiting hot flushes uterine bleeding fluid retention	breast cancer in postmenopausal women

REFERENCES

1. HEUSON, J.C., LEGROS, N., HEIMANN, R.: Influence of insulin administration on growth of the 7,12-dimethylbenz-(a)-anthracene-in-
   duced mammary carcinoma in intact, oophorectomized, and hypophy-
   sectomized rats. Cancer Res. 32, 233 (1972).
2. PEARSON, O.M.: Biological problems regarding hormonal surgery.
   In: Major Endocrine Surgery for the Treatment of Cancer of the
   Breast in Advanced Stages, p. 215 (eds. M. Dargent and Cl. Romieu).
   Lyon: Simep Edition 1967.
3. STOLL, B.A.: Endocrine therapy in malignant disease. London: W.B.
   Saunders 1972.
4. HEUSON, J.C., KENIS, Y., TAGNON, H.J.: Hormonothérapie du cancer
   mammaire. Base expérimentale, plan de traitement et perspective
   thérapeutique. Rev. méd. Bruxelles 25, 607 (1969).
5. WILSON, J.D., GLOYNA, R.E.: The intranuclear metabolism of testosterone in the accessory organs of reproduction. Recent Progr. Hormone Res. 26, 309 (1970).
6. BAULIEU, E.E., ALBERBA, A., JUNG, I., LEBEAU, M.C., MERCIER-BODARD,
   C., MILGROM, E., RAYNAUD, J.P., RAYNAUD-JAMMET, C., ROCHEFORT, H.,
   TRUONG, H., ROBEL, P.: Metabolism and protein binding of sex steroids in target organs: an approach to the mechanism of hormone
   action. Recent Progr. Hormone Res. 27, 351 (1971).
7. GORAL, J.E., WITTLIFF, J.L.: Binding characteristics of glucocorticoid receptors in normal and neoplastic mammary gland of the rat.
   Proc. amer. Ass. Cancer Res. 15, 50 (1974).
8. RICHARDSON, G.S.: Current concepts. Endometrial cancer as an estro-
   gen-progesterone target. New Engl. J. Med. 286, 645 (1972).
9. WILSON, J.D.: Recent studies on the mechanism of action of testosterone. New Engl. J. Med. 287, 1284 (1972).
10. JENSEN, E.V., BLOCK, G.E., SMITH, S., KYSER, K., DeSOMBRE, E.R.:
    Estrogen receptors and breast cancer response to adrenalectomy.
    In: Prediction of Response in Cancer Therapy, National Cancer In-
    stitute, Monograph 34, p. 55. (ed. T.C. Hall). Washington: U.S.
    Government Printing Office 1971.
11. DOUGHERTY, T.F., WHITE, A.: Effect of pituitary adrenotropic hormone
    on lymphoid tissue. Proc. Soc. Exper. Biol. Med. 53, 132 (1943).
12. PEARSON, O.H., ELIEL, L.P., RAWSON, R.W., DOBRINER, K., RHOADS,
    C.P.: ACTH- and cortisone-induced regression of lymphoid tumors
    in man. A preliminary report. Cancer 2, 943 (1949).
13. THORN, G.W., Clinical considerations in the use of corticosteroids.
    New Engl. J. Med. 274, 775 (1966).
14. MATHE, G.: The immunological approach to the treatment of cancer.
    Ann. Roy. Coll. Surg. Engl. 41, 93 (1967).
15. HARTMAN, W.H., SHERLOCK, P.: Gastroduodenal metastases from car-
    cinoma of the breast. An adrenal steroid-induced phenomenon. Cancer,
    14, 426 (1961).
16. SUGARBAKER, E.V., COHEN, A.M., KETCHAM, A.S.: Facilitated metasta-
    tic distribution of the Walker 256 tumor in Sprague-Dawley rats
    with hydrocortisone and/or cyclophosphamide. J. Surg. Oncol. 2,
    277 (1970).
17. SHAHIDI, N.T.: Androgens and erythropoesis. New Engl. J. Med. 289,
    72 (1973).
18. GARDNER, F.H., NATHAN, D.G.: Androgens and erythropoiesis. III.
    Further evaluation of testosterone treatment of myelofibrosis.
    New Engl. J. Med. 274, 420 (1966).
19. KENNEDY, B.J.: Androgenic hormone therapy in lymphatic leukemia.
    J. amer. med. Ass. 190, 1130 (1964).
20. BRODSKY, I., KAHN, B., CONROY, J.F.: The effects of androgens on
    cancer chemotherapy. In: Cancer Chemotherapy II (Eds. I. Brodsky,
    S.B. Kahn, J.H. Moyer). New York: Grune and Stratton 1972.

21. ALLEN, D.M., FINE, M.H., NECHELES, T.F., DAMESHEK, W.: Oxymetholone therapy in aplastic anemia. Blood 32, 83 (1968).
22. GORDAN, G.S., WESSLER, S., AVIOLI, L.V.: Calusterone in the therapy for advanced breast cancer. J. Amer. med. Ass. 219, 483 (1972).
23. GOLDENBERG, I.S., WATERS, N., RAVDIN, R.S., ANSFIELD, F.J., SEGALOFF, A.: Androgenic therapy for advanced breast cancer in women. J. amer. Med. Ass. 223, 1267 (1973).
24. GROUPE EUROPEEN DU CANCER DU SEIN: Le traitement hormonal du cancer du sein en phase avancée. Comparaison des résultats obtenus au moyen de la Δ-1-testololactone et du propionate de testostérone. Rev. franc. Etud. clin. biol. 7, 1067 (1962).
25. THOMAS, A.N., GORDON, G.S., GOLDMAN, L., LOWE, R.: Anti-tumor efficacy of 2α methyl dihydrotestosterone propionate in advanced breast cancer. Cancer 15, 176 (1962).
26. SEAY, D.G., BRADSHAW, J.D., NICOL, N.T.: Clinical experience with dromostanolone propionate (NSC-12198) in breast carcinoma. Cancer Chemother. Rep. 56, 89 (1972).
27, REIFENSTEIN, jr., E.C.: Hydroxyprogesterone caproate therapy in advanced endometrial cancer. Cancer 27, 485 (1971).
28. BRODER, L.E., CARTER, S.K.: Ortho para' DDD (mitotane). In: Proceedings of the Chemotherapy Conference on Ortho Para' DDD. (eds. L.E. Broder, S.K. Carter). Cancer Therapy Evaluation Branch. Bethesda: National Cancer Institute 1970.
29. LUBITZ, J.A., FREEMAN, L., OKUN, R.: Mitotane: use in inoperable adrenal cortical carcinoma. J. amer. Med. Ass. 223, 1109 (1973).
30. COLE, M.P., JONES, C.T.A., TODD, I.D.H.: A new anti-oestrogenic agent in late breast cancer. An early clinical appraisal of ICI 46474. Brit. J. Cancer 25, 270 (1971).
31. TERENIUS, L.: Anti-oestrogens and breast cancer. Europ. J. Cancer 7, 57 (1971).
32. E.O.R.T.C. Breast Cancer Group: Clinical trial of nafoxidine, an oestrogen antagonist in advanced breast cancer. Europ. J. Cancer 8, 387 (1972).
33. HEUSON, J.C., WAELBROECK-VAN GAVER, C., LEGROS, N.: Growth inhibition of rat mammary carcinoma and endocrine changes produced by 2-Br-α-Ergocryptine, a suppressor of lactation and nidation. Europ. J. Cancer 6, 353 (1970).
34. STOLL, B.A.: Brain catecholamines and breast cancer: a hypothesis. Lancet 1, 431 (1972).

Chapter 5

Classification of Chemotherapeutic Agents According to their Effect on the Cell Cycle

A. CLASSIFICATION INTO PHASE- AND CYCLE-DEPENDENT AGENTS

Antitumor agents differ in ways other than their biochemical mechanisms of action as outlined in Chap. 3. They also interfere with cell growth and replication at different phases in the cell cycle. BRUCE introduced a classification of cytotoxic agents on the basis of their effects on proliferating and non-proliferating cells (1-4). This classification was made possible by the development of a method of assay that allowed the differential determination of the effect of cytotoxic drugs on normal hematopoietic stem cells (slowly proliferating) and malignant cell populations (rapidly proliferating). Normal mice and mice bearing a transplanted lymphoma are given a therapeutic agent. Thereafter a cell suspension, made from the femurs of the normal mice, is injected into lethally irradiated mice; a similar suspension from the tumor-bearing mice is injected into non-irradiated mice. Ten days later, the recipient mice are killed and their spleens examined for colonies. The colonies in the irradiated mice are hematopoietic in nature and their number reflects the number of hematopoietic stem cells in the femoral marrow of the donor mice that survived the previous treatment. Spleen colonies in the non-irradiated mice consist of lymphoma cells and their number reflects the surviving portion of the malignant cells.

Two types of dose-response curves are obtained when various cytotoxic drugs are tested with this assay: (a) for drugs that destroy cells exponentially with increasing drug dosages (Fig. 5-1, curve A) and (b) for drugs that destroy only part of the cell population in spite of large doses (curve B). Note that rapidly proliferating cells are more sensitive to both classes of drugs than slowly proliferating ones. The character of these dose-response curves tells us something about the mechanism of action of drugs. Class A agents are called cycle-dependent, because they affect cells as long as they are in proliferative cycle but are without effect on resting cells (G_0) (Table 5-1). Class B agents, called phase-dependent agents, interfere only with cells in a particular phase of the cell cycle: G_1, S, G_2 or M (Fig. 5-2). Cells that are not in the sensitive phase at the time of drug exposure survive at any dose level, which gives the plateau-type curve at higher dosages. BRUCE initially placed nitrogen mustard (together with γ-irradiation) in a third class referred to as cycle-independent (non-specific), because it was thought to destroy tumor cells with equal efficiency regardless of whether they were in proliferative cycle (2). However, as a result of studies by VAN PUTTEN et al. (5-6), VALERIOTE et al. (7), and GOLDENBERG (8) nitrogen mustard is now classified with other alkylating agents among the cycle-dependent drugs.

The mouse spleen-colony assay is not applicable to the human situation. Fortunately, in vitro culture techniques have recently been developed

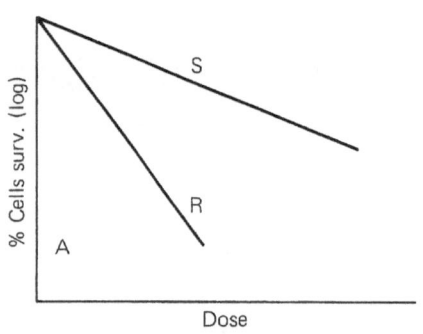
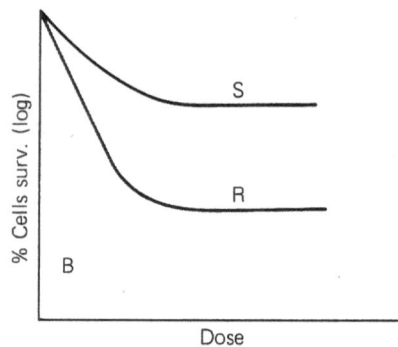

Fig. 5-1. Relationship between cell kill and dosage of cytotoxic agent.
R = rapidly proliferating cells; S = slowly proliferating cells. A.
Drugs that kill cells exponentially with increasing dosage. B. Drugs
that kill exponentially at lower dosages but reach a plateau at higher
doses. Note that for both A and B rapidly proliferating cells are more
sensitive than slowly proliferating ones

Table 5-1. Classification of cytotoxic drugs according to their effect
on the cell cycle[a]

Cycle-dependent	Phase-dependent
5-Fluoro-uracil (2, 6, 16)	Methotrexate (2, 4, 30, 34)
Imidazole carboxamide (DIC) (29)	6-Mercaptopurine (34, 35)
TIC-mustard (7)	6-MMPR (34)
BCNU (6, 13, 16, 25, 29, 30)	6-Thioguanine (34)
CCNU (6, 16, 25, 28)	5-FUDR (25, 34)
Me-CCNU	Cytosine arabinoside (4, 24, 25, 34)
Streptozotocin (25)	Hydroxyurea (24, 34, 36)
Nitrogen mustard (5, 6, 8, 16, 29, 30)	Guanazole (34)
Chlorambucil (5, 6, 16, 25, 29)	5-HP (24, 25)
Cyclophosphamide (2, 4, 6, 16, 28, 29, 30)	Procarbazine
Melphalan (5, 6, 16, 25, 29)	Azaserine (2)
TEM (6, 16, 29)	ICRF 159 (37)
Thio-TEPA (25, 29)	Vincristine (4)
Busulfan (6, 16)	Vinblastine (2,4)
Mitomycin C (25, 31, 32)	Poly-IC (30)
Actinomycin D (2, 25, 32)	Tritiated thymidine (1, 2)
Daunorubicin (33)	VM 26
Adriamycin (26, 33)	VP 16-213

[a]These results were obtained by various techniques (in vivo spleen colony, in vitro monolayer cultures, and CFU-cultures) as well as with
different cell types (normal hematopoietic stem cells, rapidly proliferating (regenerating) hematopoietic stem cells, and various types
of tumor cells (in log-phase or stationary-phase growth)).

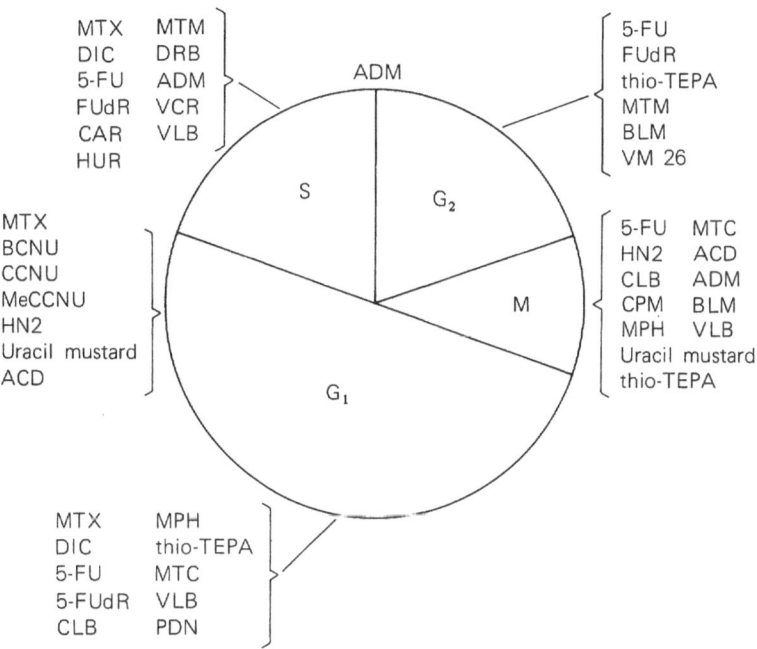

Fig. 5.2. The phases of the cell cycle where the drugs used in cancer chemotherapy exert their cytotoxic effect

ACD	*Actinomycin D*	*EPE*	*Epipodophyllotoxin-ethylidene*
ADM	*Adriamycin*	*5-FU*	*5-Fluorouracil*
ASP	*L-Asparaginase*	*HUR*	*Hydroxyurea*
BCNU	*Bis-chloroethyl nitrosurea*	*6-MP*	*6-Mercaptopurine*
BLM	*Bleomycin*	*MTX*	*Methotrexate*
CAR	*Cytosine arabinoside*	*PCZ*	*Procarbazine*
DRB	*Daunorubicin*	*6-TG*	*6-Thioguanine*
EPT	*Epipodophyllotoxin-thenylidene*	*VCR*	*Vincristine*
		VLB	*Vinblastine*

for normal hematopoietic precursor cells (committed granulocyte precursors, rather than the pluripotential hematopoietic stem cell tested in the spleen-colony assay) and for malignant cells; these techniques permit similar studies to be made on human cells (9-11). In addition, studies with synchronized cells have further delineated the phase of the cell cycle with maximal sensitivity. The results of these studies, listed in Table 5-2, are not always in complete agreement with those given in Table 5-1. The reason is that Table 5-2 cites the most sensitive phase of the cell cycle, but this does not exclude a certain sensitivity in other phases as well. Note that different results may be obtained, for example for adriamycin (Table 5-2), depending on the cell line used in the experiment. Furthermore, the modes of tumor growth (in vitro culture, or in vivo growth of ascites and solid tumors) are also important (12). For example, log-phase (rapidly proliferating) cells in culture in suspension are less sensitive to BCNU than plateau-phase cells, while in vivo solid tumors of small volume (with high growth fraction) are more sensitive than large tumor masses (few proliferating cells). BARRANCO et al. noted that in vitro plateau-phase cells were

Table 5-2. Classification of cytotoxic drugs according to their most
sensitive phase (Studies on synchronized cells)

Agent	Most sensitive phase	Cell line	Reference
5-Fluor- ouracil	All phases	DON	BHUYAN et al. ($\underline{25}$)
FUdR	All phases, except M	CHO	LOZZIO ($\underline{38}$)
	S	DON	BHUYAN et al. ($\underline{25}$)
Cytosine arabinoside	late S, early G_2	DON	KARON and SHIRAKAWA ($\underline{46}$)
	S	DON	BHUYAN et al. ($\underline{25}$)
5-Azacytidine	S	DON	BHUYAN et al. ($\underline{25}$)
Hydroxyurea	S	HELA S_3, Chinese hamster, V79	MAURO and MADOC-JONES ($\underline{27}$)
	S	Murine lymphoma in vivo	MADOC JONES and MAURO ($\underline{36}$)
5 HP	S	DON	BHUYAN et al. ($\underline{25}$)
BCNU	G_1/S and mid-S	CHO	BARRANCO and HUMPHREY ($\underline{39}$)
	G_1/S or early S	DON	BHUYAN et al. ($\underline{25}$)
CCNU	G_1/S or early S	DON	BHUYAN et al. ($\underline{25}$)
Me-CCNU	Late G_1 or G_1/S	DON	BHUYAN and FRASER ($\underline{62}$)
Strepto- zotocin	All phases	DON, L1210	LI, et al. ($\underline{45}$)
L-Aspara- ginase	G_1	Human leukemia	LAMPKIN et al. ($\underline{40}$)
Nitrogen mustard	G_1/S, M	HeLa, V79	MAURO and MADOC-JONES ($\underline{27}$)
Chlorambucil	M, G_1	DON	BHUYAN et al. ($\underline{25}$)
Melphalan	M, G_1	DON	BHUYAN et al. ($\underline{25}$)
Uracil mustard	G_1/S, M	HeLa S_3, Chinese hamster, V79	MAURO and MADOC-JONES ($\underline{27}$)
Thio-TEPA	M, G_1, G_2	DON	BHUYAN et al. ($\underline{25}$)
Mitomycin C	G_1	HeLa	DJORDJEVIC and KIM ($\underline{32}$)
	M, G_1/S	HeLa	MAURO and MADOC-JONES ($\underline{27}$)
Actinomycin D	G_1/S, M	HeLa V79	MAURO and MADOC-JONES ($\underline{27}$)
	G_1/S or early S	DON	BHUYAN et al. ($\underline{25}$)
	Early S	HeLa	DJORDJEVIC and KIM ($\underline{32}$)
Daunorubicin	All phases, max.S	HeLa	KIM and KIM ($\underline{41}$)
	All phases, max.S	Human leukemia	STRYCKMANS et al. ($\underline{47}$)
Adriamycin	Early S and M	CHO	BARRANCO and HUMPHREY ($\underline{43}$)
	S/G_2	Human lymphoma	DREWINKO ($\underline{26}$)
	S	HeLa	KIM and KIM ($\underline{41}$)

Table 5-2. (continued)

Agent	Most sensitive phase	Cell line	Reference
Mithramycin	S and G_2	DON	BHUYAN and FRASER (62)
Bleomycin	M, G_2	CHO	BARRANCO and HUMPHREY (43)
Vincristine	S	HeLa, V79 (in vitro)	MAURO and MADOC-JONES (27)
		mouse lymphoma (in vivo)	MADOC-JONES and MAURO (36)
Vinblastine	Late G_1, S, M	HeLa, V79 (in vitro)	MAURO and MADOC-JONES (27)
	S	Mouse lymphoma (in vivo)	MADOC-JONES and MAURO (36)
Prednisone	G_1	Human leukemia	ERNST and KILLMAN (44)
	G_1	Human leukemia	LAMPKIN and NAGAO (40)

much more sensitive to bleomycin and BCNU than log-phase cells (13). Opposite results were obtained by TWENTYMAN et al., using a different cell line (14, 15). These results, admittedly fragmentary and sometimes contradictory, indicate that, contrary to the classic concept, certain chemotherapeutic agents may exert a preferential cytotoxic effect on resting cells. However, the great majority of cytotoxic agents are more effective against rapidly proliferating cells than against resting cells.

The effect of various cytotoxic agents on the progression of the cell through the cycle has also to be considered. The study of this aspect of cellular interference is only just beginning and few agents have been evaluated as yet (Fig. 5-3; Table 5-3). The phase at which cells are arrested is not necessarily the phase of maximal sensitivity; for example, vincristine arrests cells in metaphase, but S phase is the most sensitive.

B. PRACTICAL APPLICATIONS OF THIS CLASSIFICATION

The characteristics of the chemotherapeutic agents under consideration, that is their cell cycle- or phase-dependent toxicity exerting differential effects on malignant and normal cells, and their interference with cell cycle traverse, should guide the mode of administration of drugs, whether given singly or in combination (16, 18, 63).

1. Phase-dependent agents will exert an increasingly toxic effect, the longer an effective concentration is maintained for the cells in the sensitive phase, as more cells have time to enter that phase (provided the drug does not prevent this entry). Given over a short period, even at a high dose level, phase-dependent drugs are not very toxic. Cells not in the sensitive phase at the time of the brief exposure are not affected and continue their progression through the proliferative cycle. The validity of this concept has been confirmed for normal hematopoietic cells with cytosine arabinoside and methotrexate (19, 20).

2. The toxicity of cycle-dependent drugs for both malignant and normal cells depends on their concentration. It is therefore logical for maximum effect to administer them intermittently at the highest dose

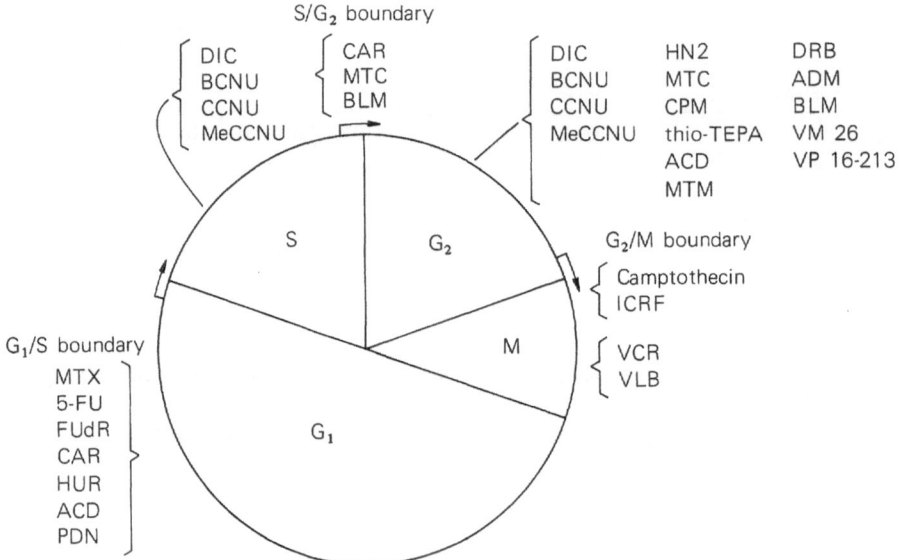

Fig. 5-3. Site of interference with cell cycle traverse (or cell cycle progression) by various chemotherapeutic agents
For abbreviations, see Fig. 5-2

Table 5-3. Influence of cytotoxic drugs on cell cycle Traverse

Agent	Cell cycle traverse	Cell line	Reference
Methotrexate	$G_1 \longrightarrow S$	H.Ep No. 2	WHEELER et al. (34)
Imidazole carboxamide (DIC)	Prolongation of G_2	L1210	SHIRAKAWA and FREI (58)
5-Fluoro-uracil	$G_1 \longrightarrow S$	H.Ep No. 2	WHEELER et al. (34)
5 FUdR	$G_1 \longrightarrow S$	H.Ep No. 2	WHEELER et al. (34)
Cytosine arabinoside	$S \longrightarrow G_2 > G_1 \longrightarrow S$	DON	KARON and SHIRAKAWA (46)
	$G_1 \longrightarrow S$	DON, L1210	BHUYAN et al. (24)
	$G_1 \longrightarrow S$	CHO	TOBEY (48)
	$G_1 \longrightarrow S$	H.Ep No. 2	WHEELER et al. (34)
5-Azacytidine	$G_1 \longrightarrow S$	CHO	TOBEY (48)
Hydroxyurea	$G_1 \longrightarrow S$	DON, L1210	BHUYAN et al. (24)
	$G_1 \longrightarrow S$	CHO	TOBEY (48)
	$G_1 \longrightarrow S$	H.Ep. No. 2	WHEELER et al. (34)
Guanazole	$G_1 \longrightarrow S$	H.Ep. No. 2	WHEELER et al. (34)
5-HP	$G_1 \longrightarrow S$	DON, L1210	BHUYAN et al. (24)
BCNU	Delays progression in all phases of cell cycle	CHO	BARRANCO and HUMPHREY (39)

Table 5-3. (continued)

Agent	Cell cycle traverse	Cell line	Reference
	Prolongation of S and G_2	L1210	SHIRAKAWA and FREI (58)
	Prolongation of S and G_2	L1210	YOUNG and DEVITA (59)
CCNU	Prolongation of S and G_2	L1210	BRAY et al. (55)
Me-CCNU	Prolongation of S	L1210	YOUNG (54)
Nitrogen mustard	G_2 block	Ehrlich	LAYDE and BASERGA (60)
Cyclophospha-amide	G_2 block	Ehrlich	PALME and LISS (61)
ICRF 159	$G_2 \longrightarrow M$	Human leukemia	SHARPE et al. (49)
Actinomycin D	$G_2 \longrightarrow M$	CHO	TOBEY et al. (52)
	$G_1 \longrightarrow S$	Mouse leukemia L5178Y	DOIDA and OKADA (53)
Daunorubicin	$S \longrightarrow M$	CHO	TOBEY (48)
Adriamycin	Delays progression in all phases of cell cycle except M	CHO	BARRANCO et al. (42)
Mithramycin	$S \longrightarrow M$	CHO	TOBEY (48)
Puromycin	$G_1 \longrightarrow S$	Mouse leukemia L5178Y	DOIDA and OKADA (53)
Vincristine	Metaphase block	HeLa	PFEIFFER and TOLMACH (57)
Vinblastine	Metaphase block	L cells	BRUCHOWSKY et al. (56)
Camptothecin	$S \longrightarrow G_2$ or $G_2 \longrightarrow M$	DON	LI et al. (45)
	$S \longrightarrow M$	CHO	TOBEY (48)
Prednisone	$G_1 \longrightarrow S$	Human acute lymphoid leukemia	ERNST and KILLMAN (44)

tolerated. Both experimental (21) and clinical studies (22, 23) have confirmed the effectiveness of this mode of administration.

3. Interference with the cell cycle traverse may reduce the effectiveness of cytotoxic drugs, since a phase-dependent agent is maximally effective only if it allows cycling cells to enter the cytotoxic phase. Cytosine arabinoside, hydroxyurea, and 5-hydroxy-2-formylpyridine thiosemicarbazone (5-HP) markedly inhibit DNA synthesis and are maximally cytotoxic to cells in S phase, but since they inhibit the progression of G_1 cells into S (Fig. 5-3), cells not in S phase are protected from their cytotoxic effects. Their protective effect can be overcome by giving the drug intermittently at intervals that permit the non-S phase cells to enter S during the drug-free period (24).

4. Some drugs give a dose-survival curve that exhibits a shoulder followed by an exponential portion (25, 26). The existence of a shoulder region is important with respect to the dose and the frequency of drug administration. If single doses are administered infrequently, then the

largest possible dose tolerated by the host should be administered to ensure that the dose is not in the region of the shoulder of the survival curve and optimal cell killing is obtained. However, if frequent small doses are administered and the shoulder region represents repair of drug damage, then repeated doses should be given within the interval required to repair the damage so that the damage will be cumulative for the malignant cells.

5. Several recommendations can be made with respect to combination chemotherapy. It would seem unreasonable to give two drugs that inhibit the same phase of the cell cycle simultaneously (25). Such therapy will probably not improve cell kill, though development of resistance may be delayed. For simultaneous administration, drugs that are most effective at different phases of the cell cycle should be selected (27). The effect on cell cycle traverse can be exploited beneficially in combinations, for example cytosine arabinoside and hydroxyurea, which block cells at the G_1-S interphase, can be combined with agents that act in M or G_1, or at the G_1-S interphase. An augmented cell kill can also be obtained by first synchronizing cells (for example vincristine, hydroxyurea, bleomycin) (see p.144), then a second drug is given at the time when the synchronized cell population is in the phase of the cell cycle with the greatest sensitivity to that drug.

6. Tumor cells in G_0 represent a special problem since they are generally not greatly affected by the drugs currently available. Hence they can contribute to the repopulation or regrowth of the tumor. Human solid tumors are largely made up of resting cells by the time a diagnosis is made, and the poor results obtained with chemotherapy in many such tumors are well known to chemotherapists. The sensitivity of such tumors to chemotherapy might improve if we could (a) develop methods to bring resting cells into cycle (recruitment), (b) develop new agents active against resting tumor cells, or (c) block cells in resting phase and prevent them from entering the proliferating pool until they are eliminated by natural cell death.

The problem of cells in G_0 requires further investigation. We mentioned in a preceding paragraph that under certain circumstances resting cells may be more sensitive to cytotoxic agents than rapidly proliferating cells. A decreased capacity for repair of the damage caused by these drugs might be invoked to explain the greater sensitivity of the resting cells. These studies indicate that factors other than cell proliferation rate influence the effectiveness of cytotoxic agents on different cell populations. The variation in intrinsic cellular sensitivity could be based upon differences in cell permeability to the drug, or on differences in repair capacity.

7. It must be appreciated that the normal tissues of the host also contain stem cells in G_0 and that these can be influenced in the same way by procedures attempting to interfere with malignant cells in G_0. The critical normal cells most sensitive to chemotherapeutic agents are those with high mitotic, or potentially mitotic activity. Of special concern are the hematopoietic cell precursors (colony-forming cells), most of which are normally in the resting state. After cytotoxic marrow damage, such cells may be recruited to a proliferative state until marrow repopulation is complete. The problems of damage to hematopoietic cells and other normal tissue, especially lymph-node tissue, are discussed in greater detail in subsequent chapters.

REFERENCES

1. BRUCE, W.R., MEEKER, B.E.: Comparison of the sensitivity of normal hematopoietic and transplanted lymphoma colony-forming cells to tritiated Thymidine. J. Nat. Cancer Inst. 34, 849 (1965)

2. BRUCE, W.R., MEEKER, B.E., VALERIOTE, F.A.: Comparison of the sensitivity of normal hematopoietic and transplanted lymphoma colony-forming cells to chemotherapeutic agents administered in vivo. J. nat. Cancer Inst. 37, 233 (1966).
3. BRUCE, W.R., The action of chemotherapeutic agents at the cellular level and the effects of these agents on hematopoietic and lymphomatous tissue. Canad. Cancer Conf. 7, 53 (1966).
4. BRUCE, W.R., MEEKER, B.E., POWERS, W.E., VALERIOTE, F.A.: Comparison of the dose- and time-survival curves for normal hematopoietic and lymphoma colony-forming cells exposed to vinblastine, vincristine, cytosine arabinosyl, and amethopterin. J. nat. Cancer Inst. 42, 1015 (1969).
5. VAN PUTTEN, L.M., LELIEVELD, P.: Factors determining cell killing by chemotherapeutic agents in vivo. II. Melphalan, chlorambucil and nitrogen mustard. Europ. J. Cancer 7, 11 (1971).
6. VAN PUTTEN, L.M., LELIEVELD, P., KRAM-IDSENGA, L.K.J.: Cell-cycle specificity and therapeutic effectiveness of cytostatic agents. Cancer Chemother. Rep. 56, 691 (1972).
7. VALERIOTE, F.A., TOLEN, S.J.: Survival of hematopoietic and lymphoma colony-forming cells in vivo following the administration of a variety of alkylating agents. Cancer Res. 32, 470 (1972).
8. GOLDENBERG, G.J., LYONS, R.M., LEPP, J.A., VANSTONE, C.L.: Sensitivity to nitrogen mustard as a function of transport activity and proliferation rate in L5178Y lymphoblasts. Cancer Res. 31, 1616 (1971).
9. PLUZNIK, D.H., SACHS, L.: The cloning of normal mast cells in tissue culture. J. Cell. Comp. Physiol. 66, 319 (1965).
10. BRADLEY, T.R., METCALF, D.: The growth of mouse bone marrow cells in vitro Aust. J. Exp. Biol. Med. Sci. 44, 287 (1966).
11. BRADLEY, T.R., ROBINSON, W., METCALF, D.: Colony production in vitro by normal polycythaemic and anaemic bone marrow Nature. 214, 511 (1967).
12. HAGEMANN, R.F., SCHENKEN, L.L., LESHER, S.: Tumor chemotherapy: efficacy dependent on mode of growth. J. nat. Cancer Inst. 50, 467 (1973).
13. BARRANCO, S.C., NOVAK, J.K., HUMPHREY, R.M.: Response of mammalian cells following treatment with bleomycin and 1,3-bis (2-chloroethyl)-1-nitrosourea during plateau phase. Cancer Res. 33, 691 (1974).
14. TWENTYMAN, P.R., BLEEHEN, N.M.: The sensitivity of cells in exponential and stationary phases of growth to bleomycin and to 1,3-bis (2-chloroethyl)-1-nitrosourea. Brit. J. Cancer 28, 500 (1973).
15. TWENTYMAN, P.R., BLEEHEN, N.M.: The sensitivity to bleomycin of spleen colony-forming units in the mouse. Brit. J. Cancer 28, 66 (1973).
16. VAN PUTTEN, L.M.: The kinetics of cell kill and cell proliferation in relation to curability of malignant disease. In: The Design of Clinical Trials in Cancer Therapy, p. 115 (ed. M. Staquet). Brussels: Editions Scientifiques Européennes 1972.
17. STRYCKMANS, P., MANASTER, J.: Kinetic aspects of leukaemia therapy. In: The Design of Clinical Trials in Cancer Therapy, p. 132 (ed. M. Staquet). Brussels: Editions Scientifiques Européennes 1972.
18. SKIPPER, H.E., SCHABEL, Jr., F.M., MELLET, L.B., MONTGOMERY, J.A., WILKOFF, L.J., LLYOD, H.H., BROCKMAN, R.W.: Implications of biochemical, cytokinetic, pharmacologic and toxicologic relationships in the design of optimal therapeutic schedules. Cancer Chemother. Rep. 54, 431 (1970).
19. FREI, E., III., BICKERS, J.N., HEWLETT, J.S., LANE, M., LEARY, W.V., TALLEY, R.W.: Dose schedule and antitumor studies of arabinosyl cytosine (NSC-63878). Cancer Res. 29, 1325 (1969).
20. KENIS, Y., MICHEL, J., DEBUSSCHER, L., LACHAPELLE, F.: Toxic and antitumor effects of methotrexate. Proc. amer. Ass. Cancer Res. 12, 44 (1971).

21. MATHE, G., SCHNEIDER, M., SCHWARZENBERG, L.: The time factor in cancer chemotherapy. Europ. J. Cancer 6, 23 (1970).
22. BERGSAGEL, D.E.: An assessment of massive-dose chemotherapy of malignant disease. Canad. Med. Ass. J. 104, 31 (1971).
23. GREEN, R.A., HUMPHREY, E., CLOSE, H., PATNO, M.E.: Alkylating agents in bronchogenic carcinoma. Amer. J. Med. 46, 516 (1969).
24. BHUYAN, B.K., FRASER, T.J., GRAY, L.G., KUENTZEL, S.L., NEIL, G.L.: Cell-kill kinetics of several S-phase-specific drugs. Cancer Res. 33, 888 (1973).
25. BHUYAN, B.K., SCHEIDT, L.G., FRASER, T.J.: Cell cycle phase specificity of antitumor agents. Cancer Res. 32, 398 (1972).
26. DREWINKO, B., GOTTLIEB, J.A.: Survival kinetics of cultured human lymphoma cells exposed to adriamycin. Cancer Res. 33, 1141 (1973).
27. MAURO, F., MADOC-JONES, H.: Age response of cultured mammalian cells to cytotoxic drugs. Cancer Res. 30, 1397 (1970).
28. VAN PUTTEN, L.M., LELIEVELD, P.: Factors determining cell killing by chemotherapeutic agents in vivo. I. Cyclophosphamide. Europ. J. Cancer 6, 313 (1970).
29. VALERIOTE, F., TOLEN, S.: Comparison of the cytotoxicity of 5-(3,3 -bis(2-chlorethyl)-1-triazeno) imidazol-4-carboxamide (NSC-82196) on normal and leukemic colony-forming cells. Cancer Chemother. Rep. 55, 43 (1971).
30. BROWN, C.H., CARBONE, P.P.: Effects of chemotherapy agents on normal mouse bone marrow grown in vivo. Cancer Res. 31, 185 (1971).
31. LAHIRI, S.K.: Response of mouse bone marrow colony-forming units in different stages of the cell cycle to in vitro incubation with mitomycin-C. Cell Tissue Kin. 6, 509 (1973).
32. DJORDJEVIC, B., KIM, J.H.: Different lethal effects of mitomycin C and actinomycin D during the division cycle of HeLa cells. J. Cell Biol. 38, 477 (1968).
33. RAZEK, A., VALERIOTE, F., VIETTI, T.: Survival of hematopoietic and leukemic colony-forming cells in vivo following the adminstration of daunorubicin or adriamycin. Cancer Res. 32, 1496 (1972).
34. WHEELER, G.P., BOWDON, B.J.M., ADAMSON, D.J., VAIL, M.H.: Comparison of the effects of several inhibitors of the synthesis of nucleic acids upon the viability and progression through the cell cycle of cultured H.Ep. no. 2 cells. Cancer Res. 32, 2661 (1972).
35. TIDD, D.M., KIM, S.C., HORAKOVA, K., MORIWAKI, A., PATERSON, A.R.P.: A delayed cytotoxic reaction for 6-mercaptopurin. Cancer Res. 32, 317 (1972).
36. MADOC-JONES, H., MAURO, F.: Age response to X rays, Vinca alkaloids, and hydroxyurea of murine lymphoma cells synchronized in vivo. J. nat. Cancer Inst. 45, 1131 (1970).
37. HELLMAN, K., FIELD, E.O.: Effect of ICRF 159 on the mammalian cell cycle: significance for its use in cancer chemotherapy. J. nat. Cancer Inst. 44, 539 (1970).
38. LOZZIO, C.B.: Lethal effects of fluorodeoxyuridine on cultured mammalian cells at various stages of the cell cycle. J. Cell Physiol. 74, 57 (1969).
39. BARRANCO, S.C., HUMPHREY, R.M.: The effects of 1,3-bis(2-chloroethyl) -1-nitrosourea on survival and cell progression in Chinese hamster cells. Cancer Res. 31, 191 (1971).
40. LAMPKIN, B.C., NAGAO, T., MAVER, A.M.: Synchronization and recruitment in acute leukemia. J. clin. Invest. 50, 2204 (1971).
41. KIM, S.H., KIM, J.H.: Lethal effect of adriamycin on the division cycle of HeLa cells. Cancer Res. 32, 323 (1972).
42. BARRANCO, S.C., GERNER, E.W., BURK, K.H., HUMPHREY, R.M.: Survival and cell kinetics effects of adriamycin on mammalian cells. Cancer Res. 33, 11 (1973).
43. BARRANCO, S.C., HUMPHREY, R.M.: The effects of bleomycin on survival and cell progression in Chinese hamster cells in vitro. Cancer Res. 31, 1218 (1971).

44. ERNST, P., KILLMANN, S.A.: Perturbation of generation cycle of human leukemic blast cells by cytostatic therapy in vivo: effect of corticosteroids. Blood 36, 689 (1970).
45. LI, L.H., FRASER, T.J., OLIN, E.J., BHUYAN, B.K.: Action of campto-thecin on mammalian cells in culture. Cancer Res. 32, 2643 (1972).
46. KARON, M., SHIRAKAWA, S.: Effect of 1ß-D-arabinofuranosylcytosine on cell cycle passage time. J. nat. Cancer Inst. 45, 861 (1970).
47. STRYCKMANS, P.A., MANASTER, J., LACHAPELLE, F., SOQUET, M.: The mode of action of chemotherapy in vivo on human acute leukemia. I. Daunomycin. J. clin. Invest. 52, 126 (1973).
48. TOBEY, R.A.: Effects of cytosine arabinoside, daunomycin, mithra-mycin, azacytidine, adriamycin, and camptothecin on mammalian cell cyle traverse. Cancer Res. 32, 2720 (1972).
49. SHARPE, H.B.A., FIELD, E.O., HELLMANN, K.: Mode of action of the cytostatic agent "ICRF 159". Nature 226, 524 (1970).
50. TOBEY, R.A.: A simple, rapid technique for determination of the effects of chemotherapeutic agents on mammalian cell-cycle traverse. Cancer Res. 32, 309 (1972).
51. TOBEY, R.A.: Arrest of Chinese hamster cells in G2 following treat-ment with the anti-tumor drug bleomycin. J. Cell Physiol. 79, 259 (1972).
52. TOBEY, R.A., PETERSON, D.F., ANDERSON, E.C., PUCK, T.T.: Life cycle analysis mammalian cells. III. The inhibition of division of chi-nese hamster cells by puromycin and actinomycin. Biophys. J. 6, 567 (1966).
53. DOIDA, Y., OKADA, S.: Effects of actinomycin D and puromycin on the cell progress from M to G1 and S stages in cultured mouse leu-kemia L5178Y cells. Cell Tissue Kin. 5, 15 (1972).
54. YOUNG, R.C.: The effect of methyl-CCNU (NSC-95441) on the cellular kinetics of normal and leukemic murine tissues in vivo. Cell Tissue Kin. 6, 35 (1973).
55. BRAY, D.A., DEVITA, V.T., ADAMSON, R.H., OLIVERIO, V.T.: Effects of 1-(2-chloroethyl)-3-cyclohexyl-1-nitrosourea (CCNU; NSC-79037) and its degradation products on progression of L1210 cells through the cell cycle. Cancer Chemother. Rep. 55, 215 (1971).
56. BRUCHOVSKY, N., OWEN, A.A., BECKER, A.J., TILL, J.E.: Effects of vinblastine on the proliferative capacity of L cells and their pro-gress through the division cycle. Cancer Res. 25, 1232 (1965).
57. PFEIFFER, S.E., TOLMACH, L.J.: Selecting synchronous populations of mammalian cells. Nature 213, 139 (1967).
58. SHIRAKAWA, S., FREI, E.III: Comparative effects of the antitumor agents 5-(dimethyltriazeno)-imidazole-4-carboxamide and 1,3-bis (2-chloroethyl)-1-nitrosourea on cell cycle of L1210 leukemia cells in vivo. Cancer Res. 30, 2173 (1970).
59. YOUNG, R.C., DEVITA, V.T.: The effect of chemotherapy on the growth characteristics and cellular kinetics of leukemia L1210. Cancer Res. 30, 1789 (1970).
60. LAYDE, J.P., BASERGA, R.: The effect of nitrogen mustard on the life cycle of Ehrlich ascites tumor cells in vivo. Brit. J. Can-cer 18, 150 (1964).
61. PALME, G., LISS, E.: Effect of alkylating agents on the life cycle of Ehrlich tumour cells, autoradiographic studies. Europ. J. Can-cer 1, 245 (1965).
62. BHUYAN, B.K., FRASER, T.J.: Cytotoxicity of antitumor agents in a synchronous mammalian cell system. Cancer Chemother. Rep. Part 1, Vol. 58, 149 (1974).
63. HILL, B.T., BASERGA, R.: The cell cycle and its significance for cancer treatment. Cancer Treat. Rev. 2, 159 (1975).

Chapter 6
General Principles of Cancer Chemotherapy. Experimental Data

Cancer chemotherapy has become a science based largely on principles derived from animal experiments; it can no longer be conducted on a trial-and-error basis. In the past two decades, considerable progress has been made in the understanding of some important factors that influence the effectiveness of chemotherapy:

1. The log-kill hypothesis

2. Cell kinetics of both normal and malignant cells

3. The mechanisms of action of different cytotoxic drugs and their effects on the cell cycle

4. The influence of drug scheduling (pharmacokinetics)

5. Drug toxicity, especially the effects on the hematopoietic and immune system

6. Selectivity of cytotoxic drugs for certain histologic cell types

7. Drug resistance

To obtain maximum tumor-cell kill, certain principles must be taken into consideration in designing a chemotherapy protocol.

A. PRINCIPLES LEARNED FROM SINGLE-AGENT THERAPY

1. A malignant tumor should be regarded as a quantity of cells that must be eliminated including the very last cell (see Fig. 2-26) (1). SKIPPER, using the transplantable L1210 leukemia in mice, showed that a single tumor cell may indeed kill the host (2, 3).

2. Working with the same model, SKIPPER learned that tumor-cell kill by cytotoxic drugs follows "first-order kinetics" (2, 3). This means that a given dose of a given drug kills, not a constant number, but a constant fraction (maximum 99 to 99.99 percent or 2 to 4 logs) of a particular tumor-cell population. The fraction killed is independent of the number of cells present and is never 100%. In practice, this means that if a certain dosage of a given drug reduces the cell number by 99 percent, the cell count will fall to 10^4 if it was 10^6, to 10^2 if it was 10^4 and to 1 if it was 10^2. It also means that there would be a 99 percent chance of eradicating the cancer if only one cancer cell were present.

3. Following the administration of a chemotherapeutic agent, the surviving cancer cells will proliferate with the same kinetics as before chemotherapy (Figs. 6-1 and 6-2) (3-5). If advanced solid tumors showing plateau-type growth are "uncrowded" by a cytotoxic treatment, the surviving cells may resume an exponential type of growth and thus grow faster (6).

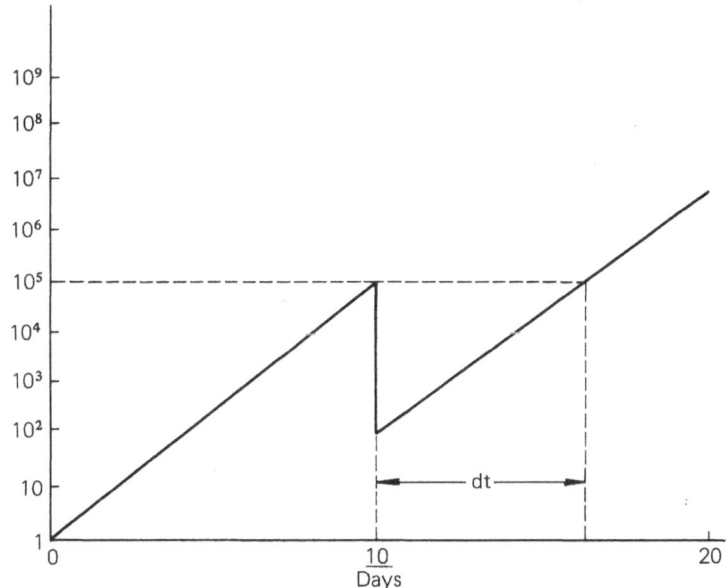

Fig. 6-1. *Study of the doubling time of L1210 leukemia cells following treatment: the tumor grows with a constant doubling time. DT = the time required for the tumor population to restore the number of cells killed by the treatment. (From SKIPPER (4))*

4. The effect of a second dose of the drug depends on the fraction of cells it is able to kill and on the number of cells present. This in turn is determined by the number of cells that survived the first treatment, the time interval between the two treatments, and the doubling time of the tumor. The possibility of drug resistance developing between treatments must also be considered (see p. 125). The time interval between two drug administrations should therefore not be chosen arbitrarily but must be reduced to its strict minimum, that is, the time required to recover. Figure 6-3 shows how the net result may favor either the host or the tumor, depending on dose and time interval.

5. There is a clear dose-response relationship, the fall in the log number of malignant cells being directly proportional to the dose of drug given, at least for cycle-dependent drugs and up to a certain dosage level for phase-dependent drugs. The level of the individual dose is limited by the toxicity of the drug to the normal cells of the host.

6. Since each dose of chemotherapeutic agent kills only a certain percentage of tumor cells, it can be anticipated that prolonged treatment

will be necessary (Fig. 6-3, A and C) to reduce the malignant cell population to a low enough number (<10^5) to be dealt with by the host's own immune defenses.

The importance of drug scheduling has been demonstrated for tumors in both animals and humans. For the same total dose of drug, high-dose intermittent schedules are as a rule more effective than daily administration of small doses (Fig. 6-4) (7-11). If combination chemotherapy is used, the sequence of the administration of the various agents

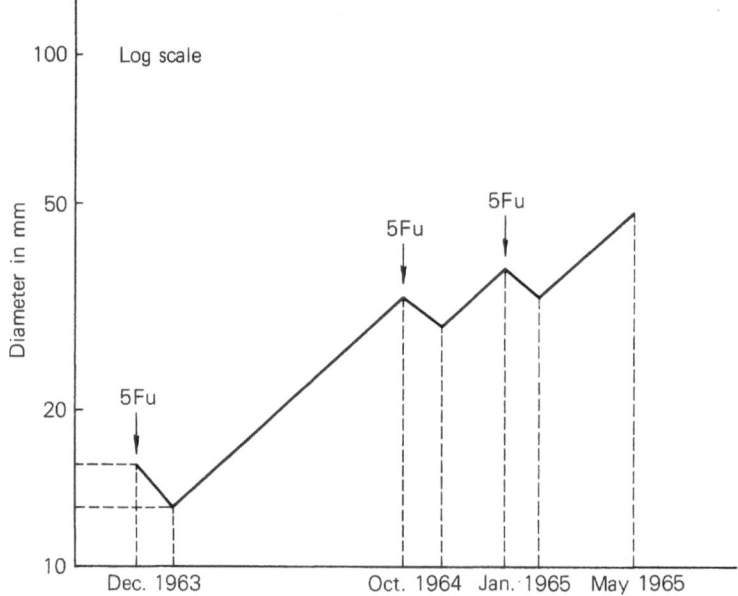

Fig. 6-2. Pulmonary metastasis of a rectal adenocarcinoma treated with 5-fluorouracil. The doubling time (DT = 70 days) is constant after each course of 5-FU. (from COMBES et al. (5))

making up the combination may alter the overall tumoricidal effect (Fig. 6-5) (12). A particular drug schedule can increase cell kill in synchronization protocols.

8. Chemotherapy should be started early; it will be more effective since the log number of tumor cells will be smaller and the growth characteristics of the tumor population will favor chemotherapy when more cells are in cycle. In large tumors, drug penetration may be hampered because of poor vascularization. With large tumors there is also a greater chance for the selection of drug-resistant clones. Furthermore, a host with a limited burden will also be in better condition to tolerate chemotherapy; higher response rates are obtained in patients whose survival prospects are good when therapy is initiated (13, 14, 65). Among other things, this may be because immune reactivity is better preserved in the earlier stages of cancer.

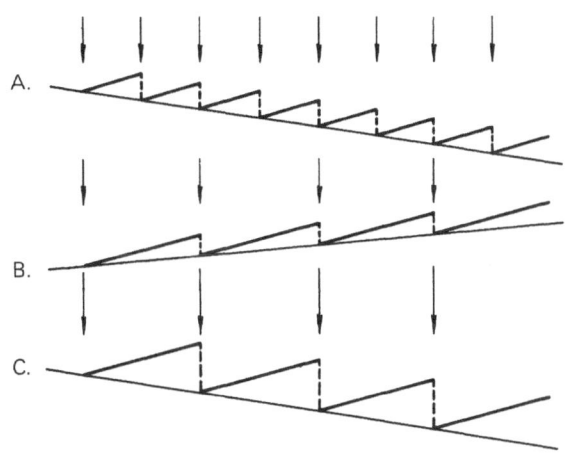

Fig. 6-3. Schematic representation of the balance between tumor growth and cytotoxic tumor destruction. Note that, for a given dose of drug, the effect may be favorable or not depending on the time interval between the drug administrations (compare A and B)

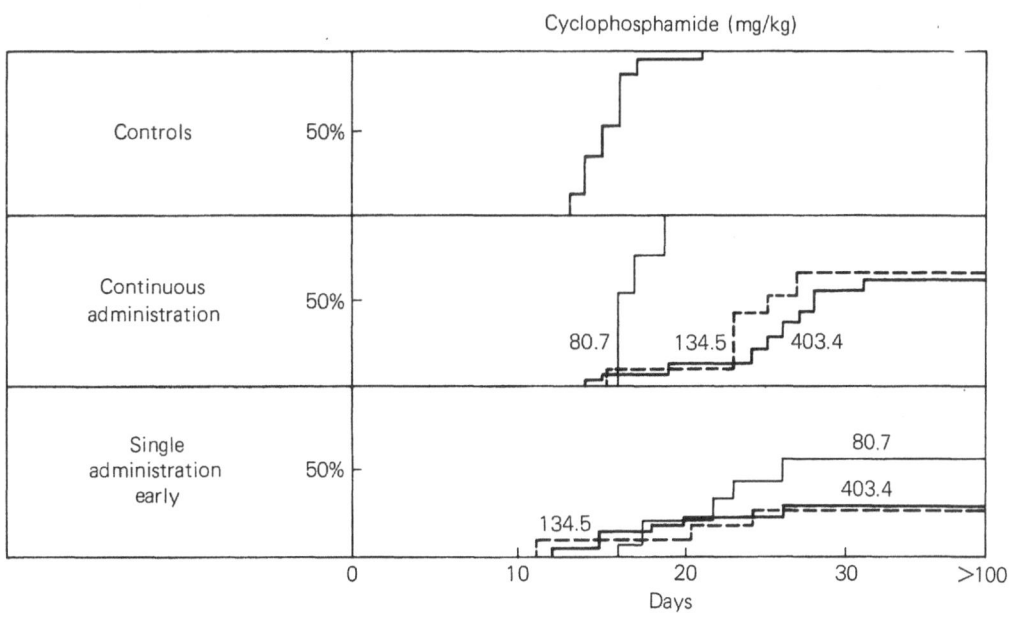

Fig. 6-4. Cumulative survival curves of animals carrying L1210 leukemia, treated with different total doses of cyclophosphamide, administered either as a single dose or as continuous treatment. For all three dose levels (80.7 mg/kg, 134.5 mg/kg, and 403.4 mg/kg), the percentage of animals surviving more than 100 days is greater with the single large dose schedule (9)

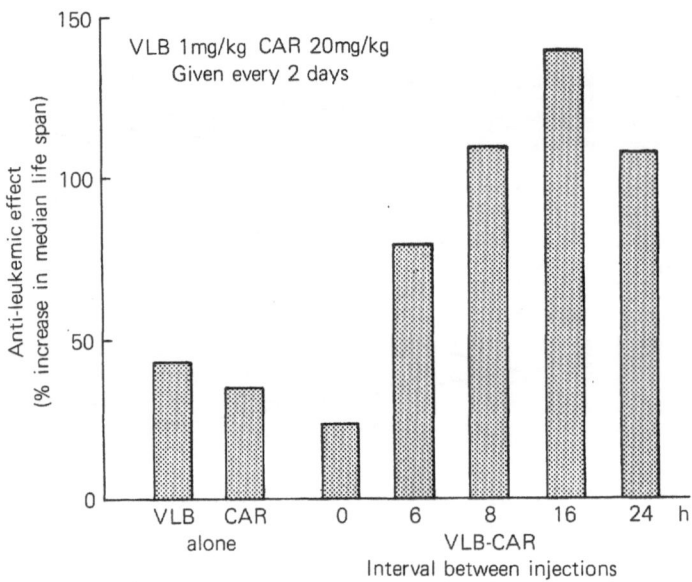

Fig. 6-5. Effect of different schedules of vinblastine (VLB) and cytosine arabinoside (CAR) on L1210 leukemia. (From VADLAMUDI et al.(12))

B. CELL KINETICS AND GROWTH CHARACTERISTICS

The design of cytotoxic therapy should take into consideration the growth characteristics of the malignancy to be treated and the effect of the different drugs on the cell cycle (8, 15-20). We have already described tumor growth as a Gompertz function (see p. 26). Early growth is exponential, the growth fraction is high and the volume doubling time short. As the cell population increases, a plateau phase will be reached with a long doubling time, increasing cell death, and a low growth fraction as many cells remain for prolonged periods in G_1 or enter G_0. This growth pattern is characteristic of most human solid tumors at the time of diagnosis. At this stage, agents that are most effective during S phase will be relatively ineffective, while drugs interacting primarily with DNA tend to be more effective. If the cell population is "uncrowded" (e.g., by surgical resection, radiotherapy, or chemotherapy with cell-phase-independent agents), the remaining cells may resume exponential growth and become more susceptible to cell-phase-dependent drugs (Fig. 6-6). Such a model has been described by SCHABEL (6) and treatment protocols based upon it have been evaluated in experimental animals and in humans (21-26).

To exploit cell kinetics intelligently, there are a number of things we need to know: the duration of the cell cycle and the S phase; the approximate number of cells at the onset of therapy; the proportion of tumor cells and normal cells entering S phase (en route to division) per unit of time; the fractional reduction of different types of normal stem cells which is life-threatening; the rate of recovery of both the host tissues and the tumor cell population; the effect of treatment on the subsequent proliferative behavior of the tumor cells and the normal cell population; the minimum cytotoxic level; and the rate at which the drug disappears from body fluids.

C. DIFFERENTIAL CELL KILL

Chemotherapy must aim at "differential cell kill", that is destroying malignant cells without irreversibly damaging normal cells. The cytotoxic drugs currently available do not distinguish between normal cells and tumor cells; rapidly proliferating cells are particularly vulnerable. Among these, the hematopoietic cells are of special concern to the chemotherapist. Hematopoietic cells are intermediate between the differentiated blood cells and the hematopoietic stem cells; they are in cycle and will be killed by both phase- and cycle-dependent drugs. However, it has been estimated that between 15 and 85 percent of the hematopoietic stem cells are in G_0 and theoretically are not sensitive to cytotoxic agents (Fig. 6-7 (27). To replace the lost hematopoietic elements, resting hematopoietic stem cells are recruited to a proliferative state and thereby made sensitive to chemotherapy until the marrow is repopulated. It is not surprising that daily administration, as was customary in the early days of chemotherapy (and is still the case for busulfan in chronic myeloid leukemia), endangers the stem cell population of the bone marrow. It can result in marrow aplasia if not stopped as soon as cytopenia begins to occur (Fig. 6-8). In contrast, intermittent therapy allows for recovery of the hematopoietic stem cells, as long as the next dose is not given until after the stem cells returned to G_0, having completed their compensatory proliferation (Fig. 6-9) (9, 28). An intermittent schedule can often be repeated for months once the maximum tolerated dose has been determined. The resulting kinetic events will repeat themselves; however, a tendency toward compounding of hematologic toxic effects with repeated courses has been observed with the nitrosoureas (61). The time interval needed between the first and the second cycles for bone-marrow restoration will remain approximately the same following subsequent treatment cycles (Fig. 6-10). That normal marrow stem cells can regenerate faster than malignant cells is evidenced by the fact that cytotoxic drugs can induce remissions in acute lymphoid leukemia, that is clearing of the leukemic cells with regeneration and restoration of the normal bone-marrow elements.

Immunocompetent cells are also damaged by chemotherapy (29). Most cytotoxic agents including corticosteroids and L-asparaginase which are not bone-marrow depressant are immunosuppressant. The degree of immunosuppression in the cancer patient on chemotherapy should be monitored (see p. 187), since it may be detrimental to the patient. Not only may he become susceptible to opportunistic infections (herpes, cytomegalic inclusion disease, Pneumocystis Carinii, and fungus infections) (30) but immunosuppression may allow his tumor to grow or disseminate (31). Indeed, there is growing evidence that immune responses, especially at the cellular level, are important in the host's defense against cancer. The majority of immunocompetent cells are in a resting state (G_0), except for those stimulated and transformed into immunoblasts or plasmablasts by a specific antigen, for example a tumor-specific antigen or microbial antigens. Thus, it is active immune responses rather than the stem-cell population that are threatened by chemotherapy. This suppression, which is temporary, is lifted shortly after chemotherapy is discontinued. Once again, low-dose daily chemotherapy is more dangerous as an immunosuppressant than high-dose intermittent therapy (Table 6-1) (8, 32). It is not surprising that azathioprine or

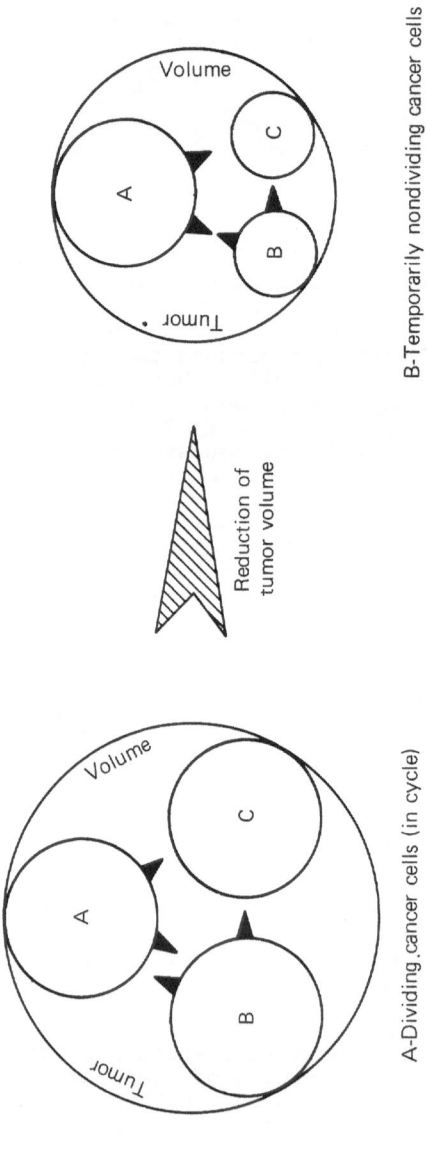

A-Dividing cancer cells (in cycle)

B-Temporarily nondividing cancer cells
(in G_0 or prolonged G_1)

C-Permanently nondividing cancer cells

Fig. 6-6. Effect of a reduction in tumor volume: a larger proportion of cells is in cycle

prednisone is prescribed in a daily schedule to produce immunosuppression sufficient to induce tolerance against allografts.

Damage to epithelial cells of the gastrointestinal tract, another rapidly proliferating tissue, is noncomfortable for the patient and may be the site of entry for serious local and systemic infections.

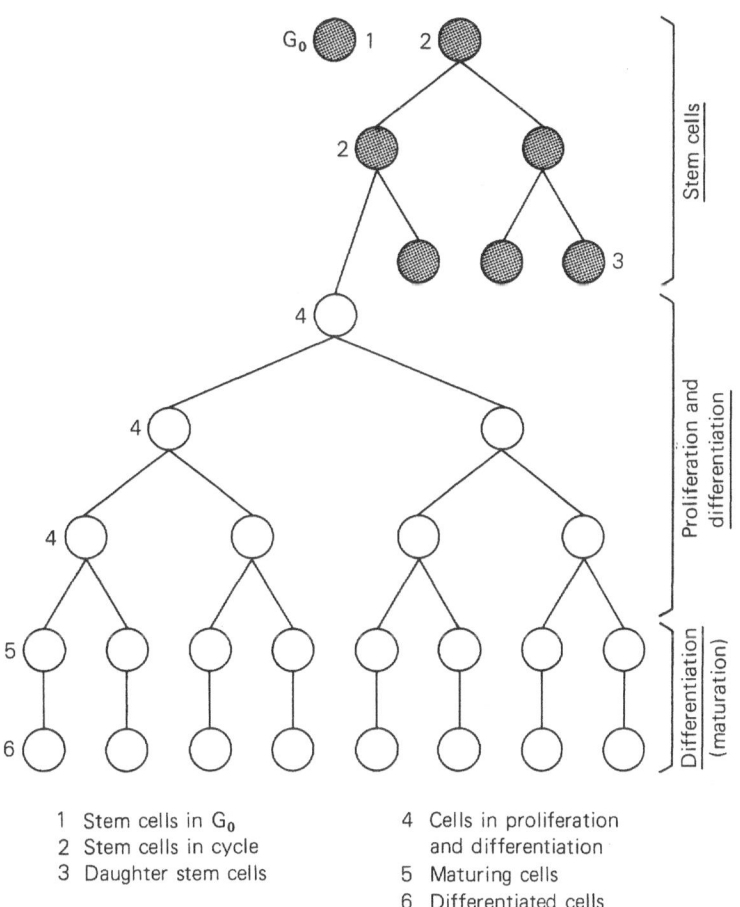

1 Stem cells in G_0
2 Stem cells in cycle
3 Daughter stem cells

4 Cells in proliferation and differentiation
5 Maturing cells
6 Differentiated cells

Fig. 6-7. Stem cells, proliferating and maturing cells of the hematopoietic system

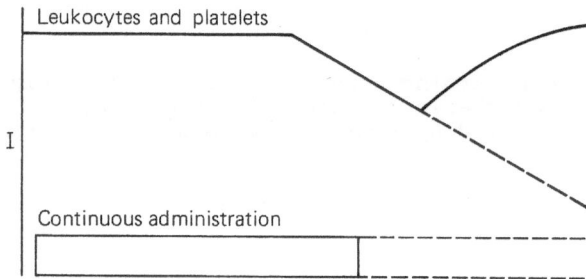

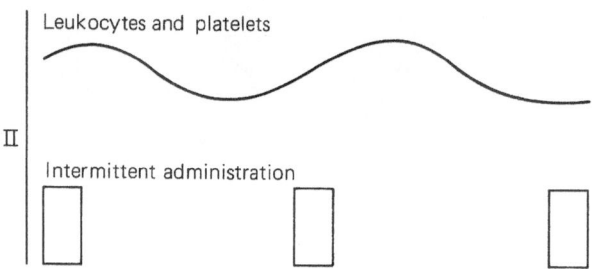

Fig. 6-8. Effect of continuous (I) versus intermittent (II) chemothera-py on the leukocyte and platelet count

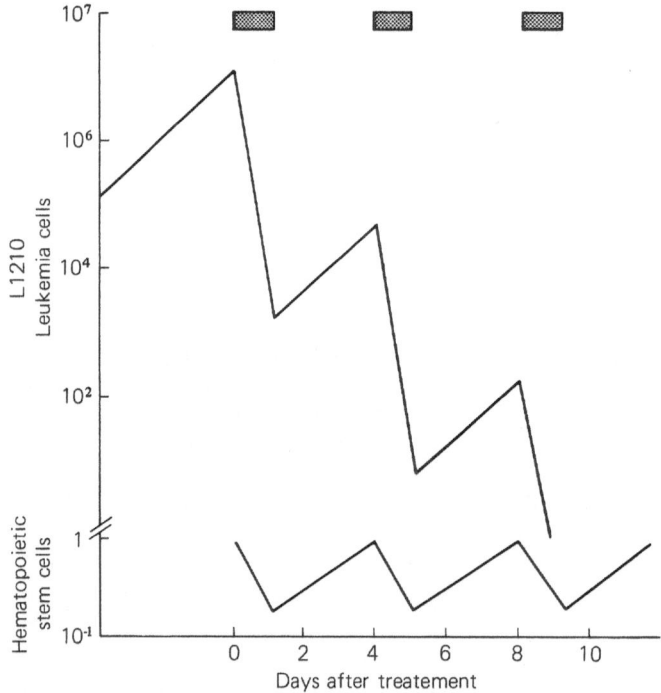

Fig. 6-9. Effect of cytosine arabinoside, administered for 24 h every 4 days, on L1210 leukemia and hematopoietic stem cells (most favorable therapeutic index). (After FREI et al. (28))

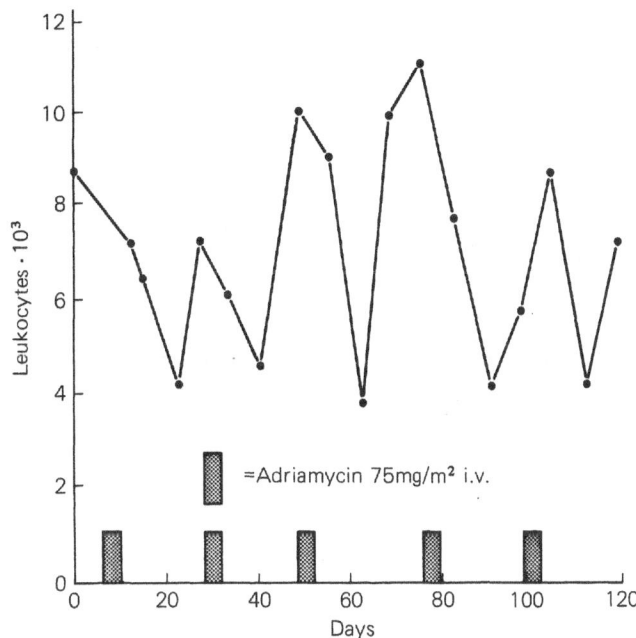

Fig. 6-10. Bronchus carcinoma treated with adriamycin once every three weeks. Each injection of adriamycin causes a similar degree of leukocyte depression without evidence of cumulative toxicity

Table 6-1. Comparison of the immunosuppressive effect of continuous and intermittent chemotherapy[a]. From SCHNEIDER et al. (32)

Detectable immunosuppressive effect

	Absent		Present	
Intermittent chemotherapy	51/57	89.4%	6/57	10.6%
Continuous chemotherapy	9/27	33.3%	18/27	66.6%

[a]Patients in whom the immunosuppressive effect of chemotherapy could not be evaluated because they failed to react to BCG both before and after chemotherapy are not included.

D. TISSUE SELECTIVITY

Many cytotoxic drugs and hormones have some degree of tissue selectivity although none shows selectivity with respect to malignant cells. For example, 5-FU is more effective in carcinomas of the gastrointestinal tract and breast cancer, both of endodermal origin; bleomycin is more effective in skin cancer and lung metastases.

Tissue selectivity may be based upon:

(a) sensitivity to particular hormones (breast, endometrium, prostate);

(b) selective accumulation in the target tissue (e.g., ^{131}I in thyroid, ^{198}Au in the RES, bleomycin in skin and lung)

(c) selective bioactivation in target tissue (e.g., diethylstilbestrol in prostate, cyclophosphamide in tissue rich in phosphamidase);

(d) selective tissue toxicity (e.g. O,P' DDD in tumors of the adrenal cortex).

This selectivity can be exploited in prescribing chemotherapy. Unfortunately, malignant tissues usually rapidly lose their sensitivity, for example to hormone action, while normal tissues remain sensitive.

E. METHODS TO AUGMENT CELL KILL ABOVE THAT OF SINGLE-AGENT THERAPY

In attempts to improve the log kill and to prevent or delay the onset of drug resistance, programs have been designed with several drugs used sequentially or in combination.

In most tumors only a portion of the cells are in cycle; even fewer cells are in the sensitive phase during the brief period when there is an effective concentration in the blood of a phase-dependent agent being given in an intermittent fashion. Therefore, combinations of drugs that act in different phases of the cell cycle, for example, G1 and M, will affect a larger number of cells. A phase-dependent drug can also be combined with a cycle-dependent agent.

However, other factors must be considered in the selection of compounds for combination. The agents to be used must be effective when used alone in the type of tumor to be treated, and should preferably have different mechanisms of action. In addition, they should have different types of toxicity. C.O.P. is a combination much used in the USA for the treatment of lymphomas; it was selected for trial because it combines three drugs, each of which is effective in lymphoma, but their major toxicities differ. Cyclophosphamide is myelosuppressive, vincristine is neurotoxic, and prednisone has the side-effects of corticosteroid therapy. Combinations of drugs with early (CAR) and late (nitrosoureas) myelotoxicity is also acceptable, (see p. 135).

However, it must be pointed out that drug combinations are not necessarily more effective than single-agent therapy. Let us assume that drug A has a response rate (RR) of 30 percent and drug B of 25 percent. When the two drugs are combined, a variety of interactions can occur: (1) addition of their effects (RR of A + B = 55 percent), (2) potentiation (e.g., A + B = 75 percent), or (3) antagonism (A + B = 20 percent) (Table 6-2) (33). Table 6-3 shows one of the few known examples of potentiation (34). The value of these data is, however, limited since they were not obtained in a randomized trial. An example of antagonism is illustrated in Fig. 6-11. The combination of methotrexate and L-asparaginase in L1210 mouse leukemia was less effective than methotrexate alone (35). Indeed, it has been shown that methotrexate is inactive in cells deficient in asparagine.

The effectiveness of new combinations should always be compared with single-agent therapy, with the same agents in sequence, or with other combinations. Experimental studies are often limited by cost, since

122

Table 6-2. Effect of 8 chemotherapeutic agents, combined two by two, on L1210 leukemia. (From HOSHINO et al. (33)

	6MP	5FU	MTC	DRB	VLB	CAR	ADM
MTX	±	+	+	±	±	+	+
6MP		+	+	±	±	++	+
5FU			++	+	+	++	+
MTC				+	+	++	++
DRB					±	++	
VLB						+	±
CAR							++

++ Synergistic effect + Simple additive effect ± Less than additive effect

MTX = methotrexate
6MP = 6-mercaptopurine
5FU = 5-fluorouracil
MTC = mitomycin C
DRB = daunorubicin
VLB = vinblastine

CAR = cytosine arabinoside
ADM = adriamycin

Table 6-3. An example of potentiation

Combination of two drugs for induction of remission in childhood ALL	
Prednisone (PDN) induces	57% CRm
6-MP	27% CRm

The combination of PDN plus 6-MP should theoretically result in:

$$57\% + 27\% \left(\frac{100-57}{100}\right) = 57\% + 11.6\% = 69\%$$

The actual induction rate is 82% (34).

very large numbers of animals are required to test not only combinations of different drugs, but also different dose levels and schedules (62). Moreover, animal data do not always apply to the human situation. Comparative clinical studies are even scarcer. A disadvantage of combinations is that the contribution of each individual drug cannot be evaluated; it is always possible that a drug may enhance the toxicity of the combination without contributing to the tumor effect. The mechanisms of antagonism and potentiation are not always understood. BROCKMAN (63), BONO (64), and VALERIOTE (66) have reviewed some of the biochemical rationales for combining antitumor drugs.

1. The effectiveness of a cytotoxic drug may be enhanced by the administration of another agent that inhibits the enzymatic degradation of the cytotoxic compound, for example the degradation of 8-azaguanine by guanine aminohydrolase is effectively inhibited by 4-amino-5-imidazole carboxamide.

2. Several agents can be combined that block sequential steps in a biosynthetic pathway. We have already referred to the combination of 6-MP and 6-MMPR which produces a dual block in purine biosynthesis.

123

3. The combination of DNA-binding agents (e.g., ADM) with alkylating agents might be effective since the repair of DNA damaged by the alkylating agent could be hampered by the presence of the compound that is bound to DNA.

4. Agents that inhibit synthesis of new DNA (e.g., CAR) could be administered together with agents (e.g., BLM) that produce breaks in DNA to result in degradation of existing DNA.

5. One would expect a therapeutic potentiation by combining alkylating agents (e.g., CPM) with compounds that inhibit repair (e.g., nitrosoureas)

6. We have already discussed in Chap. 5 the rationales for selecting drug combinations based on the effect of an agent in the cell as it passes through the proliferative cell cycle. Cell destruction can be augmented by exploiting interference with cell progression, as is done in synchronization protocols. The cells are first temporarily blocked in a particular phase of the cell cycle, where they accumulate. They will then enter subsequent phases of the cell cycle more or less simultaneously as a cohort (synchronization), so that larger numbers of cells can be killed by giving the appropriate cytotoxic drug at the proper time. In fact, several chemotherapeutic agents are themselves capable of synchronizing cells, even though they may not have any cytotoxic effect. Cell-phase-dependent agents, especially mitotic poisons, are suitable for this purpose (see p. 144).

It is also possible to increase tumor-cell kill by giving a large dose of a chemotherapeutic agent over a short period followed by an antidote to minimize systemic toxicity. This method has been used successfully with methotrexate followed by folinic acid (36).

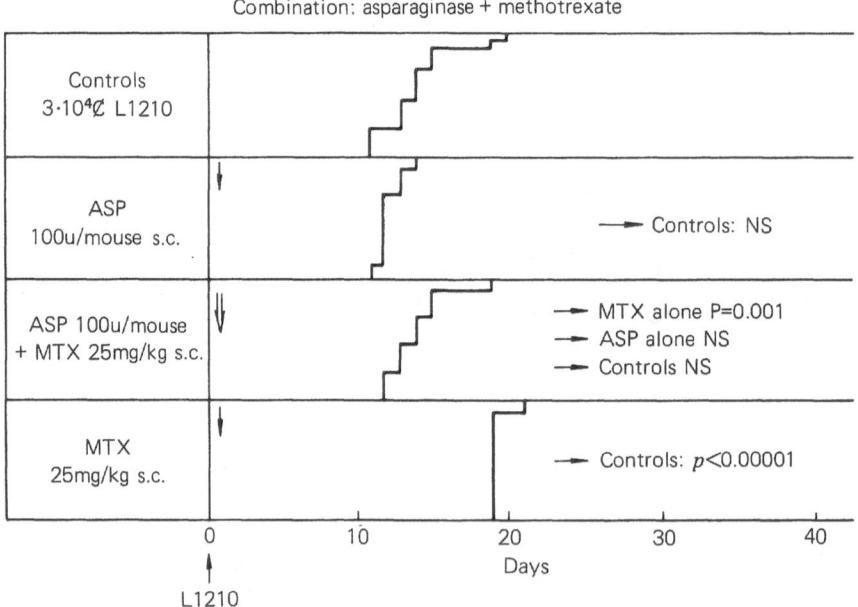

Combination: asparaginase + methotrexate

Fig. 6-11. The combination of methotrexate and L-asparaginase is less effective than methotrexate alone in L1210 mouse leukemia (From MATHÉ et al. (35))

The problem of resting cells (cells in G_0), for which we have few effective drugs, can be approached through "recruitment" into proliferative cycle. If the tumor is "uncrowded" by preliminary cell-reducing surgical resection, radiotherapy, or chemotherapy with cell-cycle-dependent drugs, a larger portion of the remaining cells will pass into cycle and become sensitive to phase-dependent drugs.

F. THE PROBLEM OF DRUG RESISTANCE

Soon after chemotherapy was introduced, it was learned that, as with antibiotic therapy, resistance may become a problem (37-39). Two types are distinguished: primary and secondary. In primary resistance a drug is ineffective from the beginning of treatment. Resistance is said to be secondary or acquired when, following an initial response, a tumor cell population emerges that is completely resistant to chemotherapy. Such an outcome may be the result of drug-induced adaptation and selection of a new phenotype, or of drug-induced mutation and selection of a new genotype (38).

Several biophysical and biochemical mechanisms of resistance have been identified:

1. The intracellular concentration of the drug is reduced because of decreased permeability of the cell membrane or altered binding of the drug to the "carrier". Such mechanisms have been described in cells resistant to methotrexate (40-42), Vinca alkaloids (43), alkylating agents (44, 45) and actinomycin D. The sensitivity of mammary tumors to hormones is determined by the presence or absence in the cytoplasm of a specific protein that binds estrogen before transporting it to the nucleus, where the estrogen exerts its effect by binding to the chromatin (46).

2. Increased or accelerated degradation of the active compound results in a lowered intracellular concentration, for example breakdown of guanine analogs by increased guanine deaminase activity. Breakdown of methotrexate (47) and alkylating agents (48) has also been suggested to account for the resistance to these agents.

3. Enzyme deficiency: many cytotoxic agents, especially purine and pyrimidine analogs, must first be converted to nucleotides before they can inhibit cellular metabolism. The enzymes required for this conversion have been found to be deficient in cells resistant to 5-FU (49-50), 6-MP (51), and cytosine arabinoside (52-54).

4. Changes in cellular metabolism alter feedback mechanisms, for example elevated pools of deoxycytidine nucleotides (d-CTP) accumulating in CAR-resistant cells compete with ara-CTP (55).

5. Changes in enzymes: in some instances, resistance is due to an increase in the activity of the target enzyme. For example, there is increased activity of folic acid reductase in methotrexate-resistant cells (56), while in other cells a variant of the target enzyme appears that has less affinity for the inhibitor, than the natural substrate. This phenomenon has been observed in 6-MP (57), 5-FU- (49), and methotrexate-resistant (58, 59) cell lines.

6. Accelerated repair is another mechanism through which resistance to alkylating agents can develop (60).

The mutation-selection mechanism is probably of most importance in the origin of resistance. This has serious implications with respect to the requirement of "total tumor-cell kill" in order to obtain a cure. Clonal evolution and instability are more frequent in solid tumors than in acute leukemias. This cytogenetic heterogeneity is likely to result in selection of drug-resistant clones. The risk of drug resistance is decreased by combining various therapeutic agents.

Finally, there may be instances of relative resistance, not related to the intrinsic qualities of the tumor cells but due to the clinical condition of the host and the advanced stage of the disease. For instance, a compromised bone-marrow reserve may not permit the administration of effective doses or, since chemotherapy follows first-order kinetics, a tumor may clinically appear to be resistant, because the tumor volume, and hence the number of cells, is excessive. Some cells may appear resistant because they receive less than average drug exposure being located in so called "tumor sanctuaries".

REFERENCES

1. MATHE, G.: La dernière cellule. Presse méd. 75, 2591 (1967).
2. SKIPPER, H.E., SCHABEL, F.M., WILCOX, W.S.: Experimental evaluation of potential anticancer agents. XIII. On the criteria and kinetics associated with "curability" of experimental leukemia. Cancer Chemother. Rep. 35, 1 (1964).
3. SKIPPER, H.E., SCHABEL, F.M., WILCOX, W.S.: Experimental evaluation of potential anticancer agents. XIV. Further study of certain basic concepts underlying chemotherapy of leukemia. Cancer Chemother. Rep. 45, 5 (1965).
4. SKIPPER, H.E.: Cellular kinetics associated with "curability" of experimental leukemias. In: Perspectives in leukemia, Vol. 1, p. 187, (eds. W. Dameshek, R.M. Dutcher). New York: Grune and Stratton 1968.
5. COMBES, P.F., DOUCHEZ, J., CARTON, M., NAJA, A.: Etude de la croissance des métastases pulmonaires humaines comme argument objectif d'évaluation du pronostic et des effets thérapeutiques. J. Radiol. Electrol. 49, 893 (1968).
6. SCHABEL, F.M.: The use of tumor growth kinetics in planning "curative" chemotherapy of advanced solid tumors. Cancer Res. 29, 2384 (1969).
7. SELAWRY, O.S., HANANIAN, J., WOLMAN, I.J., ABIR, E., CHEVALIER, L., GOURDEAU, R., DENTON, R., GUSSOFF, B., LEVY, R., BURGERT, O., MILLS, S.D., BLOM, J., JONES, B., PATTERSON, R.B., McINTYRE, O.R., HARRANI, F.I., MOON, J.H., HOOGSTRATEN, B., KUNG, F.H., SHECHE, P.R., FREI, E. III, HOLLAND, J.F.: New treatment schedule with improved survival in childhood leukemia (ALGB). J. amer. med. Ass. 154, 75 (1965).
8. MATHE, G.: Operational research in cancer chemotherapy. Chemotherapy in the strategy of cancer treatment. In: Scientific Basis of Cancer Chemotherapy, p.72. (ed. G. Mathe). Berlin-Heidelberg-New York: Springer-Verlag 1969.
9. MATHE, G., SCHNEIDER, M., SCHWARZENBERG, L.: The time factor in cancer chemotherapy. Europ. J. Cancer 6, 23 (1970).
10. SKIPPER, H.E., SCHABEL, Jr., F.M., MELLET, L.B., MONTGOMERY, J.A., WILKOFF, L.J., LLOYD, H.H., BROCKMAN, R.W.: Implications of biochemical, cytokinetic, pharmacologic and toxicologic relationship in the design of optimal therapeutic schedules. Cancer Chemother. Rep. 54, 431 (1970).
11. GOLDIN, A.: Importance of dose schedule and route of administration. In: The Design of Clinical Trials in Cancer Therapy. p. 82, (ed. M. Staquet). Brussels: Editions Scientifiques Européennes 1972.

12. VADLAMUDI, S., GOLDIN, A.: Influence of mitotic cycle inhibitors in the antileukemic activity of cytosine arabinoside (NSC-63878) in mice bearing leukemia L1210. Cancer Chemother. Rep. 55, 547 (1971).
13. CARTER, S.K.: Study design principles for the clinical evaluation of new drugs as developed by the chemotherapy programme of the NCI. In: The Design of Clinical Trials in Cancer Therapy, p. 242 (ed. M. Staquet) Brussels: Editions Scientifiques Européenne 1972.
14. GARDERE, S., HUSSAIN, S., COWAN, D.H.: Treatment of metastatic maligant melanoma with a combination of 5-(3,3-dimethyl-1-triazen)-imidazole-4-carboxamide (NSC-45388), cyclophosphamide (NSC-26271). and vincristine (NSC-67574). Cancer Chemother. Rep. 56, 357 (1971).
15. SKIPPER, H.E.: Cancer chemotherapy is many things: G.H.A. Clowes memorial lecture. Cancer Res. 31, 1173 (1971).
16. SKIPPER, H.E.: Kinetics of mammary tumor cell growth and implications for therapy. Cancer, 28 1479 (1971).
17. SKIPPER, H.E.: Kinetic behavior versus response to chemotherapy. Nat. Cancer Inst. Monogr. 34, 2 (1971).
18. VAN PUTTEN, L.M.: The kinetics of cell kill and cell proliferation in relation to curability of malignant disease. In: The Design of Clinical Trials in Cancer Therapy, p. 115 (ed. M. Staquet) Brussels: Editions Scientifiques Européennes 1972.
19. STRYCKMANS, P., MANASTER, J.: Kinetic aspects of leukaemia therapy. In: The Design of Clinical Trials in Cancer Therapy, p. 132 (ed. M. Staquet) Brussels: Editions Scientifiques Européennes 1972.
20. DE VITA, C.T.: Cell kinetics and the chemotherapy of cancer. Cancer Chemother. Rep. 2, 23 (1971).
21. TYRER, D.D., KLINE, I., VENDITTI, J.M., GOLDIN, A.: Separate and sequential chemotherapy of mouse leukemia L1210 with 1ß-D-arabino-furanosylcytosine hydrochloride and 1,3-bis(2-chlorethyl)-1-nitro-sourea. Cancer Res. 27, 873 (1967).
22. HOFFMAN, G.S., KLINE, S., GANG, M., TYRER, D.D., GOLDIN, A., MANTEL, N., VENDITTI, J.M.: Sequential chemotherapy with cyclophospha-mide (NSC 26271) and cytosine arabinoside (NSC 63878) in mice with advanced leukemia L1210. Cancer Chemother. Rep. 53, 265 (1969).
23. STRAUS, M.J., MANTEL, N., GOLDIN, A.: The effect of the sequence of administration of cytoxan and methotrexate on the life-span of L1210 leukemic mice. Cancer Res. 32, 200 (1972).
24. VAN EDEN, E.B., FAIKSON, H.C., FALKSON, G.: 1,3-bis(2-chlorethyl)-1-nitrosourea (BCNU) given concomitantly with cytosine arabino-side in the treatment of cancer. Cancer Chemother. Rep. 54, 347 (1970).
25. KINNE, D.W., HUMPHREY, E.W.: Combined therapy with cytosine ara-binoside and 1,3-bis(2)chloroethyl)1-nitrosourea (BCNU) for ad-vanced solid tumors. Cancer Chemother. Rep. 56, 53 (1972).
26. LEVITT, M., MARSH, J.C., DE CONTI, R.C., MITCHELL, M.S., SKEEL, R.T., FARBER, L.R., BERTINO, J.R.: Combination sequential chemo-therapy in advanced reticulum cell sarcoma. Cancer 29, 630 (1972).
27. BRUCE, W.R., MEEKER, B.E.: Comparison of the sensitivity of normal hematopoietic and transplanted lymphoma colony-forming cells to tritiated thymidine. J. nat. Cancer Inst. 34, 849 (1965).
28. FREI, E.III., BICKERS, J.N., HEWLWTT, J.S., LANE, M., LEARY, W.V., TALLEY, R.W.: Dose schedule and antitumor studies of arabinosyl cytosine (NSC-63878). Cancer Res. 29, 1325 (1969).
29. AL-SARRAF, M., WONG, P., SARDESAI, S., VAITKEVICIUS, V.K.: Clini-cal immunologic responsiveness in malignant disease. I. Delayed hypersensitivity reaction and the effect of cytotoxic drugs. Cancer 26, 262 (1970).
30. SIMONE, J.V., HOLLAND, E., JOHNSON, W.: Fatalities during remis-sions of childhood leukemia. Blood 39, 759 (1972).

31. SUGARBAKER, E.V., COHEN, A.M., KETCHAM, A.S.: Facilitated metasta-
    tic distribution of the Walker 256 tumor in Sprague-Dawley rats
    with hydrocartosone and/or cyclophosphamide. J. Surg. Oncol. 2,
    277 (1970).
32. SCHNEIDER, M.: Effect des chimiothérapies antimitotiques sur une
    réaction d'hypersensibilité retardée. Rev. franc. Etudes clin.
    biol. 13, 877 (1968).
33. HOSHINO, A., KATO, T., AMO, H., OTA, K.: L1210 mouse leukemia as
    an experimental system for clinical combination chemotherapy.
    Proc. VIIth International Congress Chemotherapy. Munich: Urban
    und Schwarzenberg 1971.
34. FREI, E.III, FREIREICH, E.J.: Progress and perspectives in the
    chemotherapy of acute leukemia. Advan. Chemotherapy 2, 269 (1965).
35. MATHE, G., AMIEL, J.L., SCHWARZENBERG, L., SCHNEIDER, M., HAYAT,
    M., JASMIN, C., DE VASSAL, F.: Asparaginase and immune responses:
    the place of asparaginase in a protocol envisaged to eradicate
    acute lymphoblastic leukemia. In: Symposium International sur la
    L-asparaginase", Vol. 1, p. 227. Paris: C.N.R.S. 1971.
36. SCHWARZENBERG, L., MATHE, G., HAYAT, M., DE VASSAL, F., AMIEL,
    J.L., CATTAN, A., SCHNEIDER, M., SCHLUMBERGER, J.R., JASMIN, C.,
    NGO MINH MAN: Une nouvelle combinaison de méthotrexate-acide fo-
    linique pour le traitement des cancers (leucémies et tumeurs
    solides). Presse méd. 77, 385 (1969).
37. BROCKMAN, R.W.: Mechanisms of resistance to anticancer agents. Adv.
    Cancer Res. 7, 129 (1963).
38. BROCKMAN, R.W.: Drug resistance: clinical and experimental. His-
    torical perspectives. In: Oncology 1970, Vol. II, p. 254 (eds. R.L.
    Clark, R.W. Cumley, McCay). Chicago: Year Book Medical Publishers
    1971.
39. HARRAP, K.R.: Pharmacologic disposition of anticancer agents. In:
    The Design of Clinical Trials in Cancer Therapy, p. 292. (ed. M.
    Staquet). Brussels: Editions Scientifiques Européennes 1972.
40. FISCHER, G.A.: Defective transport of amethopterin (methotrexate)
    as a mechanism of resistance to the antimetabolite in L5178Y leu-
    kemic cells. Biochem. Pharm. 11, 1233 (1962).
41. SIROTNAK, F.M., KURITA, S., HUTCHISON, D.: On the nature of a
    transport alteration determining resistance to amethopterin in
    the L1210 leukamia. Cancer Res. 28, 75 (1968).
42. KESSEL, D., HALL, T.C., DeWAYNE, R.: Modes of uptake of methotre-
    xate by normal and leukemic human leucocytes in vitro and their
    relation to drug response. Cancer Res. 28, 564 (1968).
43. CREASEY, W.A.: Modifications in biochemical pathways produced by
    the Vinca alkaloids. Cancer Chemother. Rep. 52, 501 (1968).
44. WHEELER, G.P.: Studies related to mechanisms of resistance to bio-
    logical alkylating agents. Cancer Res. 23, 1334 (1963).
45. WOLPERT, M.K., RUDDON, R.W.: A study on the mechanism of resistance
    to nitrogen mustard (HN2) in Ehrlich ascites tumor cells: compari-
    son of uptake of HN2-^{14}C into sensitive and resistant cells. Cancer
    Res. 29, 873 (1969).
46. JENSEN, E.V., BLOCK, G.E., SMITH, S., KYSER, K., DESOMBRE, E.R.:
    Estrogen receptors and breast cancer response to adrenalectomy.
    In: Prediction of Response in Cancer Therapy. (ed. T.C. Hall), 55
    (1971).
47. ROTHENBURG, S.P.: Alteration of methotrexate by leukemic cells
    loss of affinity for an anion exchange resin. Cancer Res. 29,
    2047 (1969).
48. HARRAP, K.R., HILL, B.T.: The selectivity of action of alkylating
    agents and drug resistance. III. The uptake and degradation of al-
    kylating drugs by Yoshida ascites cells in vitro. Biochem. Pharm.
    19, 209 (1970).
49. HEIDELBERGER, C.: Fluorinated pyrimidines. Progr. Nucl. Acid. Res.
    Mol. Biol. 4, 1 (1965).

50. KESSEL, D., HALL, T.C.: Nucleotide formation as a determinant of 5-fluorouracil response in mouse leukemia. Science 154, 911 (1966).
51. BROCKMAN, R.W., ROOSA, R.A., LAW, L.W., STUTTS, P.: Purine ribonucleotide phosphorylase activity and resistance to purine analogs in P388 murine lymphocytic leukaemia. J. cell.Comp.Physiol. 60, 65 (1962).
52. CHU, M.Y., FISCHER, G.A.: Comparative studies of leukemic cells sensitive and resistant to cytosine arabinoside. Biochem. Pharm. 14, 333 (1965).
53. KESSEL, D., HALL, T.C.: Transport and phosphorylation as factors in the antitumor action of cytosine arabinoside. Science 156, 1240 (1967).
54. SMITH, D.B., CHU, E.H.Y.: A genetic approach to the study of cytotoxicity and resistance to cultured Chinese hamster cells in the presence of cytosine arabinoside. Cancer Res. 32, 1651 (1972).
55. MOMPARLER, R.L., CHU, M., FISCHER, G.A.: Studies on a new mechanism of resistance of L5178Y murine leukemia cells to cytosine arabinoside. Biochem. Biophys. Acta 161, 481 (1968).
56. FRIEDKIN, M., CRAWFORD, E., HUMPHREY, S.R., GOLDIN, A.: The association of increased dihydrofolate reductase with amethopterin resistance in mouse leukemia. Cancer Res. 22, 600 (1962).
57. ROY-BURMAN, P.: Analogues of nucleic acid components. Rec. Res. Cancer Res. 25, 20 (1970).
58. BLUMENTHAL, G., GREENBERG, D.M.: Evidence for two molecular species of dihydrofolate reductase in amethopterin resistant and sensitive cells of the mouse leukemia 4946. Oncology 24, 223 (1970).
59. SKEEL, R.T., BERTINO, J.R.: Association of acquired methotrexate resistance with altered dihydrofolate reductase in acute lymphocyte leukemia. Blood 40, 934 (1972).
60. LAWLWY, P.D., BROOKES, P.: Molecular mechanism of the cytotoxic action of bifunctional alkylating agents and of resistance to this action. Nature 206, 480 (1965).
61. MOERTEL, C.G.: Therapy of advanced gastrointestinal cancer with the nitrosoureas. Cancer Chemother. Rep. Part 3, 4, 27 (1973).
62. CARTER, S.K.: Planning combined therapy - The interaction of experimental and clinical studies. Cancer Chemother. Rep. Part 2, 4, 3 (1974).
63. BROCKMAN, R.W.: Biochemical aspects of drug combinations. Cancer Chemother. Rep. Part 2, 4, 115 (1974).
64. BONO, V.H.: Biochemical rationales for the selection of combinations of chemotherapeutic agents. Cancer Chemother. Rep. Part 2, 4, 131 (1974).
65. MOERTEL, C.G., SCHUTT, A.J., HAHN, R.G., REITEMEIER, R.J.: Effects of patient selection on results of phase II chemotherapy trials in gastrointestinal cancer. Cancer Chemother. Rep. Part 1, Vol. 58, 257 (1974).
66. VALERIOTE, F., HSIU-SAN LIN: Synergistic interaction of anticancer agents: a cellular perpective. Cancer Chemother. Rep. Part 1, 59, 895 (1975).

Chapter 7

Application of the Basic Principles of Chemotherapy to Human Malignancies

Among all the recommendations made in textbooks and medical journals by those doing basic research with animal models, and by individual clinical investigators or cooperative study groups (e.g., NCI, EORTC) reporting on clinical studies, the practicing oncologist must select the treatment program best suited for his patients. This is not always an easy task, as the recommendations are often not in agreement. The treatment modalities for the different tumors are outlined in later chapters. In this chapter, we discuss in more general terms the application to the clinical situation of the principles outlined in the previous pages. It must be remembered that many of these concepts are derived from studies with animal models, and these do not necessarily resemble human malignancies. Nonetheless, much of the information gained from animal studies can be applied, and the validity of the findings verified in clinical practice (131).

In cancer patients, as in animals, early and prolonged treatment with intermittent schedules is generally to be recommended. The choice of drugs will to a great extent be determined by, on the one hand, the sensitivity of different malignant and normal tissues to the various chemotherapeutic agents and/or their mode of administration and, on the other hand, by the kinetics of normal and malignant cells. Thus, the following factors must also be taken into consideration: the histologic type, extent (stage), and rate of progression of the tumor; the effect of the tumor and/or the therapy on the general condition of the patient and the integrity of his organs, especially bone marrow, immune system, liver, and kidneys. Finally, it is important to take into consideration any prior therapy and the patient's response to it, so as to avoid prescribing drugs that are ineffective or to which he has developed resistance.

A. TUMOR SELECTIVITY

Experience has taught us that the different chemotherapeutic agents have some degree of tissue selectivity but not, unfortunately, any selectivity with respect to malignant cells (see p. 121). Table 7-1 lists the principal malignancies and the agents that have been found effective in treating them, listed roughly in decreasing order of effectiveness. This classification is relative, as not all drugs have been tested in each of these malignancies (132, 156) and most of the reported data are based on trials without controls. We would like to point out the selectivity of sex hormones for prostate, breast, and endometrial carcinoma (organs normally influenced by these hormones), and of corticosteroids for lymphoid tissue. Since o, p' DDD interferes with the synthesis of corticosteroids, it is not surprising that its antitumor

Table 7-1. Selection of effective cytotoxic agents for various malignancies

Acute lymphoid leukemia	1. Prednisone, vincristine, adriamycin or daunorubicin, methotrexate, 6-mercaptopurine, L-asparaginase, cytosine arabinoside 2. Cyclophosphamide
Acute myeloid leukemia	1. Cytosine arabinoside, adriamycin or daunorubicin, 6-thioguanine 2. Methyl-GAG, methotrexate, 6-mercaptopurine, L-asparaginase, cyclophosphamide
Acute monocytoid leukemia	VP 16-213
Chronic myeloid leukemia	1. Busulfan 2. Hydroxyurea, dibromomannitol 3. Pipobroman, piposulfan, 6-mercaptopurine
Polycythemia vera (Vaquez)	1. ^{32}P, busulfan, chlorambucil, cyclophosphamide, melphalan 2. Pipobroman, piposulfan, hydroxyurea, dibromomannitol, dibromodulcitol
Myelosclerosis with myeloid metaplasia	1. ^{32}P, busulfan, chlorambucil 2. Androgens, corticosteroids
Chronic lymphoid leukemia	1. Chlorambucil 2. Cyclophosphamide, mitoclomine, prednisone
Myeloma	1. Melphalan, cyclophosphamide 2. Prednisone 3. Procarbazine, nitrosoureas, adriamycin, vincristine
Macroglobulinemia	1. Chlorambucil, cyclophosphamide, melphalan 2. Prednisone
Hodgkin's disease	1. Procarbazine, vinblastine, nitrogen mustard, chlorambucil, cyclophosphamide 2. Prednisone, vincristine (in combination), CCNU, BCNU, adriamycin, bleomycin, VM-26, VP 16-213 3. Piposulfan, rufochromomycin, imidazole carboxamide, streptonigrin, dibromodulcitol
Non-Hodgkin lymphoma (lymphosarcoma, reticulosarcoma)	1. Cyclophosphamide, chlorambucil, vincristine, prednisone 2. Adriamycin, vinblastine, bleomycin, nitrosoureas, VM-26, procarbazine, L-asparaginase (lymphosarcoma)
Burkitt's tumor	1. Cyclophosphamide 2. Methotrexate, vincristine, cytosine arabinoside
Mycosis fungoides	1. Nitrogen mustard (topical, systemic) 2. Cyclophosphamide, BCNU, methotrexate, bleomycin, vinblastine, prednisone
Histiocytosis-X	Cyclophosphamide, vincristine, vinblastine, corticosteroids, daunorubicin, methotrexate, 6-mercaptopurine

Table 7-1. (continued)

Skin cancer	Bleomycin, topical 5-fluorouracil
Malignant melanoma	1. Imidazole carboxamide 2. Nitrosoureas, hydroxyurea, actinomycin D, dibromodulcitol, vincristine, vinblastine, procarbazine, bleomycin, cyclophosphamide
Cancer of the head and neck	1. Methotrexate, bleomycin 2. Hydroxyurea, cyclophosphamide, vinblastine, 5-fluorouracil, adriamycin, mitomycin C, nitrosoureas
Lung cancer	1. Cyclophosphamide, nitrogen mustard, methotrexate, adriamycin, hexamethylmelamine 2. Nitrosoureas, mitomycin C, hydroxyurea, procarbazine, dibromodulcitol
Cancer of the esophagus	Bleomycin, methotrexate, methyl-GAG
Cancer of the stomach	5-Fluorouracil, mitomycin C, BCNU, adriamycin
Cancer of the colon and rectum	5-Fluorouracil, mitomycin C, nitrosoureas, cyclophosphamide
Cancer of the pancreas	5-Fluorouracil, mitomycin C, streptozotocin
Primary cancer of the liver	5-Fluorouracil, adriamycin
Breast cancer	1. Adriamycin, methotrexate, cyclophosphamide, 5-fluorouracil, vincristine 2. Other alkylating agents, vinblastine, mitomycin C, nitrosoureas, hexamethylmelamine, dibromodulcitol
	1. Estrogens, tamoxifene 2. Androgens, corticosteroids 3. Progestins
Cancer of the ovary	1. Alkylating agents: chlorambucil, thio-TEPA, melphalan, cyclophosphamide 2. 5-Fluorouracil, adriamycin, methotrexate, actinomycin D, mitomycin C, hexamethylmelamine, vinblastine, procarbazine
Cancer of the endometrium	1. Progestins 2. Alkylating agents, 5-fluorouracil, hexamethylmelamine, adriamycin, hydroxyurea
Cancer of the cervix	Methotrexate, alkylating agents (chlorambucil, cyclophosphamide), hexamethylmelamine, vincristine, 5-fluorouracil, bleomycin, mitomycin C, adriamycin
Cancer of the vulva	Bleomycin
Gynecologic sarcomas	5-Fluorouracil, adriamycin

Table 7-1. (continued)

Trophoblastic disease	1. Methotrexate, actinomycin D 2. 6-Mercaptopurine, vinblastine, alkylating agents
Testicular cancers	1. Actinomycin D, vinblastine, bleomycin, alkylating agents (melphalan, chlorambucil, cyclophosphamide) 2. Adriamycin, vincristine, cis-diamminodichloroplatinum
Seminoma	Alkylating agents
Embryonal cell carcinoma	Mithramycin
Teratocarcinoma	Vinblastine (high doses)
Prostate cancer	1. Estrogens 2. Progestins, corticosteroids, Estracyt 3. Cyclophosphamide, 5-fluorouracil, adriamycin, hydroxyurea
Renal cancer	1. Progestins, androgens 2. Hydroxyurea, dibromodulcitol, cyclophosphamide, CCNU, 6-mercaptopurine, vinblastine, 5-fluorouracil
Bladder cancer	Adriamycin, VM-26, mitomycin, bleomycin, 5-fluorouracil
Thyroid carcinoma	1. Thyroid hormones 2. ^{131}I 3. Adriamycin 4. Cyclophosphamide, 5-fluorouracil, bleomycin, VP 16-213
Carcinoma of the cortex	o,p' DDD
Malignant insulinoma	1. Streptozotocin 2. Tubercidin, alkylating agents, 5-fluorouracil
Carcinoid tumors	5-Fluorouracil, cyclophosphamide, streptozotocin, methotrexate, actinomycin D
Brain tumors	1. Nitrosoureas, VM-26, procarbazine 2. Mithramycin, vincristine, methotrexate, vinblastine
Retinoblastoma	1. Alkylating agents 2. Vincristine, actinomycin D
Neuroblastoma	1. Cyclophosphamide 2. Vincristine, adriamycin 3. Actinomycin D, daunorubicin
Wilms' tumor	1. Actinomycin D, vincristine 2. Cyclophosphamide, adriamycin
Osteogenic sarcoma	1. Adriamycin, methotrexate (high dose, with folinic acid rescue) 2. Mitomycin C, alkylating agents, imidazole carboxamide

Table 7-1. (continued)

Ewing's sarcoma	1. Cyclophosphamide, adriamycin, actinomycin D, vincristine 2. Daunorubicin, BCNU
Soft-tissue sarcomas	Adriamycin, cyclophosphamide, vincristine, actinomycin D, imidazole carboxamide, mitomycin C, dibromodulcitol, methotrexate

effect is limited to certain tumors of the adrenal (1). The mitotic poison, vincristine, is useful mainly in malignancies of the lymphoid tissue, while vinblastine is recommended in Hodgkin's disease. Preliminary studies suggest that podophyllotoxin derivatives have an affinity for histiocytic malignancies (2, 3). Adriamycin and actinomycin D - agents that interfere with transcription - demonstrate an antitumor effect against soft-tissue sarcomas, while mithramycin, another drug in the same class, is used almost exclusively in embryonal carcinomas of the testis (4, 5). The selectivity of radiomimetic agents is exemplified by the affinity of procarbazine for Hodgkin's disease, and of bleomycin for epithelial carcinomas and pulmonary metastases (6). Of the group of alkylating agents, chlorambucil is traditionally used to control chronic lymphoid leukemia, while busulfan is capable of rapid normalization of the peripheral white cell count in chronic myeloid leukemia (7). Among the agents that interfere with synthesis, 6-MP and L-asparaginase obtain worthwhile response rates in acute lymphoid leukemia, cytosine arabinoside and thioguanine in acute myeloid leukemia, and 5-FU in gastrointestinal tumors. Malignant melanoma and sarcomas are the only malignancies that respond to DIC used as a single agent (8, 9). The nitrosoureas (BCNU, CCNU, and MeCCNU) are of special interest in primary and secondary tumors of the central nervous system, because they penetrate the blood-brain barrier (10). We have already mentioned that the glucosamine carrier of streptozotocin may account for its specificity for the β cells of the pancreas and for its activity in insulinomas (11).

This selectivity is not as real as may at first appear. Some drugs seem to be specific because they are virtually inactive outside the one malignancy in which they elicit responses, for example 6-MP in ALL. 5-FU is generally recommended as the drug of choice for gastrointestinal tumors, and more recently DIC for malignant melanoma, though neither treatment gives a response rate of over 20 percent; but then, no better drugs are known for these conditions.

The reputation for specificity of some other drugs is more the result of tradition than of fact. For example, melphalan is traditionally used for the treatment of myeloma, though cyclophosphamide is just as effective (12).

Finally, some reputed specificities stem from limited explorations of the tumor spectrum of the drug in question. For instance, methotrexate was for years thought to be specific for ALL, and it was not until other treatment schedules were investigated that its activity was found to extend to a number of solid tumors, thus ending a harmful reputation for selectivity (13, 14).

Despite the above reservations, the data listed in Table 7-1 are an important guide to the selection of the appropriate chemotherapy.

B. TISSUE SELECTIVITY: TOXICITY

Just as malignant tissues seem to demonstrate a degree, however relative, of selective sensitivity to various cytotoxic drugs, so do the normal tissues and organs of the host. This sensitivity is expressed in a variety of toxic manifestations associated with different classes of drugs used in cancer chemotherapy (Table 7-2).

Cytotoxic agents do not act specifically on tumor cells, they affect all cells of the host, especially those of rapidly proliferating tissues, that is bone marrow, lymphoid system, oral, gastrointestinal epithelium, skin, hair roots, germinal epithelium of the gonads, and embryonic structures. Toxic effects on these tissues and organs must be expected in cancer chemotherapy.

A number of side-effects are common to most antitumor agents. Bone marrow hypoplasia or aplasia is the most serious complication, and is caused by all cytotoxic drugs with the exception of bleomycin, vincristine (in the doses used), and hormones. Myelosuppression is usually dose-related and is especially common with alkylating agents, daunorubicin, adriamycin and agents that interfere with synthesis (purine and pyrimidine analogs). Bone marrow toxicity is usually first manifested in leukopenia. Two patterns of marrow recovery are observed (15). Following cyclophosphamide, methotrexate, 5-fluorouracil, cytosine arabinoside, adriamycin, and vinblastine, the leukocyte count falls to a nadir at about the 8th to the 10th day of treatment and returns to normal within 17 to 21 days (Fig. 7-1). Following the nitrosoureas and melphalan, the leukocyte count falls in two waves, reaching the minimum value at about the 4th week.

This dual pattern of marrow recovery, rapid or delayed, has to be taken into consideration in determining the interval between two treatments. Busulfan and melphalan in particular have caused delayed and irreversible bone marrow aplasias (16). The different hematopoietic cell lines may show some degree of selective sensitivity. For example, among the alkylating agents, cyclophosphamide is relatively platelet-sparing, while busulfan produces first a granulocytopenia and mitoclomine a lymphocytopenia (17).

Anorexia, nausea, and vomiting are frequent gastrointestinal symptoms. Stomatitis is especially common with methotrexate, 5-FU, daunorubicin, adriamycin, mitomycin, and actinomycin D; also diarrhea with 5-FU therapy. Patients on vincristine, adriamycin, cyclophosphamide, procarbazine and many other drugs are frequently bothered by alopecia. The use of a headband can often prevent hair loss (133), however, by using an inflated tourniquet at a pressure of 240 mm Hg for 20 min after injection of adriamycin we have been rarely able to prevent significant hair loss (134). All chemotherapy results in immunosuppression, especially prolonged daily treatment (see p. 117) with, in particular, 6-MP, cyclophosphamide, mitoclomine, L-asparaginase, and corticosteroids. Intermittent chemotherapy has a greater effect on circulating antibody response as compared to continuous treatment which has a relatively greater effect on cellular immunity.

Since chemotherapeutic agents interfere with cellular metabolism and proliferation, it is to be anticipated that they will interfere with fertility and fetal development. Male patients on chemotherapy may have low sperm counts or aspermia, while women may suffer menstrual irregularities, endometrial hypoplasia, amenorrhea, damage to ovaries, and decreased incidence of pregnancy (18-25).

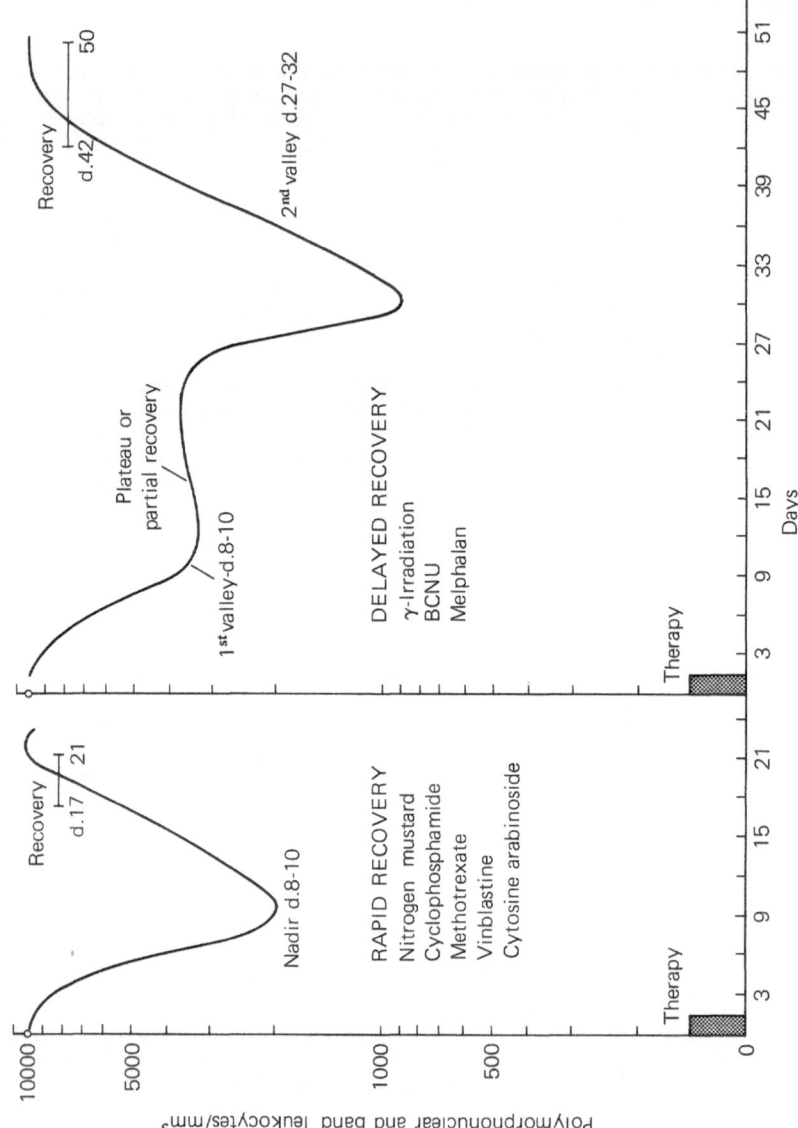

Fig. 7-1. Two patterns of bone marrow recovery, rapid and delayed, following the administration of chemotherapeutic agents. (From D.E. BERGSAGEL (15))

Table 7-2. Toxic effects of chemotherapeutic agents, classified by organ or tissue affected

Tissue or organ	Drugs
Hematopoietic tissue (Bone marrow and peripheral blood)	All drugs except vincristine (at usual doses), bleomycin and steroid hormones. Cyclophosphamide is relatively platelet-sparing
total aplasia	Busulfan, melphalan, daunorubicin, adriamycin
leukopenia (predominantly)	Cyclophosphamide
thrombocytopenia (predominantly)	Mitomycin C
granulocytopenia (predominantly)	Busulfan
lymphopenia (predominantly)	Chlorambucil, mitoclomine
Immunocompetent cells	All agents, especially in high dosages and prolonged daily therapy. In particular: 6-mercaptopurine, cyclophosphamide, mitoclomine, L-asparaginase, corticosteroids
Gastrointestinal tract	
nausea and vomiting	Through central action: alkylating agents, nitrosoureas, daunorubicin, adriamycin, methotrexate, imidazole carboxamide, cytosine arabinoside, L-asparaginase, etc. Most agents administered orally
ulceration of mucous membranes	Methotrexate, 5-fluorouracil, cytosine arabinoside, daunorubicin, adriamycin, actinomycin D, bleomycin[1], streptonigrin, mitomycin C[1], hydroxyurea
diarrhea	5-Fluorouracil, methotrexate, cytosine arabinoside, 5 azacytidine, streptozotocin, methyl-GAG, mitoclomine, piposulfan, actinomycin D
constipation, paralytic ileus	Vincristine (137)
Liver	Methotrexate[1] (62, 63), 6-mercaptopurine (1) (64), L-asparaginase (52-54), glucocorticosteroids, BCNU[1], streptozotocin (11), mithramycin (56), busulfan[1] (65).
Pancreas	
pancreatitis	L-asparaginase[1] (55, 138)
destruction of islets of Langerhans	Streptozotocin (11)
Bladder	
cystitis	Cyclophosphamide (41-44)
atony	Vincristine[2] (66)

(1) These agents produce the corresponding toxicity in only a minority of patients (generally less than 10%)
(2) Toxic manifestations have been described in exceptional cases.

Table 7-2. (continued)

Tissues or organ	Drugs
Kidneys	Methotrexate[1] ([67]), streptozotocin ([11], [90]), BCNU[1], mithramycin ([56]), mitomycin C[1] ([68]), L-asparaginase ([52], [53]), methoxyellipticine, isophosphamide[1], cis-diamminodichloroplatinum ([140])
Lungs fibrosis	Busulfan[1] ([46-49]), cyclophosphamide[2] ([69]), bleomycin[1] ([45])
allergic reaction	Methotrexate ([50])
Heart	Daunorubicin[1] ([36], [37], [141]), adriamycin[1] ([38-40]), cyclophosphamide[2] (at very high doses) ([70])
Arteries occlusions	Mithramycin[2] ([142])
cardiovascular accidents	Estrogens[1]
Skin and adnexae sclerosis, hyperkeratosis, necrosis	Bleomycin ([51])
atrophy, panniculitis	Corticosteroids[1] ([71])
hyperpigmentation	Bleomycin, busulfan, 5-FU[1], methotrexate[1], adriamycin[2] ([143], [144])
bulbous eruption	Busulfan[2] ([72])
allergic reactions	Rare; can occur with any drug, especially L-asparaginase
erythema of irradiated areas	Actinomycin D
folliculitis	Actinomycin D ([73])
alopecia	Almost all cytotoxic agents, especially cyclophosphamide, adriamycin, actinomycin D, mitomycin C, vincristine, vinblastine
facial rash ("racoon" rash)	Mithramycin ([56])
phototoxicity	Nafoxidine ([74])
Nervous system paresthesias, loss of reflexes, paresis	Vincristine ([34], [35], [86], [145], [146]), procarbazine[1], vinblastine[1] ([75])
paraplegia	Methotrexate[2] and cytosine arabinoside[2] intrathecally ([76])
somnolence, coma	L-Asparaginase ([52], [53]), nitrogen mustard[2] ([77]), procarbazine[1] ([146])
psychic disturbances	Corticosteroids[1], procarbazine[1], L-asparaginase ([52], [53]), methyl-GAG, BCNU
cerebellar ataxia	5-Fluorouracil[1] ([79], [80], [81])
orthostatic hypotension	Vincristine[2] ([87], [145]), procarbazine[2] ([146])
deafness for high frequencies	Platinum derivatives
Eye cataracts	Corticosteroids[1], busulfan[2] dibromomannitol[2] ([88])

Table 7-2). continued

Tissues or organ	Drugs
Coagulation abnormalities	L-Asparaginase ([52](#), [53](#)), mithramycin ([56](#))
Endocrine system and metabolism	
hypoglycemia	Methyl-GAG[1] ([89](#))
hyperglycemia	L-Asparaginase ([55](#)), corticosteroids, streptozotocin
hypocalcemia	Mithramycin ([57](#))
hyponatremia	Vincristine[2] ([145](#))
water intoxication	Cyclophosphamide[2] ([82](#))
alcohol intolerance	Procarbazine
pseudoaddisonism	Busulfan[2] ([83](#))
pituitary insufficiency	Busulfan[2] ([84](#))
Cushing's syndrome	Corticosteroids ([58](#))
masculinization	Androgens
feminization	Estrogens
osteoporosis	Corticosteroids, methotrexate ([85](#))
amenorrhea	Alkylating agents, especially busulfan, chlorambucil, cyclophosphamide ([20-25](#))
azoospermia	idem
Fetal abnormalities	
miscarriage	Most agents in animal experiments. In man: busulfan[2], chlorambucil[2], cyclophosphamide[2], methotrexate[2], corticosteroids[2] ([18, 19, 26](#))
Mutagenesis, carcinogenesis	Most agents in animal experiments. In man: busulfan[2], melphalan[2] and other alkylating agents (acute leukemia) ([27-33](#), [150](#)) cyclophosphamide (bladder cancer) ([152](#))
Other side-effects:	
febrile response	Bleomycin ([51](#)), L-asparaginase ([52, 53](#)), cytosine arabinoside ([86](#)), mithramycin ([4, 56](#)), actinomycin D; exceptionally, with many drugs
flu-like illness	Imidazole carboxamide ([91](#)), cytosine arabinoside ([92](#))
Anaphylactic reaction	L-Asparaginase, bleomycin

Many experimental studies have demonstrated the toxicity of antitumor agents upon the fetus ([18, 19, 26](#)). In humans, only isolated reports are available for most of the agents. It appears that these agents may induce abortion if used early in its course, and fetal anomalies during the critical first trimester but not thereafter ([18, 19, 26](#)).

Initially, little attention was paid to the possible mutagenic and carcinogenic effects of chemotherapy (Fig. 7-2) ([27, 28, 150, 151](#)). Now that long survival is becoming an increasing reality, this aspect of chemotherapy must be looked at more carefully ([135](#)). It is with concern that we read an increasing number of reports of secondary malignancies and leukemias, especially in patients with Hodgkin's disease, multiple myeloma, and other tumors treated by radiotherapy and/or chemotherapy ([29-33, 136](#)). Cyclophosphamide has been implicated in the carcinogenesis of bladder tumors ([152](#)).

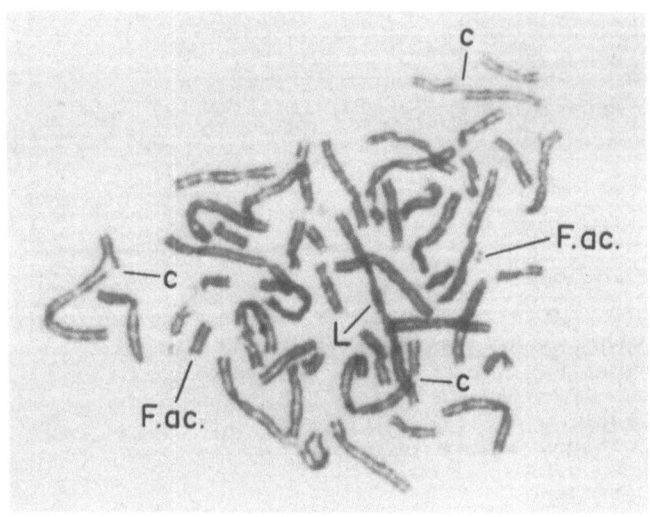

Fig. 7-2. Chromosome abnormalities induced by daunorubicin (Photograph provided by J. DE GROUCHY). F.ac: acentric fragment, c: break, L: long chromosome

Some drugs have in addition more specific toxicity (listed in Table 7-2) that may affect the nervous system, liver,kidneys, bladder, pancreas, lungs, heart, or hemostasis. Among the more common effects are the neurotoxicity of vincristine (34, 35), the cardiac toxicity of daunorubicin (36, 37), adriamycin (Fig. 7-3), (38-40, 153), the hemorrhagic cystitis due to cyclophosphamide (41-44), the pulmonary toxicity of bleomycin (45), busulfan (46-49), and methotrexate (50) (Fig. 7-4), and skin manifestations with bleomycin (Fig. 7-5) (51). A febrile response occurs in about 50 percent of patients soon after injection of bleo· mycin. Since a large number of proteins are synthesized in the liver, it is not surprising that L-asparaginase is mainly hepatotoxic (52-54). A lowering of albumin, transferrin, fibrinogen, and several other coagulation factors and the cholesterol level in the blood is commonly noted. The alkaline phosphatase and transaminases are often elevated, while liver biopsy reveals steatosis; hyperglycemia and pancreatitis are less common (55). A complex hemorrhagic diathesis is also seen with mithramycin (56); this drug in addition lowers the calcium level and because of this property it has been used to treat the hypercalcemia associated with malignancies and Paget's disease (57). The characteristic side-effects of corticosteroids and sex hormones are well known (58).

Not all complications of chemotherapy are necessarily caused directly by the cytotoxic agents. Hyperuricemia (59) or hyperkalemia (60) may follow the massive destruction of malignant cells. The former occurs especially during the treatment of lymphoid malignancies and can be prevented by allopurinol. Hypercalcemia may be seen shortly after the initiation of hormone therapy for breast cancer with bone metastases. Tumor growth may sometimes be enhanced rather than inhibited in this situation.

Toxic effects are strongly dose-dependent, but other factors are important. Patients who are elderly, debilitated, in poor general condition, or recovering from surgery tolerate chemotherapy less well. The bone

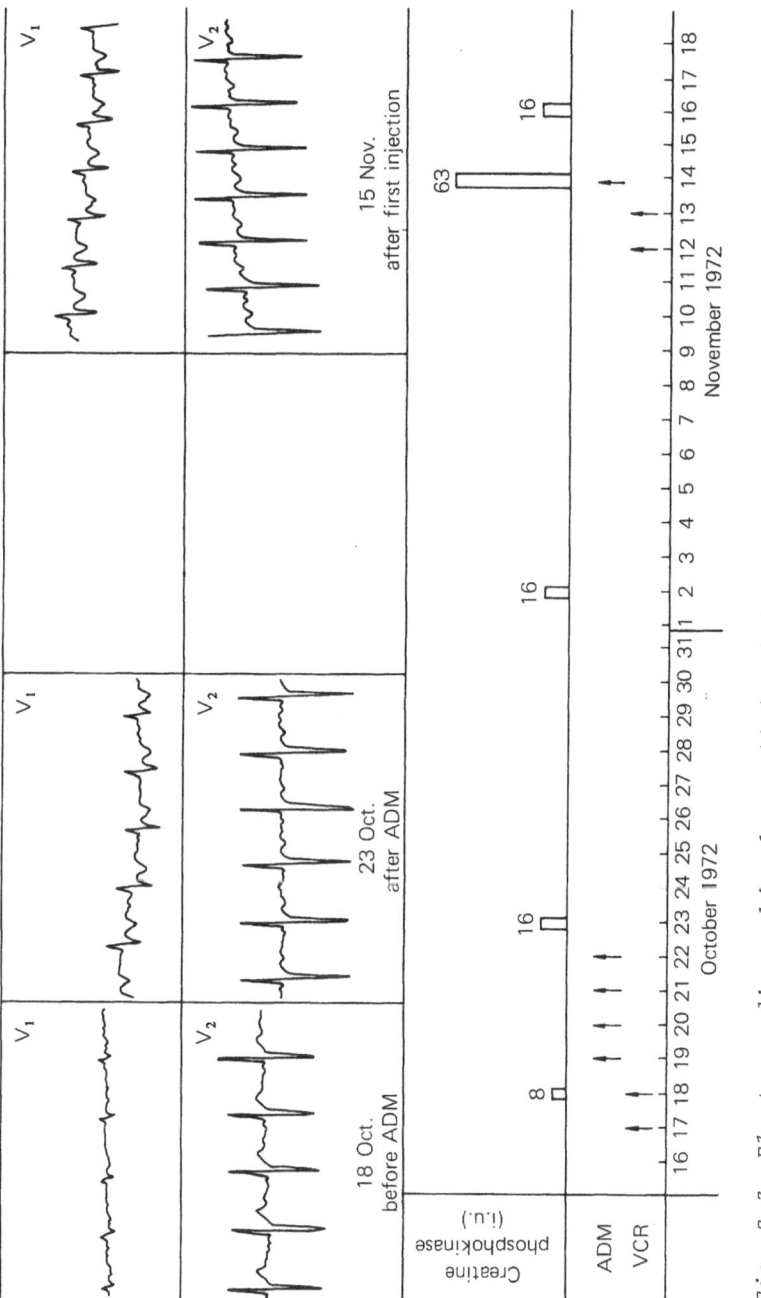

Fig. 7-3. Electrocardiographic abnormalities induced by adriamycin

marrow reserve may be reduced as a result of prior radiation and chemotherapy or tumor involvement. This too must be taken into consideration
when determining the drug dose. The integrity of liver and kidney function is important, especially if the drugs used are activated, metabolized, or excreted via these organs. Again, the function of the organs

may be altered by tumor infiltration (61), mechanical obstruction by tumor masses, prior therapy or, in the case of the kidney, by complicating hypercalcemia or hyperuricemia.

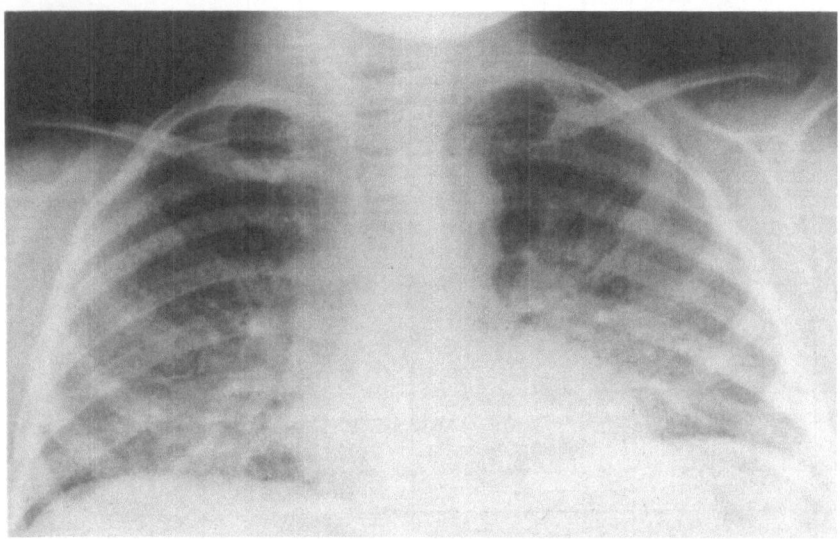

Fig. 7-4. Example of "methotrexate lung", a pulmonary infiltrative disease of undetermined etiology (50)

C. CELL KINETICS AND GROWTH CHARACTERISTICS OF THE TUMOR TO BE TREATED

The selection of a chemotherapy program must take account of the kinetic characteristics of the tumor to be treated and the normal tissues of the host. We have already pointed out that, with the exception of L-asparaginase, chemotherapeutic agents show no biochemical differences upon which to base selective destruction of the tumor-cell population. However, the work of BRUCE has shown that rapidly proliferating cells are more sensitive to both cell-phase- and cell-cycle-dependent drugs than slowly proliferating ones (93), while others have shown that a high percentage of cures can be obtained in the model situation of L1210 leukemia in mice by careful manipulation of the treatment schedule according to kinetic parameters (94). It is a major contribution of the experimental work of cell kinetics that it has taught us that high-dose intermittent therapy is safer than prolonged low-dose, daily therapy. The former not only offers more protection to normal tissues with rapid proliferation, especially the bone marrow and the immuno-competent cells, but at the same time produces a greater antitumor effect for the same total dose (see Chap. 6). It has also taught us to select drugs, cycle-dependent or phase-dependent, alone or in sequence, in accordance with the kinetic parameters of the tumor, especially the growth fraction. In sum, we have learned to administer both classes of agents in a more effective way.

A number of studies show that some of these concepts can be applied effectively in clinical medicine. For instance, methotrexate given intermittently at 30 mg/m^2 twice a week significantly prolonged the duration of remission in ALL compared to a daily dose of 5 mg/m^2, while the toxicity of both schedules was similar (95).

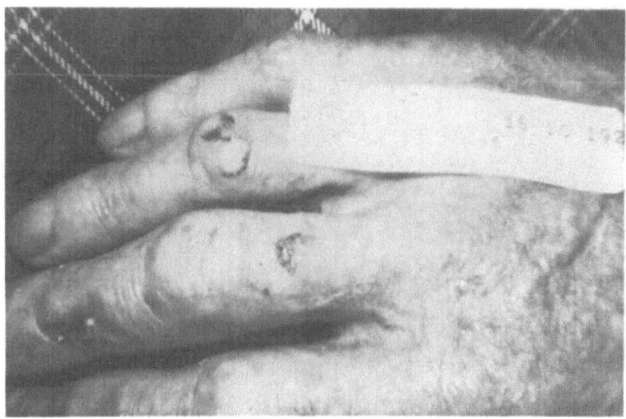

Fig. 7-5. Bleomycin skin toxicity: sclerosis and necrosis

Unfortunately, our knowledge of the kinetics of human tumors is rather superficial. They do not lend themselves to detailed kinetic studies (96). Burkitt's tumor is the only human tumor that resembles the ideal experimental model, in that the majority of the cells are in cycle (97); this is probably the reason for its unusual sensitivity to chemotherapy. Other human tumors are much more heterogeneous with respect to their kinetic parameters (98). Our appreciation of the growth characteristics of human tumors is often based on the clinical rate of progression or the doubling time (which is a very crude estimate if there is significant cell loss), and the morphological features: well-differentiated cells and rare mitotic figures in slow-growing tumors, lack of differentiation and abundant mitoses in fast-growing tumors.

For rapidly growing tumors, a program of intensive intermittent therapy with phase-dependent drugs can be designed, assuming that such tumors have a high growth fraction and a short doubling time. For instance, methotrexate can be given in doses of 75 mg/m^2 every 8 h for 6 doses (2 days), followed after 8 h by folinic acid, 16 injections of 25 mg/m^2 every 6 h to reduce the toxicity (4 days) (13, 147, 154). Further cycles are given once the patient's blood count has recovered, usually one week later. With this schedule serum concentrations can be maintained for 48 h, which kill cells in vitro. Methotrexate affects cells in S phase, so theoretically all cells passing through S phase in the relevant 48 h should be affected. This schedule is thus especially useful in rapidly proliferating tumors (Figs. 7-6 and 7-7). Such tumors can also be treated with high-dose intermittent therapy with cycle-dependent agents. Thus, cyclophosphamide at 40 mg/kg is capable of inducing long-term remissions of Burkitt's tumor, some of which will be cures (99).

D. METHODS TO AUGMENT CELL KILL

In slow-growing tumors, such intensive therapy with a single agent is theoretically less likely to be effective. Few cells are in cycle or sensitive to cycle-dependent drugs, and even fewer will be in a particular phase of the cell cycle to be affected by phase-dependent drugs. Combinations of drugs with different mechanisms of action and affecting different phases of the cell cycle have been used to augment cell kill in slow-growing tumors. They are generally less responsive than rapidly proliferating tumors, yet some encouraging results have been obtained.

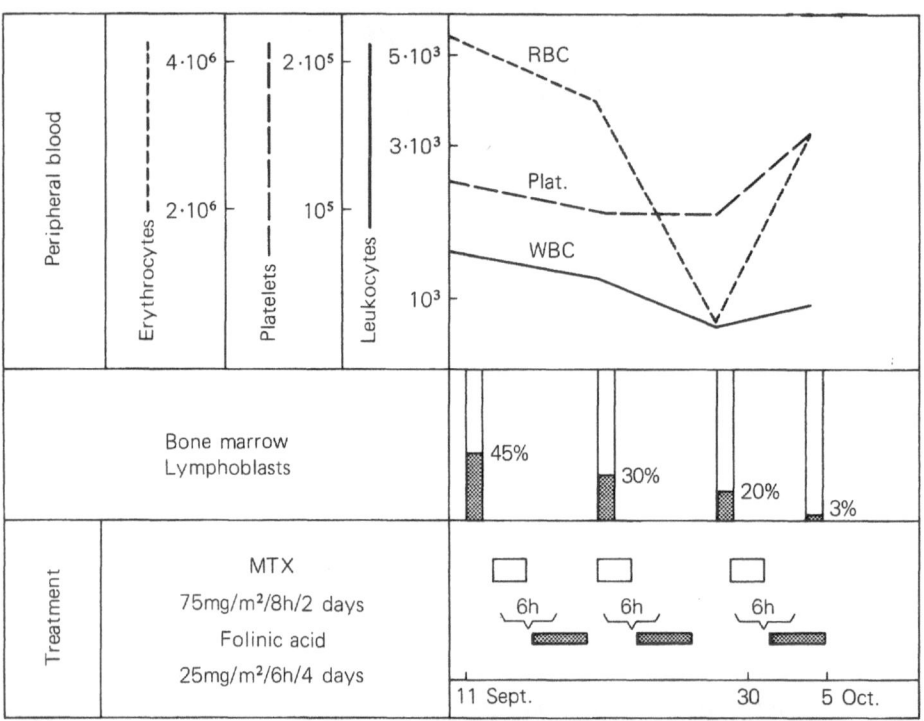

Fig. 7-6. Induction of apparent complete remission by high-dose methotrexate therapy in acute lymphoid leukemia (from SCHWARZENBERG et al. (13))

It is not our intention to review here the value of combination chemotherapy in detail, since several recent articles have already done so (100-111, 148). The more effective ones are discussed in later chapters (Table 7-3).

Application of the concept of recruitment is another approach to slow-growing tumors (see p. 125). Several clinical studies have been carried out with varying degrees of success (112-114). We have studied the effectiveness of synchronization protocols at the Institut de Cancérologie et d'Immunogénétique (ICIG). The principle is outlined on page 124 and the validity of its application has been demonstrated by KLEIN (115).

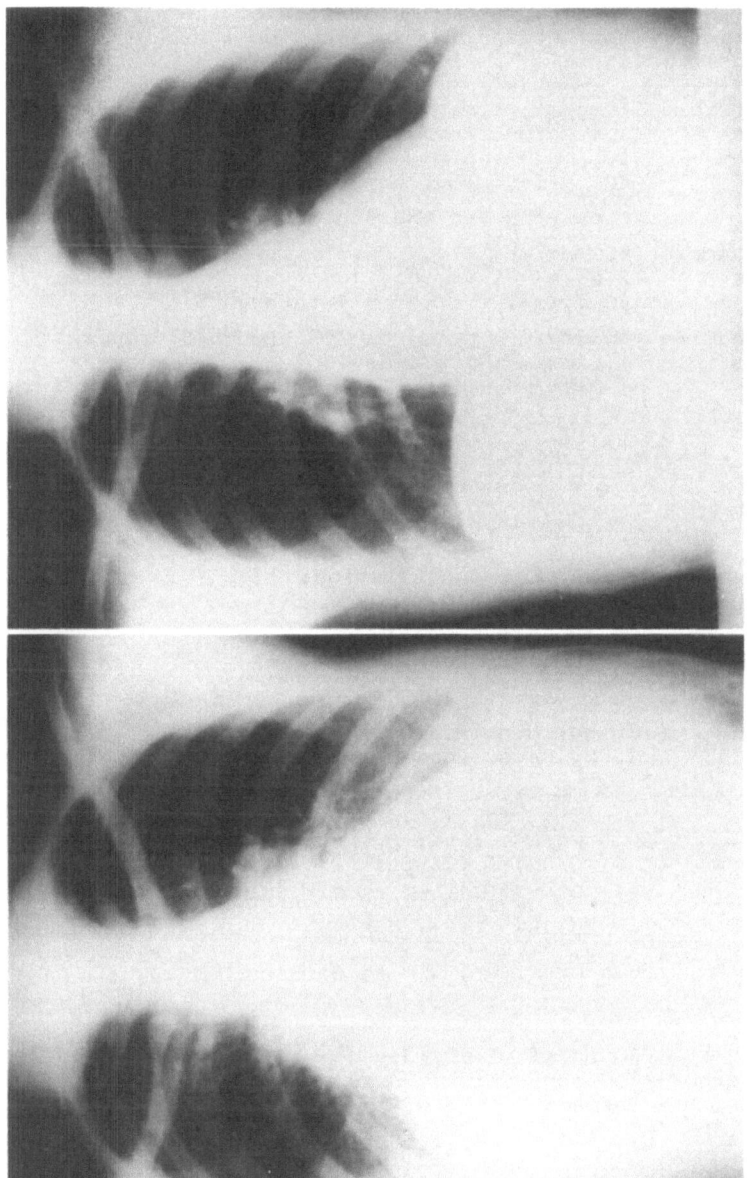

Fig. 7-7. Regression of pulmonary metastases and hepatomegaly in breast cancer following therapy with methotrexate and folinic acid

Our preliminary results have been reported by POUILLART et al. (108-110, 149). Vincristine or EPT (VM26), given on two consecutive days, results in an increase in the mitotic index, followed after about 48 h by an increase in the labeling index with tritiated thymidine, indicating

Table 7-3. Combination chemotherapy. Examples of some of the more frequently used combinations. (not necessarily designed on the basis of
kinetic considerations)

MOPP	Nitrogen mustard	6 mg/m^2, i.v., day 1 and 8	repeat
	Vincristine	1.4 mg/m^2, i.v., day 1 and 8	day 28
	Procarbazine	100 mg/m^2, p.o., day 1 through 14 x 6	
	Prednisone$^+$	40 mg/m^2, p.o., day 1 through 14	
		$^+$ only in 1st and 4th courses	
COP	Cyclophosphamide	800 mg/m^2, i.v., day 1	repeat
	Vincristine	2 mg/m^2, i.v., day 1	day 14
	Prednisone	60 mg/m^2, p.o., day 1 through 5	x 6
CVP	Cyclophosphamide	400 mg/m^2, p.o., day 1 through 5	repeat
	Vincristine	1.4 mg/m^2, i.v., day 1	day 21
	Prednisone	100 mg/m^2, p.o., day 1 through 5	
COOPER	5-Fluorouracil	12 mg/kg, i.v., daily x 4, then	
		500 mg i.v., weekly	
	Methotrexate	25-50 mg, i.v., weekly	
	Vincristine	0.035 mg/kg, i.v., weekly	
	Cyclophosphamide	2.5 mg/kg, p.o., daily	
	Prednisone	0.75 mg/kg, p.o., daily	
		ANSFIELD'S modification:	
	5-Fluorouracil	500 mg, i.v., weekly	
	Methotrexate	25 mg, i.v., weekly	
	Vincristine	1 mg, i.v., weekly	
	Cyclophosphamide	100 mg, p.o., daily	
	Prednisone	45 mg, p.o., daily x 14	
		30 mg, p.o., daily x 14	
		15 mg, p.o., daily	
COMF	Cyclophosphamide	300 mg, i.v., push day 1 and 5	repeat
	Vincristine	0.025 mg/kg, i.v., day 2 and 5	day 21
	Methotrexate	0.5 mg/kg, i.v., push day 1 and 4	
	5-Fluorouracil	10 mg/kg, i.v., push day 1 through 5	
LI	Chlorambucil	12 mg, qd, p.o., day 1 through 9	2 wks bet-
	Methotrexate	10 mg, qd, p.o., day 1 " 9	ween cour-
	Vincristine	2 mg, i.v., " 1 and 9	ses 1 and
	Actinomycin D	0.5 mg, i.v., " 3 through 7	2, then e-
			very 4-5
			weeks
GOTTLIEB	Adriamycin	60 mg/m^2, i.v., day 1	repeat
	Imidazole carbox-	250 mg/m^2, i.v., drip, day 1	day 21
	amide	through 5	
MTX-FA	Methotrexate	75-100 mg/m^2, i.m., or i.v., every	
		8 h for 48 h	
	Folinic acid	5-10 mg/m^2, i.m., (beginning 8 h after MTX)	
		every 8 h for 48 h	
KENIS	CCNU	130 mg/m^2, p.o., every 6 weeks	
	Vincristine	1.4 mg/m^2, i.v., weekly	
	Bleomycin	5-10 mg/m^2, i.v., or i.m.,	
		twice weekly	
MATHE	Cyclophosphamide	300 mg/m^2, i.v., weekly	
	Methotrexate	60 mg/m^2, rapid infusion, weekly	
	Vinblastine	6 mg/m^2, i.v., weekly	
	(Bleomycin)	(15 mg/m^2, i.m. or i.v., weekly)	
	Cyclophosphamide	300 mg/m^2, i.v., weekly	
	Vinblastine	6 mg/m^2, i.v., weekly	
	5-Fluorouracil	600 mg/m^2, i.v., weekly	

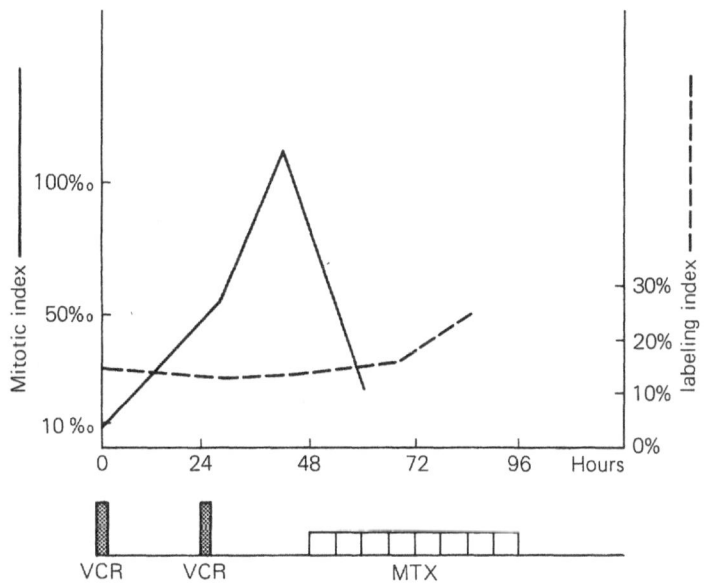

Fig. 7-8. Average mitotic index (MI) and labeling index (LI) in patients with acute lymphoid leukemia during treatment with vincristine (VCR) followed by methotrexate (MTX). The mitotic index increases following treatment with VCR, indicating arrest of cells in mitosis. This is followed by an increase in LI. (From POUILLART et al. (108))

partial synchronization of the cells that have not been killed by the mitotic poison (Fig. 7-8) (108, 109). One of a number of agents can then be selected, depending on the sensitivity of the tumors to be treated, for administration over 2 to 5 days to kill the partially synchronized cells. This is called the executor drug.

Table 7-4 lists a series of synchronization protocols that have been evaluated at the ICIG. Intermittent cycles of chemotherapy are given. Each cycle consists of 2 days of vincristine or VM-26 followed by 2 to 5 days of the executor drug. Cycles are repeated only after recovery of the bone marrow (Fig. 7-9). The approximate drug-free intervals required for such restoration are indicated in Table 7-4.

Table 7-4. Chemotherapy protocols based on synchronization with M-phase dependent agents

1. Dosages in mg/m^2 for executor drugs used as single agents:

Synchronizing agent (M-phase dependent)		Executor drugs[a]					Intervals (days)
Days 1	2	3	4	5	6	7	
VCR 1 mg	VCR 1 mg	CPM 400 mg	CPM 400 mg	CPM 400 mg	CPM 400 mg		17
	or						
EPT 60 mg	EPT 60 mg	5-FU 600 mg	5-FU 600 mg	5-FU 600 mg	5-FU 600mg		10

Table 7-4. (continued)

Synchronizing agent (M-phase dependent)	Executor drugs[a]					Intervals (days)
Days 1 2	3	4	5	6	7	
EPT is used when VCR is contraindicated or when its maximal dose has been reached, or for certain tumors that are especially sensitive to podophyllotoxin derivatives (e.g., bladder, reticulosarcoma) or for particular localizations (e.g., serous cavities, brain)	ADM 7 mg	ADM 7 mg	ADM 7 mg	ADM 7 mg		14
	MTX 15 mg/ 6 h	MTX 15 mg/ 6 h				10
	ACD 0.3 mg	ACD 0.3 mg	ACD 0.3 mg	ACD 0.3 mg		14
	PCZ 150 mg	PCZ 150 mg	PCZ 150 mg	PCZ 150 mg		10
	BNCU 70 mg	BNCU 70 mg				21
	CCNU 130 mg	CCNU 130 mg	CAR	CAR		21
	CAR 100 mg/ 12 h	CAR 100 mg/ 12 h	CAR 100 mg/ 12 h	CAR 100 mg/ 12 h		14
	MTC 5 mg	MTC 5 mg	MTC 5 mg	MTC 5 mg		21
	DIC 300 mg	DIC 300mg	DIC 300 mg	DIC 300 mg		21
			BLM 10 mg	BLM 10 mg		7
			AND[b]	AND	AND	
			EST[b]	EST	EST	
			PRO[b]	PRO	PRO	
			PDN 50 mg	PDN 50 mg	PDN 50 mg	

2. Combinations and indications:

Tumor or site	Synchronizing agent (M-phase dependent)		Executor drugs					Intervals (days)
Days	1	2	3	4	5	6	7	
Head and neck	VCR[c,d]	VCR[c]	MTX	MTX	FA BLM	FA BLM	(50 mg)	14
Esophagus	VCR[c]	VCR[c]	CPM	CPM	CPM BLM	CPM BLM		17
Gastrointestinal adenocarcinomas	VCR[c]	VCR[c]	FU MTC	FU MTC	FU MTC	FU MTC		21
Lung	VCR[c]	VCR[c]	CPM MTX	CPM MTX	CPM	CPM		21

148

Table 7-4. (continued)

Tumor or site	Synchronizing agent (M-phase dependent)		Executor drugs					Intervals (days)
Days	1	2	3	4	5	6	7	
Melanoma	VCR[c]	VCR[c]	DIC BCNU	DIC BCNU	DIC BLM	DIC BLM		21
Breast	VCR[c]	VCR[c]	CPM MTX	CPM MTX or PRO or EST and/or PDN	CPM AND PRO EST PDN	CPM AND PRO EST PDN	AND PRO EST PDN	21
Ovary	VCR[c]	VCR[c]	CPM MTX	CPM MTX	CPM	CPM		21
Cervix	VCR[c]	VCR[c]	CPM MTX	CPM MTX	CPM	CPM		21
Endometrium	VCR[c]	VCR[c]	CPM MTX	CPM MTX	CPM PRO	CPM PRO	PRO	21
Prostate	VCR[c]	VCR[c]	FU ADM	FU ADM[e]	FU EST	FU EST	EST	21
Testis	VCR[c]	VCR[c]	ACD CPM	ACD CPM	ACD (BLM	ACD BLM[f])		21
Kidney	VCR[c]	VCR[c]	BCNU	BCNU	PRO	PRO	PRO	21
Bladder	EPT	EPT	ADM	ADM	ADM	ADM		14
Brain	EPT	EPT	BCNU	BCNU				21
Sarcomas	VCR[c]	VCR[c]	ACD or ADM CPM	ACD ADM CPM	ACD ADM CPM	ACD ADM CPM	ACD	21
Acute lymphoid leukemia	VCR[c]	VCR[c]	ADM or MTX or CPM or CAR	ADM MTX CPM CAR	ADM CPM CAR ±/PDN	ADM CPM CAR PDN	PDN	
Acute myeloid leukemia	VCR[c]	VCR[c]	ADM or CAR	ADM CAR	ADM CAR	ADM CAR		
Lymphosarcoma	VCR[c]	VCR[c]	CPM	CPM	CPM PDN	CPM PDN	PDN	17
Reticulosarcoma	EPT	EPT	CPM	CPM	CPM PDN	CPM PDN	PDN	17
Hodgkin's disease	VCR[c]	VCR[c]	PCZ	PCZ	PCZ (PDN	PCZ PDN	PCZ PDN)	14

[a] see Table 3-2 for abbreviations
[b] AND = androgen preparation, PRO = progestin, EST = estrogen

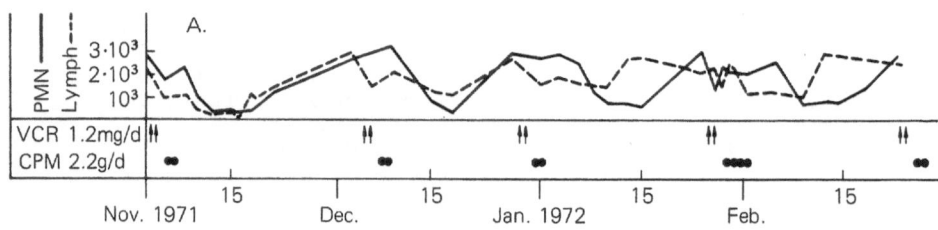

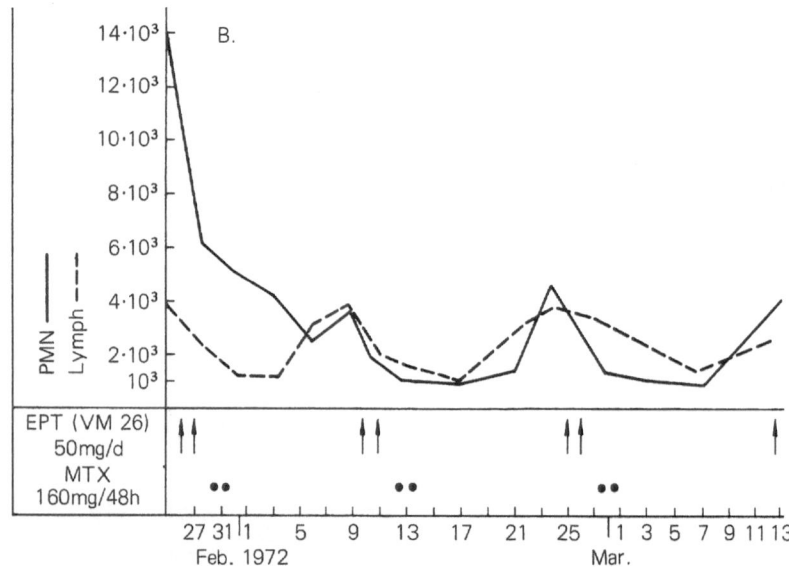

Fig. 7-9. Examples of the intervals between cycles for different synchronization protocols. A: vincristine (VCR) and cyclophosphamide (CPM), B: VM-26 and methotrexate (MTX)

Figs. 7-10 and 7-11 illustrate some responses that have been obtained with our synchronization protocols. It is noteworthy that tumor regressions have been observed in patients who had become resistant to both the synchronizing and the executor drug when used in a nonsynchronizing manner (Figs. 7-12 and 7-13).

Mitotic poisons are not the only drugs that can achieve cell synchronization. Cells can be synchronized in S phase, both in vitro and in vivo, by certain S-phase-dependent drugs (CAR, HUR) (116-119).

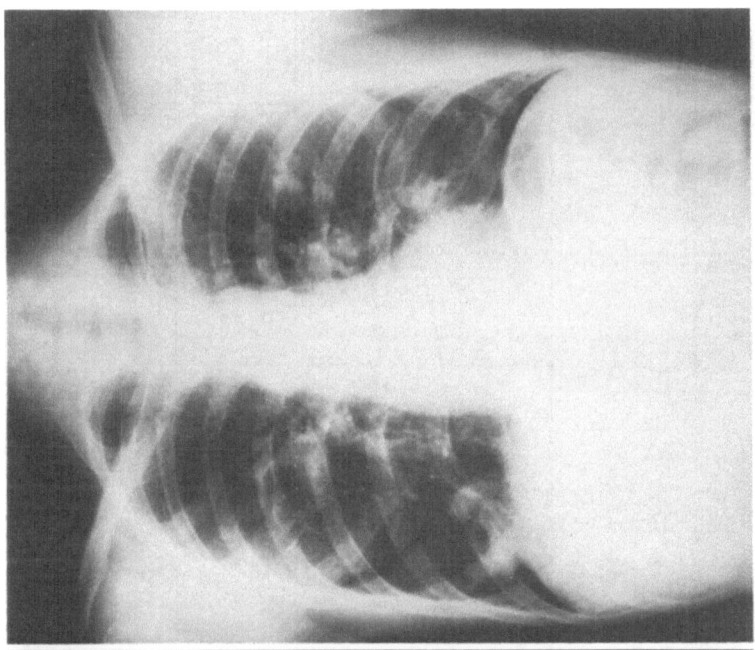

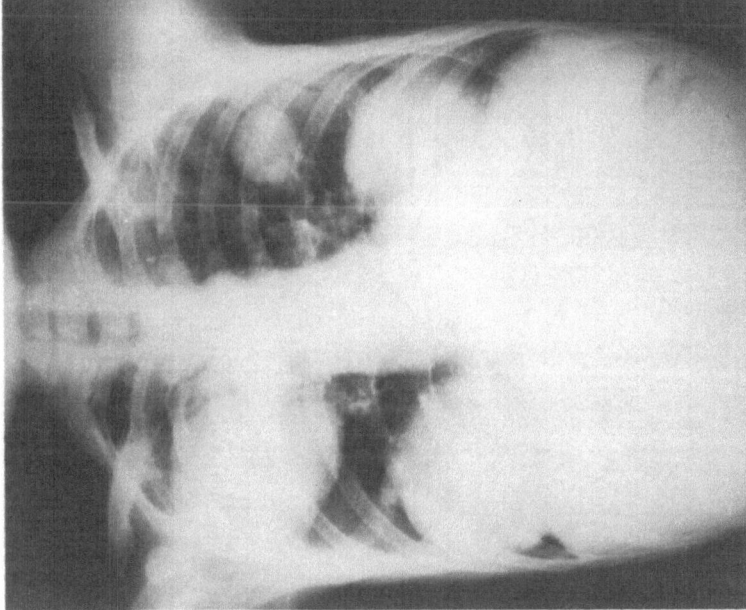

Fig. 7-10. Testicular choriocarcinoma: pulmonary metastases before and after 5 cycles of a synchronization protocol with vincristine and bleomycin

BERGSAGEL has proposed a synchronization protocol for myeloma with each cycle made up of melphalan 5 mg/m^2 daily and prednisone 20 mg/m^2 daily, both given orally for 6 days; vincristine 1 mg/m^2, i.v., on day 10 and cyclophosphamide 400 mg, i.v., on day 11. The drug-free interval between cycles is 6 weeks ([120]).

Cell kill can also be augmented in combinations by potentiation of the cytotoxic effect (see p. 122). Finally, it is possible to design com-

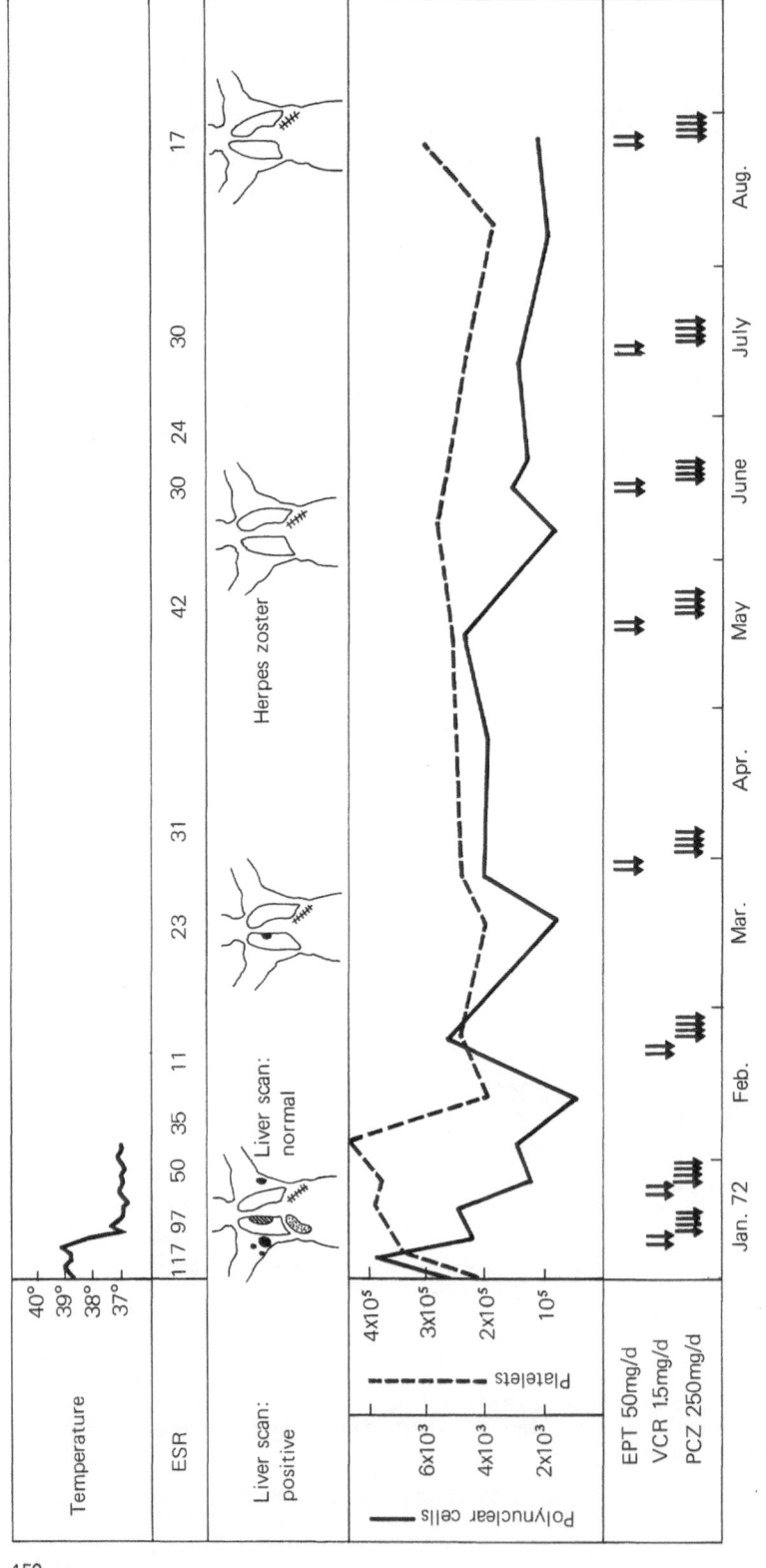

Fig. 7-11. Hodgkin's disease, Stage IV: complete remission with a synchronization protocol with vincristine and procarbazine. Vincristine was later replaced by EPT or VM-26 because of neurotoxicity

Table 7-5. Potentiation by sequential administration of two drugs (From POUILLART et al. (121)). A = potentiation or synergistic effect; B = effect less than category A but more effective than the most active agent used single; C = effect less than category A or B. A preliminary injection of vincristine (VCR) potentiates the action of cyclophosphamide (CPM), methotrexate (MTX), mitomycin C (MTC) and 5-fluorouracil (5-FU). VM-26 potentiates CPM and MTC. A synergistic effect is also obtained by CPM and CCNU and a subsequent injection of 5-FU

Second Drug

Second Drug	VCR 0.075 mg/kg	VM 26 45 mg/kg	CPM 150 mg/kg						MTX 25 mg/kg					ADC 1.65 mg/kg				MTC 0.825 mg/kg	5-FU 100 mg/kg	CARC 100 mg/kg	BCNU 2 mg/kg	CCNU 25 mg/kg
			0	8 h	24 h	40 h	48 h	72 h	0	8 h	24 h	40 h	48 h	0	8 h	24 h	48 h	24 h	24 h	24 h	24 h	24 h
VCR 0.075 mg/kg			B	A $p<0.05$	A $p<0.001$	A $p<0.01$	A	B	B	A $p<0.05$	A $p<0.05$	A $p<0.05$	A	C	C	C	C	A $p<0.02$	A $p<0.05$	B	C	?
VM 26				A $p<0.05$									B				C	A $p<0.01$	B			?
ACD													C									
CPM	A $p<0.2$																		A			
CCNU																			A			

153

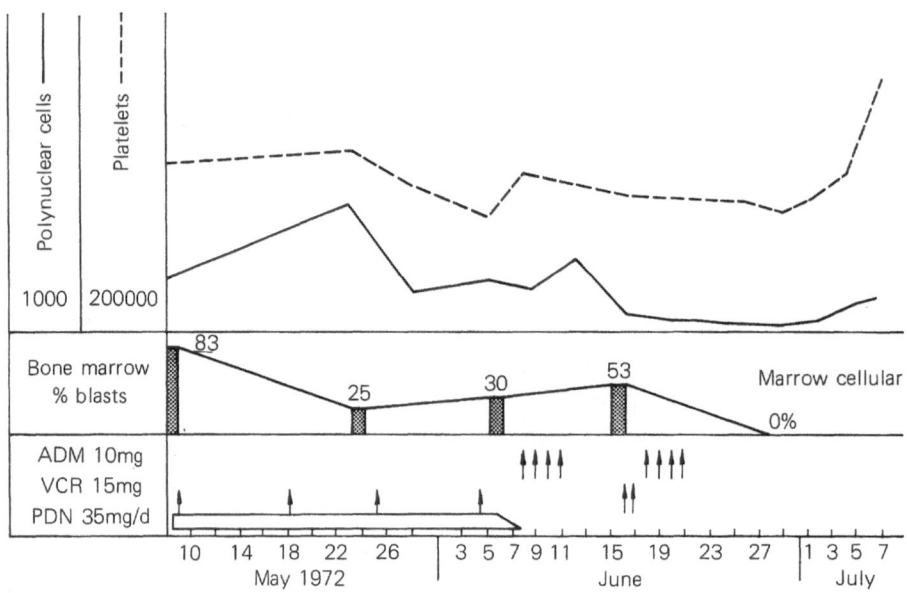

Fig. 7-12. Acute lymphoid leukemia in fourth perceptible phase resistant to vincristine (VCR) and to adriamycin (ADM) but sensitive to the combination of VCR plus ADM in a synchronization protocol

binations that exploit simultaneously phenomena of selective tumor sensitivity, selective toxicity, synchronization, and potentiation. Our knowledge of the latter phenomenon is still fragmentary. Table 7-5 shows some of the results obtained by POUILLART et al. at the ICIG (121). According to these data, and taking into consideration selective tumor sensitivity, selective toxicity and synchronization, we have designed several clinical protocols (Table 7-6). Our preliminary results for tumors, treated in adequate numbers to permit evaluation, demonstrate the therapeutic value of this approach (Table 7-7) (122, 155).

These are only a few of the combinations that can be worked out on the basis of cell kinetics. We have discussed them to exemplify the attempt to make a logical selection of drugs and schedules rather than a haphazard one, as has so often been the case (123).

Though kinetic studies have been of value in designing more rational and therefore, hopefully, more effective treatment programs, their im-

Table 7-6. Combinations based on selective tumor sensitivity, selective toxicity, synchronization, and potentiation. (POUILLART et al. (122))
VCR = 1 mg/m^2/day; VM-26 = 60 mg/m^2/day; CPM = 300 mg/m^2/day; 5-FU = 500 mg/m^2/day; CCNU = 60 mg/m^2/day

Day	1	2	3	4	5	6	Tumor site	Interval (days)
	VCR,	VCR,	CPM,	CPM,	CPM,	CPM		
			5-FU,	5-FU,	5-FU,	5-FU	Breast	21
	VCR,	VCR,	CCNU,	CCNU				
			5-FU,	5-FU,	5-FU		Lung	21
	VM26,	VM26,	CCNU,	CCNU			Brain	21

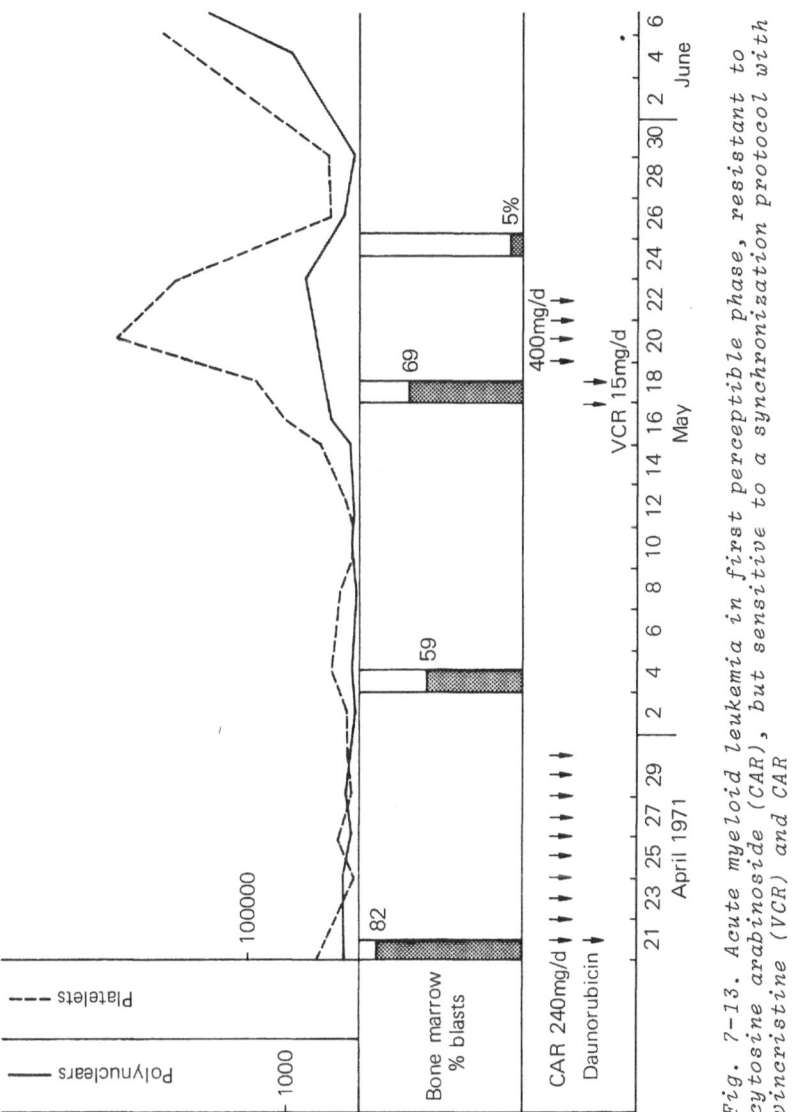

Fig. 7-13. Acute myeloid leukemia in first perceptible phase, resistant to cytosine arabinoside (CAR), but sensitive to a synchronization protocol with vincristine (VCR) and CAR

portance should not be overstressed (124). We must not forget that they are for the most part based on a experimental mouse leukemia that is not a good model for human tumors. Too much emphasis on kinetics may lead us to ignore biochemical differences (they must exist, though we have not yet identified them) and problems with drug resistance. Many clinical observations related to the different reponse rates of various malignancies cannot be explained by differences in cytokinetics. To cite only one example: ALL is highly sensitive to numerous agents while AML is almost resistant to the same agents, yet there are no character-istic differences in their cell-cycle kinetics. The pharmacologic fac-tors of drug delivery and drug metabolism are also very important de-terminants of the response rates of human malignancies, and they deserve further study.

155

Table 7-7. Clinical results with combinations based on selective tumor sensitivity, selective toxicity, synchronization, and potentiation (POUILLART et al. (122))

	Number of patients	Complete tumor regression Complete remission	Tumor regression >50%	Tumor regression <50%	Total failure
Breast cancer	27	33% (9)	41% (11)	22% (6)	4% (1)
Lung cancer	16	12% (2)	44% (7)	25% (4)	19% (3)
				Stabilization	
Brain cancer	17	30% (5)	36% (6)	15% (4)	11% (2)

It is therefore always important to compare new combinations with single-agent therapy in order to document their superior response rates. Comparative clinical studies are rare, and their results may be contradictory (125-128) (129, 130).

REFERENCES

1. LUBITZ, J.A., FREEMAN, L., OKUN, R.: Mitotane use in inoperable adrenal cortical carcinoma. J. amer. Med. Ass. 223, 1109 (1973).
2. E.O.R.T.C. CLINICAL SCREENING CO-OPERATIVE GROUP.: Epipodophyllotoxin VP 16 213 in the treatment of acute leukaemias, haematosarcomas and solid tumours. Brit. Med. J. 3, 199 (1973).
3. E.O.R.T.C. CLINICAL SCREENING CO-OPERATIVE GROUP: Clinical screening of 4-demethyl-epipodophyllotoxine-β-D-thenylidene glucoside (VM 26) in malignant lymphomas and solid tumors. Brit. med. J. 2, 744 (1972).
4. KENNEDY, B.J.: Mithramycin therapy in advanced testicular neoplasms. Cancer 26, 755 (1970).
5. HILL, G.J. II., SEDRANSK, N., ROCHLIN, D., BISEL, H., ANDREWS, N. C., FLETCHER, W., SCHROEDER, J.M., WILSON, W.L.: Mithramycin (NSC 24559) therapy of testicular tumors. Cancer 30, 900 (1972).
6. UMEZAWA, H., ISHIZUKA, M., MAEDA, K., TAKEUCHI, T.: Studies on bleomycin. Cancer 20, 891 (1967).
7. RUNDLES, R.W., GRIZZLE, Y., BELL, W.N., CORBEY, C.D., FROMMEYER, Jr., W.B., GREENBERG, B.G., HUGULEY, Jr., C.M., JAMES, G.W., JONES, Jr., R., LARSEN, W.E., LOEB, V., LEONE, L.A., PALMER, J.G., RISER, Jr., W.H., WILSON, S.J.: Comparison of chlorambucil and myleran in chronic lymphocytic and granulocytic leukaemia. Amer. J. Med. 27, 424 (1959).
8. CARTER, S.K., FRIEDMAN, M.A.: 5-(3,3-dimethyl-1-triazeno)-imidazole-4-carboxacide (DTIC, DIC, NSC-45388), a new antitumor agent with activity against malignant melanoma. Europ. J. Cancer 8, 85 (1972).
9. GOTTLIEB, J.A., BAKER, L.H., QUAGLIANA, J.M., LUCE, J.K., WHITECAR, J.P., SINKOVICS, J.G., RIVKIN, S.E., BROWNLEE, R., FREI, E.: Chemotherapy of sarcomas with a combination of adriamycin and dimethyl triazeno imidazole carboxamide. Cancer 30, 1632 (1972).
10. WALKER, M.D.: Nitrosoureas in central nervous system tumors. Cancer Chemother. Rep. Part 3, 4, 21 (1973).
11. BRODER, L.E., CARTER, S.K.: II. Results of therapy with streptozotocin in 52 patients. Ann. Int. Med. 79, 108 (1973).

12. RIVERS, S.L., PATNO, M.E.: Cyclophosphamide versus melphalan in treatment of plasma cell myeloma. J. Amer. Med. Ass. 207, 1328 (1969).
13. SCHWARZENBERG, L., MATHE, G., HAYAT, M., DE VASSAL, F., AMIEL, J.L., CATTAN, A., SCHNEIDER, M., SCHLUMBERGER, J.R., JASMIN, C., NGO MINH MAN,: Une nouvelle combinaison de méthotrexate-acide folinique pour le traitement des cancers (leucémies et tumeurs solides). Press méd. 77, 385 (1969).
14. DJERASSI, I., ROMINGER, C.J., KIM, J.S., TURCHI, J., SUVANSRI, U., HUGHES, D.: Phase I study of high doses of methotrexate with citrovorum factor in patients with lung cancer. Cancer 30, 22 (1972).
15. BERGSAGEL, D.E.: An assessment of massive-dose chemotherapy of malignant disease. Canad. Med. Ass. J. 104, 31 (1971).
16. PEROL, C., NAJEAN, Y., TANZER, J., JACQUILLAT, C., BOIRON, M., BERNARD, J.: Les aplasies du busulfan au cours des leucémies myéloides chroniques. Nouv. Rev. franc. Hématol. 7, 884 (1967).
17. FOX, M., REES, R.W.M., BENNETT, D.H.J., HENRY, L.: Investigations into lymphopenic and immunosuppressive properties of the antitumour agent, mitoclomine. Lymphology 4, 35 (1971).
18. STUTZMAN, L., SOKAL, J.E.: Use of anticancer drugs during pregnancy. Clin. Obstet. Gynec. 11, 416 (1968).
19. TOLEDO, T.M., HARPER, R.C., MOSER, R.H.: Fetal effects during cyclophosphamide and irradiation therapy. Ann. intern. Med. 74, 87 (1971).
20. MILLER, D.H.: Alkylating agents and human spermatogenesis. J. Amer. med. Ass. 217, 1662 (1971).
21. QURESHI, M.S.A., GOLDSMITH, H.J., PENNINGTON, J.H., COX, P.E.: Cyclophosphamide therapy and sterility. Lancet 2, 1290 (1972).
22. KUMAR, R., BIGGART, J.D., McEVOY, J., McGEOWIN, M.G.: Cyclophosphamide and reproductive function. Lancet 1, 1212 (1972).
23. FAILEY, K.F., BARRIE, J.U., JOHNSON, W.: Sterility and testicular atrophy related to cyclophosphamide therapy. Lancet 1, 568 (1972).
24. SHERINS, R.J., DEVITA, V.T.: Effect of drug treatment for lymphoma on male reproductive capacity. Ann. intern. Med. 79, 216 (1973).
25. WARNE, G.L., FAIRLEY, K.F., HOBBS, J.B., MARTIN, F.I.R.: Cyclophosphamide-induced ovarian failure. New Engl. J. Med. 289, 1159 (1973).
26. KARNOFSKY, D.A.: Drugs as teratogens in animals and man. Annu. Rev. Pharmacol. 5, 447 (1965).
27. FRAUMENI, J.F., MILLER, R.W.: Drug-induced cancer. J. nat. Cancer Inst. 48, 1267 (1972).
28. D'ARCY, P.F., GRIFFIN, J.P.: Drug-induced neoplasia. In: Iatrogenic Diseases. London, New York, Toronto: Oxford University Press 1972.
29. KYLE, R.A., PIERRE, R.V., BAYRD, E.D.: Multiple myeloma and acute myelomonocytic leukemia. Report of four cases possibly related to melphalan. New Engl. J. Med. 283, 1121 (1970).
30. CHAN, B.W.B., McBRIDE, J.A.: Hodgkin's disease and leukemia. Canad. Med. Ass. J. 106, 558 (1972).
31. DAVIS, Jr, H.L., PROUT, M.N., McKENNA, P.J., COLE, D.R., KORBITZ, B.C.: Acute leukemia complicating metastatic breast cancer. Cancer 31, 543 (1973).
32. KHALEELI, M., KEANE, W.M., LEE, G.R.: Sideroblastic anemia in multiple myeloma: a preleukemic change. Blood 41, 17 (1973).
33. ARSENEAU, J.C., SPONZO, R.W., LEVIN, D.L., SCHNIPPER, L.E., BONNER, H., YOUNG, R.C., CANELLOS, G.P., JOHNSON, R.E., DeVITA, V.T.: Non-lymphomatous malignant tumors complicating Hodgkin's disease. Possible association with intensive therapy. New Engl. J. Med. 287, 1119 (1972).
34. HILDEBRAND, J., COERS, Ch.: Etude clinique, histologique et électrophysiologique des neuropathies associées au traitement par la vincristine. Europ. J. Cancer 1, 51 (1965).
35. HILDEBRAND, J., KENIS, Y.: Additive toxicity of vincristine and other drugs for the peripheral nervous system. Three case reports. Acta neurol. belg. 71, 486 (1971).

36. RASKIN, M.M., RAJURKAR, M.G., ALTMAN, D.H.: Daunomycin cardiac to-
    xicity. Amer. J. Roentgenol. 118, 68 (1973).
37. BUJA, L.M., FERRANS, V.J., MAYER, R.J., ROBERTS, W.C., HENDERSON,
    E.S.: Cardiac ultrastructural changes induced by daunorubicin
    therapy. Cancer 32, 771 (1973).
38. GILLADOGA, A.C., MANUEL, C., TAN, C.C., WOLLNER, N., MURPHY, L.:
    Cardiotoxicity of adriamycin (NSC-123127) in children. Cancer Chemo-
    ther. Rep. Part 3, 6, 209 (1975).
39. LEFRAK, E.A., PITHA, J., ROSENHEIM, S., O'BRYAN, R.M., BURGESS, M.A.,
    GOTTLIEB, J.A.: Adriamycin cardiomyopathy. Cancer Chemother. Rep.
    Part 3, 6, 203 (1975).
40. MINOW, R.A., BENJAMIN, R.S., GOTTLIEB, J.A.: Adriamycin (NSC-123127)
    cardiomyopathy. An overview with determination of risk factors.
    Cancer Chemother. Rep. Part 3, 6, 195 (1975).
41. PHILIPS, F.S., STERNBERG, S.S., CRONIN, A.P., VIDAL, P.M.: Cyclo-
    phosphamide and urinary bladder toxicity. Cancer Res. 21, 1577
    (1961).
42. GODMAN, R.L., WARNER, N.E.: Hemorrhagic cystitis and cytomegalic
    inclusions in the bladder associated with cyclophosphamide therapy.
    Cancer 25, 7 (1970).
43. JOHNSON, W.W., MEADOWS, D.C.: Urinary-bladder fibrosis and telan-
    giectasia associated with long-term cyclophosphamide therapy. New
    Engl. J. Med. 284, 290 (1971).
44. PRIMACK, A.: Amelioration of cyclophosphamide-induced cystitis.
    J. nat. Cancer Inst. 47, 223 (1971).
45. DE LENA, M., GUZZON, A., MONFARDINI, S., BONADONNA, G.: Clinical,
    radiologic, and histopathologic studies on pulmonary toxicity
    induced by treatment with bleomycin (NSC-125066). Cancer Chemo-
    ther. Rep. 56, 343 (1972).
46. OLINER, H., SCHWARTZ, R., RUBIO, Jr., F., DAMESHEK, W.: Intersti-
    tial pulmonary fibrosis following busulfan therapy. Amer. J. Med.
    31, 134 (1961).
47. MIN, K.W., GYORKEY, F.: Interstitial pulmonary fibrosis, atypical
    epithelial changes and bronchiolar cell carcinoma following busul-
    fan therapy. Cancer 22, 1027 (1968).
48. FEINGOLD, M.L., KOSS, L.G.: Effects of long-term administration
    of busulfan. Report of a patient with generalized nuclear abnorma-
    lities, carcinoma of vulva, and pulmonary fibrosis. Arch. intern.
    Med. (Chic.) 124, 66 (1969).
49. KIRSCHNER, R.H., ESTERLY, Y.R.: Pulmonary lesions associated with
    busulfan therapy of chronic myelogenous leukemia. Cancer 27, 1074
    (1971).
50. CLARYSSE, A.M., CATHEY, W.J., CARTWRIGHT, G.E., WINTROBE, M.M.:
    Pulmonary disease complicating intermittent therapy with metho-
    trexate. J. Amer. med. Ass. 209, 1861 (1969).
51. E.O.R.T.C. CLINICAL SCREENING CO-OPERATIVE GROUP: Study of the
    clinical efficiency of bleomycin in human cancer. Brit. med. J. 2,
    643 (1970).
52. OETTGEN, H.F., STEPHENSON, P.A., SCHWARTZ, M.K., LEEPER, R.D.,
    TALLAL, L., TAN, C.T., CLARKSON, B.D., GOLBEY, R.B., KRAKOFF, I.H.,
    KARNOFSKY, D.A., MURPHY, M.L., BURCHENAL, J.H.: Toxicity of E. coli
    L-asparaginase in man. Cancer 25, 253 (1970).
53. HASKELL, C.M., CANELLOS, G.P., LEVENTHAL, B.G., CARBONE, P.P.,
    BLOCK, J.B., SERPICK, A.A., SELAWRY, O.S.: L-asparaginase. Thera-
    peutic and toxic effects in patients with neoplastic disease. New
    Engl. J. Med. 281, 1028 (1969).
54. PRATT, C.B., JOHNSON, W.W.: Duration and severity of fatty meta-
    morphosis of the liver following L-asparaginase therapy. Cancer,
    28, 361 (1971).
55. WHITECAR, Jr., J.P., BODEY, G.P., HILL, Jr., C.S., SAMAAN, N.A.:
    Effect of L-asparaginase on carbohydrate metabolism. Metabolism
    19, 581 (1970).

56. KENNEDY, B.J.: Metabolic and toxic effects of mithramycin during tumor therapy. Am. J. Med. 49, 494 (1970).
57. PERLIA, C.P., GUBISCH, N.J., WOLTER, J., EDELBERG, D., DEDERICK, M.M., TAYLOR, S.G. III.: Mithramycin treatment of hypercalcemia. Cancer 25, 389 (1970).
58. THORN, G.W.: Clinical considerations in the use of corticosteroids. New Engl. J. Med. 274, 775 (1966).
59. KRAKOFF, I.H.: Use of allopurinol in preventing hyperuricemia in leukemia and lymphoma. Cancer 19, 1849 (1966).
60. ARSENEAU, J.C., BAGLEY, C.M., ANDERSON, T., CANELLOS, G.P.: Hyperkalaemia a sequel to chemotherapy of Burkitt's lymphoma. Lancet 1, 10, (1973).
61. ERAS, P., SHERLOCK, P.: Hepatic coma secondary to metastatic liver disease. Ann. intern. Med. 74, 581 (1971).
62. EPSTEIN, Jr., E.H., CROFT, Jr., J.D.: Cirrhosis following methotrexate administration for psoriasis. Arch. Derm. 100, 531 (1969).
63. PODURGIEL, B.J., McGILL, D.B., LUDWIG, J., TAYLOR, W.F., MULLER, S.A.: Liver injury associated with methotrexate therapy for psoriasis. Mayo Clin. Proc. 48, 787 (1973).
64. EINHORN, M., DAVIDSOHN, I.: Hepatotoxicity of mercaptopurine. J. Amer. med. Ass. 188, 802 (1964).
65. UNDERWOOD, J.C., SHAHANI, R.T., BLACKBURN, E.K.: Jaundice after treatment of leukemia with busulfan. Brit. med. J. 1, 556 (1971).
66. GOTTLIEB, R.J., CUTTNER, J.: Vincristine-induced bladder atony. Cancer 28, 674 (1971).
67. CONDIT, P.T., CHANES, R.E., JOEL, W.: Renal toxicity of methotrexate. Cancer 23, 126 (1969).
68. LIU, K., MITTELMAN, A., SPROUL, E.E., ELIAS, E.G.: Renal toxicity in man treated with mitomycin C. Cancer 28, 1314 (1971).
69. ROSENOW, E.C. III.: The spectrum of drug-induced pulmonary disease. Ann. intern. Med. 77, 977 (1972).
70. BUCKNER, C.D., RUDOLPH, R.H., FEFER, A., CLIFT, R.A., EPSTEIN, R.B., FUNK, D.D., NEIMAN, P.E., SLICHTER, S.J., STORB, R., THOMAS, E.D.: High-dose cyclophosphamide therapy for malignant disease. Toxicity, tumor response, and the effects of stored autologous marrow. Cancer 29, 357 (1972).
71. JAFFE, N., HANN, H.W., VAWTER, G.F.: Post-steriod panniculitis in acute leukemia. N. Engl. J. Med. 284, 366 (1971).
72. DOSIK, H., HUREWITZ, D.J., ROSNER, F., SCHWARTZ, J.M.: Bullous eruption and elevated leukocyte alkaline phosphatase in the course of busulfan-treated chronic granulocytic leukemia. Blood 35, 543 (1970).
73. EPSTEIN, Jr., E.H., LUTZNER, M.A.: Folliculitis induced by actinomycin D. New Engl. J. Med. 281, 1094 (1969).
74. E.O.R.T.C. BREAST CANCER GROUP: Clinical trial of nafoxidine, an oestrogen antagonist in advanced breast cancer. Europ. J. Cancer 8, 387 (1972).
75. BROOK, J., SCHREIBER, W.: Vocal cord paralysis: a toxic reaction to vinblastine (NSC-49842) therapy. Cancer Chemother. Rep. 55, 591 (1971).
76. SAIKI, J.H., THOMPSON, S., SMITH, F., ATKINSON, R.: Paraplegia following intrathecal chemotherapy. Cancer 29, 370 (1972).
77. BETHLENFALVAY, N.C., BERGIN, J.J.: Severe cerebral toxicity after ·intravenous nitrogen mustard therapy. Cancer 29, 366 (1972).
78. MANN, A.M., HUTCHISON, J.L.: Manic reaction associated with procarbazine hydrochloride therapy of Hodgkin's disease. Canad. med. Ass. J. 97, 1350 (1967).
79. MOERTEL, C.G., REITEMEIER, R.J., BOLTON, C.F., SHORTER, R.G.: Cerebellar ataxia associated with fluorinated pyrimidine therapy. Cancer Chemother. Rep. 41, 15 (1964).
80. GOTTLIEB, J.A., LUCE, J.K.: Cerebellar ataxia with weekly 5-fluorouracil administration. Lancet 1, 138 (1971).

81. BOILEAU, G., PIRO, A.J., LAHIRI, S.R., HALL, T.C.: Cerebellar ataxia during 5-Fluorouracil (NSC-19893) therapy. Cancer Chemother. Rep. 55, 595 (1971).

82. DeFRONZO, R.A., BRAINE, H., COLVIN, O.M., DAVIS, P.J.: Water intoxication in man after cyclophosphamide therapy. Time course and relation to drug activation. Ann. intern. Med. 78, 861 (1973).

83. KYLE, R.A., SCHWARTZ, R.S., OLINER, H.L., DAMESHEK, W.: A syndrome resembling adrenal cortical insufficiency associated with long-term busulfan (Myleran) therapy. Blood 18, 497 (1961).

84. VIVACQUA, R.J., HAURANI, F.I., ERSLEY, A.: "Selective" pituitary insufficiency secondary to busulfan. Ann. intern. Med. 67, 330 (1967).

85. RAGAB, A.H., FRECH, R.S., VIETTI, T.J.: Osteoporotic fractures secondary to methotrexate therapy of acute leukemia in remission. Cancer 25, 580 (1970).

86. ROSE, M.S.: Vinca alkaloids and salivary-gland pain. Lancet 1, 213 (1967).

87. CARMICHAEL, S.M., EAGLETON, L., AYERS, C.R., MOHLER, D.: Orthostatic hypotension during vincristine therapy. Arch. intern. Med. (Chic.) 126. 290 (1970).

88. PODOS, S.M., CANELLOS, G.P.: Lens changes in chronic granulocytic leukemia: possible relationship to chemotherapy. Amer. J. Ophthal. 68, 500 (1969).

89. MIHICH, E., REGELSON, W., ENGLANDER, L.S., COSTA, G., SELAWRY, O., HOLLAND, J.F.: Hypoglycemic effects of methylglyoxal-bis-(guanylhydrazone) in animals and man. Cancer Chemother. Rep. 16, 177 (1962).

90. SADOFF, L.: Nephrotoxicity of streptozotocin (NSC-85998). Cancer Chemother. Rep. 54, 457 (1970).

91. COWAN, D.H., BERGSAGEL, D.E.: Intermittent treatment of metastatic melanoma with high-dose 5-(3,3-dimethyl-triazeno)imidazole-4-carboxamide (NSC-45388). Cancer Chemother. Rep. 55, 175 (1971).

92. ABU-ZAHRA, H., CLARYSSE, A., COWAN, D.H., HASSELBACK, R., BERGSAGEL, D.E.: Treatment of acute myeloblastic leukemia in adults: remission induction with combination of cyclophosphamide, cytarabine and vincristine. Canad. med. Ass. J. 107, 1073 (1972).

93. BRUCE, W.R., MEEKER, B.E., VALERIOTE, F.A.: Comparison of the sensitivity of normal hematopoietic and transplanted lymphoma colony-forming cells to chemotherapeutic agents administered in vivo. J. nat. Cancer Inst. 37, 233 (1966).

94. SCHABEL, Jr., F.M.: The use of tumor growth kinetics in planning "curative" chemotherapy of advanced solid tumors. Cancer Res. 29, 2384 (1969).

95. SELAWRY, O.S., HANANIAN, J., WOLMAN, I.J., ABIR, E., CHEVALIER, L., GOURDEAU, R., DENTON, R., GUSSOFF, B., LEVY, R., BURGERT, O., MILLS, S.D., BLOM, J., JONES, B., PATTERSON, R.B., McINTYRE, O.R., HAURANI, F.I., MOON, J.H., HOOGSTRATEN, B., KUNG, F.H., SHEEHE, P.R., FREI, E. III, HOLLAND, J.F.: New treatment schedule with improved survival in childhood leukemia (ALGB). J. amer. med. Ass. 194, 75 (1965).

96. FRINDEL, E., MALAISE, E., TUBIANA, M.: Cell proliferation kinetics in five human solid tumours. Cancer 22, 611 (1968).

97. COOPER, E.H., FRANK, G.L., WRIGHT, D.H.: Cell proliferation in Burkitt tumours. Europ. J. Cancer 2, 377 (1966).

98. TUBIANA, M.: The kinetics of tumor cell proliferation and radiotherapy. Brit. J. Radiol. 44, 325 (1971).

99. ZIEGLER, J.L.: Chemotherapy of Burkitt's lymphoma. Cancer 30, 1534 (1972).

100. GOLDIN, A.: Rationale of combination chemotherapy based on preclinical experiments. Cancer Chemother. Rep. Part 3, 4, 189 (1973).

101. FREI, E., FREIREICH, E.J.: Progress and perspectives in chemo-therapy of acute leukemia. Adv. Chemother. 2, 269 (1965).
102. NATHANSON, L., HALL, T.C., SCHILLING, A., MILLER, S.: Concurrent combination chemotherapy of human solid tumors: experience with a three-drug regimen and review of the literature. Cancer Res. 29, 419 (1969).
103. HENDERSON, E.S., SAMAHA, R.J.: Evidence that drugs in multiple combinations have materially advanced the treatment of human malignancies. Cancer Res. 29, 2272 (1969).
104. YOUNG, C.W.: Formal discussion: cautionary considerations of combination chemotherapy in the treatment of human malignancies. Cancer Res. 29, 2281 (1969).
105. CARTER, S.K.: Clinical trials and combination chemotherapy. Cancer Chemother. Rep. 2, 81 (1971).
106. FREI, E. III.: Combination cancer therapy: presidential address. Cancer Res. 32, 2593 (1972).
107. DeVITA, V.T., SCHEIN, P.S.: The use of drugs in combination for the treatment of cancer. New Engl. J. Med. 288, 998 (1973).
108. POUILLART, P., SCHWARZENBERG, L., MATHE, G., SCHNEIDER, M., JASMIN, C., HAYAT, M., WEINER, R., DE VASSAL, F., AMIEL, J.L., BEYER, H.P., FAJBISOWICZ, S.: Essai clinique de combinaisons chimiothérapiques basées sur la notion de tentative de synchronisation cellulaire. Nouv. Presse méd. 1, 1757 (1972).
109. POUILLART, P., SCHWARZENBERG, L., MATHE, G.: Une nouvelle approche pour les combinaisons chimiothérapiques dans le traitement des tumeurs solides: essai de synchronisation, recrutement. Ann. Méd. interne 124, 437 (1973).
110. POUILLART, P., WEINER, R., MISSET, J.-L., SCHWARZENBERG, L.: Com-bination chemotherapy based on a model of recruitment by partial synchronization. Proc. amer. Ass. Cancer Res. 14, 115 (1973).
111. RODRIGUEZ, V., BODEY, G.P., FREIREICH, E.J.: Combination chemo-therapy for lymphomas and leukemias. Disease-A-Month, (Chic.) April 1973.
112. VAN EDEN, E.B., FALKSON, H.C., FALKSON, G.: 1,3-bis(2-chloroethyl)-1-nitrosourea (BCNU) given concomitantly with cytosine arabino-side in the treatment of cancer. Cancer Chemother. Rep. 54, 347 (1970).
113. KINNE, D.W., HUMPHREY, E.W.: Combined therapy with cytosine ara-binoside and 1,3-bis(2-chloroethyl)-1-nitrosourea (BCNU) for advanced solid tumors. Cancer Chemother. Rep. 56, 53 (1972).
114. LEVITT, M., MARSH, J.C., DE CONTI, R.C., MITCHELL, M.S., SKEEL, R.T., FARBER, L.R., BERTINO, J.R.: Combination sequential chemo-therapy in advanced reticulum cell sarcoma. Cancer 29, 630 (1972).
115. KLEIN, H.O., LENNARTZ, K.J., TEICHMULLER, W., GROSS, R.: Cyto-static treatment of partially synchronized tumor cells in animals and in men. Proc. VIIth International Congress of Chemotherapy, Vol. II, Abstr. B-5/10, Prague: 1971.
116. RAJEWSKI, M.F.: Synchronisation in vivo: kinetics of a malignant cell system following temporary inhibition of DNA synthesis with hydroxyurea. Exp. Cell Res. 60, 269 (1970).
117. BARRANCO, S.C., LUCE, J.K., ROMSDAHL, M.M., HUMPHREY, R.M.: Bleo-mycin as a possible synchronizing agent for human tumor cells in vivo. Cancer Res. 33, 882 (1973).
118. LAMPKIN, B.C., NAGAO, T., MAUER, A.M.: Synchronization and recruit-ment in acute leukemia. J. clin. Invest. 50, 2204 (1971).
119. LAMPKIN, B.C., McWILLIAMS, N.B., MAUER, A.M.: Cell kinetics and chemotherapy in acute leukemia. Semin. Hemat. 9, 211 (1972).
120. BERGSAGEL, D.E.: pers. comm.
121. POUILLART, P., HOANG THY HUONG, T., BRUGERIE, E., LHERITIER, J.: Sequential administration of two oncostatic drugs: study of modali-ties for pharmacodynamic potentiation. Biomedicine 21, 471 (1974).

122. POUILLART, P., SCHWARZENBERG, L., AMIEL, J.L., MATHE, G. et al.: Combinaisons chimiothérapeutiques de drogues se potentialisant. I. Application au traitement des cancers du sein II. Application au traitement des cancers bronchiques III. Application aux tumeurs primitives du système nerveux central. Nouv. Presse Med. 4, 713-724 (1975).

123. HRYNIUK, W.M., BERTINO, J.R.: Rationale for the selection of chemotherapeutic agents. Adv. intern. Med. 15, 267 (1969).

124. HALL, T.C.: Limited role of cell kinetics in clinical cancer chemotherapy. In: Prediction of Response in Cancer Therapy. National Cancer Institute Monograph 34, p. 15. (ed. T.C. Hall). US Govt. Printing Office, Washington (1972).

125. SMALLEY, R.V., MURPHEY, S., CHAN, Y.-K., HUGULEY, Jr., C.M.: Comparison of two five-drug regimes versus sequential chemotherapy in metastatic breast carcinoma. Proc. amer. Soc. Clin. Oncol. Abstr. no. 82 (1973).

126. VAUGHN, C.B., BAKER, L.H., AL-SARRAF, M., VAITKEVICIUS, V.K.: Combination versus sequential cytotoxic chemotherapy in the treatment of advanced breast cancer. Proc. amer. Soc. Clin. Oncol. Abstract no. 87 (1973).

127. LEMKIN, S.R., DOLLINGER, M.R.: Combination vs. single drug therapy in advanced breast cancer. Proc. amer. Ass. Cancer Res. 14, 37 (1973).

128. LEONE, L.A., REGE, V.: Treatment of metastatic recurrent or inoperable carcinoma of breast with VCR/Pred/5-FU/MTX/Cyclo (reg.1) vs. VCR.Pred/5-FU (reg. II). Proc. amer. Ass. Cancer Res. 14, 125 (1973).

129. CAREY, R.W.: Comparative study of cytosine arabinoside therapy alone and combined with thioguanine, mercaptopurine, or daunomycin in acute myelocytic leukemia. Proc. amer. Ass. Cancer Res. 11, 15 (1970).

130. E.O.R.T.C. LEUKEMIA AND HEMATOSARCOMA GROUP: A comparative trial of remission: induction by cytosine arabinoside, or CAR and thioguanine, or CAR and daunorubicin, and maintenance therapy by CAR or methyl-GAG in acute myeloid leukemia. Biomed. 18, 192 (1973).

131. CARTER, S.K.: Some thoughts on experimental models and their clinical correlations. Eur. J. Cancer 9, 833 (1973).

132. CARTER, S.K., SOPER, W.T.: Integration of chemotherapy into combined modality treatment of solid tumors. I. The overall strategy. Cancer Treat. Rev. 1, 1 (1974).

133. LYONS, A.R.: Prevention of hair loss by head-band during cytotoxic therapy. Lancet 1, 354 (1974).

134. CLARYSSE, A.: unpublished observations.

135. SCHEIN, P.S., WINOKUR, S.H.: Immunosuppressive and cytotoxic chemotherapy: long-term complications. Ann. Intern. Med. 82, 84 (1975).

136. SAHAKIAN, G.J., AL-MONDHIRY, H., LACHER, M., CONNOLLY, C.E.: Acute leukemia in Hodgkin's disease. Cancer 33, 1369 (1974).

137. HOBSON, R.W., JERVIS, H.R., KINGRY, R.L., WALLACE, J.R.: Small bowel changes associated with vincristine sulfate treatment: an experimental study in the guinea pig. Cancer 34, 1888 (1974).

138. WEETMAN, R.M., BAEHNER, R.L.: Latent onset of clinical pancreatitis in children receiving L-asparaginase therapy. Cancer 34, 780 (1974).

139. DeFRONZO, R.A., ABELOFF, M., BRAINE, H., HUMPHREY, R.L., DAVIS, P.J.: Renal dysfunction after treatment with isophosphamide. Cancer Chemother. Rep. Part 1, 58, 375 (1974).

140. HARDAKER, W.T., STONE, R.A., McCOY, R.: Platinum nephrotoxicity. Cancer 34, 1030 (1974).

141. HALAZUN, J.F., WAGNER, H.R., GAETA, J.F., SINKS, L.F.: Daunorubicin cardiac toxicity in children with acute lymphocytic leukemia. Cancer 33, 545 (1974).

142. MARGILETH, D.A., SMITH, F.E., LANE, M.: Sudden arterial occlusion associated with mithramycin therapy. Cancer 31, 708 (1973).
143. ROTHBERG, H., PLACE, C.H., SHTEIR, O.: Adriamycin toxicity: unusual melanotic reaction. Cancer Chemother. Rep. Part 1, 58, 749 (1974).
144. PRATT, C.B., SHANKS, E.C.: Hyperpigmentation of nails from doxorubicin. J. Amer. Med. Ass.: 228, 460 (1974).
145. ROSENTHAL, S., KAUFMAN, S.: Vincristine neurotoxicity. Ann. Intern. Med. 80, 733 (1974).
146. WEISS, H.D., WALKER, M.D., WIERNIK, P.H.: Neurotoxicity of commonly used antineoplastic agents. New Engl. J. Med. 291, 75 and 127 (1974).
147. FREI, E., III, JAFFE, N., TATTERSALL, M.H.N., PITMAN, S., PARKER, L.: New approaches to cancer chemotherapy with methotrexate. New Engl. J. Med. 292, 846 (1975).
148. DeVITA, V.T., YOUNG, R.C., CANELLOS, G.P.: Combination versus single agent chemotherapy: a review of the basis for selection of drug treatment of cancer. Cancer 35, 98 (1975).
149. EAGAN, R.T., AHMAN, D.L., EDMONDSON, J.H.: Pilot study of a schedule for vincristine and adriamycin intended to achieve partial tumor synchronization. Proc. Am. Soc. Clin. Oncol. 16, 225 (1975).
150. SIEBER, S.M.: Cancer Chemotherapy agents and carcinogenesis. Cancer Chemotherapy Rep. Part 1, 59, 915 (1975).
151. CANELLOS, G.P., De VITA, V.T., ARSENEAU, J.C., WHANG-PENG, J., JOHNSON, R.E.C.: Malignancies complicating Hodgkin's disease in remission. Lancet 1, 947 (1975).
152. WALL, R.L., CLAUSEN, K.P.: Carcinoma of the urinary bladder in patients receiving cyclophosphamide. New Engl. J. Med. 293, 271 (1975).
153. CORTES, E.P., LUTMAN, G., WANKA, J., WANG, J.J., PICKREN, J., WALLACE, J., HOLLAND, J.F.: Adriamycin (NSC-123127) cardiotoxicity: a clinicopathologic correlation. Cancer Chemother. Rep. Part 3, 6, 215 (1975).
154. Proceedings of the high-dose methotrexate therapy meeting: december 19, 1974. Cancer Chemother. Rep. Part 3, 6, 1-82 (1975).
155. MISET, J.L., POUILLART, P., AMIEL, J.L., SCHWARZENBERG, L., HAYAT, M. et al.: Combinaison d'adriamycin de VM 26, de cyclophosphamide et de prednisone (AVmCP) pour la chimiotherapie des lymphoréticulo-sarcomes disséminés. Nouv. Presse Med. 4, 3117 (1975).
156. WASSERMAN, T.H., COMIS, R.L., GOLDSMITH, M., HANDELSMAN, H., PENTA, J.S., SLAVIK, M., SOPER, W.T., CARTER, S.K.: Tabular analysis of the clinical chemotherapy of solid tumors. Cancer Chemother. Rep. Part 3, 399 (1975).

Chapter 8
Preclinical and Clinical Evaluation of Chemotherapeutic Agents

Progress in chemotherapy in recent years has been much advanced by organized studies of different aspects of the treatment of cancer by cytotoxic drugs. Such studies have replaced the random observations out of which chemotherapy originated. Preclinical and clinical studies nowadays utilize different methods and phases to obtain their objectives. It may be useful to define them, since this will help us to understand the reports of such studies that appear in the literature.

A. CLASSIFICATION OF STUDIES ACCORDING TO OBJECTIVES (1)

1. Toxicologic and/or Tolerance Studies

Are used to determine whether a drug can be administered safely, and at what dose level. In animals, either the LD_{50} (the dose that kills 50 percent of the recipients) or the LD_{10} (kills 10 percent) is determined (2). The same experiments also reveal the major manifestations of toxicity.

2. Screening Studies

Are carried out to test which of the major categories of tumors in animals or in man are responsive to the test drug (3-6). The sensitivity of certain animal tumors resembles that of human tumors (Table 8-1) (4, 7, 19).

3. Pharmacodynamic Research

Tries to elucidate the mechanisms of action of drugs using a biochemical, biophysical, physiological, and/or morphological methodology.

4. Pharmacokinetic Research

Studies the metabolism and distribution of the agent with different modes of administration and dose levels, or in combination with other drugs. Fig. 8-1, for example, summarizes our knowledge of pharmacokinetic data for methotrexate (8-10). Information on other drugs is listed in Table 3-2. Pharmacokinetic data can be very useful. For instance, when one realizes that cyclophosphamide must be split by the liver to yield the active compound, it is clearly illogical to inject this drug intrapleurally to control a malignant effusion, or intra-arterially for local chemotherapy.

Table 8-1. Effectiveness of a series of clinically active drugs in antitumor screening systems. (After SCHEPARTZ ([4]))

Drug	Survival systems[a]		TWI systems[b]	
	L1210	Lewis lung	Ca755	Walker 256 im
Methotrexate	100	<25	66	95
Busulfan	0	–	84	80
6-Thioguanine	90	–	98	80
6-Mercaptopurine	50	<25	95	86
Nitrogen mustard	55	<25	33	62
Dactinomycin	45	<25	90	65
Chlorambucil	31	<25	75	84
Thio-TEPA	45	–	86	96
Melphalan	75	<25	71	95
Prednisone	0	<25	80	80
5-Fluorouracil	60	<25	77	72
Mithramycin	<25	<25	65	12
Cyclophosphamide	80	>100	90	90
Mitomycin C	40	–	81	95
5-Fluor-2'-deoxyuridine	52	30	70	75
Hydroxyurea	40	54	70	47
Methyl-GAG	60	–	44	44
5-(3,3-Dimethyl-1-tri-azeno)-imidazole-4-carboxamide	67	<25	95	52
Vinblastine sulfate	40	–	27	89
Cytarabine hydrochloride	94	35	86	32
Vincristine sulfate	39	–	46	80
Procarbazine hydrochloride	45	<25	–	75
1-(2-Chloroethyl)-3-cyclohexyl-1-nitrosourea	>300	–	–	93
Daunomycin	58	–	–	90
Streptozotocin	50	–	–	60
Dibromomannitol	<25	–	62	93
Bleomycin	<25	50	–	–
Carmustine	150	30	50	98

[a]In routine survival system screening, an increase in mean survival (L1210) or median survival time (Lewis lung) over controls giving an increase in lifespan (ILS) equal to or greater than 25% is regarded as sufficient to warrant further interest. A higher level of activity in subsequent testing (in which the theoretically optimal drug dose is more nearly approximated) is normally required for selection as a candidate for clinical trial.
[b]In tumor weight inhibition systems current criteria require: (a) a 58% inhibition of tumor weight relative to untreated controls (TWI) at a dose equal to or less than LD_{10} along with, (b) a therapeutic index (LD_{10} dose/minimum effective dose, MED, required for 58% TWI) equal to or greater than 2. In both systems criteria for clinical candidacy may be more stringent based upon class of compound.

5. Operational Research

Investigates the optimal modalities of administration of drugs used either alone or in combination. The result can be quantitatively ex-

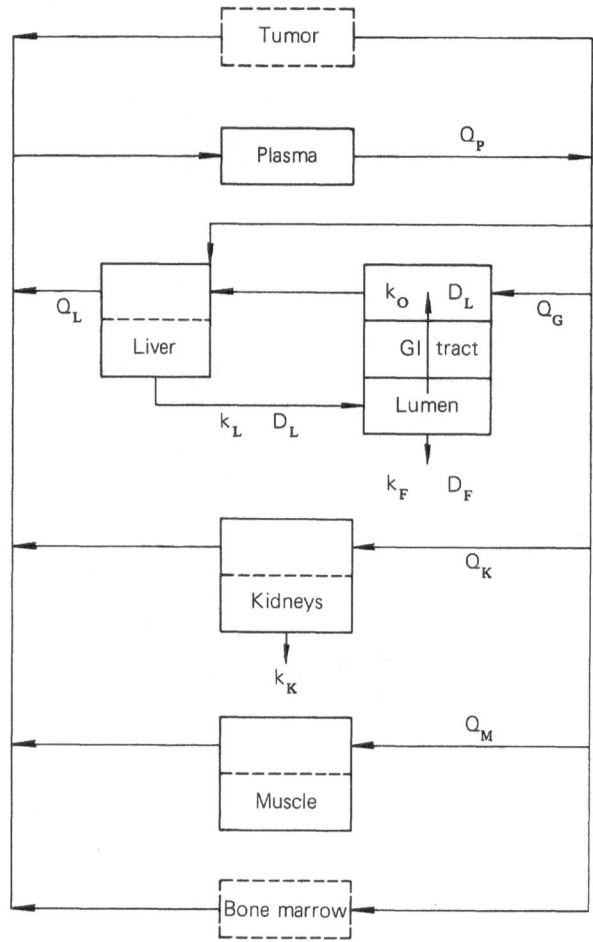

Fig. 8-1. Tissues important in methotrexate distribution. Mathematical model based on the variation of the distribution of methotrexate in mice, rats, dogs, and man at different dose levels and by different routes of administration. (From ZAHARKO et al. (8, 9) and OLIVERIO (10)) Q = blood flow rates; k = rate constants for elimination or absorption; D = delay times present before initial appearance of drug. Subscripts: P = plasma; G = small intestine; L = liver; K = kidney; M = muscle; F = feces; O = Michaelis-Menton process

expressed by the therapeutic index = $\dfrac{\text{oncostatic effect}}{\text{unwanted toxic effects}}$

6. Strategic Research

Evaluates chemotherapy in combination with the other treatment modalities of cancer: surgery, radiotherapy, and immunotherapy.

B. PHASED CLINICAL TRIALS

Clinical trials are conducted in several phases (1, 11-13).

1. Phase-I Trials

Are the bridge between preclinical and clinical studies (1, 11). Once a drug has been evaluated in animals with respect to tolerance, level and toxicity of oncostatic dose, tumor spectrum and optimal modality of administration, the drug will be given to humans, provided that some tumor effects can be anticipated from the animal studies.

Phase-I studies are primarily pharmacological, aiming to establish the dosage in man that is capable of producing a biologic effect (not necessarily an antitumor effect), to establish maximum tolerated doses and toxicity parameters, and to determine whether toxicity is predictable, treatable, and/or reversible.

Patients submitted to Phase-I studies must have malignant disease resistant to other possible forms of therapy, so that they have nothing to lose from the trial. Indeed, they may well derive some benefit from the drug to be evaluated. They should have relatively normal organ functions and an estimated survival time of at least 2 months, to permit complete evaluation of toxicity, including delayed side-effects. American Phase-I studies (NCI) do not require patients to have measurable lesions. A favorable clinical response, though gratifying and significant if it occurs, is not essential at this stage and does not determine whether a drug will subsequently move into Phase-II studies (11). In European Phase-I studies (EORTC) a qualitative antitumor effect (not just any biologic effect) is looked for, and therefore only patients with measurable lesions are included (1).

Only one patient at a time should be given the drug, to limit the risk of simultaneous toxicity in case of an unpredictable accident. The side-effects are often similar from one species to another but some species, including man, may occasionally deviate from the general pattern. This species-specific response can be either advantageous or detrimental.

The dose administered to the first patient should be one third of the minimum toxic dose of the most sensitive large animal, usually either beagle hound or rhesus monkey (11), or should not exceed one tenth of the LD_{10} for animals (1). Body surface area (BSA) expressed in square meters rather than weight in kg is used to extrapolate the correct of the LD_{10} for small animals (1). Body surface area (BSA) expressed in square there is a good correlation between the maximum tolerated dose in man (adults and children) and in different species (mouse, rat, dog, monkey) (Fig. 8-2) (7). Furthermore, BSA correlates better than weight with certain metabolic parameters, for example tissue distribution and excretion (Fig. 8-3) (10).

The first patient is kept at the initial dose level for an arbitrary period, for instance 6 weeks, less if toxicity occurs. Three patients, entered in the study at appropriate intervals, are treated at the chosen starting dosage. At this dose level there are often no significant positive or secondary effects; however, the dosage should not be escalated in the same patients but in new patients. Escalating the dose in the same patient carries a risk of cumulative toxicity and obscures the prediction of a safe starting dose for Phase-II studies. Dose escalations in subsequent patients, again entered at appropriate intervals, are carried out according to a modified FIBONACCI scheme (Table 8-2) until

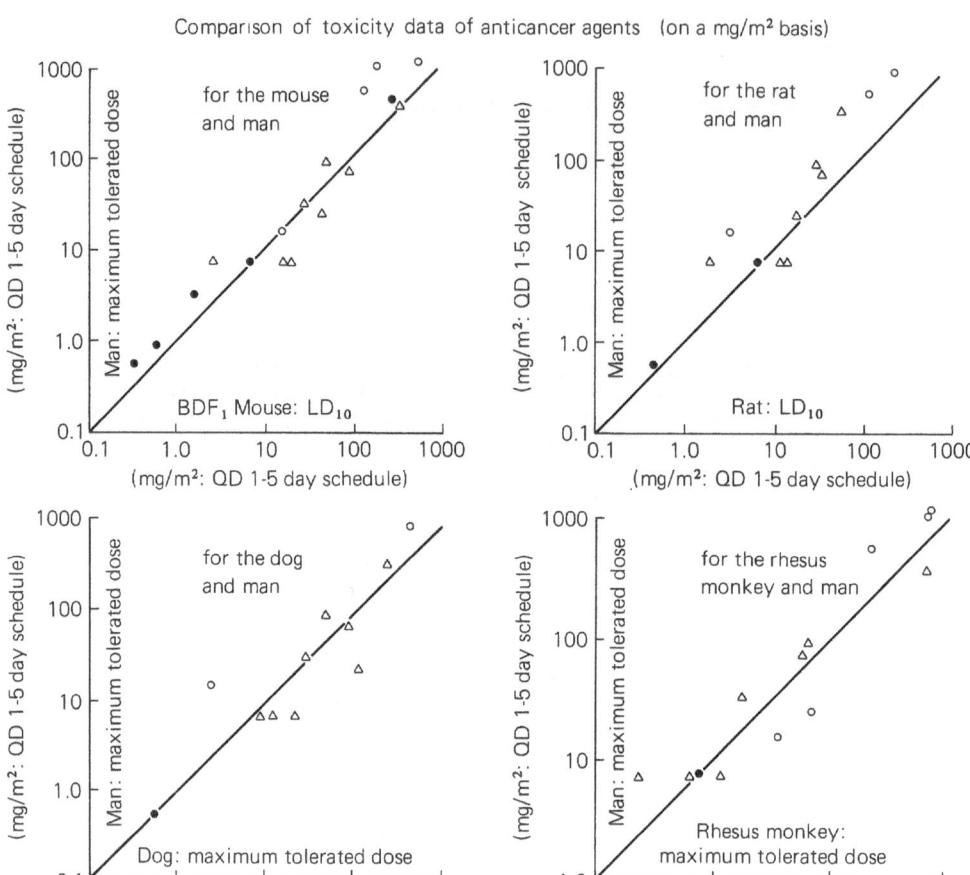

Comparison of toxicity data of anticancer agents (on a mg/m² basis)

○ Antimetabolites   △ Alkylating agents   ● Others

Fig. 8-2. Comparison of toxicity data in animals and man (From DIXON (2))

an oncostatic or toxic dose, is reached. Three patients are treated at each nontoxic and six at subtoxic levels. Experience shows that the tolerated dose will be determined within 5 + 3 dose steps. Thus, between 10 and 30+ patients will be required to define the initial dose schedule. More than one schedule, that is daily versus intermittent, can be investigated, but additional patients will be required.

2. Phase-II Trials

Traditionally screen for the antitumor activity of new agents, new methods of administration, or a new combination (the last two belong to the class of operational research) (1, 11). For screening, the NCI recommends treating a small number of patients with measurable lesions in each of 10 "signal tumors" (slow-growing: cancer of the breast, colon, lung, ovary, pancreas; fast-growing: malignant melanoma, AML, ALL, lymphomatous disease, malignant glioma) (11). The NCI prefers this kind

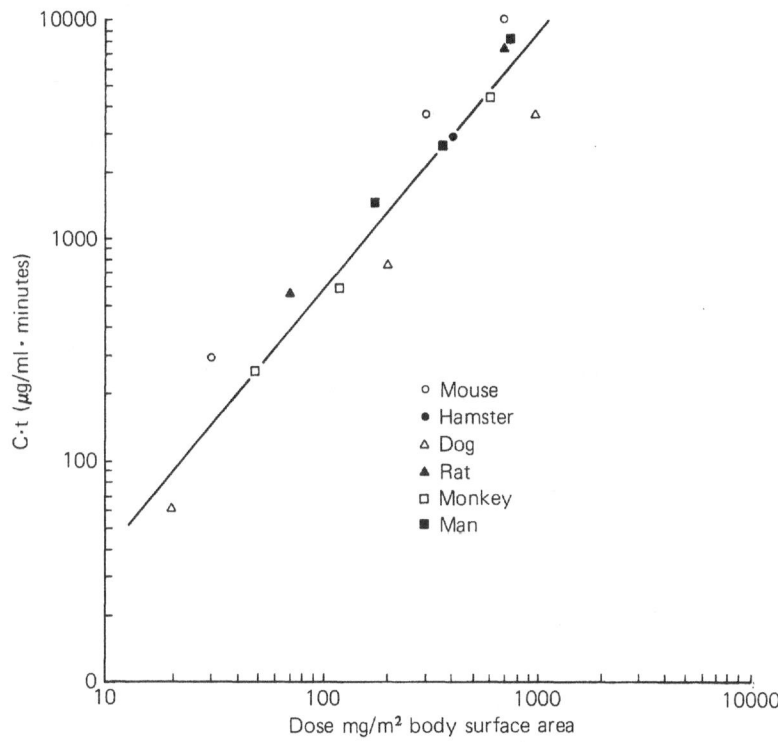

Fig. 8-3. Relationship between cyclophosphamide dosage (mg/m² body surface aera) and c x t (µg/ml x min) attained in man and animals (From OLIVERIO (10))

Table 8-2. Modified Fibonacci scheme for dose escalation in Phase-I studies (From CARTER (11))

Drug dose	Percentage increase above preceding dose level
n^a	–
2n	100
3.3n	67
5n	50
7n	40
9n	30-35
12n	30-35
16n	30-35

[a]Starting dose n (mg/m²).

of disease-oriented Phase-II trial to one in which a wide range of tumor types are treated; a few types in large enough numbers will give meaningful results. Screening studies require clearly evaluable cases in most instances, this is done by measuring lesions (see p. 181). Fifteen patients are sufficient to detect, with a risk of error of 5 percent a drug with a response rate of approximately 20 percent (14, 15).

Phase-II studies are not usually randomized. Since tumor growth, as observed in clinical stages, is constant, the slope of the growth curve during therapy can be compared with that of the period preceding the test therapy (Fig. 8-4). Placebo-treated control patients are therefore not required (13). However, some investigators insist that Phase-II studies must include control patients treated with known effective agents. This approach has been used for several years by the Cooperative Breast Cancer Group and the EORTC Breast Cancer Group. The purpose of the control group is not to compare the efficacy of the test therapy with that of established therapy (this is an objective of phase-III studies) but to check patient selection for a given study. For example, the interpretation of the value of a new hormonal agent for advanced breast cancer revealing no tumor effect in a particular study will be different according to whether the response rate in the control group treated with ethinyl estradiol is 30 percent or 0 percent. If 30 percent, it must be concluded that the test drug has not attained the critical level of activity,' since the remission rate for ethinyl estradiol is well within the normal range for this hormone. This indicates that the study group is representative of advanced breast cancers. If there is 0 percent response in the controls treated with ethinyl estradiol, no conclusion can be drawn regarding the efficacy of the new test compound because of an (inadvertent) selection of hormone-resistant patients. Many pretreatment factors in the study subjects may influence response rate and survival: age, sex, extent of the disease (clinical stage), grade of malignancy (morphological stage), pathologic variant, previous therapy, disease-free interval between primary therapy and subsequent recurrence or metastases, site of recurrence, and estimated survival time when the study is started. These factors make up the basis for patient "stratification", that is a division into subgroups that will propably respond differently to therapy (11). The comparability of groups is improved by an even distribution of factors known to affect the outcome of treatment.

Phase-II studies are crucial, since they determine whether a drug is worth further study in a particular disease. In making such a decision, one must consider in addition to the response rate other possible qualities of the drug, for example absence of bone marrow toxicity, penetration into tumor sanctuaries, and effects against cell in G_O.

3. Phase-III Trials

Compare the effects of different therapies. For example, (a) a new compound found to be active in a phase-II trial is compared with the most effective agent previously available for this particular malignancy; (b) two modes of administering the same agent are compared; (c) a drug is used singly and in combination with others (1, 11). Such studies are justified only if the difference between the two treatments is anticipated to be relatively small. A large number of patients is required; they must be randomly allocated to a treatment group to ensure that even distribution will neutralize the various factors that could influence the results. Pretreatment stratification, randomization, and crossover protocol designs (the patient is transferred from one treatment arm to the other if he fails to respond or progresses after an initial response) have several advantages. They improve the comparability of the treatment groups, remove patient selection bias, provide data on crossresistance and permit maximal utilization of patient resources. To provide the large numbers of patients required to answer a particular question within a reasonably short period, cooperative study groups have been organized. However, multi-institutional trials are difficult to manage (16). The time advantage may be lost due to differences in methods of diagnosis and treatment, and in the assessment of results. Rigid adherence to the protocol is mandatory.

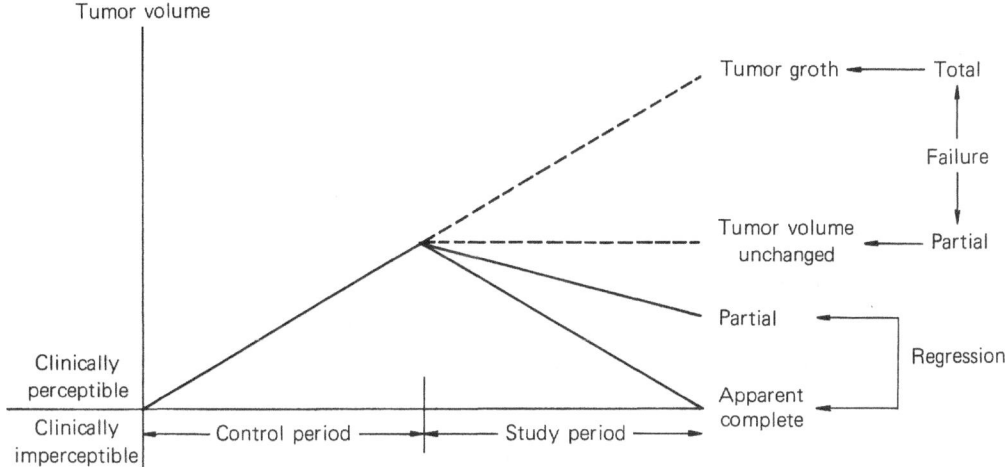

Fig. 8-4. Evaluation of response to therapy in Phase-II trial: the effect on tumor growth during the treatment (study period) is compared with tumor growth in the time interval preceding (control period) the study period

4. Phase-IV Trials

The various phases of the clinical trials we have described are usually carried out in special research institutes and large medical centers. However, observations made by practicing physicians after the drug has been made commercially available must be taken into account. This could be called Phase IV of clinical trials. For example, one of us reported a pulmonary complication with intermittent methotrexate maintenance therapy in ALL; this complication had not been described in the original study that recommended this regimen (17). Most centers treat selected patients, hence a biased population. The results of such studies may differ from those observed in general practice.

One must be aware that some investigators tend to publish only favorable results, trials in which the drug was well tolerated over the minimum period of time required to obtain the result sought for. The response rate can be significantly improved by eliminating a large number of patients as "inadequate trials" or "lost to follow-up" (usually patients who were doing badly). Some authors have thus eliminated as many as 45 percent (with 30 percent due to early death) of those entered in the study (18). The same study illustrates another problem with multi-insttutional trials: if they are not well coordinated, a large number of patients may be treated with a toxic drug before it is realized that it is ineffective (only 5 partial response in 195 patients treated).

REFERENCES

1. MATHE, G., KENIS, Y.: Logistics of clinical trials: The example of cancerology. Biomedicine 18, 181 (1973).
2. DIXON, R.L.: Laboratory of toxicology. Cancer Chemother. Rep. Part 3, 2, 61 (1971).

3. GOLDIN, A., SERPICK, A.A., MANTEL, N.: Experimental screening procedures and clinical predictability value. Cancer Chemother. Rep. 50, 173 (1966).
4. SCHEPARTZ, S.A.: Screening. Cancer Chemother. Rep. Part 3, 2, 3 (1971).
5. E.O.R.T.C. SCREENING GROUP: Handbook of materials and methods. Europ. J. Cancer 8, 185 (1972).
6. VENDITTI, J.M.: Working session report: In vivo-in vitro screening. Cancer Chemother. Rep. Part 3, 3, (1972).
7. HOMAN, E.R.: Quantitative relationship between toxic doses of antitumor chemotherapeutic agents in animals and man. Cancer Chemother. Rep. Part 3, 3, 13 (1972).
8. ZAHARKO, D.S., DEDRICK, R.L., BISSCHOFF, K.B., LONGSTRETCH, J.A., OLIVERIO, V.T.: Methotrexate tissue distribution: prediction by a mathematical model. J. nat. Cancer Inst. 46, 77 (1971).
9. ZAHARKO, D.S.: Pharmacokinetics. Cancer Chemother. Rep. Part 3, 3 21 (1972).
10. OLIVERIO, V.T.: Pharmacology in the chemotherapy drug development. Program of the NCI. Cancer Chemother. Rep. Part 3, 2, 73 (1971).
11. CARTER, S.K.: Study design principles for the clinical evaluation of new drugs as developed by the chemotherapy programme of the NCI. In: The Design of Clinical Trials in Cancer Therapy, p. 242 (ed. M. Staquet). Brussels: Editions Scientifiques Européennes 1972.
12. SANCHO, H., HAYAT, M.: Are controlled clinical trials unnecessary? Biomedicine 18, 173 (1973).
13. GEHAN, E.A., FREIREICH, E.J.: Non-randomized controls in cancer clinical trials. New Engl. J. Med. 290, 198 (1974).
14. GEHAN, E.A.: The determination of the number of patients required in a preliminary and follow-up trial of a new chemotherapeutic agent. J. Chron. Dis. 13, 346 (1961).
15. GEHAN, E.A.: Early studies of anticancer agents in humans: the question of sample size. Cancer Chemother. Rep. 16, 93 (1962).
16. STAQUET, M.: Planning and design of multi-institutional trials. In: The design of clinical trials in cancer therapy, p. 405 (ed. M. Staquet). Brussels: Editions Scientifiques Européennes 1972.
17. CLARYSSE, A.M., CATHEY, W.J., CARTWRIGHT, G.E., WINTROBE, M.M.: Pulmonary disease complicating intermittent therapy with methotrexate. J. Amer. med. Ass. 209, 1861 (1969).
18. QUAGLIANA, J.M., COSTANZI, J., O'BRYAN, R.: A phase-II study of 5-azacytidine in the treatment of solid tumors. Proc. amer. Ass. Cancer Res. 15, 121 (1974).
19. GORDON, M.H.: A stimulation of the preclinical development of anticancer drugs. Cancer Chemother. Rep. Part 3, 5, 65 (1974).

Chapter 9
Achievements and Failures of Cancer Chemotherapy

A. RESULTS OF CURRENT CHEMOTHERAPY

Thirty years ago, no therapy was available for disseminated malignancies; those that were not localized enough to be resected or irradiated invariably had a fatal outcome. Today, a normal life expectancy, in fact a cure, can be obtained with chemotherapy alone in Burkitt's tumor and choriocarcinoma, two disseminated malignancies (1, 2). Admittedly, these are two special tumors, the former having a high growth fraction (3) and the latter a favorable immunologic tumor-host relationship (4). A normal life expectancy may nowadays be attained for several other hematologic malignancies and solid tumors by combining chemotherapy with surgery and/or radiotherapy (Table 9-1). Most such tumors are relatively rare and occur predominantly in children and young adolescents; however, before the advent of chemotherapy normal life expectancy was rare in these malignancies.

In some of the more frequent tumors, for example cancer of the breast, prostate, and ovary, significant palliation and some prolongation of survival is obtained. Unfortunately, the majority of patients with inoperable cancer fall into the category where chemotherapy produces tumor regression in fewer than one third of patients. The regressions are usually of short duration and do not substantially improve survival.

These results, though modest, have permitted medical oncology to establish itself as an independent specialty with unique contribution to make to the treatment of cancer, especially in advanced malignancies and, theoretically, in earlier stages (adjuvant chemotherapy). It is a very young and dynamic specialty that has scarcely begun to realize its potential (and its shortcomings), in contrast to surgery and radiotherapy, which have already done so.

B. PROGRESS AT THE EXPERIMENTAL AND CLINICAL LEVELS

Progress has been made simultaneously at the experimental (preclinical) and clinical levels (5, 6). An extensive and costly drug-screening program supplies the clinician with a steadily increasing number of drugs for clinical use (Fig. 9-1) (7).

New agents become available as the result of: (1) empiric screening of existing and new compounds; (2) screening of agents possessing certain biological activities: histopathogenic effect, influence on growth or differentiation; (3) synthesis of compounds that might be expected to interfere with an essential molecular process, for example antimetabolites (8).

Table 9-1. Effectiveness of current chemotherapy

Condition	Response rate[1]
1. Curative (in high % of cases) Gestational trophoblastic tumors Burkitt's tumor	
2. Very sensitive to chemotherapy (high % of responses, long-term remissions, prolongation of survival and some cures, even in advanced stages often in combination with surgery and/or radiotherapy)	
Childhood acute lymphoid leukemia	> 90%
Chronic myeloid leukemia	90%
Retinoblastoma	85%
Polycythemia vera	80%
Wilms' tumor	80%
Hodgkin's disease	80%
Non-Hodgkin's lymphoma	70%
Childhood rhabdomyosarcoma	65%
Chronic lymphoid leukemia	60%
Ewing's sarcoma	60%
Testicular cancers	45 to 90%
3. Moderately sensitive to chemotherapy (frequent tumor regressions, possibly with prolongation of survival)	
Breast cancer	60%
Myeloma	60%
Soft tissue sarcomas	60%
Osteogenic sarcoma	50 to 75%
Acute myeloid leukemia	50%
Neuroblastoma	50%
Myelosclerosis with myeloid metaplasia	30 to 50%
Ovarian cancer	30 to 50%
Head and neck cancer	30 to 50%
Cervix cancer	30 to 50%
Brain tumors	30 to 50%
4. Relatively resistant to chemotherapy (tumor regressions in less than one-third; no prolongation of survival)	
Bronchus cancer	30 to 50%
Melanoma	25 to 40%
Gastro-intestinal cancer	20 to 40%
Endometrium cancer	30%
Bladder cancer	25 to 35%
Renal cancer	20%

[1] Estimates based on the more effective cytotoxic therapy

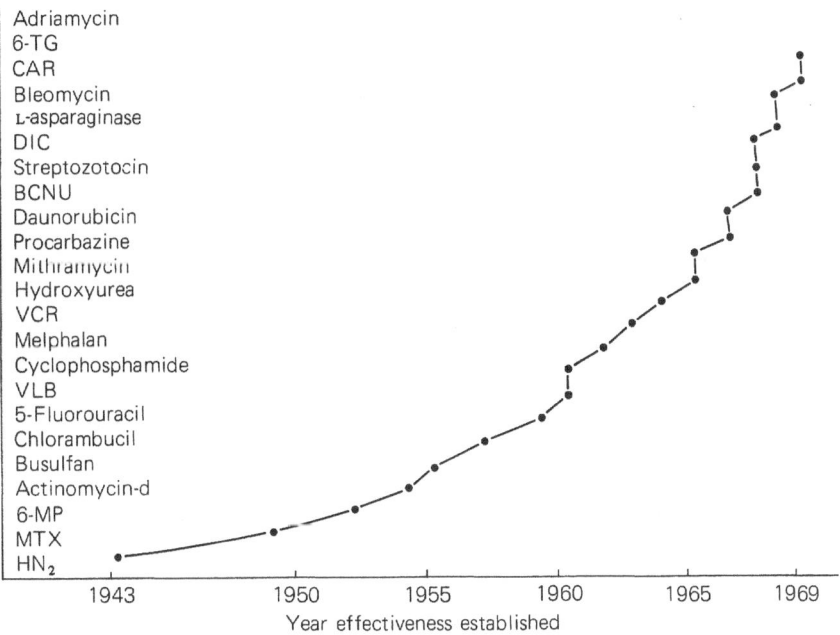

Adriamycin
6-TG
CAR
Bleomycin
L-asparaginase
DIC
Streptozotocin
BCNU
Daunorubicin
Procarbazine
Mithramycin
Hydroxyurea
VCR
Melphalan
Cyclophosphamide
VLB
5-Fluorouracil
Chlorambucil
Busulfan
Actinomycin-d
6-MP
MTX
HN₂

1943   1950   1955   1960   1965   1969
Year effectiveness established

*Fig. 9-1. Rate of discovery of clinically effective antitumor agents,
excluding hormones. For abbreviations, see p. 61. (From FREI (7))*

It is hoped that the availability of better models for screening will
improve the predictive accuracy of this program. Fast-growing, transplantable tumor systems (e.g., L1210 leukemia) do not resemble the majority of clinical tumors, which have a low growth fraction. Experimental tumors with a low growth fraction, such as the transplanted
Lewis lung tumor in mice, mimic their clinical counterparts rather better. Spontaneous virus-induced tumors (e.g., AKR leukemia and C3H mammary carcinoma) can be used to study the effects of antiviral agents
and inhibitors of reverse transcriptase, or to select drugs aimed at
preventing late relapse, and for immunotherapy (6). A program has been
established for toxicologic and pharmacokinetic studies.

Progress in the basic sciences, especially molecular biology, virology,
immunology, biochemistry, and pharmacology, and cell-kinetics and tissue-
culture studies have been of major significance in the development of
cancer chemotherapy. Pointers have been given to the development of
new drugs (e.g., L-asparaginase, rifampicin, chalones, and antiviral
agents, to name only a few), better use of existing drugs (by taking
into consideration cell-kinetic parameters), and new treatment modalities (immunotherapy). From studies in all these different fields, the
principles of cancer chemotherapy have evolved.

Methods have been worked out to test the sensitivity to various chemotherapeutic agents of human tumor cells in vitro, as well as the sensitivity (9, 10) and the recovery pattern of normal hematopoietic stem
cells (11). Considerable efforts have been made to predict tumor response and to select patients most likely to respond to a given therapy
(12, 13). For a few selected cancers (myeloma, choriocarcinoma, testicular carcinomas), the reduction of tumor cells can be monitored to well
below the clinically detectable level (10^9). It is hoped that similar
information, which is most useful for the determination of the effec-

175

tiveness and the duration of chemotherapy, will eventually be available for most tumors.

Clinicians for their part have organized and programmed their clinical investigations. Cooperative cancer chemotherapy study groups are coordinating their efforts to gather information more rapidly than individual investigators could hope to do. This approach is especially useful for the rare tumors (e.g., National Ewing Sarcoma Study).

A network of cancer centers is being developed to assure provision of the best possible treatment to the maximum number of patients (14). Such enterprises require the cooperation of a multitude of diagnostic and therapeutic disciplines to plan the immediate and long-term cancer strategy. The initial therapy will generally be given at a center which has at its disposal appropriate integrated resources in surgery, radiotherapy, chemotherapy, and immunotherapy. Cancer centers are the only institutions that can offer the necessary sophisticated support for intensive chemotherapy. Some of the advances made in this field, especially in the prevention and management of bleeding and infection, are discussed in Chap. 11. Long-term therapy, follow-up, and rehabilitation will often be possible on an out-patient basis with the active participation of the patient's own doctor under the supervision of the center. Most centers integrate basic research and clinical investigation to ensure that fundamental discoveries are applied in clinical practice and to provide those doing basic research with clinical material.

C. CAUSES OF FAILURE OF CHEMOTHERAPY

It would be quite wrong to be satisfied with present achievements. The hard fact remains that the survival of the overwhelming majority of patients with disseminated malignancies has not been significantly improved by current cancer chemotherapy. Some shortcoming in the drug, the tumor, or the patient may explain this failure.

I. Drug
1. Cell kill by chemotherapy follows first-order kinetics, and thus fails to kill 100 percent of the tumor cells.

2. Cell kill by chemotherapy is nonspecific, affecting both normal and malignant cells.

3. Few drugs are effective against resting tumor cells.

4. The cytotoxic compound may fail to reach malignant cells in "tumor sanctuaries".

5. The optimal mode of administration has not been adequately studied for most of the agents in use.

II. Tumor
1. Primary and secondary resistance is common.

2. Most human malignancies have a low growth fraction.

3. The tumor load may be excessive (e.g. 10^{12} cells)

III. Host
   Patients with far advanced tumors are often unable to tolerate
   adequate chemotherapy because of:

1.   Deficient bone marrow reserve

2.   Deficient immune defenses

3.   Deficient essential organ function (hepatic, renal, pulmonary).

In attempts to remedy these problems, the chemotherapist has resorted
to combination chemotherapy, recruitment, potentiation and synchronization protocols (see p. 144). In addition, he has had to give up the
idea that chemotherapy alone can cure cancer. Instead, he has joined
forces with the practitioners of other treatment modalities. It is to
be hoped that in future the medical oncologist will no longer be con-
sulted only when the patient carries an enormous tumor load (10^{12}),
too disseminated to be resected, is resistant to radiotherapy, and
perhaps even resistant to chemotherapy as a result of homeopathic,
single-agent daily therapy. This type of patient, all too often seen
by the chemotherapist, has a deficient bone marrow reserve and failing
immune responses and organ functions. Not chemotherapy, but a miracle
would be required to cure him. The value of chemotherapy as an adjuvant
to the initial surgery and/or radiotherapy must be investigated, especially in cancers where the cure rate after attempts at curative resection is low; preliminary reports are encouraging (see p. 238).

REFERENCES

1. BURKITT, D.P., WRIGHT, D.H.: Burkitt's lymphoma, Vol. 1. Edinburgh-
   London: E.S. Livingstone 1970.
2. LI, M.C., HERTZ, R., SPENCER, D.B.: Effect of methotrexate therapy
   upon choriocarcinoma and chorioadenoma. Proc. Soc. exp. Biol. (N.Y.)
   93, 361 (1956).
3. COOPER, E.H., FRANK, G.L., WRIGHT, D.H.: Cell proliferation in
   Burkitt tumours. Europ. J. Cancer 2, 377 (1966).
4. MATHE, G., DAUSSETT, J., HERVET, D., AMIEL, J.L., COLOMBANI, J.,
   BRULE, G.: Immunological studies in patients with placental choriocarcinoma. J. nat. Cancer Inst. 33, 193 (1964).
5. ZUBROD, C.G.: The basis for progress in chemotherapy. Cancer 30,
   1474 (1972).
6. ZUBROD, C.G.: Chemical control of cancer. Proc. nat. Acad. Sci. USA
   69, 1042 (1972).
7. FREI, E. III.: Combination cancer therapy: presidential address.
   Cancer Res. 32, 2593 (1972).
8. HANSCH, C.: Commentary: Strategy in drug design. Cancer Chemother.
   Rep. 56, 433 (1972).
9. HOOVIS, M.L., CHU, M.Y., FISCHER, G.A., CALABRESI, P.: Predictive
   system for testing drug sensitivity in human leukemias. Blood 40,
   935 (1972).
10. TISMAN, G., HERBERT, V., EDLIS, H.: Determination of therapeutic
    index of drugs by in vitro sensitivity tests using human host and
    tumor cell suspensions. Cancer Chemother. Rep. 57, 11 (1973).
11. COWAN, D.H., CLARYSSE, A., ABU-ZAHRA, H., SENN, J.S., McCULLOCH,
    E.A.: The effect of remission induction in acute myeloblastic leu-
    kemia on efficiency of colony formation in culture. Ser. Haemat.
    5, 179 (1972).

12. HALL, T.C.: Biochemical factors predicting response to chemothera-
    peutic agents. In: Cancer Chemotherapy, p. 93 (eds. I. Brodsky,
    S.B. Kahn, J.H. Moyer). New York: Grune and Stratton 1972.
13. Prediction of response in cancer therapy. (ed. T.C. Hall). National
    Cancer Institute Monograph 34. Washington: U.S. Government Printing
    Office 1972.
14. Conference on planning for cancer centers. Cancer $\underline{29}$, 819-923
    (1972).

Chapter 10
Practical Aspects of the Treatment of Cancer with Chemotherapy

A. WORK-UP OF PATIENT PRIOR TO CHEMOTHERAPY

Before one can select and outline a treatment program for a particular patient, it is necessary to do a complete, baseline work-up.

1. It is imperative to establish a <u>pathologic diagnosis</u>. Once therapy has been initiated, material for histologic examination may no longer be available, or may be altered beyond recognition by the treatment. If there was any doubt about the original diagnosis, it may then never be resolved. There is no place in modern cancer chemotherapy for therapeutic trials. The cell type (adenocarcinoma, squamous-cell carcinoma, sarcoma, etc.) is important as is the histologic grade of malignancy (Broder's classification) or the pathologic variant. It is no longer enough to make a pathologic diagnosis of, for instance, Hodgkin's disease, malignant lymphoma, or acute lymphoid leukemia. In each of these malignancies subvariants are now recognized that have not only characteristic morphologic features, but also often a characteristic natural history and different response rates to chemotherapy (<u>1</u>, <u>2</u>). If at all possible the site of origin should be determined, since the treatment often depends on this information; for example metastatic adenocarcinoma of the prostate and of the colon would be treated differently. Pathologic confirmation may also be necessary for metastatic or recurrent disease to rule out the possibility of a second malignancy or a nonmalignant disease mimicking tumor.

2. <u>The extent of the malignant process</u> (local, regional, or metastatic) must be determined. This "staging" is done by history, physical examination, roentgenograms, including angiography and lymphangiography, radioisotope scans, function studies (liver, kidney, lung), cytology, biopsy, endoscopy and, if necessary, exploratory laparotomy or thoracotomy. Which tests are selected will to a great extent be determined by the physical findings, the natural history, and particular pattern of spread of each malignancy. Staging procedures differ for a patient with Hodgkin's disease from those for a lung cancer patient. As a result of this more or less extensive work-up, the patient can be placed in a particular "stage". Unfortunately, there is little uniformity at the present time among different investigators as regards the extent of the staging work-up or the method of defining the different stages (<u>3-5</u>). For example, European groups tend to use the TNM (UICC) classification for breast cancer and American groups the "Columbia Classification". This makes comparison of the results of different studies very difficult, if not impossible.

3. Information on the duration and the <u>rate of progression</u> of the tumor is useful to formulate an impression (if based on the history) or, preferably, a quantitative expression (if serial roentgenograms or scans are available) of the growth rate of the tumor.

4. The repercussion of the malignant process on the general condition of the patient should be evaluated. This can be recorded by using Karnofsky's criteria of performance status (PS), based on useful activity and requirements for supportive measures (Table 10-1) (6). The estimated survival should also be recorded, as this parameter and the PS may influence the response to therapy (7, 8).

Table 10-1. Criteria of performance status (PS)

	%	
Able to carry on normal activity; no special care needed	100	Normal; no complaints; no evidence of disease
	90	Able to carry on normal activity; minor signs or symptoms of disease
	80	Normal activity with effort; some signs or symptoms of disease
Unable to work; able to live at home; cares for most personal needs; a varying amount of assistance needed	70	Cares for self; unable to carry on normal activity or to do active work
	60	Requires occasional assistance but is able to care for most of his needs
	50	Requires considerable assistance and frequent medical care
Unable to care for self; requires equivalent of institutional or hospital care; disease may be progressing rapidly	40	Disabled; requires special medical care and assistance
	30	Severly disabled; hospitalization is indicated although death not imminent
	20	Very sick; hospitalization necessary; active supportive treatment necessary
	10	Moribund; fatal processes progressing rapidly
	0	Dead

5. The function of essential organs such as bone marrow, liver, and kidneys should be assessed by appropriate tests, not only to rule out tumor involvement but also as a baseline for interpreting later developments and as a pointer to problems with drugs that are activated, metabolized and/or excreted via these organs. A baseline for calcium and uric acid is often indicated.

6. The study of immune responses in cancer patients has been emphasized in recent years. A number of tests are available for evaluating humoral and cellular responses to various antigens (see p. 188). Baseline studies are useful since immune responsiveness may be suppressed by chemotherapy or by progressive malignant disease. Specialized laboratories can search for evidence of an immune response to tumor-specific antigens.

7. The presence of complicating or associated medical problems, whether related to the malignancy or not, should be determined as it may affect the treatment plan (e.g., steroids should be used cautiously in a patient with diabetes) or additional specific therapy may be needed.

8. Previous therapy should be recorded. As regards surgical procedures, we note the date, place, type of surgery (e.g., total gastrectomy), the intent (cure or palliation), the gross involvement (organs, lymph nodes, blood vessels) and microscopic findings (involvement of suture line?), and the result (cure, local control, local or distant recurrence, with the date of the recurrence and the disease-free interval. Similarly, with regard to previous radiotherapy, we record the place and dates of treatments as well as the field size, dose, type of radiation (ortho-voltage, megavoltage, cobalt, etc.), fractionation, patient tolerance, and the result (cure, local control, recurrence). If the patient has received prior chemotherapy, we record the nature of the drugs, doses, schedule, dates, tolerance or toxicity, and the response (objective or subjective) and its duration. It is especially important to identify drugs that were ineffective (provided the proper dose schedule was used) or to which the patient has become resistant.

9. Finally, the investigator must determine what parameters (or indica-tor lesions) will be used as an objective criterion of tumor responsive-ness. These parameters will vary in each individual patient and with each malignancy. The various types are listed below.

(i) The diameters of clinically palpable tumors are measured with cali-pers and the tumor mass is defined as the product of the longest x widest perpendicular diameter, or by means of serial photographs. Fig. 10-1 illustrates the deceptive nature of this type of arithmetical evalua-tion of the tumor response as compared with a logarithmic scale.

(ii) Changes in tumors or metastases can be measured on comparative roentgenograms or (less well) on scans.

(iii) Involvement of organs such as the liver and kidneys is studied by serial function studies.

(iV) Certain tumors produce characteristic enzymes or other proteins or peptides that can be quantitated (9, 10). It is assumed that the quantity of enzyme or protein is proportional to the number of tumor cells. Examples are the HCG titer in choriocarcinoma (11), or testi-cular tumors and the M protein in myeloma (12, 13). Radio-immunoassays are useful in hormone-producing tumors.

(V) Leukemias are studied by monitoring the disappearance of malignant cells from the peripheral blood and bone marrow, and the regeneration of normal hematopoietic tissue.

10. All this information, obtained from various sources, is recorded on a relatively simple form. However, it becomes an extremely valuable document in the management of the patient and provides data for prospec-tive or retrospective studies (Table 10-2). The large number of pre-treatment variables included (age, sex, extent of disease, histologic variant and grade, site and treatment of primary disease, disease-free interval, site of recurrence, and previous therapy) may all influence the objective response rate and survival time with the therapy to be prescribed (7). They constitute the elements for stratification (divi-sion of subjects into subgroups likely to have a different response to therapy) and determine patient selection, an important factor when comparing results of different studies (see p. 170).

B. WHO SHOULD TREAT THE CANCER PATIENT?

The conduct of the outlined initial evaluation of the patient and the next step in the management, the selection of the proper course of

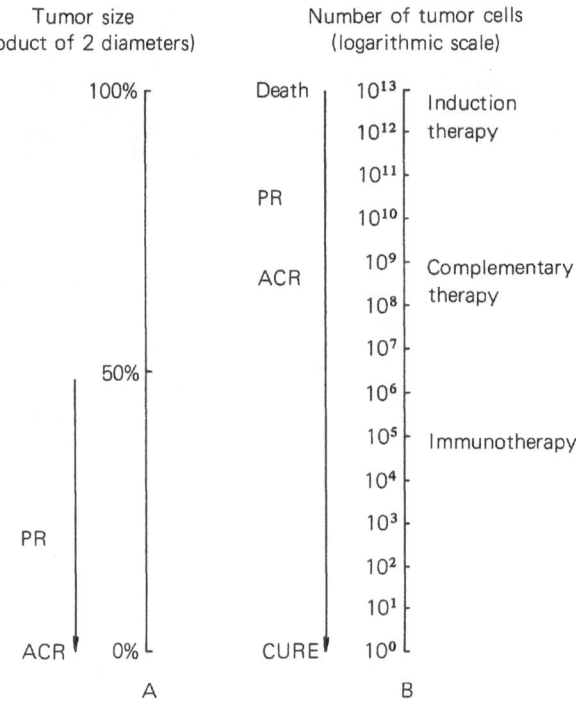

Fig. 10-1. (A.) Evaluation of tumor response by measurement of tumor
size. A reduction to less than 50% of the product of two diameters is
considered a partial response (PR). If the tumor is no longer palpable,
the patient is said to be in (apparent) complete remission (ACR). (B.)
Evaluation of the tumor response on a logarithmic scale places ACR in
proper perspective

treatment, will be facilitated if the physician in charge is familiar
with natural history or behavior of the malignancy to be treated. This
will permit him to orient his management toward the total treatment
of the patient from diagnosis to either death or cure. He must anticipate the occurrence of local or systemic relapses, problems with tumor
sanctuaries, or complications due to the disease or the treatment and
undertake timely and appropriate steps toward their prevention. Not
only must he know what each of the four treatment modalities has to
offer at every stage of each malignancy, he should also be an all-round
physician who can detect the significance of a minor abnormality of the
nervous system, liver or renal function, or any other system at an early
stage. Indeed, tumor involvement or the complications of therapy do not
spare any organ or function of the human body. Especially heavy demands
will be made on his knowledge of pharmacology, toxicology, immunology,
hematology and microbiology (14-16). He must think like a research
scientist in terms of the concepts outlined in earlier chapters, and
at the same time be human and capable of acting as psychologist or psy-
chiatrist, helping his patient to adjust to and cope with a chronic and
often fatal illness. Finally, he must be satisfied with small rewards
and not lose courage or hope in the face of repeated failures. It is
fair to say that it requires a special breed of man to make a medical
oncologist.

Table 10-2. Record of initial evaluation

DIVISION OF MEDICAL ONCOLOGY

Hosp. No - - - - - - - - - - - -
Name: - - - - - - - - - - - -
Birth date: - - - - - Sex - - -
Date initial work-up: - - - - -
Wt: - - Kg   Ht: - - m BSA:- -m^2

RECORD OF INITIAL EVALUATION

Summary of history:

Diagnosis: 1. Site of primary: - - - - - - - - - - - - - - - - - -
           2. Histology: cell type:- - - - - - - - - - - - - - - - -
                         grade:- - - - - - - - - - - - - - - - - - -
                         variant:- - - - - - - - - - - - - - - - - -

Work-up: list pertinent tests and results:

    1. Hematology:
    2. Chemistry:
    3. Biopsies:
    4. X-rays:
    5. Scans:
    6. Special procedures:

Stage: - - - - - - - - - - - (classification used: - - - - - - - -)

       Organs involved:- - - -, - - - -, - - - -, - - - -, - - - -

       Performance status: - - - - - - - - (Karnofsky)

       Estimated survival prior to treatment: - - - - - - - - - - -

Growth rate: - - - - - - - - - - - - (estimated from history, serial
                                      X-rays)

Immune responsiveness: Test: - - - - - - -   Result: - - - - - - - - -
                             - - - - - - -   - - - - - - - - -
                             - - - - - - -   - - - - - - - - -

Parameters (indicator lesions): 1. - - - - - - - - - - - - - - - - - -
                                2. - - - - - - - - - - - - - - - - - -
                                3. - - - - - - - - - - - - - - - - - -

Previous treatment: 1. Surgery:
                    2. Radiotherapy:
                    3. Chemotherapy:

Associated illnesses: - - - - - - - - - - - - - - - - - -
                      - - - - - - - - - - - - - - - - - -

Proposed - Rx: -
                -

C. FACTORS THAT INFLUENCE THE SELECTION OF THERAPY

Now that we have defined the qualities and qualifications of the man
who should manage cancer patients, at least those not curable from the
onset by surgery or radiotherapy, let us consider the decision-making
itself. The final selection of a treatment program for a particular
patient will depend on a number of variables associated with the malignant disease itself - the host, the treating physician, the treating
institution, and on the objectives of the treatment.

The most important determinants of treatment selection lie in the malignancy to be treated: site of origin, cell type, grade or histologic
variant, extent, growth rate, previous therapy, and possible resistance.
One must consider the responsiveness of the particular tumor class in
general to various drugs and combinations as reported in the literature.
It is much easier to be dogmatic about the treatment of choriocarcinoma
or Burkitt's tumor, for which we have highly effective treatment programs, than about lung cancer, which is not responsive to any degree
worth mentioning to any of the agents or combinations currently available.

The general condition and the estimated survival of the patient may pre-
clude therapy. He may suffer from severe cachexia, infection, uncontrol-
lable effusions, marked impairment of bone marrow, hepatic or renal
function, or he may have serious associated illnesses. the patient must
be motivated to cooperate with the demands of intensive chemotherapy.
Such therapy cannot be undertaken unless regular supervision and follow-up visits are guaranteed. It is sometimes necessary to select a
simpler and less effective therapy for an uncooperative patient, a patient who lives too far away, or one who cannot afford the cost of drugs
and hospitalization.

The treatment will also depend on the expertise of the primary physician
and whether he is a participant in cooperative studies, and on the quality and cooperation of physicians in the community, whose help is often
required in carrying out certain aspects or phases of the treatment.

Finally, the treating institution is important. More aggressive therapy
can be carried out with greater safety in a specialized cancer center,
preferably closely associated with, if not part of, a major medical
center where the necessary ancillary diagnostic and treatment services
are readily available (17). Facilities for isolation and replacement
of blood components are especially important in addition to most of the
services to hand in the majority of the major hospitals in the USA. In
general, we recommend that patients be entered as often as possible on
protocol studies that are designed to answer specific questions. Most
studies as organized by the American cooperative groups under the aus-
pices of the NCI and the European cooperative groups (EORTC) are intended to provide information that will be useful for the patient and
for other patients with similar disease, while not being harmful. The
strict requirements of these studies for proper monitoring of the tumor
response and toxicity manifestations offer the patient the assurance
of a careful and close follow-up.

D. OBJECTIVES OF CHEMOTHERAPY

The objectives of chemotherapy are to a great extent determined or limited by the factors described in the preceding paragraph. When seeing

a new patient, the medical oncologist must always consider whether the patient is indeed beyond the stage of cure by surgery or radiotherapy. If the answer is "yes", his aim should be, for the diseases listed in Table 9-1, 1 cure and return to normal life by means of chemotherapy, or, for the malignancies listed in Table 9-1, 2 and 3, prolongation of useful survival by holding the disease in check for as long as possible. There is still a long list of diseases, unfortunately the more common ones, where the objective can be no more than a temporary tumor regression, hopefully associated with palliation of symptoms and better quality of life (Table 9-1, 4). However, the results of current chemotherapy programs are so encouraging that there are few patients with inoperable cancer who should not be given the benefit of a chemotherapeutic trial. If the therapy is properly conducted, the chances the patient will benefit outweigh the risks. If follow-up observations indicate that the patient is not benefiting from the treatment, it can always be changed or discontinued, and little or no harm will have been done.

Chemotherapy, of course, always involves careful balancing of the therapeutic advantages for the patient against the toxic side-effects. The degree of discomfort, that we are willing to impose on our patients depends to a great extent on our objectives. It seems legitimate to subject a child with ALL to a prophylactic series of uncomfortable intrathecal injections and irradiation of the brain if this (in addition to other therapy) means the difference between a reasonable chance of cure or death from subsequent CNS leukemia.

E. WHEN SHOULD CHEMOTHERAPY BE USED?

The answer to this question is in theory simple: treatment should be started as soon as the diagnosis of advanced cancer has been established. The number of tumor cells can only increase. Rare indeed are the tumors that undergo temporary spontaneous regressions (18). In practice one must adapt to individual needs, but as a general rule we recommend early treatment. It may be necessary first to control an infection or a complicating diabetes, or to correct anemia with transfusions. It would be wrong, however, to withhold chemotherapy, for example from a leukemic patient, because of neutropenia or thrombocytopenia. The only way to correct these abnormalities is to institute therapy that will be effective in clearing the infiltrated bone marrow, so allowing regeneration of the normal hematopoietic elements.

It is difficult to be dogmatic about the indications for adjuvant chemotherapy. Most of the earlier studies on this subject were inconclusive or contradictory (19). More recent trials have already proven that adjuvant chemotherapy is effective in Wilms' tumor, in osteogenic sarcoma, probably in Ewing's sarcoma, in stages II B and III B of Hodgkin's disease, and in breast cancer.

F. TREATMENT PROTOCOL: RECORDING TUMOR RESPONSE AND TOXICITY

Once it has been decided to treat a patient and the proper regimen has been selected, it is essential to keep proper records of the drugs administered and the patient's response. The best method is to use "flowsheets" specially designed for the purpose, as regularly used by cooperative groups (Table 10-3). The drug or drugs to be administered

Table 10-3. Solid tumor flowsheet

DIVISION OF MEDICAL ONCOLOGY		FLOWSHEET						
	Date							
	Day on study							
RX (a)	1							
	2							
	3							
	4							
	5							
	6							
	7							
	8 Transfusion							
	9 Radiation							
PB	10 hgb GM%							
	11 hct vol%							
	12 retics %							
	13 plats (10^3)							
	14 wbc (10^3)							
	15 PMN %							
	16 L %							
	17 M %							
	18 E %							
	19 ESR %							
BM	20 Cell.							
	21							
Lab.	22 Creatinine							
	23 BUN							
	24 uric acid							
	25 Ca							
	26 Bil D/T							
	27 Alk. ptase							
	28 y-GT							
	29 SGOT							
	30 SGPT							
	31 LDH							
	32 TSP/Alb							
	33							
	34							
Phys.	35 Wt							
	36 T							
	37							
	38							
Param.	39							
	40							
	41							
	42							
	43 New lesions							
Sympt.	44 PS							
	45							
	46							

Hosp. No – – – – –
Name – – – – – – –
Diagnosis – – – –
Stage – – – – – –
Protocol – – – – –

Progress notes and remarks

Table 10-3. (continued)

Tox. (b)	47 48 49 50						
Resp. (c)	51 Objective 52 Subjective						

a Record amount of drug administered.

b Describe under remarks and rate severity: 0 = none, 1 = mild, 2 = moderate, 3 = severe, 4 = fatal.

c Rate response as: C(complete), P(partial), M(mixed), N(no change), or I(increasing disease).

are listed as well as the dose (nowadays preferably expressed in mg/m^2 BSA rather than in mg/kg body weight, see Fig. 10-2), [+] route of administration, frequency and duration. For some drugs with cumulative toxicity, for example bleomycin, adriamycin, or daunomycin, there should be a predetermined total dose that must not be exceeded. The presence of "poor risk" factors may require less than the standard dose of cytotoxic agents. Patients suspected of having a reduced bone marrow reserve as a result of extensive prior radiotherapy or chemotherapy, and patients with severe neutropenia, thrombocytopenia, or impairment of hepatic or renal function, or aged above 65, qualify for a dose reduction.

The drugs are recorded on the days that they are adminstered together with incidental therapy, for example radiotherapy for palliation of localized bone pain, corticosteroids for cerebral edema, intrathecal injections, transfusions and any other procedures or therapy that may alter the patient's response or interfere with the evaluation of that response. The flowsheets also contain spaces for serial blood counts and important chemical tests, especially BUN, liver function studies, alkaline phosphatase, calcium, uric acid, and serum proteins.

The patient's response is recorded under the headings: objective response (serial measurements of tumor masses, M protein, HCG titers, etc.) and subjective response, which is difficult to quantitate. Each assessment covers the period between the time of the examination and the previous visit.

There are several in vitro and in vivo tests the clinician can use to evaluate both cellular and humoral immunity, and these are also recorded on the flowsheets (20, 21). Small lymphocytes of thymic origin are associated with cell-mediated immune responses, including the rejection of cancer cells. To test existing sensitivity, delayed hypersensitivity skin tests are most useful (Table 10-4). If the patient's cellular immune responses are intact, erythema and induration > 5 mm in

---

[+] The conversion factor from mg/kg to mg/m^2 is approximately 35-40 for non-obese adult patients.

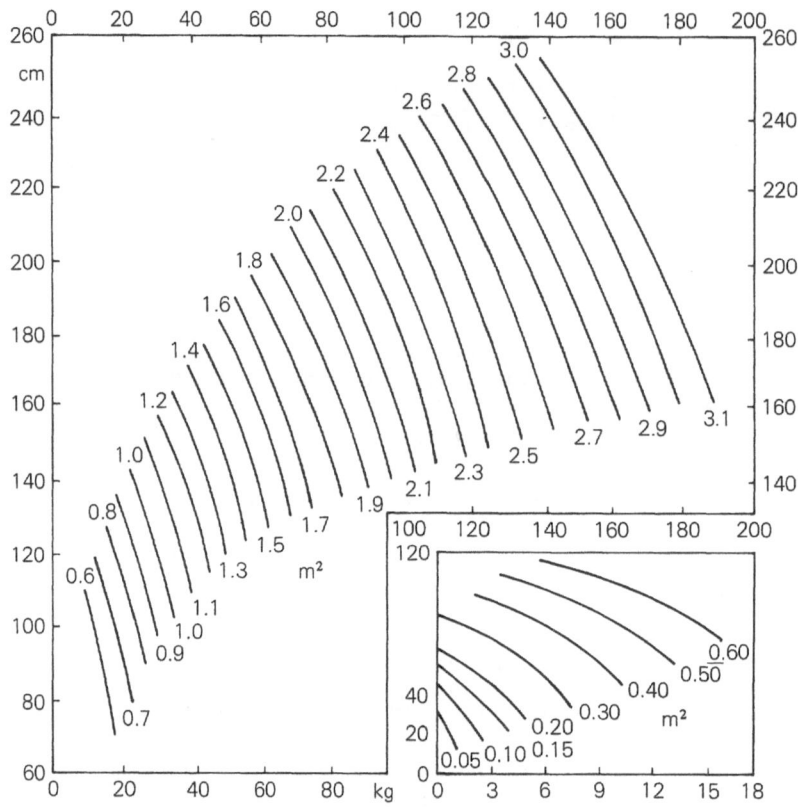

Fig. 10-2. Estimation of body surface area from height and weight (Eli Lilly)

Table 10-4. Clinical evaluation of immune responsiveness

I. Skin tests

    A. Active sensitization: 2,4-Dinitrochlorobenzene   (DNCB)

    B. Prior sensitization: skin-test antigens

        1. Tuberculin, PPD, first and intermediate strength
        2. Candida albicans
        3. Mumps
        4. Dermatophyton

II. In vitro tests

    Lymphocyte transformation in response to

        1. Phytohemagglutinin[a]
        2. Pokeweed[b]
        3. PPD
        4. Allogenic lymphocytes

[a] Transforms only T lymphocytes
[b] Transforms T and B lymphocytes

diameter will develop 48 to 72 h after intradermal application of the antigens. An adult who is unreactive to all 4 of the antigens can be assumed to be anergic. These tests can be repeated at regular intervals during treatment (Fig. 10-3) (22). To test primary immune response (to a new antigen), active sensitization with dinitrochlorobenzene (DNCB) is used. This test has the advantage that a negative reaction to this single allergen can be equated with immune impairment. Unfortunately, the test is time-consuming since 2 applications are necessary, the first to immunize the patient, and the second to evaluate the patient's response.

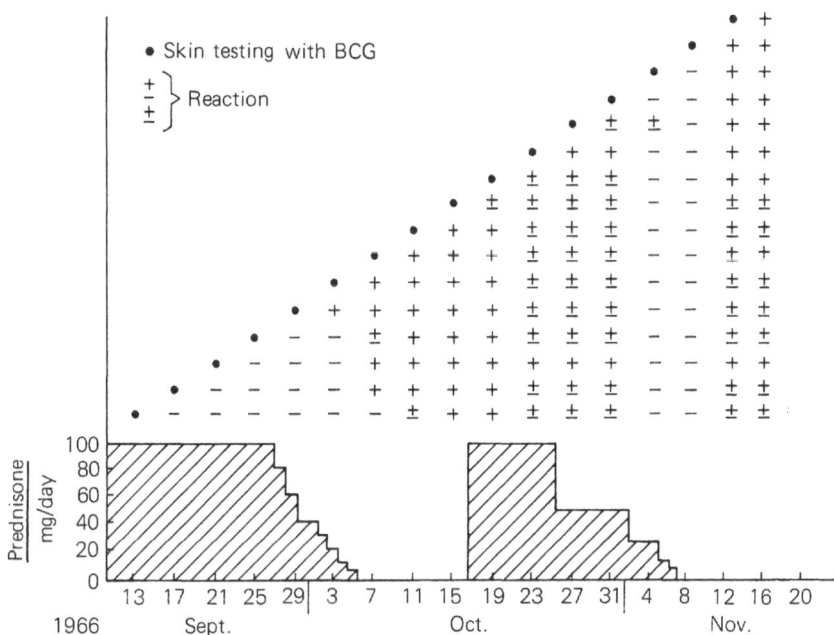

Fig. 10-3. Effect of prednisone on the immune responses to BCG. (From MATHE et al. (22))

The reactivity of T lymphocytes can also be tested in vitro by stimulating them to undergo blast-cell transformation with phytohemagglutinin, a mutagen specific for this cell line.

The role of antibodies (humoral immunity) in the defense against the cancer cells is complex. Antibodies directed against tumor cells can be either "cytotoxic" (complement-fixing antibodies) or "enhancing" (blocking antibodies). The latter may be responsible for the phenomenon of tumor enhancement. The study of tumor-directed antibodies is complicated and can only be carried out in research institutes.

Changes in weight (provided the patient does not have edema or ascites) and performance status reflect changes in general condition.

Special flowsheets are often used for leukemic patients. The size of lymph nodes and spleen, changes in the blood counts and number of blasts in the peripheral blood and bone marrow, as well as the marrow cellularity are the most important parameters in hematologic malignancies. The use of semilogarithmic charts is recommended because they show the rate at which the count falls, which is more important than the absolute level.

In evaluating toxicity, it is sometimes difficult to determine whether certain alterations in blood counts or chemistry (e.g., transaminases, bilirubin, etc.) are side-effects of the therapy or due to progressive disease. A short break in the chemotherapy may give the answer. The toxic manifestations of drugs were described in Chap. 7. With all chemotherapy, it is most important to obtain blood counts (Hct, WBC and, platelets) at certain intervals, depending on the drug and how it is given (daily vs. intermittent doses), and on the disease. More frequent counts are necessary in leukemias or when the bone marrow reserve is reduced by tumor involvement or previous therapy. Bone marrow toxicity is usually first manifested by leukopenia. With intermittent therapy, the low point of the white blood count may occur early (days 8 to 10) or late (day + 28), depending on the drug (see Fig. 7-1) (23). Most oncologists prefer to obtain some degree of toxicity, especially suppression of the neutrophil count, because this is an indication that the doses used are pharmacologically active and maximally tolerated. BROSS et al., however, have questioned whether there is any relationship between tumor response and degree of host toxicity (24-26). The preferential effect of some drugs on platelets must be kept in mind (see p. 135). A relatively stable hematocrit does not mean that chemotherapy is not myelosuppressive. Because of the long lifetime of the red blood cells, anemia is a late sign of bone marrow toxicity.

Table 10-5 shows a check list for toxic manifestations that occur specifically with particular agents and the tests used to monitor their early appearance.

G. DURATION OF THERAPY: INDICATIONS FOR A CHANGE IN THERAPY

Once a patient has received a particular drug regimen for a certain period of time, referred to as an "adequate trial" in protocol study terminology, the physician in charge must decide whether or not the patient is deriving any benefit from the treatment or in other words, whether to continue that treatment or try another one. Benefit is very relative and must be judged in terms of the results or the objectives listed in Table 9-1.

A particular regimen should be discontinued if the disease progresses despite an adequate trial to toxic levels. If the disease neither progresses nor regresses, the treatment may be continued as long as the disease remains stable, especially in the case of a tumor that was growing rapidly before treatment was initiated, or a malignancy for which no other effective chemotherapy is available. Under those circumstances, even if there is a slow progression of the disease. What constitutes an adequate trial depends on the type of drug used, the treatment schedule, and the disease treated (whether slowly or rapidly proliferating). With drugs given at high doses every 2 or 3 weeks, for instance, it should be possible to determine whether a tumor shows some sensitivity after 1 to 3 cycles. Incidently, the response, as judged from measurements of the diameter of tumor masses, may be deceptive. The size of a tumor mass may not change significantly for some time, since cells effectively killed by drugs may continue through several cycles before dying and swell before final dissolution (Fig. 10-4) (27).

Table 10-5. Checklist for "specific" toxicity of chemotherapeutic agents

Drugs	Clinical manifestations	Tests
Cyclophosphamide	Dysuria, hematuria	Urinalysis
Busulfan	Pulmonary	Chest X-ray (fibrosis)
Methotrexate	Stomatitis, Pulmonary	BUN, creatinine Liver function Chest X-ray (infiltrates)
6-MP	Icterus	Liver function
Cytosine arabinoside	Fever, flu-like illness	
5-FU	Stomatitis	
DIC	Flu-like illness	
Vincristine	Loss of reflexes, Muscle weakness	
Actinomycin D	Stomatitis	
Mithramycin	Rash (facial flush), Bleeding, CNS reactions	Coagulation tests, platelets, Ca Liver function Renal function
Bleomycin	Fever, Skin: dyskeratosis, Pulmonary Anaphylaxis	Chest X-ray (pneumonitis, fibrosis) Pulmonary function
Adriamycin Daunorubicin	Stomatitis, Arrhythmia, Congestive failure	Serum CPK ECG Chest X-ray (cardiomegaly)
L-Asparaginase	Rash, Anaphylaxis	Serum proteins, albumin, fibrinogen BUN, glucose Liver function Coagulation tests

No-one will deny that, in patients who respond, chemotherapy should be continued for as long as the patient continues to improve. It is much more difficult to decide how long to continue treatment in a patient who has obtained a complete remission. This is happening more frequently with several malignancies (Table 9-1), and studies designed to answer this question are still in progress. The task would be easier if there were some means of quantitating the number of tumor cells persisting in the body after the clinical manifestations of the malignancy have disappeared. Quantitation of chemical products (e.g., HCG in choriocarcinoma) or immunologic materials (tumor antigens such as the carcinoembryonic antigen in gastrointestinal malignancies) may in the future help to determine the optimal duration of chemotherapy (33). A retrospective method based on the "duration of unmaintained remissions" (28) is illustrated in Figs. 10-5 and 10-6 (23).

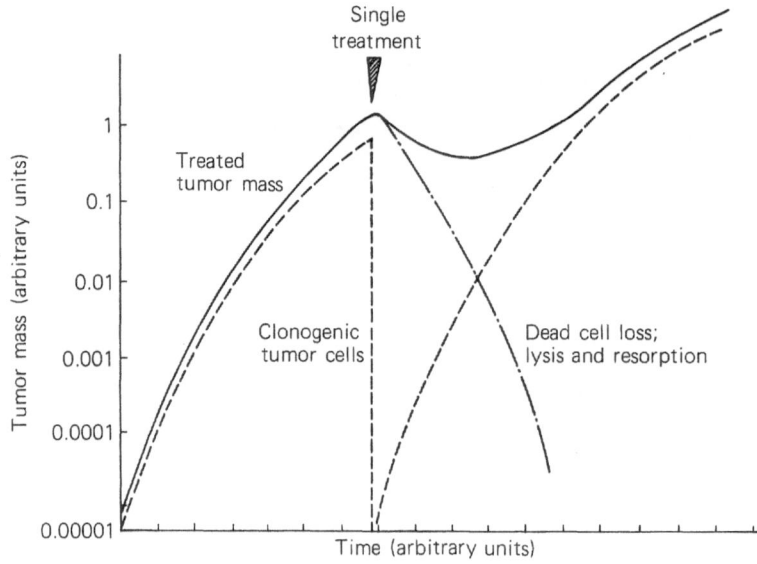

Fig. 10-4. Changes in tumor volume inaccurately reflect tumor response. As illustrated, a very effective treatment (a 5 log reduction of clonogenic tumor cells) is reflected by only a 50% regression in tumor volume. (From SKIPPER (27))

H. FINAL EVALUATION OF THERAPY

The final aspect of a treatment program is the recording of the response, both objective and subjective, at the end of the trial (Table 10-6).

Several systems are used. Karnofsky's classification in several categories, O, I, and II with subclasses (e.g., I-A, I-B, I-C, etc.), is cumbersome because these numerals are not descriptive of the response and the user has either to memorize them or make constant reference to a table (Table 10-7) (29).

Most of the American cooperative studies classify their responses in terms of complete remission, partial response, and failure, as defined in Table 10-8 (7). However, this classification fails to distinguish between the two important parameters in the evaluation of response: (1) the tumor itself, of which we measure the extent of the "regression" and its duration, and (2) the patient, in whom we determine the degree of "remission" of the "pathologic state" caused by the tumor (30, 31). The response in these two parameters is not necessarily concordant. For instance, an apparent complete tumor regression may be accompanied by complete remission, incomplete remission, or no remission at all, perhaps even death through a complication of the disease or the treatment. The classification used by the EORTC (Table 10-9) distinguishes between these two parameters. Thus, the response of a patient with lung cancer whose tumor mass disappears during therapy with a new agent, but who dies in aplasia, is not classified as complete remission (31), yet the potential activity of the drug in lung cancer is duly recognized. We urge that there be more uniformity in systems for staging diseases as well as for reporting results. More could then be learned from comparisons of different studies.

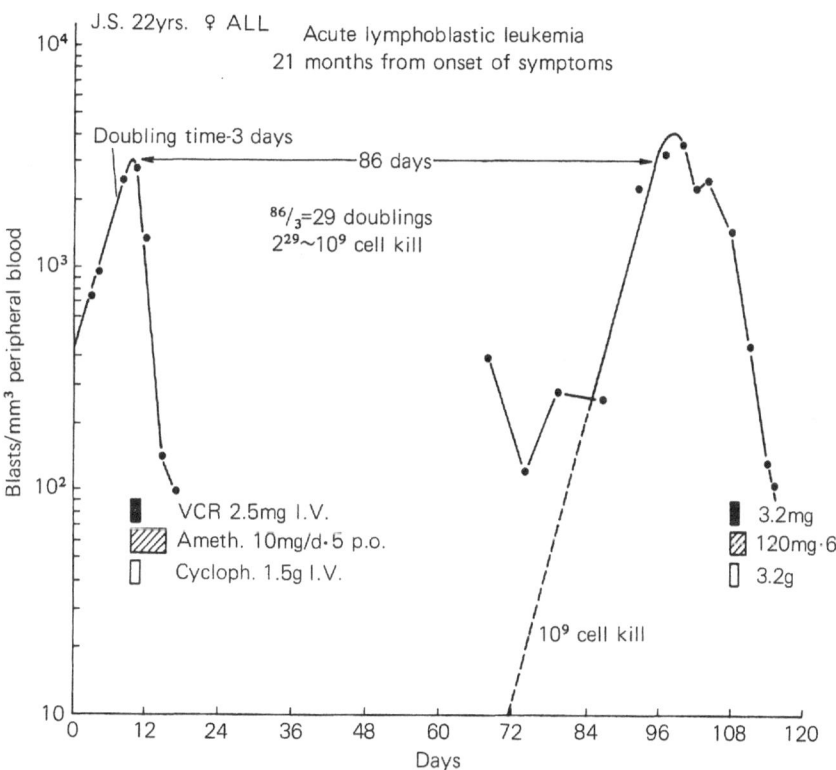

Fig. 10-5. Estimation of the leukemic cell kill in acute lymphoblastic leukemia. The total number of leukemic blast cells per mm³ of peripheral blood was determined at intervals before and after treatment with a combination of vincristine (VCR), amethopterin (ameth.), and cyclophosphamide (cycloph.). Prior to treatment and during relapse the leukemic blasts increased with a doubling time of three days. It took 86 days for the leukemic blasts to recover to the pre-treatment value, indicating that the treatment reduced these cells by the equivalent of 86 ÷ 3, or 29 doublings. 2^{29} is equivalent to a 10^9 cell kill. The extrapolation of the line plotting the rate of increase of leukemic blasts during relapse back to the time of treatment also indicates a 10^9 cell kill. (From BERGSAGEL (23))

The response to a particular regimen can also be evaluated by determining the prolongation of survival (7). This method is most valuable when there are no measurable lesions, for instance, in adjuvant therapy studies, but it has several disadvantages. A larger number of patients is required to neutralize various nontherapeutic factors that may affect survival. Moreover, the fact that no therapy may be given subsequent to the initial test drug creates serious ethical problems. This method allows evaluation only a posteriori, after death, but we need to know while patients are still alive whether a therapy is ineffective or harmful. Tumor regression does not necessarily mean prolonged survival. In rapidly fatal malignancies, such as lung carcinoma, answers are obtained whithin a couple of years. In malignancies that run a more protracted course, or where a high cure rate is obtained, one can attempt to evaluate the benefit of a treatment modality by determining the "disease-free" intervals following therapy. For instance, it has been determined that patients with Hodgkin's disease who remain

Table 10-6.

DIVISION OF MEDICAL ONCOLOGY

Hosp. No –

Name –

Diagnosis – primary site –
– cell type – – – – – – – – – – – – – – –

Stage –

Protocol –

OFF STUDY SUMMARY

TREATMENT SUMMARY	Dates		Dose schedule	Amount each dose	Total amount administered
	first dose	last dose			

REPONSE

OBJECTIVE

☐ complete
☐ partial
☐ >50%
☐ <50%
☐ mixed
☐ statu quo
☐ failure (progressive disease)
☐ inadequate trial

If CR or PR

Parameter _____
Duration _____

SUBJECTIVE

☐ good
☐ fair
☐ none
☐ worse
☐ not evaluable

Parameter _____
Duration _____

Table 10-6. (continued)

SIDE EFFECTS	attributed to			severity			life		effect on therapy
	drug	Ca.	other	mild	mod.	severe	threat.	irrev.	measures required

---

OFF STUDY SUMMARY

Date off study _____

☐ study completed

☐ study terminated early reason: _____

☐ Death
☐ Toxicity
☐ Refused further therapy
☐ Lost to follow up
☐ Other _____

SURVIVAL STATUS

☐ Alive: further chemotherapy planned

☐ yes

☐ no

Death: data of death _____

Autopsy
☐ yes
☐ no
☐ unknown

Cause of death:
☐ tumor
☐ infection
☐ drug
☐ other
☐ unknown

195

Table 10-7. Evaluation of response to therapy. (From KARNOFSKY (<u>29</u>))

Categories of response

Category 0	No clinically useful effect on the course of the disease
0-0	Disease-progresses-no objective or subjective benefit.
0-A[+]	Subjective benefit without favorable objective changes.
0-B[+]	Favorable objective changes without subjective benefit.
0-C	Subjective benefit and favorable objective changes in measurable criteria, but of less than 1 month's duration; then the disease progresses.
Category I	Clinical benefit with favorable objective changes in all measurable criteria of the disease
I-A[+]	Distinct subjective benefit with favorable objective changes in all measurable criteria for one month or more.
I-B[+]	Objective regression of all palpable or measurable neoplastic disease for one month or more in a relatively asymptomatic patient, who is able to carry on his usual activities without undue difficulty. The observed tumor regression should be unequivocal and it is suggested that all lesions be reduced at least 50% in bulk. This category applies as long as the regression persists, and ends if any lesion, old or new, recurs.
I-C	Complete relief of symptoms, if any, and regression of all manifestations due to active disease for 1 year or more. The relation to the frequency of therapy is not relevant, if the disease does not recur between courses of therapy.

[+]Categories apply as long as improvement from baseline persists. Superscript shows duration of response in months. Example: $0-A^4$ or $I-B^3$.

Category II	Interruption or slowing in the progression of the disease without definite evidence of subjective or objective improvement.

No criteria are presently available to classify this type of response. Statistical evidence of prolongation of survival time in specific patterns of cancer may some day be applicable.

Table 10-8. Definitions of tumor response commonly used in clinical trials (<u>7</u>)

Complete remission:
Disappearance of all clinical evidence of active tumor (recognizable tumor masses and/or biochemical changes directly related to the tumor). (Some studies specify: disappearance of all subjective evidence of disease).

Partial remission:
50% or greater reduction in measurable tumor (of one or more lesions) in the absence of progression or occurrence of new lesions elsewhere).

Stable disease:
Steady state or response less than the partial remission. No increase in size of any lesion or appearance of new lesions.

Progressive disease:
Occurrence of any new lesion or increase of any measurable lesion >50%, irrespective of regression elsewhere.

Table 10-9. Proposed evaluation of response to therapy (30).

Treatment	Diagnosis	Number of patients treated	Complete regression		Partial regression >50%		Partial regression <50%		Failure	Toxic cost	
			With complete remission	Without complete remission	With partial remission	Without remission	With partial remission	Without remission		Lethal	Non lethal

Definitions

Complete regression: The disappearance of tumor cells to the limits of clinical and laboratory investigation (imperceptible disease)

The tumor

Partial regression: The measurable reduction of tumor cells by clinical and laboratory parameters
(perceptible disease)

Complete remission: The disappearance of signs and symptoms of disease to the limits of clinical and
laboratory examination of the patient

The patient

Partial remission: The measurable amelioration of signs and symptoms of disease by clinical and
laboratory examination of the patient

197

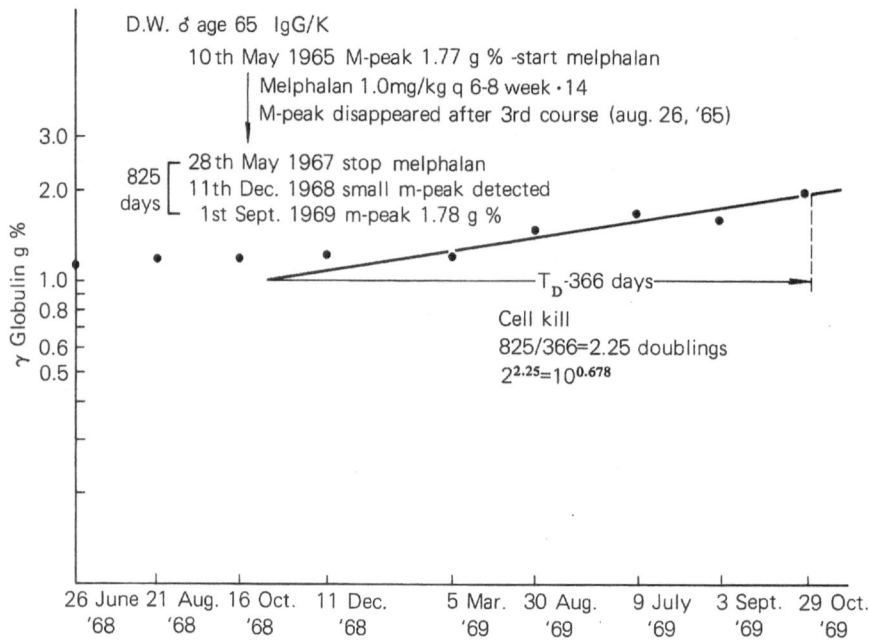

Fig. 10-6. Method of calculating the log cell kill in multiple myeloma
by serial determinations of the serum M protein. Melphalan was stopped
after 14 courses. The M protein reappeared 2 years later and increased
slowly with doubling time of 366 days. The period from the end of therapy until the serum protein increased to the pretreatment level was 825
days. From these data it is possible to estimate that the 14 course
of melphalan therapy reduced the tumor size by the equivalent of the
number of cells formed in 2.25 doublings, or 67.8%, which is less than
one log. (From BERGSAGEL (12))

relapse-free for 5 years after radiotherapy have a 95 percent chance
of being permanently cured (32).

REFERENCES

1. LUKES, R., CRAVES, L., HALL, T., RAPPAPORT, H., RUBIN, P.: Report on
   nomenclature Commitee. Cancer Res. 26 (part 1), 1311 (1966)
2. MATHE, G., POUILLART, P., WEINER, R., HAYAT, M., STERESCO, M., LA-
   FLEUR, M.: Classification and subclassification of acute leukemias
   correlated with clinical expression, therapeutic sensitivity and
   prognosis. In: Recent Results in Cancer Research, Vol. 43, p. 6.
   Nomenclature, Methodology and Results of Clinical Trials in Acute
   Leukemia (eds. G. Mathê, P. Pouillart, L. Schwarzenberg) Berlin-Heidelberg-New York: Springer 1973.
3. UNION INTERNATIONALE CONTRE LE CANCER. T.N.M. classification of
   malignant tumours. Geneva: G. de Buren S.A. 1968
4. Clinical oncology (ed. UICC). Berlin-Heidelberg-New York: Springer-
   Verlag 1973
5. RUBIN, P. A unified classification of cancers: an oncotaxonomy with
   symbols. Cancer 31, 963 (1973)

6. KARNOFSKY, P.A., BURCHENAL, J.H.: The clinical evaluation of chemotherapeutic agents in cancer. In: Evaluation of Chemotherapeutic
   Agents, p. 191 (ed. C.M. Macleod). New York: Columbia Univ. Press
   1949
7. CARTER, S.K. Study design principles for the clinical evaluation
   of new drugs as developed by the chemotherapy programme of the NCI.
   In: The Design of Clinical Trials in Cancer Therapy, p. 242. (ed.
   M. Staquet) Brussels: Editions Scientifiques Européennes 1972
8. MOERTEL, C.G., SCHUTT, A.J., HAHN, R.G., REITEMEIER, R.J.: Effects
   of patient selection on results of Phase II chemotherapy trials in
   gastrointestinal cancer. Cancer Chemother. Rep. Part 1, _58_, 257
   (1974)
9. OMENN, G.S.: Ectopic polypeptide hormone production by tumors. Ann.
   intern. Med. _72_, 136 (1970)
10. BODANSKY, O.: Biochemical tests for cancer. CA, _23_, 275 (1973)
11. BAGSHAWE, K.D.: Choriocarcinoma. Baltimore: Williams and Wilkins
    1969
12. BERGAGEL, D.E.: Multiple myeloma: clinical course and treatment.
    In: Oncology, 1970, Vol _4_, p. 453 (eds R.L. Clark, R.W. Cumley,
    McCay) Chicago: Year Book Medical Publishers 1971
13. SALMON, S.E.: Immunoglobulin synthesis and tumor kinetics of multi-
    ple myeloma. Seminars in Hemat. _10_, 135 (1973)
14. KENNEDY, B.J., CALABRESI, P., CARBONE, P.P., FREI, E. III, HOLLAND,
    J.F., OWENS, Jr., A.H., SLEISENGER, M.H., BECK, J.C.: Training pro-
    gram in medical oncology. Ann. intern. Med. _78_, 127 (1973)
15. KENNEDY, B.J.: Oncology in medicine. Ann. intern. Med. _73_, 637
    (1970)
16. MATHE, G.: Le rôle de l'interniste en cancérologie clinique. Le
    nécessaire service de médecine cancérologique interne dans le cen-
    tre hospitalier universitaire. In: Entretiens de Bichat 1973. Le
    Praticien face aux problèmes du cancer, p. 59. Paris: L'Expansion
    Ed. 1973
17. E.O.R.T.C. Leukaemia and Hematosarcoma Co-op. Group: A controlled
    trial in acute myeloid leukaemia, comparing CAR, CAR combined with
    THG and CAR combined with DRB. Absence of difference. Biomedicine
    _18_, 192 (1973)
18. EVERSON, T.C., COLE, W.H.: Spontaneous Regression of Cancer. Phila-
    delphia: W.B. Saunders 1966
19. KENIS, Y.: Chemotherapy of residual disease in solid tumours. Rev.
    Europ. Etudes Clin. et Biol. _16_, 103 (1971)
20. SCHNEIDER, M.: Effet des chimiothérapies antimitotiques sur une
    réaction d'hypersensibilité retardée (BCG). Rev. franc. Etudes clin.
    biol. _13_, 877 (1968)
21. AISENBERG, A.C.: Value of immunologic testing. J. amer. Med. Ass.
    _222_, 1301 (1972)
22. MATHE, G.: Operational research in cancer chemotherapy. Chemotherapy
    in the strategy of cancer treatment. In: Scientific Basis of Cancer
    Chemotherapy, p. 72 (ed. G. Mathé), Berlin-Heidelberg-New York:
    Springer, 1969
23. BERGSAGEL, D.E.: An assesment of massive-dose chemotherapy of malig-
    nant disease. Canad. Med. Ass. J. _104_, 31 (1971)
24. BROSS, I.D.J., RIMM, A.A., SLACK, N.H., AUSMAN, R.K., JONES, Jr.,
    R.: Is toxicity really necessary? I. The question. Cancer _19_, 1780
    (1966)
25. BROSS, I.D.J., RIMM, A.A., SLACK, N.H., AUSMAN, R.K., JONES, Jr.,
    R.: Is toxicity really necessary? II. Source and analysis of data.
    Cancer _19_, 1785 (1966)
26. BROSS, I.D.J., RIMM, A.A., SLACK, N.H., AUSMAN, R.K., JONES, Jr.,
    R.: Is toxicity really necessary? III. Theoretical aspects. Cancer
    _19_, 1796 (1966)
27. SKIPPER, H.E.: Kinetic mammary tumor cell growth and implications
    for therapy. Cancer _28_, 1479 (1971)

28. FREI, E., FREIREICH, E.J.: Progress and perspectives in chemotherapy of acute leukemia. Adv. Chemother. 2, 269 (1965)
29. KARNOFSKY, D.A.: Meaningful clinical classification of therapeutic responses to anti-cancer drugs. Clin. Pharmacol. Ther. 2, 709 (1961)
30. MATHE, G., WEINER, R.: Criteria for short-term results in the treatment of acute leukemia. In: Recent Results in Cancer Research, Vol. 43, p. 110. Nomenclature, Methodology and Results of Clinical Trials in Acute Leukemia (eds. G. Mathé, P. Pouillart, L. Schwarzenberg). Berlin-Heidelberg-New York: Springer 1973
31. MATHE, G., KENIS, Y.: Logistics of clinical trials. The Example of Cancerology. Biomedicine 18, 181 (1973)
32. KAPLAN, H.S.: Prognostic Significance of Relapse Free Interval after Radiotherapy for Hodgkin's Disease. Cancer 22, 1131 (1968)
33. RAVRY, M., MOERTEL, C.G., SCHUTT, A.J., GO, V.L.W.: Usefulness of serial serum carcinoembryonic antigen (CEA) determinations during anti-cancer therapy or long-term follow-up of gastrointestinal carcinoma. Cancer 34, 1230 (1974)

Chapter 11

Management of Complications in the Course of Malignant Disease

The course of cancer patients is often plagued with complications due
to disease or its treatment. Since they may seriously compromise the outcome of therapy and the comfort of the patient, it is most important
to be familiar with their proper management.

A. INFECTIONS

Infections are especially common in acute leukemias, where they are
the cause of death in 70% of patients (1 - 5, 126). Infection is also the
most common cause of death in patients with solid tumors (3). Suppression of the myeloid, immune and reticulo-endothelial systems, caused
by the disease and further aggravated by chemotherapy, weakens the patient's defense mechanisms. Mucosal ulcerations, catheters (intravenous,
bladder), and various medical and surgical procedures become sites of
entry for infection. Frequent use of antibiotics may alter the host's
bacterial flora, and a hospital is a most dangerous environment for
this type of patient (6-8).

The majority of infections are bacterial, predominantly Pseudomonas and
other Gram-negative pathogens, such as E. coli, Klebsiella, Enterobacter-
Serratia group, and Proteus. The frequency of Gram-positive infections,
especially with Staphylococcus aureus, has declined with the advent of
penicillinase-resistant antibiotics. More exotic organisms may put the
diagnostic skills of clinicians and microbiologists to the test. Fungal
infections must always be suspected (9-10), (especially candidiasis and
aspergillosis (11), less often mucormycosis (12-13), cryptococcosis and
histoplasmosis), also higher bacteria (nocardiasis (14), tuberculosis)
and protozoa (Pneumocystis carinii (15, 16, 112), toxoplasmosis (17, 18).
Herpes simplex, Herpes zoster and cytomegalic inclusion disease are
common viral infections (19-21). Multiple organisms may be isolated from
blood cultures (22).

The oropharynx, skin, anorectal area (23, 24), lung (25, 26), blood, and
urinary tract are the most common sites of infection. The usual clinical
manifestations of infection are often absent in granulocytopenic patients, who tend to have fever without any other localizing signs or
symptoms. What would normally be an abcess may not be purulent, radiologic evidence of pneumonitis may be sparse, and infected sputum, urine,
exudates, or cerebrospinal fluid may lack granulocytes. Adequate specimens for pathologic and microbiologic examination (tracheal aspirate,
lung biopsy) can be difficult to obtain because of associated thrombocytopenia.

Prophylactic antibiotic therapy is not recommended for leukopenic patients. It can alter the normal flora and favor resistant organisms.
However, potential portals of entry for infection should be watched,
and it is good practice to carry out regular bacteriologic checks in
patients (especially those with acute leukemia) who are or may become
granulocytopenic as a result of intensive chemotherapy (1, 27). Cultures are obtained from various areas of the skin (axillae, perineum,
anus, vagina), nose, gingiva, oropharynx, urine, stool, sputum, and room
air to check for aerobes, anaerobes, and fungi. The purpose of these
checks is threefold: (1) to treat carriers of pathogens (for instance,
Staphylococcus aureus, Pseudomonas) prophylactically with local or systemic antibiotics, depending on the site of the positive culture; (2)
to exclude actual infection; and (3) to identify the flora of the host
and his environment. This information will help the clinician to select
provisional initial antibacterial therapy if the patient's clinical appearance suggests an infection, which cannot always await the results
of bacteriologic studies.

In the event of actual infection, the bacteriologic survey is repeated.
In addition, several blood cultures are obtained as well as cultures
of any obvious lesion or inflammatory exudate. Cultures of bone marrow
and cerebrospinal fluid may also be indicated (28). Gram stains of the
appropriate material may provide some guidance as to the nature of the
infection. Serum should be saved for possible serologic diagnosis and
specimens for special fungal, protozoal, and virological identification
should be collected. Once these procedures having been done, most oncology services dealing with patients with weakened defenses will treat
de novo febrile episodes quickly and vigorously, preferably with bac-
teriocidal antibiotics given in high doses parenterally. Patients with
adequate granulocyte levels who have no localizing signs or clues as
to the specific organisms are best treated by gentamycin, with or without a cephalosporin or a penicillinase-resistant penicillin. This broad-
spectrum combination should be effective against most Gram-negative organisms, including Proteus and Pseudomonas species, as well as coagu-
lase-positive Staphylococci (1). In granulocytopenic patients, carbenicillin and a cephalosporin make up an adequate combination with a similar broad spectrum including Pseudomonas, these organisms being especially lethal in neutropenic patients. Patients who respond promptly to
initial antibiotic therapy should continue to receive this therapy for
7-10 days (29). Gentamycin is less effective at low granulocyte levels
but may have to be added to carbenicillin and cephalosporin in patients
who fail to respond to this combination after 4 days of therapy (29).
BLOOMFIELD and KENNEDY used the triple combination as initial empirical
therapy of febrile episodes occurring in adults with acute leukemia (113)
Gentamycin plus carbenicillin should be used only with proven Pseudomonas infections (30-32). This combination is less active against other
Gram negative infections, for example E. Coli, Klebsiella, and Staphylococcus, than gentamycin alone. This choice of antibiotics may have to
be changed in the future, as the number of strains resistant to these
antibiotics will undoubtedly increase (33).

The patient must be frequently questioned and examined for localizing
symptoms and signs throughout the febrile episode and the initially
chosen antibiotic combination may have to be adjusted according to the
sensitivity of the causative organism, if indeed one is identified.

Amphotericin B, in spite of its many side-effects, remains the drug
of choice for fungal infections (34, 114). Pneumocystis carinii infections are best treated with pentamidine (35, 112) and Nocardia with
long-term sulfonamide therapy (14). Cytosine arabinoside seemed promising in disseminated Herpes zoster infections, but a recent controlled
study has questioned its value (36-39).

Some specialized cancer centers are equipped with "life islands" or pathogen-free rooms to protect neutropenic patients against hospital-acquired (exogenous) infections (Fig. 11-1 and 11-2) (1, 40-44, 127). Protection against the patient's own bacterial flora (endogenous infections) is provided by sterilization of the skin and oropharynx with topical antiseptics and of the gastrointestinal tract with oral, nonabsorbable antibiotics. A commonly used combination is vancomycin, gentamycin, and nystatin (45). These two methods have effectively reduced the incidence and fatality rate of severe infections. The control of infections in neutropenic patients has in recent years been greatly improved by the use of leukocyte transfusions (Table 11.1) (1, 46, 128). The incidence of infection is correlated with the severity of the neutropenia (47). When WBC counts fall below 100 granulocytes/mm^3, patients have severe infections 45 percent of the time. Large numbers of granulocytes, sufficient to raise the WBC count of neutropenic patients, can be obtained either from patients with chronic myelogenous leukemia (9^{10} to 10^{11} cells) in relapse through leukaphoresis, or from normal donors with the use of the NCI-IBM continuous-flow blood-cell separator (48-50). A newer simpler technique based on the adherence of granulocytes to nylon filters (Leukopaks, Fenwall) may make the procurement of granulocytes possible for most hospital blood banks (51, 115). The best results are obtained by using HL-A-matched donors (52).

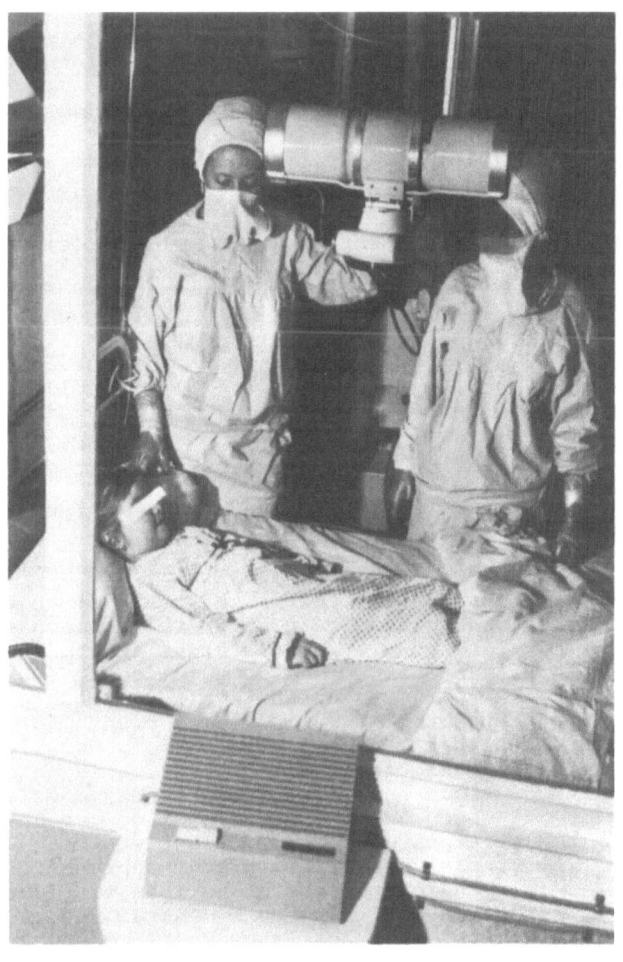

Fig. 11-1. Interior of a pathogen-free room at the Institute of Cancerology and Immunogenetics, Paul Brousse Hospital, Villejuif, France

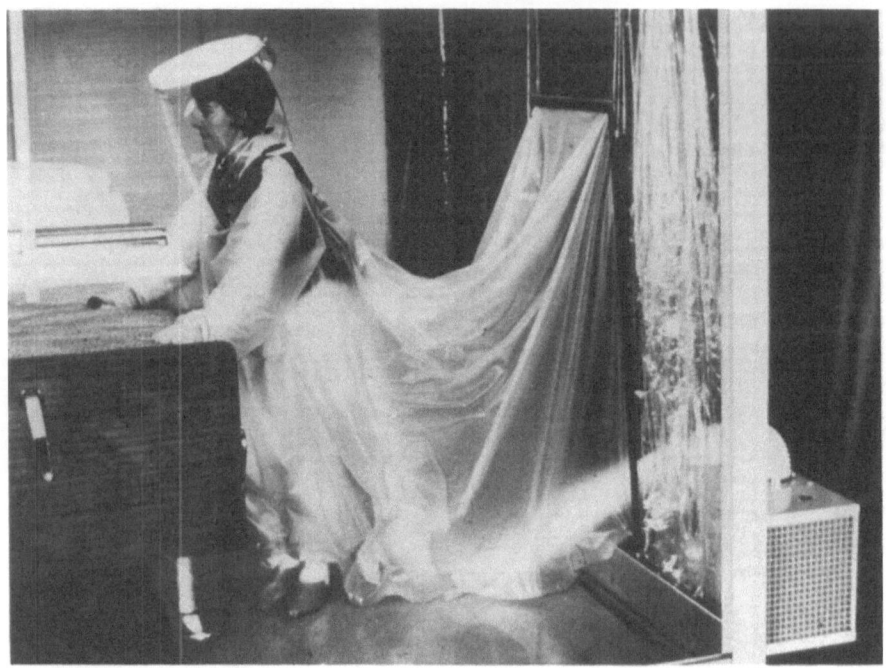

Fig. 11-2. Access to a patient in a protected environment

Table 11-1. Effectiveness of white blood cell transfusions in severe neutropenia (SCHWARZENBERG et al. (46))

Number of white cell transfusions	Number of transfused granulocytes	Results in 315 patients	
		Infection controlled	Increase in white blood count
990	749×10^{11}	164 (52%)	120 (38%)

B. BLEEDING

Bleeding disorders are the second most common cause of death in hematologic malignancies. The most prevalent mechanism is a fall in the number of platelets, but qualitative abnormalities of platelets, the presence of M proteins, and coagulation defects may also induce abnormal bleeding. There is a quantitative relationship between frequency and severity of hemorrhage and platelet count (53). Although there is no magic number that can be called safe, generally no bleeding need be anticipated until the platelet count falls below 30,000. A rapid fall is more dangerous than chronic thrombocytopenia. The incidence of major bleeding has been greatly reduced since the development of techniques for platelet transfusion (54). Platelets from HL-A-matched sibling donors are the most effective (55). The presence of fever, infection, splenomegaly, and antiplatelet-antibodies reduces the benefit of platelet transfusions (56). The more general use of platelet transfusions is still inhibited by the large number of donors required, the short life-span of the transfused platelets (5 to 10 days), inadequate storage techniques, the presence of platelet antibodies, the complexity of HL-A typing, and the rarity of HL-A identity among unrelated donors (50). Incidentally, it is good practice to prevent menorrhagia by inducing amenorrhea with progestational agents. Abnormalities of coagulation and hemostasis are also common in malignant disease and may cause hemorrhage or more rarely thrombosis (57). Intravascular coagulation and secondary fibrinolysis have been reported in almost all types of malignancy, but especially in carcinoma of the prostate and leukemia. A great deal has been learned in recent years about the diagnosis and the management of these conditions (58, 116). Several cytotoxic agents cause bleeding problems, notably L-asparaginase and mithramycin (59, 60).

C. ANEMIA

Varying degrees of anemia are often present in cancer patients, especially in the more advanced stages. Different physiopathologic mechanisms may be involved (Table 11-2) (57, 61, 62). Since some of these mechanisms are correctable, it is recommended that an attempt be made to determine the etiology of any significant degree of anemia instead merely transfusing the patient.

Table 11-2. Causes of anemia in malignant disease

---

1. Blood loss: e.g., GI, GU tract

2. Hemolysis: autoimmune
              overactivity of RES
              erythrophagocytosis
              hypersplenism
              micro-angiopathic

3. Tumor involvement of the bone marrow

4. Dyserythropoietic anemia:
              anemia of chronic disease
              sideroblastic anemia
              erythroid hypoplasia, e.g., thymoma

5. Deficiency states:
              iron
              folic acid
              B12
              protein

6. Myelosuppression due to cytotoxic therapy

D. HYPERCALCEMIA

Hypercalcemia, another complication of cancer, is generally caused by the presence of osteolytic bone metastases (63-65). More rarely, the underlying mechanism is a parathyroid hormone-like (PTH) polypeptide or a substance with vitamin D-like activity produced by the tumor (63, 66). The osteolytic type, most commonly seen in myeloma, breast cancer, and leukemia, has positive bone X-rays and scans and responds to steroids, whereas the hormonal type does not, but a radioimmunoassay for parathyroid hormone may be abnormally high. The latter type is most prevalent in squamous-cell cancers, especially of the lung, and is not necessarily associated with disseminated disease. Substances other than parathyroid hormone and metabolites of vitamin D may be implicated. The possibility that prostaglandins stimulate bone resorption has been considered (63, 129). Indomethacin could control this type of hypercalcemia by decreasing prostaglandin synthesis (117, 129). Immunobilization of the patient because of bone pain or a pathologic fracture, or the initiation of hormone therapy in breast cancer, may be a precipitating or contributory factor. The serum calcium influences a number of physiological processes: the stability and excitability of cell membranes and nervous tissues, muscle contraction, gastric secretion and activation of enzymes (e.g., of the pancreas), and coagulation. Hypercalcemia is accompanied by decreased glomerular filtration and alterations in tubular function with a clinical picture of diabetes insipidus. Cancer patients who begin to complain of weakness, anorexia, nausea, vomiting, constipation, polyuria and polydypsia, and muscular weakness must be suspected of having hypercalcemia. If the condition is confirmed, they must be treated immediately to prevent subsequent stupor, confusion, coma, or renal failure. Note that many of these symptoms are similar to those of advancing disease.

General therapeutic measures to prevent hypercalcemia or recurrences include avoidance of immobilization, maintenance of adequate hydration and salt intake, limitation of calcium intake (dairy products), oral phosphates and proper therapy for the underlying malignancy (Table 11-3).

For immediate control of milder cases, infusions of physiologic saline with corticosteroids are usually successful if the hypercalcemia is due to lytic metastases. The potent diuretics, ethacrinic acid or furosemide, may also increase calcium excretion and are a useful adjunct, especially when large amounts of fluid are administered to patients with cardiovascular disease (130). Sodium sulfate has been recommended for accelerated calcium diuresis (67). If these measures fail, mithramycin should be tried at dose levels lower than for its anti-tumor effect (68, 69). Mithramycin can also be used in cases with increased PTH-like activity. The usefulness of calcitonin is still under investigation (70, 71, 118).

Intravenous inorganic phosphate has been recommended for rapid lowering of calcium in patients with severe impairment of renal function (72). Serious side-effects can occur, especially extra-skeletal precipitation of calcium (73, 74). This problem does not occur with oral phosphates, provided they are not given until the hypercalcemia has been corrected.

When estrogens, androgens, or progestational agents have precipitated hypercalcemia, hormone therapy should be discontinued, even though it is realized that tumor regression may occasionally occur with continued estrogen therapy (75). However, the occurrence of this complication suggests that the tumor is hormone-dependent, and ablative procedures can be considered.

E. HYPERURICEMIA

Hyperuricemia used to be a serious complication of the treatment of leukemia and lymphomas in particular. There is no excuse for the occurrence of hyperuricemia in present-day chemotherapy, since allopurinol (76, 77) effectively prevents it (Table 11-4). Nucleic-acid purines are liberated during rapid destruction of tumor cells by effective chemotherapy. Oxidation of these purines leads to the production of excess

Table 11-3. Management of hypercalcemia
_____

General measures: to prevent hypercalcemia or recurrences

1. Avoid immobilization.
2. Insure adequate hydration, adequate salt intake.
3. Restrict calcium intake: milk, cheese, butter (of limited
   usefulness).
4. Treat underlying malignancy.
5. Discontinue hormone therapy if it precipitated hypercalcemia.
6. Oral phosphate therapy: 1.0-3.0 g P; q.d. in divided doses:
          Neutra - Phos® (4 capsules = 1 g P)
          Fleet Brand Phospho-soda® (10 ml = 1.5 g P)

          Adjust dose to avoid diarrhea.
          May be ineffective if aluminium hydroxide preparations
          are given simultaneously.

Measures for immediate control

   Objectives: 1. Restoration of extracellular fluid volume: isotonic
                   saline.
                2. Reduction of Ca in extracellular fluid.
                3. Correction of associated abnormalities: renal,
                   cardiac.

A. Milder cases:

   1. Infusion of physiologic saline for rehydration and increased
      urinary calcium excretion (Na competitively inhibits tubu-
      lar reabsorption of Ca). The amount depends on the degree
      of dehydration: clinical signs, weight, hemoconcentration.

   2. Corticosteroids: if hypercalcemia due to osteolytic metas-
      tases
          - Solucortef 250-500 mg/l every 8 h initially, or
          - Prednisone 30-100 mg qd, p.o., start with high dose
            and taper gradually.

   3. Especially useful in patients with cardiac disease. Add
          - furosemide or
          - ethacrynic acid to saline infusions.

B. More severe cases:

   4. Isotonic Na sulfate may be used for rapid calcium diuresis.
      The sulfate anion further inhibits tubular reabsorption by
      chelating the filtrated calcium. K sulfate and Mg sulfate
      are best added to the infusion to prevent their depletion.
      Each liter will lower Ca concentration about 1 mg/100 ml.
      Thus 5 liters may be required.
      R/ 1 l every 3-6 hrs (depending on clinical condition;
                            cardiac and renal function must be
                            adequate).

C. If there is no response to A 1 and 2 (+ 3) or A 2 and B 4:
   and for hypercalcemia due to PTH-like activity:
      R/ mithramycin
          - 0.025 µg/kg i.v.
          - repeat if no fall in serum Ca within 24-48 h, or if Ca
            returns to hypercalcemic levels.

D. In cases of renal failure:
      Hemo- or peritoneal dialysis with Ca-free media may be
      necessary.
_____

Table 11-4. Management of hyperuricemia

A. Prophylactic:
    1. ensure adequate hydration
    2. R/ allopurinol: 300 - 800 mg q.d., in divided doses,
       beginning at least 2 days prior to intensive chemotherapy.

B. Curative:
    a. if there is hyperuricemia, without renal failure:
       1. force fluids: 3-4 l per day
       2. R/ allopurinol: 200 mg, q.i.d.
       3. Alkalinization of urine: pH > 7.0
          R/ NaHCO3 5 - 10 g, q.d., p.o., and/or
          R/ acetazolamide: 0.5 - 1.0 gm, q.d., p.o., plus
          K supplement: 40 - 80 meq. q.d. (78)

    b. if there is acute acid nephropathy:
       - without oliguria: R/ same as B.a.
       - if oliguric: measures B a 1 - 3 are dangerous;
         R/ cautious diuresis with mannitol: 12.5 - 25 g, i.v.
         over 5-10 min with subsequent alkalinization if diuresis
         is successful

         cystoscopic manipulation: operative removal of stones or
         crystal deposits from ureters of renal pelvis

         peritoneal or hemo-dialysis.

uric acid and this can precipitate in the urinary tract, causing uric acid nephropathy and renal failure. Allopurinol, an isomer of hypoxanthine, inhibits xanthine oxidase, the enzyme responsible for the conversion of hypoxanthine to xanthine and then to uric acid. Allopurinol reduces serum and urine uric acid, and the resulting (lesser) increase in serum and urine non-uric acid oxypurines is seldom of any consequence, although a rare case of urinary xanthine stones has been reported (79). Allopurinol also blocks the metabolism of 6-MP to 6-thiouric acid (see page 62) and thus enhances its effect and toxicity. It is therefore recommended that the dose of 6-MP be reduced to one third of the usual dose when allopurinol is given at the same time.

F. MALIGNANT EFFUSIONS

Malignant effusions are not uncommon during the course of solid tumors (80-82). Pleural effusions occur most frequently in breast and lung cancer and in lymphomas, while ascites is especially prevalent with ovarian carcinomas. Effusions are caused by (1) the presence of tumor implants on serous surfaces, (2) a large number of free-floating viable tumor cells (like experimental ascites tumors) inducing a secondary inflammatory response, or (3) obstruction of veins or lymphatics by tumor masses (e.g., mediastinal, retroperitoneal) providing a transudate. Since effusions are often a source of great distress and discomfort to the patient, palliation is worthwhile. The selection and aggressiveness of therapy will depend on the pathophysiology of the effusion, the extent and progression of the underlying disease, and the experience of the treating physician. First, an attempt must be made to determine the nature of the effusion by the proper tests, because not all effusions in cancer patients are of malignant etiology (83). Infections, pulmonary infarction, congestive heart failure, and hypoproteinemia, among other causes, should be considered in the differential diagnosis.

Table 11-6. Agents for intracavitary instillation

	Dose	Pros and Cons	Contraindications	Possible Side-Effects
Nitrogen mustard (HN-2)	10-mg vial Pleural space: 0.4 mg/kg, but max.= 30 mg 0.2 mg/kg if marrow depression Premedicate as for systemic administration	Easy administration Inexpensive Readily available	Fluid loculation Neutropenia Thrombocytopenia	N + V Variable systemic absorption, possible marrow depression Fever (rare) "Reactive" effusion, may require 1-2 additional taps
ThioTEPA	15-mg vial 0.8 mg/kg	Less irritating than HN2; preferable for pericardial and peritoneal instillation Less effective than HN2 if an adhesive pleuritis is required	Fluid loculation	Rare
Quinacrine (Atebrine®)	200-mg ampoule, dissolved in 10 ml of saline Pleural space: 100-200 mgO q.d. or q.o.d. Ascites: 200-400 mgO q.d. or q.o.d. until sterile pleuritis or peritonitis (usually 3-5 doses) Ofirst inject 1/2 dose to test for idiosyncrasy	More irritating (effective) than HN2 and thioTEPA More acute toxicity Use only in otherwise resistant effusions No hematopoietic depression; useful when marrow reserve limited	Fluid loculation Use cautiously in patients predisposed to seizure disorder (e.g., cerebral metastases)	Local pain (50%), $\frac{+}{-}$ 24 h Fever (very common) Transient hypotension Transient ileus (after intraperitoneal instillation) Fibrothorax: difficult interpretation of subsequent chest x-rays

Table 11-6. (continued)

	Dose	Pros and Cons	Contraindications	Possible Side-Effects
Colloidal 32P (32CrPO4)	Pleural space: 5 – 10 mCi Ascites: 10 – 15 mCi	Advantages over 198Au: – produces β particles only; safer, no isolation required – physical half-life: 14.3 days; easier to obtain – less expensive – essentially no side-effects	Fluid loculation Open or draining fistula Better tolerated by leukopenic patients than HN2	Essentially no side-effect Minimal systemic absorption; minimal radiation sickness, marrow depression
Colloidal 198Au	Pleural space: 75–100 mCi Ascites: 150–225 mCi	Disadvantages: – β and γ emitter (γ has no therapeutic effect, irradiation hazard, requires isolation of patient) – physical half-life: 2.7 days; difficult to obtain, must be ordered just prior to use – expensive	Fuid loculation Open or draining fistula Presence of large tumors May be used in leukopenic patients	Mild radiation sickness after 3-4 days Nausea, diarrhea after peritoneal injection

Table 11-5. Steps in the management of malignant effusions

I   Diagnostic tap
     Determine:

          1. Nature of fluid: exudate or transudate (83).
          2. Cytology: presence of tumor cells.

II   Treat the underlying malignancy

          1. Systemic chemotherapy for disseminated cancer.
          2. Radiotherapy for localized, obstructing masses; rarely,
             surgery for localized, obstructing masses.

III General measures for control of effusions

          1. Diuretics: may control or slow down reaccumulation of
                         serosus effusions
             R/ 25 mg spirolactone q.i.d. plus
             0.5 g chlorothiazide t.i.d. or 40 mg furosemide q.d.
          2. Salt-free albumin, 25 mg q.d., i.v., if severe hypoalbu-
             minemia; effect is usually short-lived.

IV   Specific measures for control of effusions

          1. First try 1-3 paracenteses.
          2. If unsuccessful and malignant cells are present in the
             effusion, in the absence of loculations:

             A. try: local instillation of:
                     nitrogen mustard for pleural effusions
                     ThioTEPA for pericardial effusions
                                   ascites

             B. if above unsuccessful, try either:

                1. instillation of radioactive isotopes
                2. instillation of quinacrine (Atabrine®)
                3. a surgical procedure to obliterate the pleural
                   space:

                   - closed chest drainage for 4-7 days
                   - talc poudrage
                   - pleurectomy: fluid reaccumulation after closed
                                  chest drainage and patient in good
                                  condition with estimated survival
                                  of > 6 months
                   - decortication: when fibrothorax produces severe
                                    respiratory insufficiency and pa-
                                    tient in good condition with esti-
                                    mated survival > 6 months.

The treatment must always include a primary attack on the underlying
malignancy with systemic chemotherapy for disseminated disease, and
radiotherapy, or possibly surgery for localized obstructive masses that
cause transudates (Tables 11-5 and 11-6). General measures such as diuretics, or salt-free albumin in the case of hypoproteinemia, are rarely
of much benefit though they may sometimes retard reaccumulation of
fluid. One or more aspirations may sometimes suffice to control effusions and are recommended as the initial therapy in addition to the
primary treatment mentioned above. If frequent taps are required, more
aggressive local therapy should be instituted, aiming at the destruction of tumor cells, if present, and the obliteration of the pleural
space. We first try local instillation of cytotoxic agents. Nitrogen

mustard is the preferred therapy for pleural effusions, and thioTEPA, because it is less irritating, for intrapericardial and intraperitoneal instillations. If two or more injections fail, one can either try quinacrine (Atabrine) (84, 85), which is more irritant and causes more side-effects, especially local pain and fever, or resort to instillation of isotopes. The latter exert their effect primarily through radiation and secondarily through obliterative fibrosis. Isotopes are used in the form of colloidal suspensions, which are phagocytosed by the mesothelial cells lining the cavity, therefore systemic absorption is not significant and leukopenia is rare. A third option is a surgical procedure, either a closed chest drainage (86) with (119) or without intrapleural chemotherapy, talc poudrage (87), or a more extensive procedure such as pleurectomy or decortication (88, 120), depending on the general condition of the patient and the prognosis of the underlying malignancy.

Intracavitary instillations should not be used if the fluid is loculated. To instill any of the above-mentioned agents, the following procedure should be followed: first, most of the fluid is removed. After the instillation, the patient must frequently change position (prone, supine, right and left sides, and knee-chest position) to assure adequate distribution of the agent. This must be done rapidly when nitrogen mustard is used, since alkylation occurs within 5 min. An attempt should be made to keep the pleural space free of fluid, by repeated taps if necessary, until pleural adhesions develop; otherwise pockets of fluid, difficult to remove, will develop and the visceral pleura will become thickened and retract, thereby limiting pulmonary expansion. In addition to the drugs listed in Table 11-6, some authors have used 5-fluorouracil or bleomycin (89, 90, 121).

G. INTRACRANIAL HYPERTENSION

Cancer patients often present symptoms indicative of CNS derangement. The differential diagnosis includes cerebral metastases, meningeal involvement, bleeding, intracranial hypertension caused by necrosis and edema in and around metastases, infections (e.g., Cryptococcus), multifocal leukoencephalopathy, and side-effects of chemotherapy (L-asparaginase, procarbazine, mithramycin). Cerebral metastases are usually multiple (in 70 percent of cases) and most commonly associated with breast, bronchus, and gastrointestinal tumors and malignant melanoma.

The immediate work-up requires, besides a careful physical examination, X-rays of the skull, a brain scan, and EEG. A cautious lumbar puncture may also be indicated, especially in leukemic patients. Special studies (arteriography, pneumoencephalography) may be considered later, especially if the patient is thought to have a single metastasis for which surgery may be contemplated.

If control of intracranial hypertension is urgent, hypertonic solutions are used (91). Hypertonic urea, 0.5 - 1.0 g/kg is effective in 20-30 min and reduces pressure for approximately 6 h. Mannitol 20 percent in distilled water, 1.5 - 2.0 g/kg given over 20-30 min has been more popular in recent years. It reduces CSF pressure for 2 - 4 h. Rebound swelling of the brain may occur. Parental fluid administration must be watched: 5 percent dextrose in water may further increase intracranial pressure. Saline solutions should be used instead (5 percent glucose in normal or half-normal saline).

Corticosteroids are useful if the situation is less urgent, or to maintain initial control obtained with hypertonic solutions (122). Dexamethasone, 10 mg i.v., followed by 4 mg every 6 h, is given for several days until symptoms subside. The dose is then gradually tapered and switched to an oral preparation. Some patients may require a maintenance dose of 2-4 mg dexamethasone daily.

Further measures are usually required in addition to this symptomatic therapy. Whole-brain irradiation is the best method currently available for multiple brain metastases (92-94, 123, 124). Surgery may be justified in selected patients in good general condition, with single metastatic lesions (95, 125). Currently available cytotoxic agents that cross the blood-brain barrier, for example nitrosoureas, are not effective enough to be depended upon for control of intracranial hypertension. Intrathecal chemotherapy and radiotherapy are effective in CNS leukemia (see p. 257).

H. SPINAL CORD COMPRESSION

Pressure on the spinal cord or its blood supply may be caused by an epidural mass or by a vertebral metastasis causing collapse of the vertebral column (96). The patient usually presents with some paresthesias or motor difficulties in the lower extremities and urethral or rectal sphincter dysfunction; 80% suffer from back pain at the level of the lesion. Since involvement is usually extradural, a mixture of root and spinal cord symptoms often develops. The onset of symptoms may be acute or gradual but often one is dealing with a medical emergency, if permanent hemiplegia is to be prevented. The sudden onset of paraplegia (vascular?) and presence of paraplegia for over 36 h, or complete paraplegia are poor prognostic features.

A myelogram is necessary to determine the level and the extent of the involvement as clinical findings are unreliable. Radiotherapy is the primary treatment in radiosensitive tumors: lymphoma, Hodgkin's disease, neuroblastoma, Ewing's sarcoma. A rapidly acting agent (e.g., nitrogen mustard 0.4 mg/kg) and/or corticosteroids in cases of cytopenia, may be given simultaneously with commencement of radiotherapy to obtain a more rapid tumor regression and to prevent tumor swelling due to radiotherapy (97). The indications for laminectomy and surgical decompressions are not well defined (96, 98). This should be considered as the primary therapy in radioresistant tumors, in the absence of a histologic diagnosis or in cases of vertebral collapse, to be followed by postoperative radiotherapy.

I. SUPERIOR VENA CAVA OBSTRUCTION

This syndrome most often is seen in malignant lymphoma, Hodgkin's disease, and lung cancer (98-100). Edema of the head and neck and cerebral disturbances (drowsiness, stupor, coma, and seizures) develop if the venous pressure remains elevated. The onset of symptoms is acute or subacute. Since the cardiac output is often low, the patient is at risk of sudden death from cardiovascular collapse. Therapy must therefore be instituted within hours of recognition, sometimes even without histologic confirmation, provided a block has been demonstrated angiographically and other signs of tumor are present on the chest X-ray. An upright position, fast-acting diuretics (e.g., ethacrinic acid, i.v.), a low-salt diet, and steroids are symptomatic measures of limited value. The mainstay of curative therapy consists of prompt radiotherapy, initially in small doses, until the elevated pressure subsides. Many oncologists prefer to administer a fast-acting alkylating agent such as nitrogen mustard prior to radiotherapy to obtain more rapid tumor shrinkage and avoid aggravation of symptoms by radiation-induced tumor swelling.

K. EMOTIONAL PROBLEMS OF CANCER PATIENTS

Cancer remains the most feared of all diseases. Following the initial
shock that often overwhelms the patient when he hears the diagnosis
(we are talking of advanced cancers), anxiety (80 percent), depression
(75 percent) (101-106), anger (44 percent), and guilt (36 percent) are
the more common emotional reactions. Several defense mechanisms are
used to overcome this anxiety and feeling of helplessness. It is important to be aware of these adaptational psychosomatics in order to understand the patient's behavior. Most patients resort to denial, either
of having cancer, or of the probability of death from cancer. Some patients who have previously been responsible for the care of dependents
may transfer most of their anxiety to others to escape the helplessness
of not being able to control their own fate. Others reject the dependent
role and become very difficult to treat when their illness becomes dis-
abling. Cancer may be equated to less serious diseases that the patient
has survived, which reassures him that he can do it again. Still others
identify with the physician, who will actively combat the cancer while
they remain passive, and depend upon others to take care of them and
fight their battle. Magical thinking may attribute special, if not impossible, powers to the treating physician and the wonderful advances
in medicine. Some patients become very dependent through a mechanism
of regression (reverting to an earlier development stage). Others blame
their physicians (projection) for the misfortune that has overcome them.
Sublimation can make a helpless cancer patient helpful, kind, and phi-
lanthropic.

Many doctors still debate whether to tell their patients the true nature
of their disease (105, 107, 108, 131, 132). Most cancer patients will
know sooner or later. One cannot subject the patient to the extensive
diagnostic work-up and staging procedures and carry out a treatment that
often employs radiotherapy or long-term and probably complicated chemotherapy schedules without his guessing the reason for all this medical
ado. Uncertainty is much more difficult to deal with than the truth.
There is no other branch of medicine where a close relationship between
a physician and patient is so important. The patient's complete confidence, trust and respect can only be obtained by telling him the diagnosis honestly, sincerely, and sympathetically. In addition, it gives
the patient an opportunity to arrange his financial affairs and make
his peace with his Maker. The question is not so much whether to tell,
but rather how much and how. The truth can be conveyed by installments:
thus, a mass becomes a tumor and then a malignancy as the work-up proceeds. It is usually not difficult to sense how much the patient wants
to know, and it is good practice to find out from the patient or his
relatives, what he thinks he has and his estimation of the prognosis
before breaking the news. Cancer is often already suspected. Most patients wish to know the essentials; only a few, with a strong denial
defense, desire little information.

No patient with incurable cancer should ever be told how many months
or weeks he has to live, even if he asks. After all, "no one has the
gift of prophecy". If we anticipate that the disease could run a fatal
course within a given period, we can mention this as a possibility, adding: "in the worst of circumstances, if the treatment does not work
at all" (which will seem unlikely to the patient). This gives him an
opportunity to make the necessary arrangements. Responsible members of
the family should be told the details of the prognosis. It is most important, once the nature of the disease has been revealed, to maintain
the patient's hope, even in hopeless cases. This is best done by discussing and emphasizing the proposed treatment and taking a "give us a
chance" and "let's see what happens" attitude. In most cases, we can

always truthfully add: "we have seen worse cases than yours get better and live for so many years". This gives the patient an idea of prognosis under the best of circumstances. It will help him through the initial period of shock and reactive depression and create an atmosphere of free communication and trust that will enable him to overcome his fears and give him the strength to face his problem. Isolation of the patient with cancer will thus be avoided.

The patient should be treated in an atmosphere of hope and optimism combined with realism. He is encouraged to continue his usual occupations and hobbies as far as possible, while hospitalization, medical visits, and other restrictions of his freedom and independence (e.g., catheters) are kept to a minimum (133). The assistance of his family, visiting nurses, and social workers may be invaluable (108). It is important to have a single physician in charge from the start, who directs the entire effort.

Induction of a remission is accompanied by elation (101, 105, 109). Depression will recur with subsequent relapse. Finally, the patient makes a realistic adjustment to the reality of approaching death by shortening of his goals and planning. The physician must be able to cope with expressions of elation as well as the anger, resentment, and hostility of the patient or his family. He must have the courage to assume the responsibility for the patient to the very end, allowing the patient to die in physical, emotional, and psychological peace and dignity, instead of in loneliness, abandonment or rejection (104, 108, 110, 134). Finally, accepting his own limitations, he himself, rather than the family should decide when to withhold further active therapy ("pull out the plugs"), when the patient's condition finally appears irreversible.

REFERENCES

1. LEVINE, A.S., GRAW, Jr., R.G., YOUNG, R.C.: Management of infections in patients with leukemia and lymphoma. Current concepts and experimental approaches. Semin Hematol. 9, 141 (1972).
2. REMINGTON, J.S.: The compromised host. Hosp. Practice, 59 (April 1972).
3. ARMSTRONG, D.: Life-threatening infections in cancer patients, CA, 23, 138 (1973).
4. ARMSTRONG, D., YOUNG, L.S., MEYER, R.D., BLEVINS, A.H.: Infectious complications of neoplastic disease. Med. Clin. N. Amer. 55, 729 (1971).
5. E.O.R.T.C.: Symposium on optimal antimicrobial therapy in patients with cancer. Europ. J. Cancer 9, 395-458 (1973).
6. SELDEN, R., LEE, S., WANG, W.L.L., et al.: Nosocomial Klebsiella infections: intestinal colonization as a resevoir. Ann. Intern. Med. 74, 657 (1971).
7. SCHIMPFF, S.C., YOUNG, V.M., GREENE, W.H., VERMEULEN, G.D., MOODY, M.R., WIERNIK, P.H.: Origin of infections in acute nonlymphocytic leukemia. Significance of hospital acquisition of potential pathogens. Ann. Intern. Med. 77, 707 (1972).
8. FELTS, S.K., SCHAFFNER, W., MELLY, M.A., KOENIG, M.G.: Sepsis caused by contaminated intravenous fluids. Epidemiologic clinical and laboratory investigation of an outbreak in one hospital. Ann. Intern. Med. 77, 881 (1972).
9. BODEY, G.P.: Fungal infections complicating acute leukemia. J. Chronic. Dis. 19, 667 (1966).

10. HART, P.A., RUSSELL, Jr., E., REMINGTON, J.S.: The compromised host and infection: II. Deep fungal infection. J Infect Dis. 120, 169 (1969).
11. YOUNG, R.C., BENNETT, J.E., VOGEL, C.L., CARBONE, P.P., DeVITA, V.I.: Aspergillosis: The spectrum of the disease in 98 patients. Medicine 49, 147 (1970).
12. STRAATSMA, B.R., ZIMMERMAN, L.E., GASS, J.D.M.: Phycomycosis: a clinicopathologic study of fifty-one cases. Lab. Invest. 11, 963 (1962).
13. MEYER, R.D., ROSEN, P., ARMSTRONG, D.: Phycomycosis complicating leukemia and lymphoma. Ann. intern. Med. 77, 871 (1972).
14. YOUNG, L.S., ARMSTRONG, D., BLEVINS, A., LIEBERMAN, P.: Nocardia asteroides infection complicating neoplastic disease. Amer. J. Med. 50, 356 (1971).
15. BRADSHAW, M., MYEROWITZ, R.L., SCHNEERSON, R., WHISNANT, J.K., ROBBINS, J.B.: Pneumocystis carinii pneumonitis. Ann. intern. Med. 73, 775 (1970).
16. GOODELL, B., JACOBS, J.B., POWELL, R.D., DeVITA, V.T.: Pneumocystis carinii: The spectrum of diffuse interstitial pneumonia in patients with neoplastic disease. Ann. intern. Med. 72, 337 (1970).
17. VIETZKE, W.M., GELDERMAN, A.H., GRIMLEY, P.M., VALSAMIS, M.P.: Toxoplasmosis complicating malignancy. Experience at the National Cancer Institute. Cancer, 21, 816 (1968).
18. REMINGTON, J.S.: Toxoplasmosis: recent developments. Ann. Rev. Med. 21, 201 (1970).
19. GOFFINET, D.R., GLATSTEIN, E.J., MERIGAN, T.C.: Herpes zoster-Varicella infections and lymphoma. Ann. intern. Med. 76, 235 (1972)
20. SCHIMPFF, S., SIRPICK, A., STOLER, B., RUMACK, B., MELLIN, H., JOSEPH, J., BLOCK, J.: Varicella-zoster infections in patients with cancer. Ann. Int. Med. 76, 241 (1972).
21. CAPPEL, R., KLASTERSKY, J.: Viral infections in patients with malignant diseases. Europ. J. Cancer 8, 175 (1972).
22. BODEY, G.P., NIES, B.A., FREIREICH, E.J.: Multiple organism septicemia in acute leukemia. Analysis of 54 episodes. Arch. Intern. Med. (Chic.) 116:266 (1965).
23. SEHDEV, M.K., DOWLING, Jr., M.D., SEAL, S.H., STEARNS, Jr., M.W.: Perianal and anorectal complications in leukemia. Cancer 31, 149 (1973).
24. SCHIMPFF, S.C., WIERNIK, P.H., BLOCK, J.B.: Rectal abscesses in cancer patients. Lancet, 2, 844 (1972).
25. LURIE, H.I., DUMA, R.J.: Opportunistic infections of the lungs. Human Path. 1, 233 (1970).
26. BODEY, G.P., POWELL, R.D., HERSH, E.M., YETERIAN, A., FREIREICH, E.J.: Pulmonary complications of acute leukemia. Cancer 19, 781 (1966).
27. KLASTERSKY, J.: Prevention of infectious complications and testing of antimicrobial drugs in cancer patients. In: The Design of Clinical Trials in Cancer Therapy, p. 385 (ed. M. Staquet). Brussels: Editions Scientifiques Européennes 1972.
28. HUGHES, W.T.: Leukemia monitoring with fungal bone marrow cultures. J. amer. med. Ass. 218, 441 (1971).
29. RODRIGUEZ, V., BURGESS, M., BODEY, G.P.: Management of fever of unknown origin in patients with neoplasms and neutropenia. Cancer 32, 1007 (1973).
30. KLASTERSKY, J., CAPPEL, R., DANEAU, D.: Therapy with carbenicillin and gentamicin for patients with cancer and severe infections caused by gram-negative rods. Cancer 31, 331 (1973).
31. SCHIMPFF, S., SATTERLEE, W., YOUNG, V.M., et al.: Empiric therapy with carbenicillin and gentamicin for febrile patients with cancer and granulocytopenia. New Engl. J. Med. 284, 1061 (1971).

32. WINTERS, R.E., CHOW, A.W., HECHT, R.H., HEWITT, W.L.: Combined use of gentamicin and carbenicillin. Ann. intern. Med. 75, 925 (1971).

33. FINLAND, M.: Changing patterns of susceptibility of common bacterial pathogens to antimicrobial agents. Ann. intern. Med. 76, 1009 (1972).

34. ANDRIOLE, V.T., KRAVETZ, H.M.: The use of amphotericin B in man. J. amer. med. Ass. 180, 269 (1962).

35. WESTERN, K.A., PERERA, D.R., SCHULTZ, M.G.: Pentamidine isethionate in the treatment of Pneumocystis carinii pneumonia. Ann. intern. Med. 73, 695 (1970).

36. HRYNIUK, W., FOERSTER, J., SHOJANIA, M., CHOW, A.: Cytarabine for Herpesvirus infections. J. amer. med. Ass. 219, 715 (1972).

37. DAVIS, C.M., VAN DERSARL, V., COLTMAN, Jr., C.A.: Failure of cytarabine in Varicella-Zoster infections. J. amer. med. Ass. 224, 122 (1973)

38. HALL, T.C., WILFERT, C., JAFFE, N., et al.: Treatment of Varicella-Zoster with cytosine arabinoside. Trans. Am. Assoc. Physicians 82, 201 (1969).

39. STEVENS, D.A., JORDAN, G.W., WADDELL, T.F., MERIGAN, T.C.: Adverse effect of cytosine arabinoside on disseminated zoster in a controlled trial. New Engl. J. Med. 289, 873 (1973).

40. SCHNEIDER, M., SCHWARZENBERG, L., AMIEL, J.L., CATTAN, A., SCHLUMBERGER, J.R., DE VASSAL, F., JASMIN, C., ROSENFELD, C., MATHE, G.: Pathogen-free isolation unit. Three year's experience. Brit. med. J. 1, 836 (1969).

41. MATHE, G.: Operational research in cancer chemotherapy. Chemotherapy in the strategy of cancer treatment. In: Scientific Basis of Cancer Chemotherapy, p. 72 (ed. G. Mathé). Berlin-Heidelberg-New York: Springer-Verlag 1969.

42. BODEY, G.P., FREIRICH, E.J., FREI, E., III.: Studies of patients in a laminar air flow unit. Cancer 24, 972 (1969).

43. KLASTERSKY, J., CAPPEL, R., DEBUSSCHER, L., LACHAPELLE, F.: Preliminary studies of the effectiveness of a patient isolation unit and of prophylactic antibiotics in therapy of acute leukemia. Acta clin. belg. 26, 191 (1971).

44. LEVINE, A.S.: Interdisciplinary session report. Germ-free biology and the patient with malignant disease: clinical and preclinical studies. Cancer Chemother. Rep. Part 3, 4, 61 (1973).

45. PREISLER, H.D., GOLDSTEIN, I.M., HENDERSON, E.S.: Gastrointestinal "sterilization" in the treatment of patients with acute leukemia. Cancer 26, 1076 (1970).

46. SCHWARZENBERG, L., MATHE, G., AMIEL, J.L., CATTAN, A., SCHNEIDER, M., SCHLUMBERGER, J.R.: La réanimation hématologique. Le traitement symtomatologique de l'agranulocytose par les transfusions de globules blancs. Presse Méd. 74, 1057 (1966).

47. BODEY, G.P., BUCKLEY, M., SATHE, Y.S., et al.: Quantitative relationships between circulating leukocytes and infection in patients with acute leukemia. Ann. Intern. Med. 64, 328 (1966).

48. SCHWARZENBERG, L., MATHE, G., POUILLART, P., WEINER, R., LACOUR, J., GENIN, J., SCHNEIDER, M., De VASSAL, F., HAYAT, M., AMIEL, J.L., SCHLUMBERGER, J.R., JASMIN, C., ROSENFELD, C.: Hydroxyurea, leucaphoresis, and splenectomy in chronic myeloid leukaemia at the problastic phase. Brit. med. J., 1, 700 (1973).

49. BUCKNER, D., GRAW, Jr., R.G., EISEL, R.J., et al.: Leukapheresis by continuous flow centrifugation (CFC) in patients with chronic myelocytic leukemia (CML). Blood 33, 353 (1969).

50. HENDERSON, E.S., GRAW, R.G., ANDERSON, R.M., YANKEE, R.A., OPELZ, G., LALEZARI, P., MERYMAN, H.T.: Obstacles to routine transfusion support of myelosuppressive patients. Cancer Chemother. Rep. Part 3, 4, 51 (1973).

51. HERZIG, G.P., ROOT, R.K., GRAW, Jr., R.G.: Granulocyte collection by continuous-flow filtration leukaphoresis. Blood 39, 554 (1972).
52. GRAW, Jr., R.G., GOLDSTEIN, I.M., TERASAKI, P.I.: Histocompatibility testing for leucocyte transfusion. Lancet 2, 77 (1970).
53. GAYDOS, L., FREIREICH, E.J., MANTEL, N.: Quantitative relation between platelet count and hemorrhage in patients with acute leukemia. New. Engl. J. Med. 266, 905 (1962).
54. HAN, T., STUTZMAN, L., COHEN, E., et al.: Effect of platelet transfusion on hemorrhage in patients with acute leukemia: an autopsy report. Cancer 19, 1937 (1966).
55. GRUMET, F.C., YANKEE, R.A.: Long-term platelet support of patients with aplastic anemia. Ann. Intern. Med. 73, 1 (1970).
56. FREIREICH, E.J., KLIMAN, A., GAYDOS, L.A., et al.: Response to repeated platelet transfusion from the same donor. Ann. Intern. Med. 59, 277 (1963).
57. CROWTHER, D., BATEMAN, C.J.T.: Hematologic aspects of systemic disease: malignant diseases. Clinics in Hematology 1, 447 (1972).
58. PECK, S.D., REIQUAM, C.W.: Disseminated intravascular coagulation in cancer patients: supportive evidence. Cancer 31, 1114 (1973).
59. HASKELL, C.M., CANELLOS, G.P., LEVENTHAL, B.G., CARBONE, P.P., BLOCK, J.B., SERPICK, A.A., SELAWRY, O.S.: L-asparaginase. Therapeutic and toxic effects in patients with neoplastic disease. New Engl. J. Med. 281, 1028 (1969).
60. KENNEDY, B.J.: Metabolic and toxic effects of mithramycin during tumor therapy. Amer. J. Med. 49, 494 (1970).
61. KELLER, J.W., MAJERUS, P.W., FINKE, E.H.: An unusual type of spiculated erythrocyte in metastatic liver disease and hemolytic anemia. Ann. intern. Med. 74, 732 (1971).
62. LOHRMANN, H.P., ADAM, W., HEYMER, B., KUBANEK, B.: Microangiopathic hemolytic anemia in metastatic carcinoma. Ann. intern. Med. 79, 368 (1973).
63. POWELL, D., SINGER, F.R., MURRAY, T.M., MINKIN, C., POTTS, Jr., J.T.: Nonparathyroid humoral hypercalcemia in patients with neoplastic diseases. New Engl. J. Med. 289, 176 (1973).
64. WALSER, M.: Treatment of hypercalcemias. Mod. Treat. 7, 662 (1970).
65. KESSINGER, A., LEMON, H.M., FOLEY, J.F.: Hypercalcemia of malignancy. Geriatrics 27, 97 (1972).
66. GOLDSMITH, R.S.: Medical intelligence. Current concepts. Differential diagnosis of hypercalcemia. New Engl. J. Med. 274, 674 (1966).
67. CHAKMAKIAN, Z.H., BETHUNE, J.E.: Sodium sulfate treatment of hypercalcemia. New. Engl. J. Med. 275, 862 (1966).
68. MUGGIA, F.M., HEINEMANN, H.O.: Hypercalcemia with neoplastic disease. Ann. Intern. Med. 73, 281 (1970).
69. CORTES, E.P., HOLLAND, J.F., MOSKOWITZ, R., DEPOLI, E.: Effects of mithramycin on bone resorption in vitro. Cancer Res. 32, 74 (1972).
70. PAK, C.Y., WILLS, M.R., SMITH, G.W., BARTTER, F.C.: Treatment with thyrocalcitonin of the hypercalcemia of parathyroid carcinoma. Clin. Endocr. Metab. 28, 1657 (1968).
71. HILL, Jr., C.S., QUAIS, S.G., LEISER, A.E.: Long-term administration of calcitonin for hypercalcemia secondary to recurrent parathyroid carcinoma. Cancer 29, 1016 (1972).
72. GOLDSMITH, R.S., INGBAR, S.H.: Inorganic phosphate treatment of hypercalcemia of diverse etiologies. New Engl. J. Med. 274, 1. (1966).
73. SHACKNEY, S., HASSON, J.: Precipitous fall in serum calcium, hypotension and acute renal failure after intravenous phosphate therapy for hypercalcemia. Ann. Intern. Med. 66, 906 (1967).
74. CAREY, R.W., SCHMITT, G.W., KOPALD, H.H., et al.: Massive extraskeletal calcification during phosphate treatment of hypercalcemia. Arch. Intern. Med. (Chig.) 122, 150 (1968).

75. SWAROOP, S., KRANT, M.J.: Rapid estrogen-induced hypercalcemia. J. amer. med. Ass. 223, 913 (1973).
76. KRAKOFF, I.H.: Use of allopurinol in preventing hyperuricemia in leukemia and lymphoma. Cancer 19, 1489 (1966).
77. DeCONTI, R.C., CALABRESI, P.: Use of allopurinol for prevention and control of hyperuricemia in patients with neoplastic disease. New Engl. J. Med. 274, 481 (1966).
78. HERRINGTON, R.T., FALLON, H.J.: Uric acid nephropathy in leukemia. The use of acetazolamide in its management. New Engl. J. Med. 266, 934 (1962).
79. GREENE, M.L., FUJIMOTO, W.Y., SEEGMILLER, J.E.: Urinary xanthine stones - a rare complication of allopurinol therapy. New Engl. J. Med. 280, 426 (1969).
80. SILVERBERG, I.: Management of effusions. Oncology 24, 26 (1969).
81. FRACCHIA, A.A., KNAPPER, W.H., CAREY, J.T., FARROW, J.H.: Intrapleural chemotherapy for effusion from metastatic breast carcinoma. Cancer 26, 626 (1970).
82. DOLLINGER, M.R.: Management of recurrent maignant effusions. CA. 22, 138 (1972).
83. LIGHT, R.W., MACGREGOR, I., LUCHSINGER, P.C., BALL, W.C.: Pleural effusions: the diagnostic separation of transudates and exudates. Ann. intern. Med. 77, 507 (1972).
84. DOLLINGER, M.R., KRAKOFF, I.H., KARNOFSKY, D.A.: Quinacrine (Atabrine) in the treatment of neoplastic effusions. Ann. intern. Med. 66, 249 (1967).
85. BORJA, E.R., PUGH, R.P.: Single-dose quinacrine (Atabrine) and thoracostomy in the control of pleural effusions in patients with neoplastic diseases. Cancer 31, 899 (1973).
86. LAMBERT, C.J., et al.: Treatment of malignant pleural effusions by closed trochar tube drainage. Ann. Thorac. Surg. 3, 1 (1967).
87. STARKEY, G.W.B.: Recurrent malignant pleural effusions. New Engl. J. Med. 270, 436 (1964).
88. BEATTIE, Jr., E.J.: Treatment of malignant pleural effusions by partial pleurectomy. Surg. Clin. N. Amer. 43, 99 (1963).
89. WATNE, A.L., COVEY, T.H.: Hormones, chemotherapy and the breast cancer patient. Oncology 26, 317 (1972).
90. CUNNINGHAM, T.J., OLSON, K.B., HORTON, J., WRIGHT, A., HUSSAIN, M., DAVIES, J.N.P., HARRINGTON, G.A.: A clinical trial of intravenous and intracavitary bleomycin. Cancer 29, 1413 (1972).
91. MATSON, D.D.: Treatment of cerebral swelling. New Engl. J. Med. 272, 626 (1965).
92. HINDO, W.A., DeTRANA, F.A. III, LEE, M.S., HENDRICKSON, F.R.: Large-dose increment irradiation in treatment of cerebral metastases. Cancer 26, 138 (1970).
93. GREEN, N., GEORGE, F. III: Total brain therapy: technical considerations. Radiology 96, 429 (1970).
94. HORTON, J., BAXTER, D.H., OLSON, K.B., The Eastern Cooperative Oncology Group: The management of metastases to the brain by irradiation and corticosteroids. Amer. J. Roentgenol. 111, 334 (1971).
95. HAAR, F., PATTERSON, Jr., R.H.: Surgery for metastatic intracranial neoplasm. Cancer 30, 1241 (1972).
96. MULLINS, G.M., et al.: Malignant lymphoma of the spinal epidural space. Ann. Intern. Med. 74, 416 (1971).
97. SILVERBERG, I.J., JACOBS, E.M.: Treatment of spinal cord compression in Hodgkin's disease. Cancer 27, 308 (1971).
98. ULTMANN, J.E., MORAN, E.M.: Clinical course and complications in Hodgkin's disease. Arch. intern. Med. (Chig.) 131, 332 (1973).
99. LEVITT, S.H., JONES, T.K., KILPATRICK, Jr., S.J., BOGARDUS, Jr., C.R.: Treatment of malignant superior vena caval obstruction. A randomized study. Cancer 24, 447 (1969).

100. OLUMIDE, A.A., OSUNKOYA, B.O., NGU, V.A.: Superior mediastinal compression: a report of five cases by malignant lymphoma. Cancer, 27, 193 (1971).
101. ABRAMS, R.D.: The patient with cancer: his changing pattern of communication. New Engl. J. Med. 274, 317 (1966).
102. DAY, E.: The patient with cancer and the family. New Engl. J. Med. 274, 883 (1966).
103. BINGER, C.M., ABLIN, A.R., FEUERSTEIN, R.C., KUSHNER, J.H., ZOGER, S., MIKKELSEN, C.: Childhood leukemia. Emotional impact on patient and family. New Engl. J. Med. 280, 414 (1969).
104. PECK, A.: Emotional reactions to having cancer. Amer. J. Roentgen. 114, 591 (1972).
105. BURGERT, Jr., E.O.: Emotional impact of childhood acute leukemia. Mayo Clin. Proc. 47, 273 (1972).
106. CRARY, W.G., CRARY, G.C.: Emotional crisis and cancer. CA 24, 36 (1974).
107. HORSLEY, J.S. III: Speak truthfully to the cancer patient. Surgery, Gynecol. and Obstet. 129, 804 (1969).
108. LIRETTE, W.L., KEENAN, W.D., CLEMENTS, Th.M., GAINES, R.K., IBARRA, J.D.: Management of patients with terminal cancer. Postgrad. Med. 47, 202 (1970).
109. HOLLAND, J.: Acute leukemia: psychological aspects of treatment. In: Cancer Chemotherapy, Boerhaave series for postgraduate medical education, p. 292 (eds. F. Elkerbout, P. Thomas, A. Zwaveling) Leiden: Leiden Univ. Press (1971).
110. MILTON, G.W.: The care of dying. Med. J. Austr. 2, 177 (1972).
111. INAGAKI, J., RODRIGUEZ, V., BODEY, G.P.: Causes of death in cancer patiens. Cancer 33, 568 (1974).
112. WALZER, P.D., PERL, D.P., KROGSTAD, D.J., RAWSON, P.G., SCHULTZ, M.G.: Pneumocystis pneumonia in the United States. Epidemiologic, diagnostic, and clinical features. Ann. intern. Med. (Chic.) 80, 83 (1974).
113. BLOOMFIELD, C.D., KENNEDY, B.J.: Cephalothin, carbenicillin, and gentamycin combination therapy for febrile patients with acute non-lymphocytic leukemia. Cancer 34, 431 (1974).
114. YOUNG, R.C., BENNETT, J.E., GEELHOED, G.W., LEVINE, A.: Fungemia with compromised host resistance. Ann. intern. Med. 80, 605 (1974).
115. HIGBY, D.J., YATES, J.W., HENDERSON, E.S., HOLLAND, J.F.: Filtration leukapheresis for granulocyte transfusion therapy. New Engl. J. Med. 292, 761 (1975).
116. Symposium on the intravascular coagulation-fibrinolysis syndrome. Mayo clin. Proc. 49, 635-679 (1974).
117. BRERETON, H.D., HALUSHKA, P.V., ALEXANDER, R.W., MASON, D.M., KEISER, H.R., DeVITA, V.T.: Indomethacin-responsive hypercalcemia and renal-cell adenocarcinoma. New. Engl. J. Med. 291, 83 (1974).
118. VAUGHN, C.B., VAITKEVICIUS, V.: The effects of calcitonin in hypercalcemia in patients with malignancy. Cancer 34, 1268 (1974).
119. ANDERSON, C.B., PHILPOTT, G.W., FERGUSON, T.B.: The treatment of malignant pleural effusions. Cancer 33, 916 (1974).
120. MARTINI, N., BAINS, M.S., BEATTLE, E.J.: Indications for pleurectomy in malignant effusion. Cancer 35, 734 (1975).
121. LIPPMAN, A.J., COHEN, F.B., CUSTODIO, M.C.: A clinical trial of intracavitary bleomycin. Proc. Am. Soc. Clin. Oncol. 16, 247 (1975).
122. GUTIN, P.H.: Corticosteroid therapy in patients with cerebral tumors: benefits, mechanisms, problems, practicalities. Semin. Oncol. 2, 49 (1975).
123. HENDRICKSON, F.R.: Radiation therapy of metastatic tumors. Semin. Oncol. 2, 43 (1975).
124. YOUNG, D.F., POSNER, J.B., CHU, F., NISCE, L.: Rapid-course therapy of cerebral metastases: results and complications. Cancer 34, 1069 (1974).

125. RANSOHOFF, J.: Surgical management of metastatic tumors. Semin. Oncol. 2, 21 (1975).
126. DILWORTH, J.A., MANDELL, G.L.: Infections in patients with cancer. Semin. Oncol. 2, 349 (1975).
127. PREISLER, H.D., BJORNSSON, S.: Protected environment units in the treatment of acute leukemia. Semin. Oncol. 2, 369 (1975).
128. HIGBY, D.J., HENDERSON, E.S.: Granulocyte transfusions for infection during neutropenia. Semin. Oncol. 2, 361 (1975).
129. SEYBERTH, H.W., SEGRE, G.V., MORGAN, J.L., SWEETMAN, B.J., POTTS, J.T., OATES, J.A.: Prostaglandins as mediators of hypercalcemia associated with cancer. New Engl. J. Med. 293, 1278 (1975).
130. FILLASTRE, J.P., HUMBERT, G., LEROY, J.: Treatment of acute hypercalcemia with furosemide. Current Ther. Research 15, 641 (1973).
131. CREECH, R.H.: The psychologic support of the cancer patient: a medical oncologist's viewpoint. Semin. Oncol. 2, 285 (1975).
132. BAHNSON, C.B.: Psychologic and emotional issues in cancer: The psychotherapeutic care of the cancer patient. Semin. Oncol. 2, 293 (1975).
133. LUCE, J.K., DAWSON, J.J.: Quality of life. Semin. Oncol. 2, 323 (1975).
134. KONIOR, G.S., LEVINE, A.S.: The fear of dying: How patients and their doctors react. Semin. Oncol. 2, 311 (1975).

Chapter 12
Local and Regional Chemotherapy

A. LOCAL APPLICATIONS AND INSTILLATIONS

Certain parts of the body are well suited to local treatment with cytotoxic therapy by application of ointments and lotions, or direct injections into tumors, cavities, arteries, lymphatics, and the subarachnoid
space.

Applications of 5 percent 5-FU ointment for 3 to 6 weeks have given
very good results with precancerous skin lesions, certain types of spino-
cellular and basocellular epitheliomas of the skin, xeroderma pigmentosum, and a few metastatic lesions (1-3). This form of treatment is especially indicated for extensive actinic keratosis, multiple superficial
basal-cell carcinomas and multiple squamous-cell carcinomas in situ.
Apparently complete and lasting remissions can be obtained. It should
not be used with nodular basal-cell carcinomas or infiltrative squamous-
cell carcinomas. Mycosis fungoides has been treated successfully with
local applications of aqueous solutions of nitrogen mustard (4).

Antitumor drugs can be injected directly into large tumor masses that
are readily accessible (5). Special needles with multiple openings, or
a so-called "jet injector" have been developed for this purpose (6).
The most experience has been accumulated with thioTEPA, but local necrosis and infections are disadvantages of this form of treatment.

Instillation of cytotoxic compounds into the bladder has been especially
useful for diffuse papillary lesions that have not invaded beyond the
subepithelium (7, 8).

Rousselot instilled 5-FU into the lumen of the tumor-bearing segment
of the bowel, sequestered between tapes. He hoped that the drug would
be absorbed into the mesentery of the segment to be removed, thereby
improving the survival of patients with positive lymph nodes (9, 10).
He combined this treatment with systemic intravenous 5-FU for 3 days
to kill any tumor cells in the circulation. Using this technique, he
was able to raise the 5-year survival rate of Dukes' C carcinoma (positive lymph nodes) from 27 percent to 64 percent.

We refer to page 208 for a discussion of the intrapleural, intrapericardial, and intraperitoneal instillation of cytotoxic agents and radioactive isotopes for the control of malignant effusions. These agents
have also been introduced into the chest or abdominal cavity before
closure (11). Five-year survival rates of 90 percent have been reported
for Stage-I carcinoma of the ovary when either ^{198}Au or ^{32}P was left
in the abdominal cavity, compared to a 67 percent 5-year survival rate
for surgery without isotopes (12, 13).

222

The technique of lymphangiography has led to the intralymphatic injection of radioactive colloidal isotopes (e.g., ^{198}Au) that become fixed in the lymph nodes. Doses of 20,000 to 50,000 rads can be delivered to individual lymph nodes (14, 15).

The treatment of CNS leukemia with intrathecal chemotherapy is discussed on page 257. Intrathecal chemotherapy has also been able to induce some regressions in cerebral tumors (16, 17). RUBIN et al. developed a method of perfusing the ventricles for brain tumors and CNS leukemia (18).

B. INTRA-ARTERIAL CHEMOTHERAPY: Perfusion and Infusion

In order to obtain higher and hence more effective concentrations of cytotoxic agents in the tumor tissue, it appeared logical to inject the drug into the artery feeding the tumor tissue (19, 20). Tumors refractory to systemic chemotherapy have been found to respond to local intraarterial therapy (21). Various proposals were made to reduce systemic toxicity, especially myelosuppression: (1) to use fast-acting agents, like nitrogen mustard, that are largely cleared from the blood in the first capillary bed; (2) to use an antidote to the cytotoxic drug in the systemic circulation, for example folinic acid for methotrexate; or (3) to isolate the arterial and venous circulation of the tumor from the systemic circulation during perfusion with cytotoxic agents. Two techniques have evolved in intra-arterial chemotherapy, perfusion and infusion.

In perfusion the drug is introduced via a cannulated regional artery and the venous return is collected and recirculated through a pump oxygenator, a small heart-lung machine (Fig. 12-1) (22-26). The oxygenator was added on the assumption that oxygen plays a significant role in the tumor response to many agents, and the pumps assure circulation in the extracorporeal circuit (22). An anticoagulant must, of course, be added. Various types of pumps, oxygenators, and catheters (e.g., ballon-tipped to occlude vessels) have been designed to simplify the procedure. Some physicians have eliminated the oxygenator altogether, replacing it by a simple hand-operated pump (27). Since it has been shown that cancer cells demonstrate a selective sensitivity to temperature (28), heat exchangers have been added to warm the perfusing blood (29). Warming of the blood can be combined with general hypothermia (30).

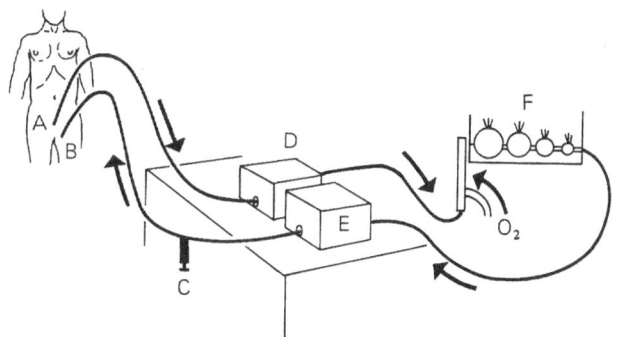

Fig. 12-1. Diagram of intra-arterial perfusion with extracorporeal circulation. (From BRULE et al. (25)), (A) vein, (B) artery, (C) site for injection of agents, (D) venous pump, (E) arterial pump, (F) oxygenator and heat exchanger

Not all parts of the body are equally suited for isolation of the circulation (23-26). Major vessel occlusion by clamping or balloon-tipped catheters must be supplemented by some form of tourniquet to reduce leakage through collaterals. This is relatively easy in the extremities, but special tourniquets had to be designed to occlude abdominal vessels. Nevertheless, some leakage of the cytotoxic drug into the systemic circulation cannot be prevented; the extent varies with anatomic region and can be evaluated with ^{51}Cr-labeled red blood cells or Evans blue. Alkylating agents (nitrogen mustard, mannitol mustard, melphalan, thio-TEPA) and antibiotics (mitomycin C, actinomycin D) have most often been used (Table 12-1). Since perfusions do not last more than 45 to 120 min, phase-dependent antimetabolites are not suitable. Vasodilators can be injected prior to infusion to obtain maximal dilatation of the vascular bed.

Table 12-1. Doses of drugs commonly used in intra-arterial perfusion

| Drug | Head and neck | Pelvis | Extremities | |
			Upper	Lower
Nitrogen mustard	10 mg/m^2	30 mg/m^2	15 mg/m^2	30 mg/m^2
Melphalan		50 mg/m^2	35 mg/m^2	50 mg/m^2
ThioTEPA	20 -30 mg/m^2	35 mg/m^2	20 mg/m^2	30 mg/m^2
5-Fluoro-uracil		700 mg/m^2	500 mg/m^2	700 mg/m^2

The technique of perfusion must be carried out by a specialized team. Its use is limited to a single short-term session or to infrequent intermittent treatments.

Infusion is the much simpler technique of intra-arterial injection of a cytotoxic agent, without any attempt to prevent residual drug carried by the venous return from entering the systemic circulation (Fig. 12-2) (23-25, 31-33). It has the distinct advantage that it can be continued for weeks or even months (34), long enough to permit many cells to pass through the sensitive phase of cell phase-dependent antimetabolite. Methotrexate has the additional advantage that supralethal doses can be infused, because folinic acid protects the patient against systemic toxicity (33). Prolonged intraarterial infusion has also been used to administer agents that might potentiate the effect of concomitant radiotherapy (35, 36).

A catheter can be introduced by direct percutaneous puncture, surgical exposure of the artery, or retrograde catheterization. Whatever the approach, it is essential to check the position of the catheter and the extent of the irrigated field. This is best done by infusing fluorescein: the infused area fluoresces intensely when exposed to ultraviolet light. This method gives a better indication of the local effect than an arteriogram with vigorous injection of a bolus of contrast medium. The catheter must be securely fixed in place, since it will be left in for prolonged periods in patients who are often ambulatory. Various types of pumps, some adapted for ambulatory use, or motor-driven syringes are available to administer the drug (23, 37-41)

Various anatomic regions can be treated (23, 24). The external carotid and its branches are infused for tumors of the head and neck, floor

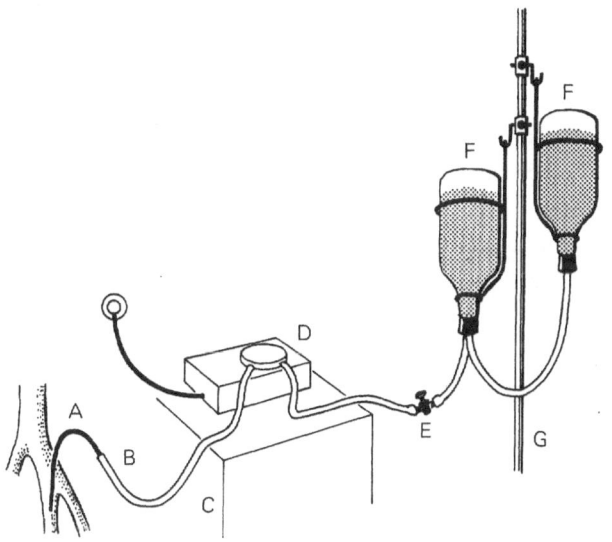

Fig. 12-2. Diagram of continuous intra-arterial infusion. (From BRULE et al. (25)), (A) polyethylene catheter in place in artery, (B) catheter connection with tubing, (C) tubing, (D) infusion pump assuring constant, continuous flow, (E) flow regulator, (F) standard intravenous bottles in tandem, (G) variable height stand

of the mouth, tongue, lip, and cheek. Retrograde catheterization via the superficial temporal artery is the safest route. The superior thyroid artery, percutaneous puncture of the common carotid artery, or surgical exposure are alternative approaches. The internal carotid artery has been used to treat brain tumors (42).

The liver can be infused via the right gastroepiploic, right gastric, or gastroduodenal arteries, at laparotomy or by retrograde catheterization (23, 43-45). BEVAN approached the liver through the umbilical vein and noted regressions of colon metastases, though it has been claimed that the hepatic artery is more important than the portal vein in supplying blood to tumors of the liver (46). The approach to the pancreas is through the gastroduodenal artery via the gastroepiploic artery, while the stomach is reached through the left gastric and gastroepiploic arteries (32). Pelvic cancers are treated by catheterization of the aorta (47) or the hypogastric arteries.

Arterial infusions have also been carried out in the upper extremity (subclavian, brachial, acromiothoracic artery) and lower extremities (retrograde catheterization of iliac or femoral artery) (32). There are also some reports of infusions of the lungs and the breast (42, 48-50).

Antimetabolites are most often used in infusion (Table 12-2). Methotrexate, usually with citrovorum factor intramuscularly, is the drug favored for head and neck infusions, 5-FU and 5-FUdR for liver infusions. Bleomycin infusions have recently been introduced for squamous-cell carcinomas (51, 52), dimethyl-triazeno-imidazole-carboxamide for malignant melanoma (53), and adriamycin for various solid tumors (54).

Complications due either to technical problems or to pharmacologic effects are common in perfusion and infusion procedures. Technical difficulties include inability to cannulate the artery, catheter clotting,

Table 12-2. Dosages of drugs for intra-arterial infusion

Methotrexate	3 - 5 mg/m^2/d
MTX + citrovorum factor	50 mg/m^2/d + 5 mg/m^2 every 5 h
5-Fluorouracil	200 - 800 mg/m^2/d
5-Fluorodeoxyuridine	15 - 30 mg/m^2/d
ThioTEPA	7 - 10 mg/m^2/d
Nitrogen mustard	2 - 6 mg/m^2/d
Melphalan	70 - 80 mg/m^2/d
Vinblastine	5 mg/m^2/d

dislodgement or kinking, and leakage of infusate into subcutaneous tissues (10 to 20 percent). Damage to the vessels, expressed in the form of thrombosis, spasm, dislodging of arteriosclerotic plaques, subintimal dissection, rupture, and (rarely) aneurysm formation, has been described. Bleeding (6 to 14 percent) and infection of catheter site (9 to 20 percent) are common. Bleeding may also occur in necrotic tumors. Hemiparesis, often transient, and death due to air embolism are feared complications of injections into the internal carotid system.

Pharmacologic effects may be systemic or limited to the treated area. The common local toxic manifestations are irritation of the skin, ranging from erythema to necrosis, discoloration, mucositis, and alopecia. Nausea, vomiting, and diarrhea may occur, especially with infusion of antimetabolites, but myelosuppression is the most serious systemic side-effect.

Problems with leakage into the systemic circulation have often limited the use of perfusions to the extremities, in particular for malignant melanoma. STEHLIN noted an incidence of 6.4 percent of recurrences in the extremities treated by perfusions, compared to 34 percent after conventional therapy (55), but not all surgeons share his enthusiasm (56). Perfusion as an adjuvant to wide excision, with or without lymph node dissection, as the primary treatment for curable melanoma remains an experimental technique, and reports of improved clinical results are not convincing. Perfusions are useful for recurrent melanoma and some other extremity cancers that would require sacrifice of much of the functioning tissue, if not amputation (57, 58). The high leak factor in the head and neck, pelvis, and abdominal viscera makes perfusion less valuable in these locations; infusion techniques are appropriate. Most infusions have in fact been carried out for squamous carcinomas of the head and neck area and for metastases of the liver. Very few controlled studies are available, so that the place of infusion chemotherapy remains uncertain. What is needed are prospective studies in which a series of patients treated by prolonged intra-arterial infusion is compared with another group treated by systemic administration of the same drug.

Thus, intra-arterial perfusion and infusion therapy must still be considered experimental procedures, to be carried out by experienced and critical investigators who are willing to give them a trial in controlled studies. These procedures are complex and often require lengthy hospitalization and a tremendous technical effort. Tumor regression (in 30 to 80 percent depending on the criteria used) is usually brief and the survival rate and the length of survival have not been improved, even though spectacular regressions are occasionally induced. The benefit is generally palliative, with significant relief of pain in up to 75 percent of patients (43).

These results may improve when more effective agents become available. However, it is not enough to introduce the drug into the artery supplying the tumor; it must be moved into the cell. Very little is known about the mechanism involved in this transport. Regional therapy, like systemic chemotherapy, cannot be expected to be very effective in large tumor masses, which contain vast numbers of cells, are poorly vascularized, and may well have grown beyond the field supplied by the perfused artery. Patients treated by local and regional techniques often have far-advanced disease that has relapsed following surgery and radiotherapy (32). It would be more logical to use regional therapy as an adjuvant to surgery or radiotherapy earlier in the course of the disease when the tumor mass is smaller and before the vascular supply has deteriorated (58, 59). The whole idea of regional therapy, at least if we hope for a cure, is that it should be done before any microscopic hematologic dissemination has yet taken place.

REFERENCES

1. KLEIN, E.: Tumors of skin. VIII. Local chemotherapy of metastatic neoplasms. N.Y. St. J. Med. 68, 877 (1968).
2. SERRI, F. (ed.): International conference on 5 % fluorouracil ointment in dermatology. Dermatologica 140, Suppl. 1 (1970).
3. ZACKHEIM, H.S., FARBER, E.M.: Topical antimetabolites. Annu. Rev. of Medic. 21, 59 (1970).
4. VAN SCOTT, E.J., KALMANSON, J.D.: Complete remissions of mycosis fungoides lymphoma induced by topical nitrogen mustard (HN2). Control of delayed hypersensitivity to HN2 by desensitization and by induction of specific immunologic tolerance. Cancer 32, 18 (1973).
5. BATEMAN, J.C.: Palliation of cancer in human patients by maintenance therapy with NN'N''-triethylene thiophosphoramide and N-(3-oxapentamethylene)-N'N'-diethylene phosphoramide. Ann. N.Y. Acad. Sci. 68, 1057 (1958).
6. LAWTON, R.L.: Jet injection of drugs into malignant neoplasms. Cancer chemother. Rep. 37, 57 (1964).
7. ABBASSIAN, A., WALLACE, D.M.: Intracavitary chemotherapy of diffuse non-infiltrating papillary carcinoma of the bladder. J. Urol. (Baltimore) 96, 461 (1966).
8. VEENEMA, R.J.: The role of thiotepa instillations in bladder cancer. J. Amer. med. Ass. 206, 2725 (1968).
9. ROUSSELOT, L.M., COLE, D.R., GROSSI, C.E., CONTE, A.J., GONZALEZ, E.M., PASTERNACK, B.S.: A five year progress report on the effectiveness of intraluminal chemotherapy (5-fluorouracil) adjuvant to surgery for colorectal cancer. Amer. J. Surg. 115, 140 (1968).
10. ROUSSELOT, L.M., COLE, D.R., GROSSI, C.E., CONTE, A.J., GONZALEZ, E.M., PASTERNACK, B.S.: Adjuvant chemotherapy with 5-fluorouracil in surgery for colorectal cancer. Dis. Colon. Rect. 15, 169 (1972).
11. JONES, R.F., SMITH, A.L., JONES, R.C.: Effects of topical chemotherapy in cancer surgery. A clinical study. Cancer 22, 1250 (1968).
12. KEETTEL, W.C., FOX, M.R., LONGNECKER, D.S., LATOURETTE, H.B.: Prophylactic use of radioactive gold in the treatment of primary ovarian cancer. Am. J. Obstet. Gynecol. 94, 766 (1966).
13. HILARIS, B.S., CLARK, D.G.C.: The value of postoperative intraperitoneal injection of radiocolloids in early cancer of the ovary.. Am. J. Roentgenol. 112, 749 (1971).
14. ARIEL, I.M., RESNICK, M.I., GALEY, D.: The intralymphatic administration of radioactive isotopes and cancer chemotherapeutic drugs. Surgery 55, 355 (1964).

15. CHIAPPA, S., MUSUMECI, R., USLENGHI, C.: Endolymphatic radiotherapy in malignant lymphomas. Recent Results in Cancer Research, Vol. 37. Berlin-Heidelberg-New York: Springer-Verlag 1971.
16. NEWTON, Jr., W.A., SAYERS, M.P., SAMUELS, L.D.: Intrathecal methotrexate (NSC-740) therapy for brain tumors in children. Cancer Chemother. Rep., 52, 257 (1968).
17. WILSON, C.B., NORRELL, Jr., H.A.: Brain tumor chemotherapy with intrathecal methotrexate. Cancer 23, 1038 (1969).
18. RUBIN, R.C., OMMAYA, A.K., HENDERSON, E.S., BERING, E.A., RALL, D.P.: Cerebrospinal fluid perfusion for central nervous system neoplasms. Neurology (Minneap.) 16, 680 (1966).
19. KLOPP, C.T., ALFORD, T.C., BATMAN, J., BERRY, G.N., DEMETZ, A.: Fractionated intra-arterial cancer chemotherapy with methyl-bis amine hydrochloride; a preliminary report. Ann. Surg. 132, 811 (1960). (1960).
20. BIERMAN, H.R., SHIMKIN, M.B., BYRON, Jr., R.L., MILLER, E.R.: The effects of intra-arterial administration of nitrogen mustard. Fifth International Cancer Congress, Paris 1950 (Abstr. of Papers) p. 186 (1950).
21. GOLDSTEIN, D.P., COUCH, N.P., HALL, T.C.: Infusion therapy in the treatment of patients with choriocarcinoma and related trophoblastic tumors. Sur. Forum 18, 426 (1967).
22. CREECH, Jr., O., KREMENTZ, E.T., RYAN, R.F., REEMTSMA, K., WINBLAD, J.N.: Experiences with isolation-perfusion technics in the treatment of cancer. Ann. Surg. 148, 616 (1958).
23. LAWRENCE, Jr., W.: Current status of regional chemotherapy. Part I: Technics. N.Y. St. J. Med. 63, 2359 (1963).
24. LAWRENCE, Jr., W.: Current status of regional chemotherapy. Part II: Results. N.Y. St. J. Med. 63, 2518 (1963).
25. BRULE, G., THOMAS, M.: La chimiothérapie locale des cancers. Rev. franc. clin. biol. 7, 978 (1962).
26. STRAWITZ, J.G.: Cancer chemotherapy using isolation perfusion. In: Cancer Chemotherapy, p. 443 (eds. I. Brodsky, S.B. Kahn, J.H. Moyer) New York: Grune and Stratton 1972.
27. ARIEL, I.M.: A simplified method of isolation perfusion of anticancer drugs. Amer. J. Surg. 104, 82 (1962).
28. CAVALIERE, R., CIOCATTO, E.C., GIOVANELLA, B.C., HEIDELBERGER, C., JOHNSON, R.O., MARGOTTINI, M., MONDOVI, B., MORICCA, G., ROSSI-FANELLI, A.: Selective heat sensitivity of cancer cells. Cancer 20, 1351 (1967).
29. STEHLIN, J.S.: Hyperthermic perfusion with chemotherapy for cancers of the extremities. Surg. Gynec. Obstet. 129, 305 (1969).
30. SHINGLETON, W.W., PARKER, R.T., MAHALEY, S.: Abdominal perfusion for cancer chemotherapy. Ann. Surg. 152, 583 (1960).
31. SULLIVAN, R.D., MILLER, E., SYKES, M.P.: Antimetabolite-metabolite combination cancer chemotherapy. Effects of intra-arterial methotrexate-intramuscular citrovorum factor therapy in human cancer. Cancer 12, 1248 (1959).
32. ROGERS, L.S.: Cancer chemotherapy by continuous intra-arterial infusion. Cancer 17, 1365 (1964).
33. SULLIVAN, R.D., SEMEL, C.J.: Arterial infusion cancer chemotherapy for solid tumors. In: Cancer Chemotherapy, p. 453 (eds. I. Brodsky, S.B. Kahn, J.H. Moyer) New York: Grune and Stratton 1972.
34. MENDELSOHN, M.L.: Chronic infusion of tritiated thymidine into mice with tumors. Science 135, 213 (1962).
35. YONEMOTO, R.H., BYRON, R.L., JACOBS, M.L.: Combined irradiation, intra-arterial chemotherapy, and surgery for the treatment of sarcomas of the extremities. Surgery 61, 355 (1967).
36. SEALY, R., HELMAN, P.: Treatment of head and neck cancer with intra-arterial cytotoxic drugs and radiotherapy. Cancer 30, 187 (1972).

37. KRANT, M.J., HALL, T.C., LLOYD, J.B., PATTERSON, W.B.: Utilization of an air-free pump for intra-arterial infusion. Cancer Chemother. Rep. 14, 39 (1961).
38. WATKINS, E.: Chronometric infusor - an apparatus for protracted ambulatory infusion therapy. New Engl. J. Med. 269, 850 (1963).
39. REYNOLDS, D.T., PATTERSON, W.B.: An arterial infusion pump for ambulatory patients. Surgery 56, 509 (1964).
40. ARIEL, I.M., PACK, G.T.: Intra-arterial chemotherapy for cancer metastatic to liver. Arch. Surg. 91, 851 (1965).
41. BURNS, G.I., GAINS, E.: The chemoinfusor, a new apparatus for maintaining continuous intra-arterial infusion chemotherapy. Brit. J. Surg. 60, 375 (1973).
42. MILLER, E.: Arterial infusion in cancer chemotherapy. In: Chemotherapy of Cancer, p. 251 (ed. Pl. A. Plattner). Amsterdam-London-New York: Elsevier 1964.
43. MASON, J.H., EDIGER, A.J., WEBB, R.S.: Intra-arterial infusion cancer chemotherapy. Clin. N. Amer. 48, 79 (1968).
44. BRENNAN, M.J., TALLEY, R.W., DRAKE, E.H., VAITKEVICIUS, V.K., POZANSKI, A.K., BRUSH, B.E.: 5-Fluorouracil treatment of liver metastases by continuous hepatic artery infusion via Cournand catheter: results and suitability for intensive postsurgical adjuvant chemotherapy. Ann. Surg. 158, 405 (1963).
45. SULLIVAN, R.D., ZUREK, W.S.: Chemotherapy for liver cancer by protracted ambulatory infusion. J. Amer. med. Ass. 194, 481 (1965).
46. BEVAN, P.O.: Cytotoxic perfusion of the liver via the umbilicial vein for liver metastases in carcinoma of the colon. Brit. J. Surg. 60, 369 (1973).
47. KRAKOFF, I.H., SULLIVAN, R.D.: Intra-arterial nitrogen mustard in the treatment of pelvic cancer. Ann. intern. Med. 48, 839 (1958).
48. WIRTANEN, G.W., ANSFIELD, F.J.: Bronchial artery infusion in bronchogenic carcinoma. Cancer Chemother. Rep. 52, 263 (1968).
49. FRECKMAN, H.A.: Chemotherapy of breast cancer by regional intra-arterial infusion. Cancer 26, 560 (1970).
50. HUMPHREY, L.J., JEWELL, W.R.: Chemotherapy for recurrent carcinoma of the breast. Oncol. 26, 223 (1972).
51. HUNTINGTON, M.C., DuPRIEST, R.W., FLETCHER, W.S.: Intra-arterial bleomycin therapy in inoperable squamous cell carcinomas. Cancer 31, 153 (1973).
52. CVITKOVIC, E., CURRIE, V., OCHOA, M., PRIDE, G., KRAKOFF, I.H.: Continuous intravenous infusion of bleomycin in squamous cancer. Proc. amer. Ass. Cancer Res. 15, 179 (1974).
53. EINHORN, L.H., McBRIDE, C.M., LUCE, J.K., CAOILI, E., GOTTLIEB, J.A.: Intra-arterial infusion therapy with 5-(3,3-dimethyl-1-triazeno)imidazole-4-carboxamide (NSC 45388) for malignant melanoma. Cancer 32, 749 (1973).
54. HASKELL, C.M., SILVERSTEIN, M.J., RANGEL, D.M., HUNT, J.S., SPARKS, F.C., MORTON, D.L.: Multimodality cancer therapy in man: a pilot study of adriamycin by arterial infusion. Cancer 33, 1485 (1974).
55. STEHLIN, Jr., J.S., CLARK, R.L.: Melanoma of the extremities. Amer. J. Surg. 110, 366 (1965).
56. PATTERSON, W.B.: Contributions of surgeons to clinical cancer chemotherapy. Oncology 26, 277 (1972).
57. GOLOMB, F.M.: Perfusion of melanoma. Oncology 26, 197 (1972).
58. LAWTON, R.L., GULESSERIAN, H.P., SHARZER, L.A.: Intra-arterial infusion. A seven-year study. Oncology 26, 259 (1972).
59. SNOW, G.B.: Intra-arterial chemotherapy combined with radiotherapy or surgery in tumors of the head and neck area. In: Cancer Chemotherapy, p. 192 (eds. G. Elkerbout, P. Thomas, A. Zwaveling). Leiden: Leiden University Press 1971.

Chapter 13
Strategy of Cancer Treatment

A. THE ROLE OF EACH OF THE FOUR TREATMENT MODALITIES IN THE TREATMENT OF CANCER

Oncologists now have four therapeutic modalities at their disposal to treat cancer: surgery, radiotherapy, chemotherapy, and immunotherapy.

Surgery. its role and indications are listed in Tables 13-1 and 13-2. As LOGAN CLENDENING cogently said: "Surgery does the ideal thing - it separates the patient from his disease." The major indication for surgery is localized disease but, as we point out later in this chapter, incomplete resection of inoperable tumors may be used to reduce the total tumor cell number in an interdisciplinary approach.

Table 13-1. Role of surgery in the treatment of cancer

---

1. Biopsy to establish a pathologic diagnosis.

2. Cancer prevention: excision of premalignant lesions.

3. Localized tumors: curative

4. Advanced tumors:
   to reduce the log number of tumor cells
   occasionally, resection of solitary metastases
   palliation: relief or prevention of ulceration, obstruction,
                bleeding, pain
   ablative hormonal manipulation

5. Special surgical techniques:
   infusion
   perfusion
   chemosurgery
   cryotherapy
   cautery
   laser

Radiotherapy kills cells through its ionizing effect. All tissues are affected but cancer cells are more susceptible than normal cells. It is recommended for localized radiosensitive tumors (Tables 13-3 and 13-4). Some localized tumors can, however, be treated equally well by surgery or radiotherapy and the choice may be dictated by practical considerations such as expertise, availability, time and cost involved, functional result, and age and general condition of the patient.

Table 13-2. Tumors treated primarily by surgery

The earlier stages of the following tumors are treated primarily by surgery. Some of these tumors can be treated with equal success by radiotherapy. Surgery may be complemented by adjuvant radiotherapy or adjuvant chemotherapy.

Breast

Lung

GI: lower esophagus, stomach, small bowel, colon, rectum, pancreas

Gyn: ovary, endometrium, cervix (in situ, Ia), vulva, vagina

GU: kidney, bladder, prostate

Skin

H + N: eye, salivary gland, lip, tongue, larynx, thyroid

Malignant melanoma

Solf-tissue sarcomas

Brain

Table 13-3. Role of radiotherapy in the treatment of cancer

1. Localized radiosensitive tumors: curative

2. Adjuvant to "curative" surgery, if high risk of local or regional failure

3. Advanced radiosensitive tumors:
   to reduce the log number of tumor cells
   palliation: relief or prevention of pain, obstruction, fracture, intracranial hypertension

4. Preoperatively: to render inoperable tumors resectable

Chemotherapy has been used from the onset in disseminated cancers (Table 13-5), because it is the only modality capable of killing tumor cells anywhere in the body (74). Chemotherapy, either with single drugs or drug combinations, can cure some patients with at least two different kinds of cancer (Table 9-1). It is most effective when the tumor cell population is small. When used optimally, it has the potential for eradicating metastatic foci of early disease.

Immunotherapy is based on the existence of tumor specific antigens and of an immune response to them (97-99). Both these aspects have been demonstrated in experimental tumors and in human malignant disease. Numerous clinical observations indicate that immunologic mechanisms influence the development and the growth of malignant tumors. The occurrence of tumors in patients receiving immunosuppressive therapy, in patients with immunologic deficiencies and the rare cases of spontaneous regression of cancer attest to their importance.

Immunotherapy follows "zero-order" kinetics, that is a specific number of immunocompetent cells or antibodies is required for the lysis of each tumor cell. Its major advantage is that all tumor cells, including the last one, can be destroyed (in contrast to chemotherapy, which follows "first-order" kinetics). It is thus of central importance to cure (75).

Table 13-4.

Radiocurable tumors	Radiotherapy useful

A. Highly radiosensitive:

  1. Embryonal origin

    seminoma (testicular)

    dysgerminoma (ovary)

    Wilms' tumor[a]

  2. Lympho-reticulo-endothelial

    lymphosarcoma[a]

    Hodgkin's disease[a]

    Ewing's sarcoma[a]

    Reticululosarcoma of bone[a]

  3. Neurogenic:

    neuroblastoma

    retinoblastoma

B. Moderately radiosensitive, often curable
(several of these tumors can be treated
with equal success by surgery)

  GI: esophagus (upper 2/3), anus

  GYN: cervix, vagina

  GU: bladder, urethra, penis, prostate

  Skin: mainly on face, including lip, eyelid

  H + N: oral cavity, nasopharynx and oropharynx,
intrinsic larynx (limited), exophytic
supraglottic larynx

  CNS: Pituitary adenoma, medulloblastoma,
brain stem

  Reticulosarcoma

(Here surgery is generally the primary therapy,
often combined with adjuvant radiotherapy. Radiotherapy is also indicated for control of inoperable,
residual or recurrent disease.)

Breast

Lung

GI: rectum

GYN: ovary, endometrium, vulva, vagina (occasionally)

GU: kidney, testicular – other than seminoma

H + N: salivary gland, paranasal sinuses, advanced
oropharynx, larynx, hypopharynx, thyroid,
chemodectomas

Soft-tissue sarcomas

CNS: gliomas, pituitary tumors, spinal cord
tumors

Tumors only occasionally favorably influenced by
radiotherapy

1. Osteogenic sarcoma

2. Chondrosarcoma

3. Malignant melanoma

4. Adenocarcinoma of pancreas

---

[a] often used in combination with chemotherapy.

Table 13-5. Role of chemotherapy in treatment of cancer

1. Advanced tumors.

2. Used prior to surgery to render unresectable tumors operable.

3. Adjuvant to "curative" surgery:

   A. Short-term: to kill malignant cells released at surgery in:
wound	local recurrence
circulation	hematogenous metastases

   B. Long-term: to kill subclinical metastases already present when "curative" surgery is attempted.

4. Preceding radiotherapy to reduce large tumor masses, thereby improving the effectivenss of radiation;

   in conjunction with radiotherapy to obtain a radio-sensitizing effect.

5. Regional perfusion of localized tumors

   in anatomic regions that cannot be approached by surgery
   occurring in maximally irradiated areas.

Experience has shown that either of these four methods used as single treatment modality can cure but a minority of all cancer patients. Surgery and radiotherapy salvage only approximately one patient in three. They are local modalities that eliminate tumor cells only where they are applied. Both have reached a plateau in their ability to eradicate solid tumors. They fail at the site of the primary tumor, surgery because of an incomplete resection of microscopic tumor extensions (marginal recurrence) or wound implantation, radiotherapy because of the relative radioresistance of cells in the tumor core due to intracellular hypoxia (central recurrence). Most failures however following surgery or radiotherapy are the result of clinically undetected disseminated metastases. It is against these microscopic seedings that chemotherapy and immunotherapy are most likely to have a curative effect. We anticipate that chemotherapy and/or immunotherapy used as an adjuvant following surgery or radiotherapy of the primary tumor will significantly improve the cure rates of these two therapeutic modalities. The limitations of chemotherapy were discussed in Chapter 9. The effect of chemotherapy depends on the total number of tumor cells present. Because of the first-order kinetics rule it is more effective against small tumor populations. The growth fraction is low in large tumor masses; in other words, the majority of cells are out of cycle and hence less sensitive to cytotoxic agents. Furthermore, drug penetration is less adequate in large tumor masses and drug-resistant clones are more likely to be selected out of a large, heterogenous tumor population. The curative potential of chemotherapy can thus be augmented by a preliminary surgical or radiotherapeutic tumor reduction.

Immunotherapy, likewise, can destroy not more than microscopic amounts of tumor. The best results today have been obtained when immunotherapy is used to eliminate malignant cells following preliminary reductions by other forms of therapy (4-6).

Table 13-6 summarizes the indications and limitations of the various modalities and indicates how they complement each other. Three types of treatment failures are recognized: (1) recurrence at the site of

Table 13-6. Indications for and limitations of each of the four treatment modalities for cancer

	Major indication (type of cancer)	Major limitations and causes of failures
Surgery	localized	1. Local extension 2. Occult metastases
Radiotherapy	Localized, radiosensitive	1. Dose-limiting toxicity 2. Radioresistance (primary and secondary) 3. Occult metastases
Chemotherapy	Advanced, metastatic Occult metastatic	1. First-order kinetics rule: fails to kill 100% of tumor cells; effect dependent on total cell number 2. Lack of specificity: systemic toxicity and immunodepression 3. Effect dependent on GF of tumor: ineffective against resting cells 4. Ineffective against tumor sanctuaries 5. Chemoresistance (primary and secondary)
Immunotherapy	Residual	1. Cannot eradicate more than 10^5 cells 2. Immunoresistance (primary and secondary) 3. Still experimental

the primary tumor, (2) metastatic spread, (3) host failure, that is incompetent immune mechanisms. The type of treatment failure tends to be different for the various tumors. For example, glioblastomas and head and neck tumors recur mainly locally, while most lung and breast cancers fail because of distant spread.

A mainly empirical approach has taught us that the use of more than one therapeutic modality, simultaneously or in sequence, can increase the cure rate of a large number of tumors (1-4, 74-76). The experience with Wilms' tumor is a good example. Cancer strategy has not been studied much in experimental animals. A large number of combinations has to be evaluated when four different forms of therapy can be combined simultaneously or in sequence. It is not easy to formulate specific guidelines for their combined use. Surgery and radiotherapy are primarily used to eliminate the primary tumor or bulky tumor masses. Chemotherapy is most effective against microscopic metastases, while immunotherapy can kill the last tumor cell once the tumor cell number has been reduced to less than 10^5 by other treatment modalities. Chemotherapy or radiotherapy can also be used to render unresectable tumors operable (77).

Three clinical situations are considered in this discussion of cancer strategy: (1) disseminated cancers, (2) localized tumors that cannot be completely excised or cured by radiotherapy, (3) localized tumors that can be cured by surgery and/or radiotherapy.

B. CANCER TREATMENT STRATEGY FOR DISSEMINATED TUMORS

It is customary to start with chemotherapy. Unfortunately, as explained earlier, large tumor masses are not very sensitive to chemotherapy. It is not surprising that most tumors at this stage show no regression, or only temporary, partial regression. A few (apparent) complete remissions have been noted but even these are temporary, with the possible exception of Burkitt's tumor and choriocarcinoma (see Table 9-1). Systemic chemotherapy, when prescribed for metastatic disease, is sometimes combined with radiotherapy or surgery of the primary tumor to prevent or palliate local complications, for example hemoptysis or atelectasis in lung tumors, hematuria in renal tumors, obstruction in malignancies of the gastrointestinal tract.

The use of surgery or radiotherapy in disseminated malignancies for the main purpose of reducing the number of tumor cells is a relatively new concept. It was deduced from the first-order kinetics rule that implies that chemotherapy alone cannot cure cancer, and from kinetic considerations that indicate that cytotoxic drugs are more effective in small tumor masses (Fig. 13-1). This approach has considerably improved the response rate and given prolongation of survival in Ewing's sarcoma (78), Wilms' tumor (79), and osteogenic sarcoma (80, 81), among others.

Another novel approach in the management of disseminated cancers is the addition of immunotherapy to kill the last cell in those rather rare tumors where chemotherapy has successfully induced a complete remission. There is no form of cancer for which more treatment modalities have been combined in an attempt to cure the patient than childhood ALL (6-8). The initial attack is by combination chemotherapy ("induction" therapy) to induce a complete remission, that is, the reduction of the initial load of leukemic cells from 10^{12} (1 kg) to 10^9 (1 gm). Rapid relapse nearly always occurs without additional therapy. "Maintenance" therapy can delay relapse, sometimes considerably, as it kills cells that enter the mitotic cycle, but it has no effect on resting leukemic stem cells (G_0 or prolonged G_1). Furthermore, a population of resistant cells is selected and with successive relapses the patient becomes resistant to most agents known to be effective in ALL. Therefore, once a complete remission has been obtained, it is logical to prescribe "complementary cell-reducing" chemotherapy in an attempt to reduce the number of leukemic cells from 10^9 to 10^5, the tumor load that can be handled by immunotherapy (Fig. 13-2). Encouraging results have been obtained with such programs at the ICIG, at the cost of far less toxicity than Pinkel's "total therapy" protocols, which rely on chemotherapy and radiotherapy (9). His maintenance therapy is associated with a 10 percent mortality of patients in complete remission (10, 11). The efficacy of a sequential chemotherapy-immunotherapy protocol has been confirmed in AML (12, 13).

C. CANCER TREATMENT STRATEGY FOR LOCALIZED TUMORS, NOT CURABLE BY SURGERY AND/OR RADIOTHERAPY

Localized inoperable tumors are conventionally treated by radiotherapy or, if they are radioresistant, by chemotherapy. This initial therapy is often prescribed in the hope that it will induce sufficient tumor regression to permit supsequent surgical resection, for example in cancer of the head and neck, carcinoma of the ovary (82) or rectosigmoid (77) (Fig. 13-3).

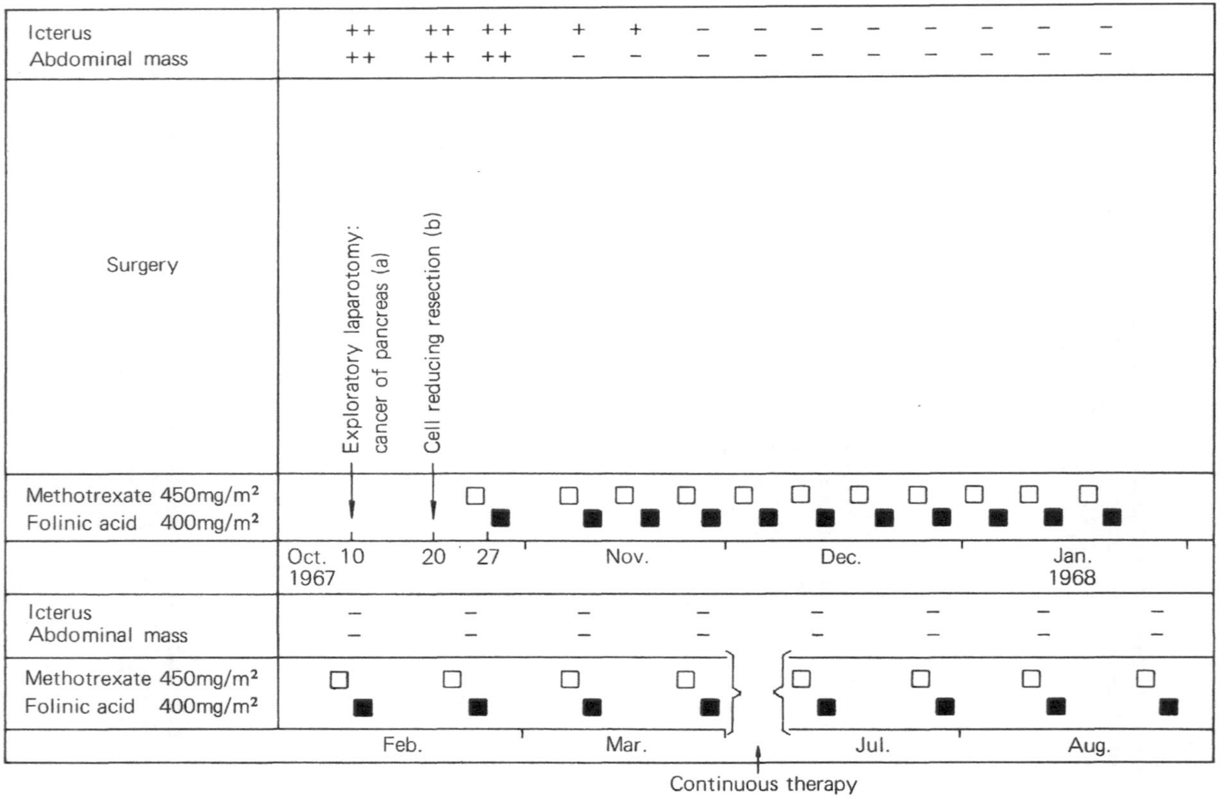
Icterus
Abdominal mass
++ ++ ++ + + – – – – – – – –
++ ++ ++ – – – – – – – – – –
Surgery
Exploratory laparotomy:
cancer of pancreas (a)
Cell reducing resection (b)
Methotrexate 450mg/m²
Folinic acid 400mg/m²
Oct. 10 20 27 Nov. Dec. Jan.
1967 1968
Icterus
Abdominal mass
Methotrexate 450mg/m²
Folinic acid 400mg/m²
Feb. Mar. Jul. Aug.
Continuous therapy

Fig. 13-1. Example of cell-reducting surgery in a case of cancer of the pancreas. Prior to surgery, the methotrexate-folinic acid combination failed to relieve the obstructive jaundice. After surgery the same combination resulted in a complete remission of 10 months duration. (From MATHE et al. (2))

a) Cancer of the pancreas: adenopathy around the origin of the mesenteric vein; thrombosis of the portal vein, b) duodenopancreatectomy, gastrojejunal terminolateral anastomosis, choled jejunal anastomosis, dissection of the portal vein and resection of a 6 cm thrombus

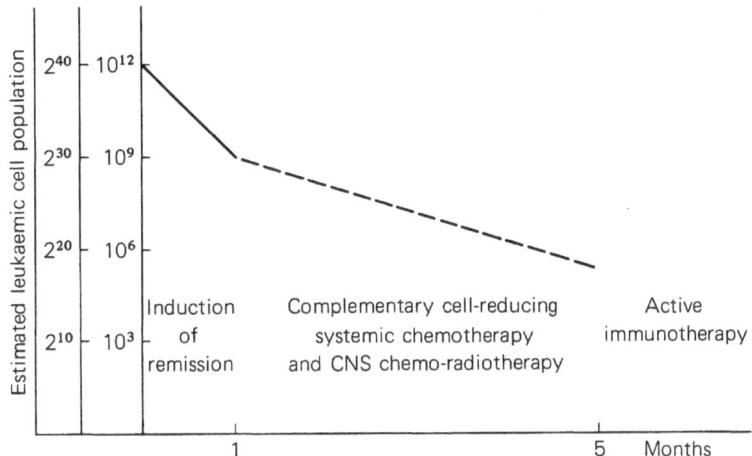

Fig. 13-2. *Principle underlying our treatment of acute lymphoid leukemia.*
Therapy consists of three successive phases: (a) chemotherapy to induce
a "complete" remission at the end of which the patient still harbors
10^9 *cells; (b) complementary cell-reducing chemotherapy (systemic and*
intrathecal) and radiotherapy to the central nervous system (CNS); (c)
active immunotherapy to eradicate the cells not killed by chemotherapy

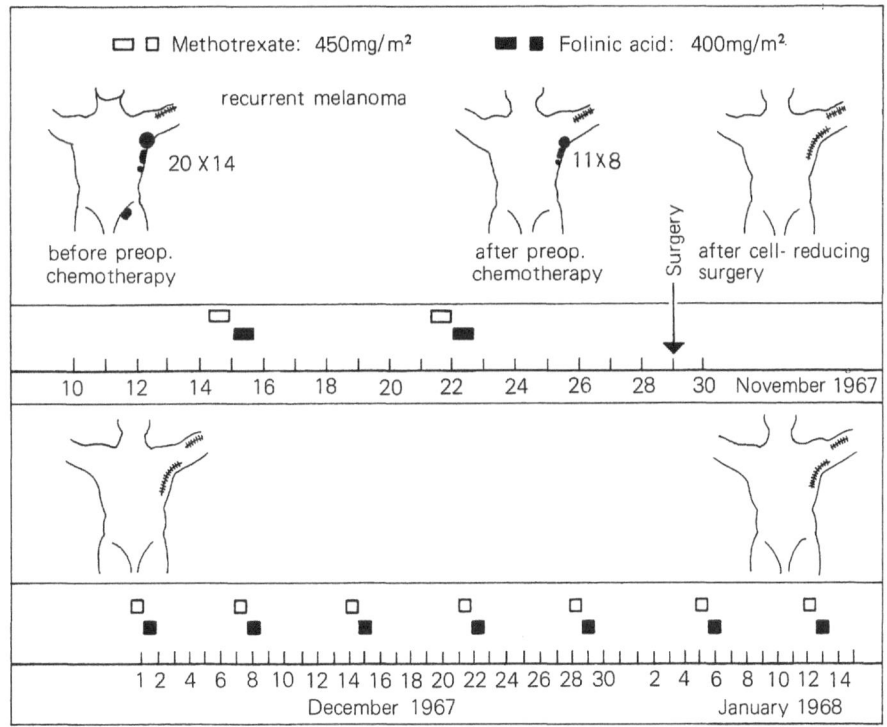

Fig. 13-3. *Inoperable recurrent malignant melanoma. Chemotherapy per-*
mitted subsequent cell-reducing surgery. This procedure was followed
by further chemotherapy. (From MATHE et al. (2))

Since chemotherapy alone is unlikely to be very effective in large tumor masses, the following sequence seems logical for localized, unresectable and radioresistant tumors: incomplete resection to reduce the tumor mass from for example 10^{12} to 10^9 cells, followed by chemotherapy to reduce the residual tumor by 2 or 4 orders of magnitude to a number (10^5) that can be eliminated by immunotherapy ($\underline{2}$). In radiosensitive tumors the sequence could be: radiotherapy, chemotherapy, immunotherapy. The combination of surgery, radiotherapy, chemotherapy (with immunotherapy still under investigation) can control locally advanced Wilms' tumor ($\underline{79}$), neuroblastoma ($\underline{82}$), and rhabdomyosarcoma ($\underline{84}$), among other forms ($\underline{82, 89}$).

D. CANCER TREATMENT STRATEGY FOR LOCALIZED TUMORS, CURABLE BY SURGERY OR RADIOTHERAPY

Surgery is obviously the treatment of choice in tumors that are sufficiently localized to be completely excised. However, additional therapy may be indicated in at least two different situations.

The surgeon may wonder whether the functional and esthetic result could be improved without affecting the cure rate obtainable by more radical surgery by using a less extensive surgical procedure supplemented by another treatment modality. HAYWARD tried to answer this question for operable breast cancer by comparing the results of simple tumorectomy followed by radiotherapy with those of radical mastectomy ($\underline{14}$). The mortality in the two randomized groups was identical but the limited-surgery group had a slightly higher incidence of local recurrences. This study indicates that a certain number of women would not be placed at risk by less extensive and less mutilating surgery. Less mutilating operations have also been proposed in childhood rhabdomyosarcoma ($\underline{84}$).

Many a surgeon has been frustrated by the sight of recurrent local disease or distant metastases after what he considered to have been curative primary surgery. For example, only 25 percent of patients who underwent "curative" surgery for lung cancers are alive after 5 years, hence the idea of "adjuvant" chemotherapy ($\underline{15-17}$). This is systemic chemotherapy given as complementary treatment following radical surgery or radiotherapy intended to rid the patient of a localized malignancy. Comparative trials are especially desirable in cancers that have a low cure rate after attempts at curative resection, that is cancer of the gastrointestinal tract, prostate, bladder, lung, breast (especially if positive axillary lymph nodes or medial-quadrant lesions are present), soft-tissue sarcomas and malignant melanoma.

Two mechanisms are thought to be responsible for failures after primary surgery in these tumors: (1) malignant cells are implanted in the operative field, causing local recurrences, or malignant cells find their way into the peripheral blood or lymphatics during the surgical manipulations and initiate distant metastases. Indeed, tumor cells have been observed in the peripheral blood, and especially in the venous blood draining the tumor area, at the time of surgery ($\underline{18}$); (2) it is also possible that microscopic metastases were already present when the primary surgery was performed. Two types of adjuvant chemotherapy have therefore been evaluated: short-term, to kill malignant cells liberated into the circulation or the wound at the time of surgery, and long-term, to eradicate subclinical metastases that may already be present when curative surgery is attempted. Chemotherapy would be expected to be more effective in combating these microscopic foci of tumor cells than later on against clinically detectable metastases ($\underline{100}$).

The value of adjuvant chemotherapy has been established in animal experiments by COLE (19), SHAPIRO et al. (20), and SHIMKIN et al. (21). Their studies confirmed that anticancer agents are less effective against large masses, that tumor cells circulating in the blood are especially sensitive to chemotherapy, and that surgery and chemotherapy are more effective in combination than either is alone.

The results of early clinical studies have been much less convincing and often contradictory. Effects were reported to be beneficial, nonexistent, or even harmful. The few clinical trials with lung, breast, stomach, colorectal and head and neck cancers have not been encouraging (Fig. 13-4; Tables 13-7 and 13-8). No consistent increase in survival time was seen with the majority of solid tumors. A beneficial effect has been reported in certain subgroups of patients, especially in breast cancer (22, 23). Several studies have shown that patients receiving chemotherapy following curative resections of lung and breast cancer actually had a higher recurrence rate than untreated controls (Fig. 13-5) (23-26). The importance of conducting controlled clinical trials is well illustrated by these reports. The problem is that the drugs used in these protocols have a tumor response of only 30 percent at best, and they may be more effective as immunosuppressants than as cytotoxic agents. Since immune reactions seem important in controlling tumor cells, the deleterious effect of adjuvant chemotherapy could be due to its immunosuppressive action. Perhaps the results of adjuvant chemotherapy could be improved by carrying out long-term (because of the cell characteristics of solid tumors) intermittent (because it is less immunosuppressive and allows for bone marrow recovery) combination chemotherapy, including agents that are effective against tumor sanctuaries. Until the value of systemic adjuvant chemotherapy is clearly confirmed by controlled clinical trials, it seems reasonable to use it only in patients who are likely to relapse in spite of attempted curative surgery (preferably in the context of an organized trial). Preliminary reports with long-term adjuvant chemotherapy with more effective cytotoxic agents or combinations following local therapy of the primary tumor seem to yield superior results in the treated patients compared

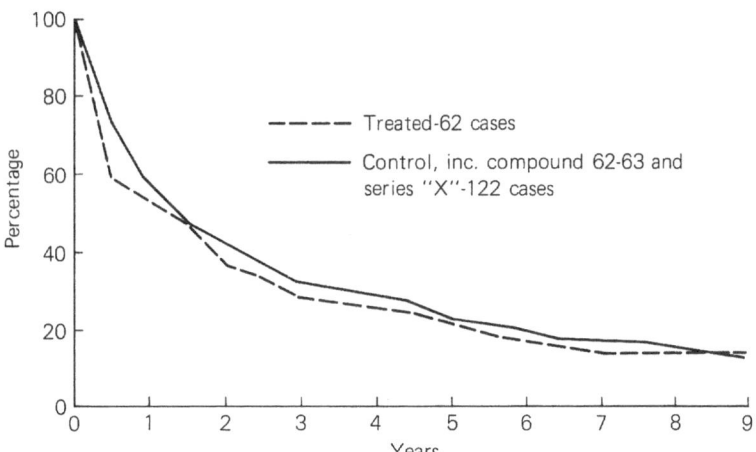

Fig. 13-4. Survival curves of patients who underwent "curative" resection for lung cancer, followed by adjuvant chemotherapy with nitrogen mustard or placebo (controls). Adjuvant chemotherapy had no beneficial effect. (From HIGGINS et al. (46))

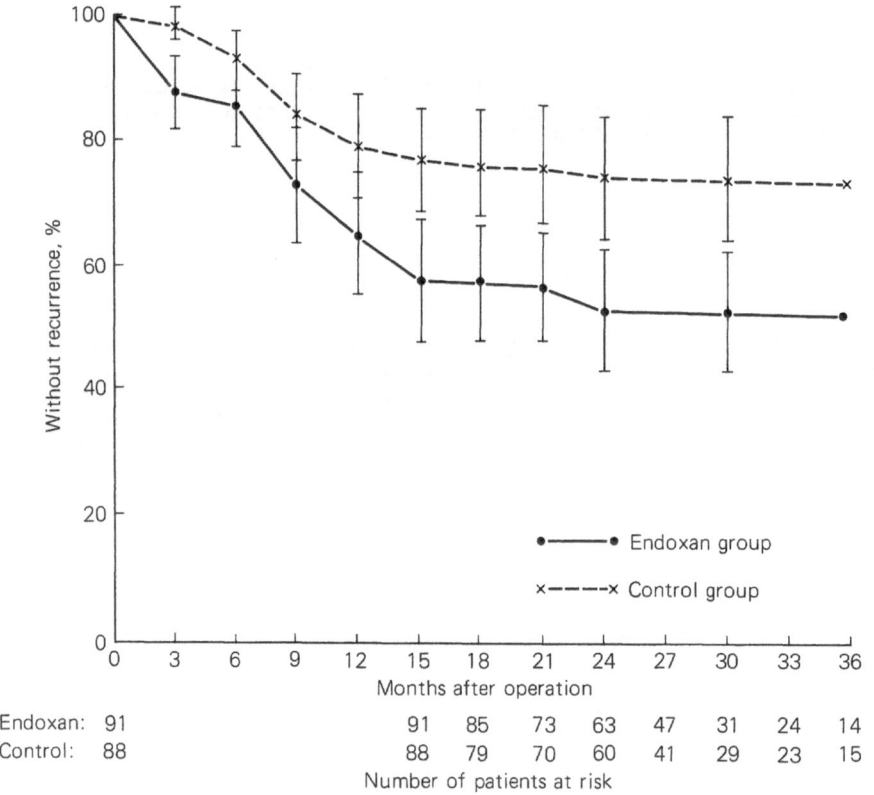

| Endoxan: | 91 | | | | 91 | 85 | 73 | 63 | 47 | 31 | 24 | 14 |
| Control: | 88 | | | | 88 | 79 | 70 | 60 | 41 | 29 | 23 | 15 |

Number of patients at risk

Fig. 13-5. An example of the unfavorable effect of long-term adjuvant chemotherapy with cyclophosphamide (Endoxan) following radical surgery for bronchus carcinoma. The higher recurrence rate in the treated group may be the result of suppression of the immune defenses by the drug (From BRUNNER et al. (26))

to untreated controls, especially in Wilms' tumor (79, 85), osteogenic sarcoma (86, 87, 88), Ewing's sarcoma (78, 89), Hodgkin's disease (90), and in breast cancer (91-93). The current trend is to try as adjuvant therapy, drugs or combinations of drugs, that have been shown to be effective in patients with advanced disease, provided they have also proven safe (74). Indeed, until there are tests to quantitate cells at the subclinical level (below 10^9) cells, therapeutic decisions must remain guesswork, and treatment, that can have serious side-effects, may be administered to patients who are in fact, cured.

Hormones have also been used as adjuvant to surgery in breast and prostate cancers. No beneficial effect could be demonstrated in breast cancers, and estrogen therapy reduced the duration of survival in certain stages of prostate carcinoma due to dose-related cardiovascular complications (27).

Immunotherapy as an adjuvant to surgery, radiotherapy, or chemotherapy has the theoretical advantage that it is capable of killing the last cell. Its value is currently under study (28-31, 94, 95).

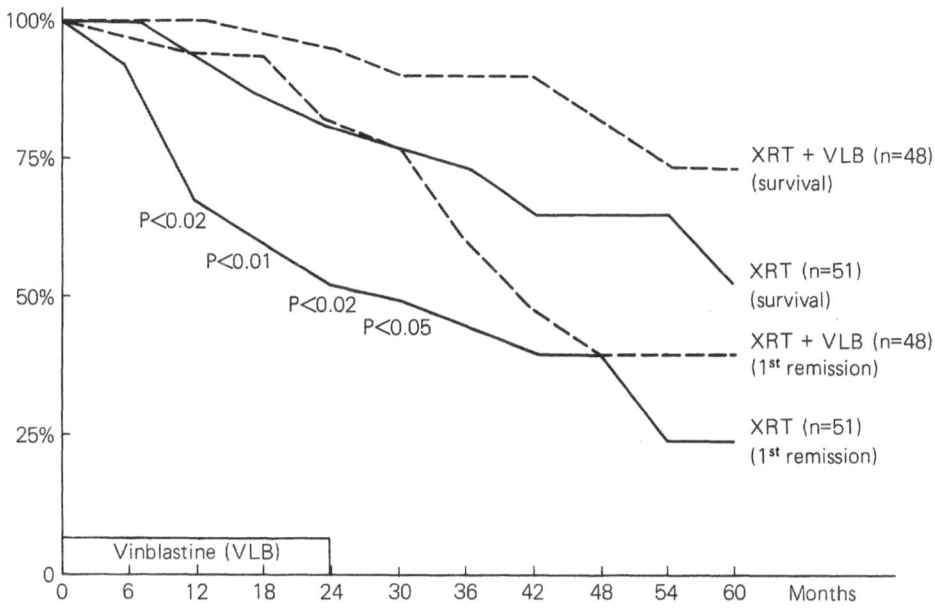

Fig. 13-6. Influence of long-term (2 years) adjuvant chemotherapy with vinblastine (VLB) following radiotherapy (XRT) on survival and duration of first remission of Stage I and II Hodgkin's disease, mixed cellularity (EORTC trial) (32)

The same considerations apply to localized radiosensitive tumors that can be cured by radiotherapy. Since esthetic and functional damage is less of a problem, the dose required to eradicate the tumor can be given. Combination of radiotherapy with other treatment modalities is considered to improve the cure rate. Radiotherapy effective in cancers of the uterus and of the head and neck area has been complemented by surgery. Chemotherapy in combination with radiotherapy may be useful in seminoma, teratoma, Wilms' tumor, Ewing's sarcoma, neuroblastoma, reticulosarcoma, and Hodgkin's disease. For example, the EORTC radiochemotherapy group reported that complementary therapy with vinblastine for 2 years significantly prolonged the duration of the first remission and of survival of patients with Stage I and II Hodgkin's disease but only for one histologic type, mixed cellularity (Fig. 13-6, 32).

Chemotherapy has also been used concomitantly with radiotherapy in the hope of obtaining a potentiating effect (96). COHEN noted that 5-FU potentiated low-dose radiotherapy (33). Indeed, 2000 r plus 5-FU was as effective in bronchus carcinoma as 4000 r, while both were more effective than 2000 r. A number of drugs have been evaluated for a potentiating effect on radiotherapy but with inconsistent results.

Table 13-7. Results of trials with adjuvant chemotherapy (Comparative trials: surgery with and without chemotherapy)

Site of tumor	Drug +/-	Result	Reference
Stomach cancer	FUDR	No difference	STERLIN et al. (34)
	thio-TEPA	No difference	DIXON et al. (35)
	thio-TEPA	No difference	V.A. Surgical adjuvant

241

Table 13-7. (continued)

Site of tumor	Drug +/-	Result	Reference
			Cancer Chemotherapy Group (36)
	nitromin or cyclophos-phamide	No difference	BLIXENKRONE-MØLLER (37)
Colon-rectum cancer	5-FU	Prolonged survival of treated patients	HIGGINS et al. (38).
	FUdR	No difference	HIGGINS and WHITE (39)
	thio-TEPA	No difference	DWIGHT et al. (40)
	thio-TEPA	Prolonged survival of certain treated subgroups	HIGGINS and WHITE (39) HOLDEN et al. (41) DIXON et al. (35)
	nitromin or cyclophos-phamide	Prolonged survival of treated patients	BLIXENKRONE-MØLLER (37)
	5-FU into lumen of bowel + systemic	Prolonged survival of treated patients	ROUSSELOT et al. (42)
Lung cancer	nitrogen mustard	No difference	HUGHES et al. (44)
	nitrogen mustard	No difference	SLACK (45)
	cyclophos-phamide	No difference	HIGGINS et al. (46)
	cyclophos-phamide or busulfan	No difference	MRC Working Party (25)
	cyclophos-phamide	Shortened disease-free interval (and probably survival) of treated patients	BRUNNER et al. (26)
	vinblastine	No difference	CROSBIE et al. (47)
Breast cancer	thio-TEPA	More recurrences among the treated group; disease-free interval shorter in treated group with positive axillary nodes	DONEGAN (48)
	thio-TEPA	Disease-free interval and survival prolonged in treated subgroup of premeno-pausal women > 4 positive axillary nodes	FISHER (22, 23)
	5-FU	No difference	FISHER (22)
	nitrogen mustard	Disease-free interval prolonged in treated subgroup of pre-menopausal women with negative axillary nodes	MRAZEK and McDONALD (49)
	cyclophos-phamide	Fewer recurrences in treated patients	NISSEN-MEYER et al. (50)

Table 13-7. (continued)

Site of tumor	Drug +/-	Result	Reference
	melphalan	disease-free interval prolonged statistically significant for premenopausal women	FISHER et al. (91)
	CPM, MTX, 5-FU	preliminary data: fewer recurrences in treated patients	BONADONNA et al. (92)
Prostate cancer	diethylstilbestrol	Shortened survival of treated patients	V.A. Coop. Urological Research Group (27)
Bladder cancer	5-FU	No difference	PROUT et al. (51)
Wilms' tumor	Actinomycin D (1 course) Actinomycin D (maintenance)	Prolonged survival in maintenance group	WOLFF et al. (52)

Table 13-8. Results of trials with adjuvant chemotherapy (comparative trials: radiotherapy with and without chemotherapy)

Site of tumor	Drug +/-	Result	Reference
Oral cavity	5-FU MTX (intra-arterially)	Prolonged survival Increased survival at 6 months in treated group but no difference at 2 years	ANSFIELD et al. (53) RICHARD (54)
	Nitrogen mustard	More frequent control of primary tumor and adenopathy in treated group	RICHARDS and CHAMBERS (55)
Hypopharynx Nasopharynx Larynx	5-FU	No difference	ANSFIELD et al. (53)
Stomach cancer	5-FU	Prolonged survival of treated group	MOERTEL et al. (56, 57)
Pancreas carcinoma	5-FU	Prolonged survival of treated group	MOERTEL et al. (56, 57)
Colon, rectum cancer	5-FU	Prolonged survival of treated group	MOERTEL et al. (56, 57)
Lung cancer	MTX or, 5-FU 5-FU or actinomycin D	No difference No difference	HOSLEY et al. (58) HALL et al. (59)
	5-FU (15 mg/kg/d)	Prolonged survival of treated group	GOLLIN et al. (60, 61)

Table 13-8. (continued)

Site of tumor	Drug +/-	Result	Reference
Lung cancer	5-FU (10 mg/kg/d)	No difference	CARR et al. (62)
	XRT (2000 rads) XRT (2000 rads)+ 5-FU XRT (4000 rads)	2000 rads + 5-FU is more effective than 2000 rads alone and as effective as 4000 rads	COHEN et al. (33)
	Nitrogen mustard	No difference	KRANT et al. (63)
	Nitrogen mustard	No difference	DURRANT et al. (64)
	Nitromin	No difference	EWING et al. (65)
	Cyclophospha-mide	No difference	E.O.R.T.C. (66)
	Cyclophospha-mide	Prolonged survival of treated group	BERGSAGEL (67)
	Vinblastine	No difference	COY (68)
Breast cancer	5-FU	No difference	VERMUND et al. (69)
	Cyclophospha-mide	Shortened survival of treated group	FINNEY (24)
Ovarian carcinoma	5-FU or cyclo-phosphamide	No difference	VERMUND et al. (69)
Bladder cancer	5-FU	No difference	EDLAND et al. (70)
Glio-blastoma	5-FU	No difference	EDLAND et al. (71)
	BCNU	Prolonged survival of treated group	WALKER and GEHAN (72)
Cerebral metastases	Prednisone	No difference	HORTON et al. (73)
Hodgkin's disease	Vinblastine	Prolonged disease-free survival and for some subgroups improved survival	E.O.R.T.C. (32)
	M.O.P.P.	Preliminary data: prolonged disease-free interval	ROSENBERG and KAPLAN (90)

REFERENCES

1. MATHE, G.: La dernière cellule. Presse méd. 75, 2591 (1967).
2. MATHE, G.: Operational research in cancer chemotherapy. Chemotherapy in the strategy of cancer treatment, In: Scientific Basis of
   Cancer Chemotherapy, p. 72 (ed. G. Mathé). Berlin-Heidelberg-New
   York: Springer-Verlag 1969.
3. MATHE, G.: Active immunotherapy. Advanc. Res. 14, 1 (1971).
4. MARTIN, D.S.: The necessity for combined modalities in cancer
   therapy. Hosp. Practice 129 (Jan. 1973).
5. MATHE, G.: Immunothérapie active de la leucémie L1210 appliquée
   après la greffe tumorale. Rev. franc. Etud. clin. biol. 13, 881
   (1968).
6. MATHE, G., POUILLART, P., SCHWARZENBERG, L., AMIEL, J.L., SCHNEIDER,
   M., HAYAT, M., DE VASSAL, F., JASMIN, C., ROSENFELD, C., WEINER,
   R., RAPPAPORT, H.: Attempts at immunotherapy of 100 patients with
   acute lymphoid leukemia: some factors influencing results. Nat.
   Cancer Inst. Monogr. 35, 361 (1972).
7. MATHE, G., AMIEL, J.L., SCHWARZENBERG, L., SCHNEIDER, M., CATTAN,
   A., SCHLUMBERGER, J.R., HAYAT, M., DE VASSAL, F.: Active immunotherapy for acute lymphoblastic leukemia. Lancet 1, 697 (1969).
8. MATHE, G.: Strategy for the treatment of acute lymphoid leukemia.
   In: 13th International Congress of Pediatrics. p. 21. Vienna: Wiener
   Med. Akad. Publ. 1971.
9. PINKEL, D., HERNANDEZ, K., BORELLA, L., HOLTEN, C., SAR, R., SAMOY,
   G., PRATT, C.: Drug dosage and remission duration in childhood lymphocytic leukemia. Cancer 27, 247 (1971).
10. SIMONE, J., AUR, J.A., HUSTU, H.O., PINKEL, D.: "Total therapy"
    studies of acute lymphocytic leukemia in children. Current results
    and prospects for cure. Cancer 30, 1488 (1972).
11. SIMONE, J.V., HOLLAND, E., JOHNSON, W.: Fatalities during remissions
    of childhood leukemia. Blood 39, 759 (1972).
12. POWLES, R., KAY, H.E.M., McELWAIN, T.J., ALEXANDER, P., CROWTHER, D.,
    HAMILTON-FAIRLEY, G., PIKE, M.: Immunotherapy of acute myeloblastic
    leukaemia in man. In G. Mathé, R. Weiner: Investigation and stimula-
    tion of immunity in cancer patients. Heidelberg, Paris, Springer-
    Verlag, CNRS, 1974.
13. VOGLER, W.R., CHAN, Y.K.: Effect of BCG in prolongation of remis-
    sions in acute myeloblastic leukemia. Proc. amer. Ass. Cancer Res.
    15, 164 (1974).
14. HAYWARD, J.: Communication, 5th plenary session, EORTC (1971).
15. KENIS, Y.: Chemotherapy of residual disease in solid tumours. Rev.
    Europ. Etudes Clin. et Biol. 16, 103 (1971).
16. PATTERSON, W.B.: Contributions of surgeons to clinical cancer
    chemotherapy. Oncology 26, 277 (1972).
17. KARRER, K.: Importance of dose schedules in adjuvant chemotherapy.
    Cancer Chemother. Rep. 56, 35 (1972).
18. ENGELL, H.C.: Cancer cells in the circulating blood. Clinical study
    of the occurrence of cancer cells in peripheral blood and in venous
    blood draining the tumour area at operation. Acta chir. Scand. 201,
    1 (1955).
19. COLE, W.H., PACKARD, D., SOUTHWICK, H.W.: Carcinoma of the colon
    with special reference to prevention of recurrence. J. Amer. med.
    Ass. 515, 1549 (1954).
20. SHAPIRO, D.M., FUGMANN, R.: A role for chemotherapy as an adjuvant
    to surgery. Cancer Res. 17, 1098 (1957).
21. SHIMKIN, M.B., MOORE, G.E.: Adjuvant use of chemotherapy in the
    surgical treatment of cancer. J. Amer. med. Ass. 167, 1710 (1958).
22. FISHER, B.: Systemic chemotherapy as an adjuvant to surgery in the
    treatment of breast cancer. Cancer 24, 1286 (1969).

23. FISHER, B.: Surgical adjuvant therapy for breast cancer. Cancer
    30, 1556 (1972).
24. FINNEY, R.: Adjuvant chemotherapy in the radical treatment of car-
    cinoma of the breast - a clinical trial. Amer. J. Roentgenol. 111,
    137 (1971).
25. MEDICAL RESEARCH COUNCIL WORKING PARTY: Study of cytotoxic chemo-
    therapy as an adjuvant to surgery in carcinoma of the bronchus.
    Brit. med. J. 2, 421 (1971).
26. BRUNNER, K.W., MARTHALER, TH., MULLER, W.: Unfavorable effects
    of long-term adjuvant chemotherapy with endoxan in radically opera-
    ted bronchogenic carcinoma. Europ. J. Cancer 7, 285 (1971).
27. VETERANS ADMINISTRATION CO-OPERATIVE UROLOGICAL RESEARCH GROUP:
    Treatment and survival of patients with cancer of the prostate.
    Surgery 124, 1011 (1967).
28. BLUMING, A.Z., VOGEL, C.L., ZIEGLER, J.L., MODY, N., KAMYA, G.:
    Immunological effects of BCG in malignant melanoma: two modes of
    administration compared. Ann. intern. Med. 76, 405 (1972).
29. ZIEGLER, J.L.: Chemotherapy of Burkitt's lymphoma. Cancer 30,
    1534 (1972).
30. SOKAL, J.E., AUNGST, C.W., SNYDERMAN, M.: Prolongation of remission
    in stage I and II lymphoma by BCG vaccination. Proc. amer. Ass.
    Cancer Res. 15, 13 (1974).
31. BAKEMEIER, R.F., DeVITA, V.T.: Combination chemotherapy and immuno-
    therapy of Hodgkin's disease. Preliminary report. Proc. amer. Ass.
    Cancer Res. 15, 183 (1974).
32. E.O.R.T.C. Radio-chemotherapy Cooperative Group: A randomized study
    for irradiation and vinblastine in stages I and II of Hodgkin's
    disease. Preliminary results. Europ. J. Cancer 8, 353 (1972).
33. COHEN, J.L., KRANT, M.J., SHNIDER, B.I., MATIAS, P.I., HORTON,
    J., BAXTER, D.: Radiation plus 5-fluorouracil (NSC-19893): clinical
    demonstration of additive effect in bronchogenic carcinoma. Cancer
    Chemother. Rep. 55, 253 (1971).
34. STERLIN, O., WOLKOFF, J.S., AMADEO, J.M., KEEHN, R.J.: Use of
    5- fluorodeoxyuridine (FUDR) as an adjuvant to the surgical manage-
    ment of carcinoma of the stomach. Cancer 24, 223 (1969).
35. DIXON, W.J., LONGMIRE, Jr., W.P., HOLDEN, W.D.: Use of triethylene-
    thiophosphoramide as an adjuvant to the surgical treatment of gas-
    tric and colorectal carcinoma: ten-year follow-up. Ann. Surg. 173,
    26 (1971).
36. VETERANS ADMINISTRATION CQ-OPERATIVE SURGICAL ADJUVANT STUDY GROUP:
    Use of thioTEPA as an adjuvant to the surgical management of car-
    cinoma of the stomach. Cancer 18, 291 (1965).
37. BLIXENKRONE-MØLLER, N.: Long-term results of operable cancer of the
    gastro-intestinal tract. Acta Chir. Scand. 133, 157 (1967).
38. HIGGINS, G.A., DWIGHT, R.W., SMITH, J.V., KEEHN, R.J.: Fluorouracil
    as an adjuvant to surgery in carcinoma of the colon. Arch. Surg.
    102, 339 (1971).
39. HIGGINS, G.A., WHITE, G.E.: Adjuvant chemotherapy and cancer surgery.
    In: Surgery Annual 1969, p. 305 (ed. P. Cooper) 1969.
40. DWIGHT, R.W., HIGGINS, G.A., KEEHN, R.J.: Factors influencing sur-
    vival after resection in cancer of the colon and rectum. Amer. J.
    Surg. 177, 512 (1969).
41. HOLDEN, W.D., DIXON, W.J., KUZMA, J.W.: The use of triethylenethio-
    phosphoramide as an adjuvant of the surgical treatment of colorectal
    carcinoma. Ann. Surg. 165, 481 (1967).
42. ROUSSELOT, L.M., COLE, D.R., GROSSI, C.E., CONTE, A.J., GONZALEZ,
    E.M., PASTERNACK, B.S.: A five-year progress report on the effective-
    ness of intraluminal chemotherapy (5-fluorouracil) adjuvant to sur-
    gery for colon rectal cancer. Amer. J. Surg. 115, 140 (1968).

43. ROUSSELOT, L.M., COLE, D.R., GROSSI, C.E., CONTE, A.J., GONZALEZ, E.M., PASTERNACK, B.S.: Adjuvant chemotherapy with 5-fluorouracil in surgery for colorectal cancer. Dis. Colon. Rect. 15, 169 (1972).
44. HUGHES, Jr., F.A., HIGGINS, G., BEEBE, G.W.: Present status of surgical adjuvant lung-cancer chemotherapy. J. Amer. med. Ass. 196, 131 (1966).
45. SLACK, N.H.: Bronchogenic carcinoma: nitrogen mustard as a surgical adjuvant and factors influencing survival. Cancer 25, 987 (1970).
46. HIGGINS, G.A., HUMPHREY, E.W., HUGHES, F.A., KEEHN, R.J.: Cytoxan as an adjuvant to surgery for lung cancer. J. surg. Oncol. 1, 221 (1969).
47. CROSBIE, W.A., KAMDAR, H.H., BELCHER, J.R.: A Controlled trial of vinblastine sulphate in the treatment of cancer of the lung. Brit. J. Dis. Chest 60, 28 (1966).
48. DONEGAN, W.: Prolonged surgical adjuvant chemotherapy with thio-TEPA for mammary carcinoma: A progress report. Tenth International Cancer Congress, Houston. Chicago: Year Book Medical Publisher 1970.
49. MRAZEK, R.G., McDONALD, G.O.: Surgery plus chemotherapy in the treatment of breast carcinoma. Tenth International Congress of Cancer, Houston. Chicago: Year Book Medical Publishers 1970.
50. NISSEN-MEYER, R., KJELLGRAN, K., MANSSON, B.: Preliminary report from the Scandinavian adjuvant chemotherapy study group. Cancer Chemother. Rep. 55, 561 (1971).
51. PROUT, G.R., SLACK, N.H., KEEHN, R.J.: Irradiation and 5-fluorouracil as adjuvants in the management of invasive bladder carcinoma. A cooperative group report after 4 years. J. Urol. (Baltimore) 104, 116 (1969).
52. WOLFF, J.A., KRIVIT, W., NEWTON, Jr., W.A., D'ANGIO, G.J.: Single versus multiple dose dactinomycin therapy of Wilms' tumor. New Engl. J. Med. 279, 290 (1968).
53. ANSFIELD, F.J., RAMIREZ, G., DAVIS, H.L., KORBITZ, B.C., VERMUND, H., GOLLIN, F.F.: Treatment of advanced cancer of the head and neck. Cancer 25, 78 (1970).
54. RICHARD, J.M.: Chimiothérapie avec infusion artérielle dans les tumeurs de la tête et du cou. Corso Superiore sulla Chemiotherapia dei Tumori, p. 505. Milano 1970.
55. RICHARDS, Jr., G.J., CHAMBERS, R.G.: Hydroxyurea: a radiosensitizer in the treatment of neoplasms of the head and neck. Amer. J. Roentgenol. 105, 555 (1969).
56. MOERTEL, C.G., CHILDS, D.S., REITEMEIER, R.J., COLBY, M.Y., HOLBROOK, M.A., KAHN, R.G.: A controlled evaluation of combined 5-fluorouracil and supervoltage radiation therapy for gastrointestinal carcinoma. Proc. Amer. Ass. Cancer Res. 10, 60 (1969).
57. MOERTEL, C.G., CHILDS, D.S., REITEMEIER, R.J., COLBY, M.Y., HOLBROOK, M.A.: Combined 5-fluorouracil and supervoltage radiation therapy of locally unresectable gastro-intestinal cancer. Lancet 2, 865 (1969).
58. HOSLEY, H.F., MARANGOUDAKIS, S., ROSS, C.A., MURPHEY, W.T., HOLLAND, J.F.: Combined radiation - chemotherapy for bronchogenic carcinoma - pilot study. Cancer Chemother. Rep. 16, 467 (1962).
59. HALL, T.C. et al.: A clinical pharmacology study of chemotherapy and X-ray therapy in lung cancer. Amer. J. Med. 43, 186 (1967).
60. GOLLIN, F.F., ANSFIELD, F.J., VERMUND, H.: Clinical studies of combined chemotherapy and irradiation in inoperable bronchogenic carcinoma. Amer. J. Roentgenol. 92, 22 (1964).
61. GOLLIN, F.F., ANSFIELD, F.J., VERMUND, H.: Continued studies of combined chemotherapy and irradiation in inoperable bronchogenic carcinoma. Cancer Chemother. Rep. 51, 189 (1967).
62. CARR, D.T., CHILDS, Jr., D.S., LEE, R.E.: Radiotherapy plus 5-FU compared to radiotherapy alone for inoperable and unresectable bronchogenic carcinoma. Cancer 29, 375 (1972).

63. KRANT, M.J. et al.: Comparative trial of chemotherapy and radiotherapy in patients with non-resectable cancer of the lung. Amer. J. Med. 35, 363 (1963).
64. DURRANT, K.R., ELLIS, F., BLACK, J.M., BERRY, R.J., RIDEHALGH, F.R., HAMILTON, W.S.: Comparison of treatment policies in inoperable bronchial carcinoma. Lancet 1, 715 (1971).
65. EWING, D.P., McEWEN, B.W., ATKINSON, L.: Combined chemotherapy and radiotherapy in carcinoma of the lung. Med. J. Aust. 2, 397 (1965).
66. GROUPE COOPERATEUR D'ESSAIS THERAPEUTIQUES SUR LES CANCERS BRONCHO-PULMONAIRES, O.E.R.T.C.: Résultats d'un essai thérapeutique clinique sur une association radiothérapie et chimiothérapie dans les cancers broncho-pulmonaires. Europ. J. Cancer 4, 437 (1968).
67. BERGSAGEL, D.E., JENKIN, R.D.T., PRINGLE, J.E., WHITE, D.M., FETTERLY, J.C.M., KLAASEN, D.J., McDERMOT, R.S.R.: Lung cancer: clinical trial of radiotherapy alone vs. radiotherapy plus cyclophosphamide. Cancer 30, 621 (1972).
68. COY, P.: A randomized study of irradiation and vinblastine in lung cancer. Cancer 26, 803 (1970).
69. VERMUND, H., GOLLIN, F.F., ANSFIELD, F.J.: Clinical studies of 5-fluorouracil as adjuvant to radiotherapy. Front. Radiat. Ther. Oncol. 4, 132 (1969).
70. EDLAND, R.W., WEAR, Jr., J.B., ANSFIELD, F.J.: Advanced cancer of the urinary bladder. An analysis of the results of radiotherapy alone vs. radiotherapy and concomitant 5-fluorouracil; a prospective randomized study of 36 cases. Amer. J. Roentgenol. 108, 124 (1970).
71. EDLAND, R.W., JAVID, M., ANSFIELD, F.J.: Glioblastoma multiforme. An analysis of the results of postoperative radiotherapy alone versus radiotherapy and concomitant 5-fluorouracil. Amer. J. Roentgenol. 111, 337 (1971).
72. WALKER, M.D., GEHAN, E.A.: An evaluation of 1-3-bis(2-chloroethyl)-1-nitrosourea (BCNU) and irradiation alone and in combination for the treatment of malignant glioma. Proc. Amer. Ass. Cancer Res. 13, 67 (1972).
73. HORTON, J., BAXTER, D.H., OLSON, K.B., The Eastern Cooperative Oncology Group: The management of metastases to the brain by irradiation and corticosteroids. Amer. J. Roentgenol. 111, 334 (1971).
74. CARTER, S.K., SOPER, W.T.: Integration of chemotherapy into combined modality treatment of solid tumor. I. Overall strategy. Cancer Treat. Rev. 1, 1 (1974).
75. MARTIN, D.S., FUGMAN, R., STOLFI, R., HAYWORTH, P.: Rationale of combined modality therapy for cancer. Cancer Chemother. Rep. Part 2, 4, 13 (1974).
76. JOHNSON, R.E.: Symposium theme: a conceptual approach to integrated cancer therapy. Cancer 35, 1 (1975).
77. POTTER, J.F., Preoperative irradiation and surgery for certain cancers. Cancer 35, 84 (1975).
78. POMERY, T.C., JOHNSON, R.E.: Combined modality therapy of Ewing's sarcoma. Cancer 35, 36 (1975).
79. WOLFF, J.A.: Advances in the treatment of Wilms' tumor. Cancer 35, 901 (1975).
80. BEATTLE, E.J., MARTINI, N., ROSEN, G.: The management of pulmonary metastases in children with osteogenic sarcoma with surgical resection combined with chemotherapy. Cancer 35, 618 (1975).
81. ROSEN, G., TEFT, M., MARTINEZ, A., CHAM, W., MURPHEY, M.L.: Combination chemotherapy and radiation therapy in the treatment of metastatic osteogenic sarcoma. Cancer 35, 622 (1975).
82. BRADY, L.W.: Combined modality therapy of gynecologic cancer. Cancer 35, 76 (1975).

83. KOOP, C.E., SCHNAUFER, L.: The management of abdominal neuroblastoma. Cancer 35, 905 (1975).
84. JOHNSON, D.: Trends in surgery for childhood rhabdomysarcoma. Cancer 35, 916 (1975).
85. EVANS, A.E.: The success and failure of multimodal therapy for cancer in children. Cancer 35, 48 (1975).
86. JAFFE, N., FREI, E., TRAGGIS, D., BISHOP, Y.: Adjuvant methotrexate and citrovorum factor treatment of osteogenic sarcoma. New Engl. J. Med. 291, 994 (1974).
87. CORTES, E.P., HOLLAND, J.F., WANG, J.J., SINKS, L.F., BLOM, J., SENN, H., BANK, A., GLIDEWELL, O.: Amputation and adriamycin in primary osteosarcoma. New Engl. J. Med. 291, 998 (1974).
88. ROSEN, G., TAN, C., SANMANEECHAI, A., BEATTLE, E.J., MARCOVE, R., MURPHEY, M.L.: The rationale for multiple drug chemotherapy in the treatment of osteogenic sarcoma. Cancer 35, 936 (1975).
89. HUSTU, H.O., FINKEL, D., PRATT, C.B.: Treatment of clinically localized Ewing's sarcoma with radiotherapy and combination chemotherapy. Cancer 30, 1522 (1972).
90. ROSENBERG, S.A., KAPLAN, H.S.: The management of staged I, II and III Hodgkin's disease with combined radiotherapy and chemotherapy. Cancer 35, 55 (1975).
91. FISHER, B., CARBONE, P., ECONOMOU, S.G., FRELICK, R., GLASS, A., et al.: L-Phenylalanine mustard in the management of primary breast cancer. New Engl. J. Med. 292, 117 (1975).
92. BONADONNA, G., BRUSAMOLINO, E., VALAGUSSA, P., VERONESI, U.: Adjuvant study with combination chemotherapy in operable breast cancer. Proc. Am. Soc. Clin. Oncol. 16, 254 (1975).
93. RAMINEZ, R.: Combined chemotherapy-radiotherapy as an adjuvant to mastectomy in patients with positive nodes. Proc. Am. Soc. Clin. Oncol. 16, 224 (1975).
94. GUTTERMAN, J.U., MAVLIGIT, G., McBRIDE, C., FREI, E. III., FREIREICH, E.J., HERSH, E.M.: Active immunotherapy with BCG for recurrent malignant melanoma. Lancet 1, 1208 (1973).
95. SOKAL, J.E., AUNGST, C.W., SNYDERMAN, M.: Delay in progression of malignant lymphoma after BCG vaccination. New Engl. J. Med. 291, 1226 (1974).
96. GOFFINET, D.R., BAGSHAW, M.A.: Clinical use of radiation sensitizing agents. Cancer Treat. Rev. 1, 15 (1974).
97. VARIOUS AUTHORS: Tumor immunology. Sem. Oncol. 1, 291-431 (1974).
98. VARIOUS AUTHORS: Immunology and Virology. CA-Cancer J. for Clinicians 25, 187-234 (1975).
99 BLUMMING, A.Z.: Current status of clinical immunotherapy. Cancer Chemother. Rep. Part 1, 915 (1975).
100. MATHE, G.: Les nouvelles frontières de la chimiothérapie des cancers. Nouv. Presse Med. 4, 3113 (1975).

Chapter 14
Acute Lymphoid Leukemia

It is in the treatment of childhood acute lymphoid leukemia (ALL) that
cancer chemotherapy and cancer strategy have attained their highest
degree of sophistication and some of their most impressive results. Up
to 25 years ago ALL was invariably fatal, with a median survival after
diagnosis of only 2 months. Now it is highly responsive to chemotherapy
and remissions can be induced in almost all previously untreated children. With some regimens currently under study in specialized leukemia
centers, 40 to 50 percent of affected children have a leukemia-free
survival of 5 years. It is hoped and anticipated that a considerable
percentage, if not most, of those children will be permanently cured.

In this chapter we review, in more or less historical fashion, how this
progress has come about. It is clear that the treatment of acute lymphoid leukemia can no longer be undertaken with the simple aim of palliation, that is prolongation of comfortable survival, while relapse
and death are accepted as inevitable (1, 2). Instead, treatment must
be planned from the onset with cure, in other words total disease eradication as the aim. Some investigators rely mainly on intensive chemotherapy in an attempt to accomplish this goal, but our group at the
I.C.I.G. uses moderately intensive chemotherapy followed by active immunotherapy to kill the last malignant cell.

Acute lymphoid leukemia, a disease affecting mostly children, presents
from the onset as a disseminated malignancy. The clinical picture is
dominated by two syndromes: (1) infiltration, by malignant lymphoid
cells, of predominantly the hematopoietic and lymphoid tissues; however,
any organ can be infiltrated and some areas, particularly the central
nervous system (CNS), pose special treatment problems; (2) insufficiency
of the normal hematopoietic and lymphoid elements with such life-threatening complications as infection due to neutropenia, with or without
immune incompetence and bleeding caused by a deficiency in platelets.
These complications are the immediate cause of death in the majority
of patients with acute leukemia. The treatment must include means to
suppress the malignant process, while supporting the marrow insufficiency either prophylactically or therapeutically. The role of germ-
free environments, and leukocyte and platelet transfusions was discussed in Chap. 11. In reporting results, authors should state the degree of correction of both abnormalities (3). The term regression describes the disappearance of the leukemic infiltrate from the tissues,
including the bone marrow; if there is also hematologic recovery, the
term complete remission is appropriate. A treatment that is excellent
in terms of tumor-cell regression may well be too toxic for the patient,
producing intolerable levels of hematopoietic and immune insufficiency.
Agents which have these drawbacks should not necessarily be rejected
for the treatment of acute leukemia. Correctly placed in a strategic
protocol designed to eradicate the tumor cell population, they may make
a useful contribution, since the leukemic cells are sensitive to therapy

To speak of regressions and remissions is to describe short-term results; these are clearly defined situations that can be achieved within a month or even a week. In treating acute leukemia, we seek to cure the patient. Cure is judged by the length of time the patient survives and by his freedom from perceptible disease; evaluation is therefore a long-term process.

It is important to make a firm diagnosis and to establish the morphologic variant, as this affects both prognosis and selection of treatment.

The majority of cases (80-90 percent) can be confirmed by examination of the blood and especially of the bone marrow. We are currently studying the value of cytochemistry, electron microscopy, cell culture on agar and in suspension, and the determination of antigenic and immunogenic characteristics (4, 88).

On the basis of increasing degree of cell differentiation we can distinguish 5 subclasses of acute lymphoid leukemia (Colour plates 1 and 2, 4; 5-6, 89): a prolymphoblastic, a lymphoblastic, further subdivided on the basis of cell diameter into macro- and microlymphoblastic, and prolymphocytic. The incidence of the various forms differs with age, but all are more frequent in younger patients, particularly the microlymphoblastic variety. We recently described a new variant, the immunoblastic acute lymphoid leukemia (90). We distinguish two clinical presentations: a so-called primary immunoblastic lymphoid leukemia with infiltration of the bone marrow by immunoblasts at the first examination of the patient; the other, labelled early leukemic immunoblastic lymphosarcoma, in which the bone marrow is invaded by immunoblasts a few weeks after the detection of a lymphoid mass. Although a remission is frequently obtained, the course is rapidly fatal.

Progress has been made in the treatment of acute leukemia since an increasing number of cytotoxic agents of varying effectiveness has become available. Lessons have been learned from protocol studies designed to answer specific questions. Finally, the principles of chemotherapy derived from experimental models have been transferred to clinical medicine.

A. CHEMOTHERAPY

Chemotherapy is the mainstay in the treatment of acute leukemia, even when the protocol combines different treatment modalities. It is used: (1) to bring the number of leukemic cells below what is clinically detectable (10^9), that is, to induce a remission; (2) to "maintain" remission; and (3) to bring the cell number still lower ("complementary cell-reducing" chemotherapy) to the level (10^5-10^6) susceptible to elimination by subsequent immunotherapy.

1. Induction of Remission

Since FARBER in 1948 obtained the first remissions with aminopterin (7), some ten different compounds have been found to be capable of inducing regression, if not remission in a variable percentage of cases (Table 14-1). Prednisone (PDN), vincristine (VCR) and adriamycin (ADM) are the most effective agents. Daunorubicin (DRB), adriamycin, cyclophosphamide (CPM), and cytosine arabinoside (CAR) tend to induce regressions rather than remissions; they are myelotoxic agents that have

Table 14-1. Drugs capable of inducing remissions in ALL[a]

Drugs	% of apparent complete remissions				Tend to induce regression > remission
	< 20 years age Personal experience	Range reported in lit.	> 20 years Personal experience	Range reported in lit.	
Prednisone	66 %	19-76 %	32 %	36-50 %	
Vincristine	50 %	44-57 %	30 %	40 %	
Adriamycin	50 %	12-37 %	37 %		++
Daunorubicin	40 %	33-50 %			++++
6-Mercaptopurine		27-42 %		8- 9 %	
Methotrexate	40 %[b]	22-31 %	30 %[b]	0-16 %	
Cytosine arabinoside	30 %	18-30 %	20 %	5-11 %	++
L-Asparaginase	30 %	36-67 %		23-25 %	
Cyclophosphamide		3-76 %		8 %	+++

[a] Results obtained when the drugs are used in the most effective schedule. Only drugs inducing remissions in more than 25 % of patients are included. The different series are not necessarily comparable; results are influenced by the phase of the disease treated (initial phase vs. subsequent relapse) and by the type of treatment center (special leukemia center vs. general hospital). Furthermore, all authors do not use the same criteria to evaluate their results. Some of these results have been reported previously (8-12, 110).
[b] High-dose MTX with folinic acid rescue (13).

little selectivity for leukemic cells. These agents tend to leave the marrow in a state of prolonged hypoplasia or aplasia; they should be used to induce remission only in cases that are resistant to more selective agents.

Single agents induce remissions in no more than 50 percent of patients, therefore, once several effective agents became available, combinations were evaluated. The treatment of choice for induction in previously untreated ALL is the time-honored combination of vincristine and prednisone. Remissions are generally induced in less than one month in 90 percent of children. This combination is well tolerated, especially by the bone marrow, an important consideration in view of the bone-marrow insufficiency associated with the clinically perceptible phase of leukemia. Adding daunorubicin to the combination of vincristine and prednisone induced remission in 100 percent of children and 75 percent of adults (14). Despite this improved response rate, we do not recommend the routine use of this triple combination because of the serious risk of marrow suppression and cardiac toxicity associated with daunorubicin. Furthermore, neither the ALGB (15, 16) nor PINKEL (17) were able to show that the addition of daunorubicin (nor of L-asparaginase) improved the duration of remissions induced by the combination prednisone-vincristine. Adding 6MP plus MTX (POMP) (18) or CPM plus ASP (19) to the standard PDN-VCR combination for induction increases the toxicity, but is less effective. The Medical Research Council suggests that L-asparaginase be introduced only after evidence of bone marrow regeneration since this agent causes significant myelosuppression when added to VCR + PDN for induction (91). We prescribe adriamycin (rather than the more toxic daunorubicin) for patients who fail to respond to the PDN-VCR combination (18). MURIEL et al. found no significant difference between PDN-VCR-DRB or PDN-VCR-ADM for induction (92). Tables 14-2 and 14-3 list the response rates obtained by this approach according to age and morphological variant. Not all investigators adopt this cautious yet effective approach. SPIERS at the Hammersmith Hospital in London uses a fourfold combination, COAP (Cyclophosphamide, Oncovin, Ara-C, Prednisone),to induce remissions in ALL (1, 12). The myelosuppressive agents cyclophosphamide and cytosine arabinoside are added to VCR + PDN. They claim that the use of this considerably more toxic combination is justified by the higher response rate (not higher than with our sequential PDN-VCR ± ADM) and the lower risk of selecting resistant cell lines at a time when the leukemic-cell body burden is at its maximum. A recent analysis of St. Jude's Hospital experience led to the conclusion that either a third drug (e.g. L-ASP) should be used during remission induction or some form of intensification therapy early during the period of remission (113)

Table 14-2. Results of drug combinations for induction of remission in ALL

	% of complete remissions	
	children	adults
1. PDN + VCR	90	50
2. PDN + VCR + ADM (for those who fail to respond to 1)	100	75
3. PDN + VCR + ASP	100	80

Table 14-3. Complete remission obtained in ALL with PDN + VCR and PDN + VCR + ADM. (First perceptible phase, all age group) (MATHE et al. (89))

Morphologic type	% complete remissions	
	PDN + VCR	PDN + VCR + ADM
Microlymphoblastic	100	100
Prolymphocytic	96	100
Macrolymphoblastic	87	87
Prolymphoblastic	37	43
Immunoblastic	0/5	

2. Maintenance Therapy

The patient in "remission" is not cured, despite the remarkable absence of abnormalities, both clinically and on examination of the bone marrow. Extensive cytologic, histologic, and radiologic investigations reveal residual disease (21), which will cause a relapse if the induction therapy is not followed by complementary chemotherapy. The time of relapse depends on the degree of cell kill effected by the induction chemotherapy (see Fig. 14-1, from (22)). The size of the residual tumor is esti-

Table 14-4. Effect of induction chemotherapy and complementary chemotherapy on duration[a] of remission

Induction chemotherapy	Complementary chemotherapy	Median total remission duration (in weeks)	References
VCR	0	6	KARON et al., 1966 (28)
VCR	VCR	9	KARON et al. 1966 (28)
PDN	0	8- 9	FREIREICH et al. 1963 (29), WOLF et al., 1967 (31)
PDN	PDN	9-12	HYMAN, et al., 1959 (27)
PDN	6-MP	33	FREIREICH et al., 1963 (29)
PDN + VCR	MTX, daily	12-13	SELAWRY et al., 1965 (30)
PDN + VCR	MTX, intermittent, for 94 days	68	SELAWRY et al. 1965 (30)
PDN + VCR	MTX, intermittent, for 8 months	50	HOLLAND and GLIDEWELL 1970 (32)
PDN + VCR	MTX, intermittent, plus periodic PDN-VCR reinforcement, for 8 months	58	HOLLAND and GLIDEWELL 1970 (32)
PDN + VCR	MTX, intermittent, until relapse	>100	HOLLAND and GLIDEWELL 1970 (32); HOLLAND 1971 (33)
PDN + VCR	MTX, intermittent, + 6MP until relapse	>100[b]	HOLLAND, 1971 (33)
PDN + VCR	1) "intensive chemotherapy" MTX, 6MP, CPM 2) "Continuation" therapy with MTX, 6MP, CPM, VCR[c] for 3 years or until relapse	60 (full dose) 24 (half dose)	PINKEL et al., 1971 (17)
PDN + VCR + MTX i.t. PDN + DRB	1) intermittent chemotherapy CAR[d] + TG + MTX i.t. (16 weeks) 2) Consolidation ASP + BCNU + MTX i.t., etc.[e]	>100	DOWLING, et al., 1973 (34)

Table 14-4. (continued)

Induction chemotherapy	Complementary chemotherapy	Median total remission duration (in weeks)	References
PDN + VCR	MTX, intermittent, plus PDN + VCR reinforcements until relapse	100[b]	HOLLAND and GLIDEWELL 1970 (32)
PDN + 6MP	6MP, VCR, MTX, CPM	64	GEORGE et al., 1966 (35)
"VAMP"		35	FREIREICH et al., 1964 (36)
"BIKE"		35	FREIREICH et al., 1965 (37)
"POMP"		58	HENDERSON et al., 1966 (38)

a Data reported in the literature up to September 1972.
b The number of patients in remission at 1 and 2 years is slightly higher with this schedule than for patients receiving MTX, alone
c MTX 20 mg/m², weekly; 6MP 50 mg/m² qd.; CPM 200 mg/m² qd.; 6MP 50 mg/m², weekly; VCR 1 mg/m², weekly.
d 125-150 mg/m² infusion qh 12 x 12-20; for 3 cycles.
e See Fig. 14-3.

mated from the time from cessation of therapy to relapse. Relapse is
assumed to represent a cell load of 10^{11} cells and the doubling time
of leukemic cells is taken to be 4 days (23). It has been calculated
that PDN + VCR reduces the leukemic cell load from 0.1 to 1.0 kg (10^{11}-
10^{12}) to 0.1 to 1.0 g (10^8-10^9). At first glance this may appear a remarkable cell kill with little more needing to be done. However, as
explained in Chap. 10, the arithmetical representation of cell kill by
chemotherapy is deceptive. Since the cytotoxic effect of therapy follows

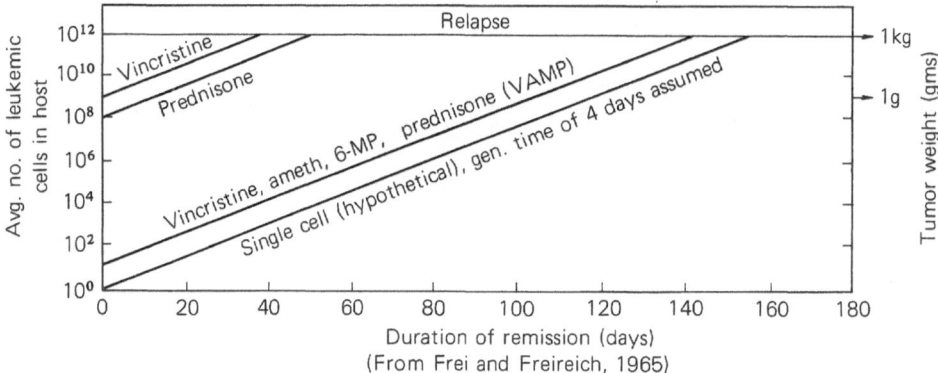

(From Frei and Freireich, 1965)

*Fig. 14-1. Estimation of tumor cell kill and extent of residual disease
from the duration of unmaintained remission (assuming a cell-cycle time
of 4 days). (From FREI and FREIREICH (22)). In the hypothetical case
where only one leukemic cell survives, relapse should occur in 150
days. This method neglects the existence of immune reactions against
tumor antigens*

first-order kinetics, a logarithmic scale must be used to put things
in perspective (24-26). It is then clear (see Fig. 10-1) that this
seemingly effective therapy (PDN + VCR) has killed only 2-3 logs while
8-9 remain to be eradicated. These concepts led first to "maintenance
therapy" and later to "consolidation" or "complementary cell-reducing
chemotherapy". It was soon realized that, in spite of an almost miracu-
lous clinical improvement - some of the earlier remissions were thought
to be cures - relapse is the rule if therapy is discontinued after remission. The attempt was first made to maintain the state of remission by
prolonging the induction therapy. It was argued that therapy that reduces
the cell load from 10^{12} to 10^8 in one month (e.g. prednisone) would reduce it to 10^4 after 2 months, and to one cell after 3 months of therapy.
However, clinical trials showed that this was not so: neither prednisone
(27) nor vincristine (28) continued beyond the induction period could
significantly prolong the duration of remission. Selection of resistant cell lines was blamed for these failures. This led to the idea of
selecting different drugs to maintain remission and to effect the induction. Various trials showed that some drugs, such as the corticosteroids,
VCR, DRB, ADM, and L-asparaginase, are more effective in inducing remission while others, for example maintenance agents such as 6MP (29) and
MTX (30), are more capable of prolonging remission. MTX given daily was
not very effective but, when given every 4 days, it considerably prolonged the duration of remission. Table 14-4 summarizes these findings.
Further trials by the ALGB demonstrated that remission lasts longer
when MTX therapy is continued until relapse than when it is stopped
after 8 months (33). Combining 6MP with intermittent MTX for mainte-

nance slightly improved the median duration of remission (16). A comparative study of intensive dosing of 6MP and MTX used sequentially vs. continuous low-dose administration of the same agents is under way (16). In addition to <u>prolonged therapy with single agents</u> or <u>combinations</u> to maintain remission, other approaches have been evaluated, for instance, using agents <u>sequentially after successive relapses</u>, so saving other drugs for subsequent remissions (39, 40), or in <u>predetermined cycles</u> in the hope of suppressing leukemic cells of different sensitivities (41, 42).

The maintenance agents are S-phase dependent; it was therefore reasoned that their action may be limited to maintaining the leukemic cell population below a clinically detectable level. They would kill cells as they entered the cell cycle (S-phase) while leaving cells in G_0 or prolonged G_1 intact. This led to the idea of adding to maintenance therapy (e.g., MTX + 6MP) repeated <u>cycles of inducing agents</u> (PDN + VCR) (ALGB) to evoke even longer remission (16, 32, 33). BERNARD's suggestion of adding daunorubicin to the combination of PDN and VCR reinforcements was according to the ALGB of no benefit (16). It may even have been responsible for a reduced survival in childhood ALL around 1968, whereas the rate had been rising steadily since 1960 (Fig. 14-2) (15).

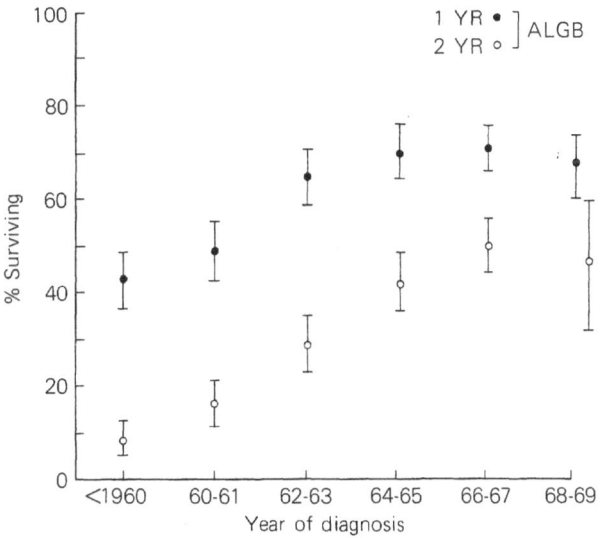

Fig. 14-2. *Survival in acute lymphoid leukemia for patients under the age of 20, diagnosed between 1960 and 1969. (From HOLLAND and GLIDEWELL (15)). (The slight decline noted around 1967 may have been related to the introduction of daunorubicin)*

Another approach initiated in the mid-1960's was the use of combinations of the <u>largest possible number of agents</u> for both induction and maintenance therapy. Combinations including VCR, PDN, 6MP, and MTX were introduced under the acronyms POMP (38) and VAMP (36), as well as 6MP, MTX, and CPM, known as BIKE (37). These programs were less effective, as shown by the results reported by the ALGB (regimen D), the Memphis group (PINKEL et al., see below) (17, 44) and our own group's experience with immunotherapy (45). The conclusion to be drawn from these trials is that the intensity of therapy is less important than its duration, however impressive the cell kill (to 10^1 cells) (see Fig. 14-1).

SPIERS modified the multi-agent approach by using 3 different super-
combinations (POMP, CART, and COAP) in sequence for a total of 132 weeks
(12). The rationale of this protocol is to ensure early and repeated
exposure to every first-line drug, and not saving any drugs to treat
subsequent relapses. No long-term follow-up is yet available for this
study, which was begun in 1970.

A serious problem to be discussed at this point is the management of
acute leukemia with CNS involvement. As the duration of remission became
progressively longer, the incidence of CNS leukemia rose, to over 50
percent in some series (46). CNS leukemia frequently occurs in patients
who appear to be otherwise in complete remission; it is often followed
rapidly by hematologic relapse. CNS leukemia is primarily an arachnoid
disease that secondarily affects the brain parenchyma (47). Since the
treatment of established CNS involvement has usually only a palliative
effect, attempts were made to prevent this common complication (46, 47).
All major studies agree in recommending prophylactic CNS therapy early
in remission. This step has dramatically improved the survival of children with ALL (16, 46-50, 92, 93, 114). Two modes of therapy are available
: irradiation and intrathecal chemotherapy, the two have also been combined. Methotrexate and cytosine arabinoside (94) can be injected intrathecally. Controlled studies by PINKEL showed that "craniospinal" irradiation at 2400 rads (but not 500 to 1200 rads) early in remission were
as effective as 2400 rads "cranial" irradiation plus intrathecal MTX
(5 doses of 12 mg/m^2) (44, 46, 47). However, the regimen that included
irradiation of the spinal axis caused considerably more myelosuppression,
often necessitating interruption of maintenance therapy. Hence, the combination of cranial irradiation (2400 rads) plus a series of intrathecal
injections seems to be the prophylaxis of choice. Our own results are
given in Table 14-5 (50, 93). Prophylactic intrathecal MTX also proved
highly effective in studies of the ALGB (16); however, it was found to
be inadequate by HITTLE et al., at least for children whose initial WBC
is above 20,000 (95). The Southwest Oncology Group compared the effectiveness of intrathecal chemotherapy (MTX, CAR, + hydrocortisone) vs.
the combination of intrathecal therapy plus cranial irradiation and
concluded that cranial irradiation offers no advantage in CNS leukemia
prevention, length of bone marrow remission or survival when added to
an effective intrathecal regimen (96). The group at St. Jude's Hospital
is of the opinion that radiotherapy should be part of CNS therapy (47).

Table 14-5. Effect of prophylactic CNS therapy. (From MATHE et al. (93))

	No meningeal involvement	Meningeal involvement
No CNS therapy	50	26
MTX alone	28	9
MTX + irradiation	23	3
Irradiation alone	0	3
MTX + CAR	2	0
MTX + CAR + irradiation	30	2

Both immediate (fever, headache, vomiting, somnolence, pleocytosis,,
alopecia, paraplegia) and long-term side-effects (effect on spinal
growth, CNS parenchymatous degeneration, intracerebral calcifications)
of various forms of CNS therapy have been reported (51-55, 93,97-100)
but the severity and relative frequency of these side-effects are not
yet fully appreciated.

The value of systemic agents that "penetrate the blood-brain barrier", such as the nitrosoureas and dibromodulcitol (56), in the prophylaxis and therapy of CNS leukemia is still under evaluation. The efficacy of BCNU has been disappointing (57). Some authors advocate intraventricular administration of MTX to ensure reliable drug distribution (57), while others are abandoning this approach because of complications (59). Intrathecal cytotoxic agents and/or radiotherapy are also used to treat symtomatic meningeal involvement (101).

Other organs may harbor leukemic cells in spite of apparent drug-induced hematologic remissions and therefore be a source for relapse. These so-called "sanctuaries" include the testes, kidney, gastrointestinal tract, lungs, and lymph nodes (21, 60, 102-104).

Several protocol studies are currently in progress to evaluate the prolonged use (2-3 years) of multiple drug combinations and CNS prophylaxis. Among the more aggressive protocols are those of the Memorial Hospital in New York, St. Jude's Children's Research Hospital in Memphis, and the Hammersmith Hospital in London.

DOWLING et al. induce a remission with VCR, PDN, and DRB (Fig. 14-3) (34, 105). This treatment is followed by complementary chemotherapy, which consists of a series of intermittent cycles of CAR plus 6TG, followed by L-asparaginase and BNCU. During this initial part of the protocol MTX is given intrathecally. The third phase (consolidation) consists of the sequential use of 6TG, CPM, HUR, DRB, MTX (systemic and intrathecal), BCNU, CAR, and VCR, and is continued for at least 3 years. The authors are encouraged by their initial results. All but one of 75 children achieved complete remission, lasting from 1 to 42 months (105). Twelve patients relapsed within 1-31 months following induction and 2 died in remission (serum hepatitis). A much longer follow-up period is required before we can be sure whether the addition of certain drugs, which individually are not very effective against ALL, does more than add toxicity to the combination.

PINKEL's "total therapy" at St. Jude's Hospital includes three phases: (a) "remission induction" with prednisone and VCR in the customary doses for 4 to 6 weeks, with or without daunorubicin, followed by (b) a week of intensive chemotherapy with 6MP, $1gm/m^2$ i.v. qd x 3, followed by MTX, 10 mg/m^2 i.v. qd x 3, followed by CPM, 600 mg/m^2 i.v. x 1; there is a 2-week interval before beginning (c) "continuation therapy" which runs for 3 years if there is no relapse (17, 44, 46). It consists of 6MP (50 mg/m^2, p.o. qd) MTX (20 mg/m^2, p.o. qw) and cyclophosphamide (200 mg/m^2, p.o. qw); every 70 days there is a reinducer course of PDN (40 mg/m^2, p.o., qd x 15) and VCR (1.5 mg/m^2, i.v. qw x 3). Various programs of CNS therapy were also investigated, as discussed in a previous paragraph. Half the patients were randomly selected to receive only half of the indicated doses (17). A number of conclusions were drawn from these studies.

1. Daunorubicin did not add to the induction regimen.

2. One week of intensive chemotherapy early in remission did not improve the results.

3. Prophylactic CNS therapy is of value.

4. The higher doses were more effective.

The logarithmic curves for complete remission within each series of patients are biphasic; they show an initial linear fall, indicating a

INTENSIVE "L-2" TREATMENT PROTOCOL FOR ACUTE LYMPHOBLASTIC LEUKEMIA

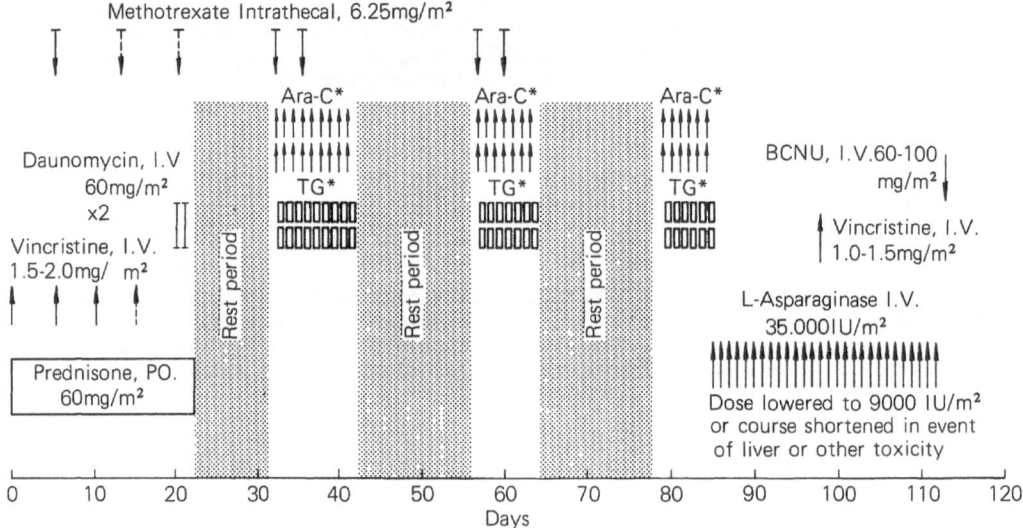

Methotrexate Intrathecal, 6.25mg/m²

Ara-C*   Ara-C*   Ara-C*

Daunomycin, I.V.
60mg/m²
x2

Vincristine, I.V.
1.5-2.0mg/ m²

Prednisone, PO.
60mg/m²

TG*   TG*   TG*

Rest period   Rest period   Rest period

BCNU, I.V.60-100
mg/m²

Vincristine, I.V.
1.0-1.5mg/m²

L-Asparaginase I.V.
35.000IU/m²

Dose lowered to 9000 IU/m²
or course shortened in event
of liver or other toxicity

0   10   20   30   40   50   60   70   80   90   100   110   120

Days

*Ara-C=Arabinosylcytosine I.V. at 125-150mg/m² q. 12 hrs. for 12-20 doses

TG=Thioguanine P.O. at 100-125mg/m² q. 12 hrs. for 12-20 doses

INTENSIVE CHEMOTHERAPY FOR ACUTE LYMPHOBLASTIC LEUKEMIA AND LEUKOSARCOMA IN CHILDREN AND ADULTS (L-2 PROTOCOL)

Part II

REMISSION MAINTENANCE THERAPY

DRUG	DOSE mg/kg	
Thioguanine (TG)	10	p.o.
Cyclophosphamide (CYT)	20	i.v.
Hydroxyurea (HU)	80	p.o.
Daunomycin (Daun)	1.5	i.v.
Methotrexate (MTX)	10mg/dose	p.o.
1,3-Bis(2-Chloroethyl)-1-nitrosourea (BCNU)	2	i.v.
Arabinosylcytosine (Ara-C)	5	i.v.
Vincristine (VCR)	0.075	i.v.
Methotrexate Inthrathecal (MTX)	6.25mg/m²	IT

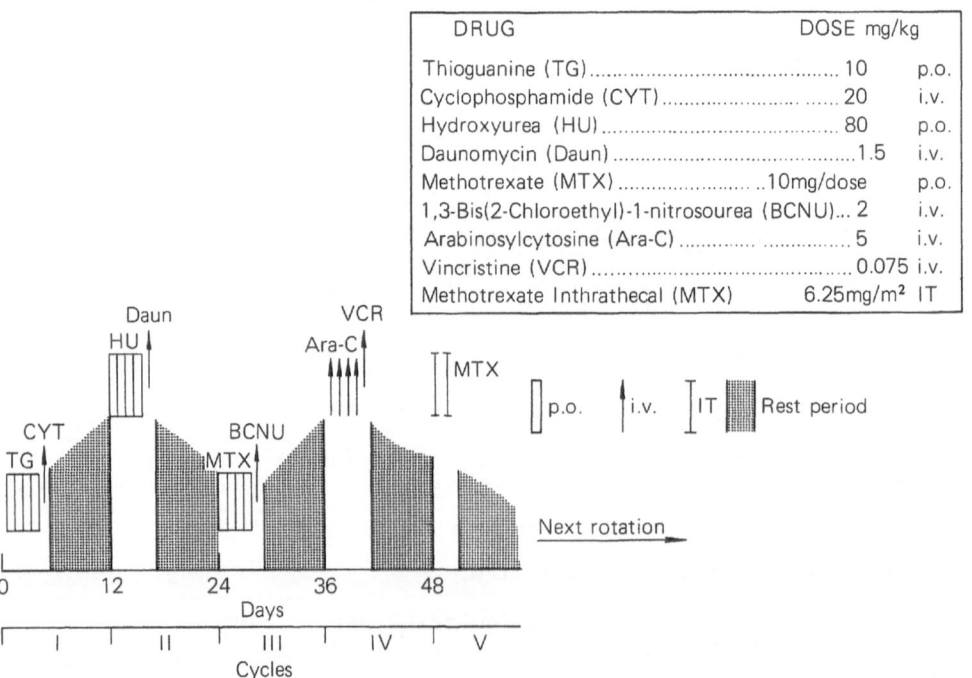

Daun   VCR
HU   Ara-C

CYT   BCNU
TG   MTX

MTX

p.o.   i.v.   IT   Rest period

Next rotation

0   12   24   36   48

Days

I   II   III   IV   V

Cycles

constant relapse rate, followed by a plateau, representing patients in continuous remission. These curves predict that 50 percent of the patients treated in recent years will enjoy long-term, leukemia-free survival (44) and confirm the value of prolonged maintenance therapy. Studies in progress are trying to determine whether the advantages of multiple chemotherapy during remission outweigh the disadvantages of dosage reduction of the more effective agents.

We have already discussed the protocols of the ALGB (16) and of SPIERS at Hammersmith Hospital (1, 12). Some of these intensive and prolonged treatment programs have been carried out at heavy cost. PINKEL and BERNARD reported 10 percent mortality of patients in remission, mainly due to opportunistic infection related to hematopoietic and immune depression (17, 46, 61, 62). Now that long-term survivors and, hopefully, cures are becoming more frequent, we have to pay attention to the delayed toxicity of chemotherapy. Interference with fertility and fetal development, and the mutagenic and carcinogenic potential of cytotoxic therapy are discussed on page 135.

B. STRATEGY

1. Immunotherapy

A different approach to the total eradication of the leukemic cell population was developed at the ICIG. This approach does not rely entirely on the chemotherapy to kill the last cell, but combines several treatment modalities in a strategic approach to the cure of leukemia (9, 45, 63, 64, 65). This seems logical, since chemotherapy rarely kills the last cell because of its first-order kinetics (24-26). It is appropriate in this context to refer to the experiments of SKIPPER (66) and POLLARD et al. (67) with spontaneous AKR murine leukemia, the best animal model for human lymphoid leukemia. These workers used intensive chemotherapy, to which the leukemic cells show great sensitivity, and apparently eradicated the whole tumor cell population. Yet the animals all relapsed, either because the last cell escaped to repopulate the host, or because the leukemia, which is known to be due to Gross virus, was reinduced. This phenomenon would not be affected by chemotherapy. Viruses have long been suspected as possible etiologic factors in human leukemia, and THOMAS et al. (68) reported the leukemic transformation of human bone-marrow-grafts in leukemic patients in remission treated by total body irradiation and marrow transplantation.

The principle of a series of treatment protocols started at the ICIG in 1964 has been the same throughout: (1) remission-induction chemotherapy, (2) complementary cell-reducing chemoradiotherapy, and (3) active immunotherapy (see Fig. 13-2). Clinical studies were not undertaken until the validity of this principle had been established.

(i) Experimental Data
Our experimental models of active immunotherapy employed immune stimulation after the establishment of disease in subcutaneously grafted L1210 (69), i.v. grafted Rauscher and $E_{\varrho}K_1$ leukemia (70), and spontaneous AKR leukemia (71). Active immunotherapy was found to be effective if the

◁*Fig. 14-3. The L-2 protocol of Dowling* et al. *(34). An example of therapy using multiple drugs and combinations and CNS prophylaxis over extended periods (at least 3 years)*

tumor load was < 10^5 cells at the onset of active immunotherapy. A higher tumor burden (> 10^5 cells) could not be treated effectively by immunotherapy; there had first to be preliminary cell reduction by chemotherapy (72). Active immunotherapy can be either nonspecific - general stimulation of the immune reactions of the host by "adjuvants of immunity", of which BCG seemed to be the most effective, or specific - use of irradiated tumor cells to stimulate reactions directed against tumor-associated antigens (63).

Criteria derived from these animal models were applied to man. ALL was the first human malignancy to be treated by immunotherapy, since in 1964 it was one of the few malignancies in which necessary preliminary cell reduction could be effected by chemotherapy. The fact that DORE et al. (73) and YOSHIDA and IMAI (74) detected autologous antibodies against leukemic cells in the serum of some patients provided additional support for an immunologic approach. Further evidence for the immune reactivity against tumor-associated antigens in ALL patients has been the demonstration of the transformation in vitro of the patient's lymphocytes stimulated by their own leukemic cells (75) and by the toxicity of the patient's lymphocytes for their leukemic cells (76) (cellular immunity).

(ii) Clinical Trials
The above experiments indicated that the optimum condition for effective active immunotherapy was that the patient should have the smallest possible number of leukemic cells. Therefore, an apparent complete remission was induced by chemotherapy, after which attempt was made to reduce the tumor cell load still further by sequential complementary systemic chemotherapy. In addition, the CNS was treated with intrathecal chemotherapy and irradiation. At one time surgery was added to the therapeutic strategy: splenectomy was carried out during remission in patients who had demonstrated splenomegaly during the initial perceptible phase, in order to remove the "last leukemic cell" left in the spleen by chemotherapy. This procedure was subsequently abandoned, since the first remission lasted no longer in splenectomized than in non-splenectomized patients (77).

The effectiveness of the general approach was apparent from our first clinical trial, started in 1964 (78). Thirty patients with ALL received the same induction and complementary chemotherapy and CNS prophylaxis (Fig. 14-4). They were then divided into 4 groups at random. The controls received no further therapy; the second group was treated with BCG scarifications[1], the third group with both intradermal and subcutaneous leukemic cells obtained from a pool of allogeneic donors suffering from ALL, and the fourth group received both forms of immunotherapy. Figure 14-5 compares the duration of remission after termination of chemotherapy in controls and patients treated by immunotherapy (grouped

---

[1] BCG was applied by skin scarifications every 4th day for the first month, and then every 7th day. Twenty cutaneous scratches, each 5 cm long were arranged in a square, and 2 ml of a suspension containing 75 mg/ml of living bacteria, was applied to the scarified area. Irradiated allogeneic tumor cells were injected intradermally each week for 3 months and then each month at a dose of 4×10^7. These cells were pooled from the peripheral blood of leukemic patients, and the leukemic cells of the recipient were specifically excluded. These cells were prepared from circulating blood by leukaphoresis and stored at -70°C in dimethyl sulfoxide. During the first 6 injections, the cells were treated with a 4 percent solution of formaldehyde to inactivate a hypothetical virus; for the ensuing injections, the cells were irradiated in vitro with 4000 rads.

together, since there were no significant differences between the 3 subgroups) with that of various chemotherapy protocols. All the control patients relapsed.

The first part of the actuarial curve for the duration of complete remission after termination of chemotherapy is identical in patients treated by immunotherapy and controls. These early relapses probably represent a population in whom chemotherapy had failed to reduce the number of leukemic cells below the number that could be adequately controlled by active immunotherapy (10^5 log). The slope of the curve then levels out for immunotherapy patients. A few late relapses are seen, probably in patients in whom the disease was temporarily controlled but either the "last" malignant cells were not destroyed or immuno-resistance developed. Between 2 and 3 years, the curve reaches a plateau, representing 7 of the 20 original patients who received immunotherapy. Although not yet a cure, this plateau represents a statistical expression of cure expectancy in 35 percent of ALL patients, since no relapses occurred between 3 and 13 years (111).

Compared with the chemotherapy programs VAMP, BIKE, and the ALGB regimen D, for which similar follow-up data exist, it can be seen that the superiority of active immunotherapy lies, not in the median duration of remission due to the less intensive nature of our complementary cell-reducing chemotherapy but in the percentage of patients reaching the plateau phase, and thus hopefully cured. Moreover, this result was obtained without any fatalities due to toxicity.

Over 200 patients have so far been treated according to our stated principle, though over the years some modifications have been made to intro-introduce new effective agents or to answer different questions. (Fig. 14-6) (107). For instance, in one protocol active immunotherapy was combined with chemotherapy (vincristine) and compared to controls

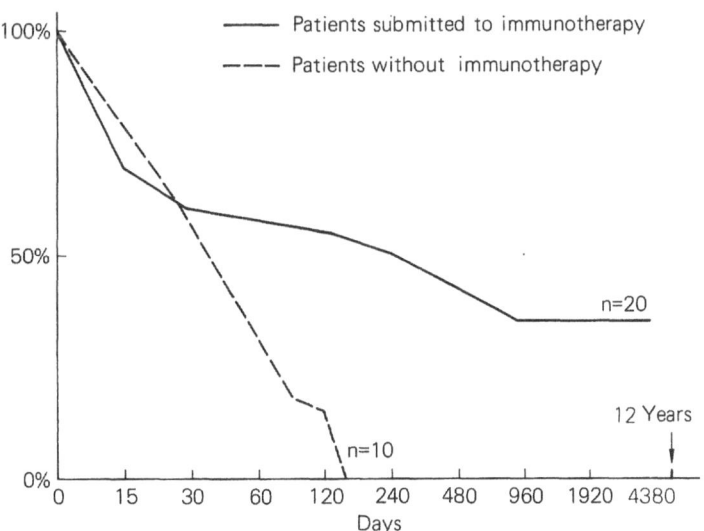

Fig. 14-4. Cumulative total duration of complete remission in patients with acute lymphoid leukemia treated by active immunotherapy after termination of chemotherapy (initial trial, initiated in 1964) (78). Note that the time scale is geometric

treated by immunotherapy alone (79). The results of the combined treatment were inferior. Simultaneous chemotherapy has adverse effect, probably because of its immunosuppressive effect.

During these studies several prognostic factors were recognized, the most important one being the cytologic type. We recently reviewed the first 100 acute lymphoid (and undifferentiated) leukemias treated with immunotherapy that could be cytologically typed as we possessed the slides obtained at the time of initial presentation of the disease (111, 112) (Table 14-6; Fig. 14-7). In contrast to the late relapses occurring in patients treated with maintenance chemotherapy (115, 116), no relapses are observed after 48 months in our immunotherapy-treated patients (Fig. 14-8). Second remissions are obtained in 94% of patients who relapse while on immunotherapy and their life expectancy following a second remission is as high as after the first one. The median survival is longer than 5 years (Fig. 14-9).

Age, an important prognostic factor in patients maintained with chemotherapy (115), does not influence the survival of our patients (Fig. 14-10). While there is no difference in survival between sexes at 3 years, there is one in favor of female patients at 4 years (Fig. 14-11). Patients with large tumour volumes (V+) more than 20,000 leukemic cells in the peripheral blood and/or presenting enlarged lymph nodes, and/or splenomegaly, and/or hepatomegaly (Fig. 14-12), or CNS involvement (Fig. 14-13) fare less well than patients without these characteristics.

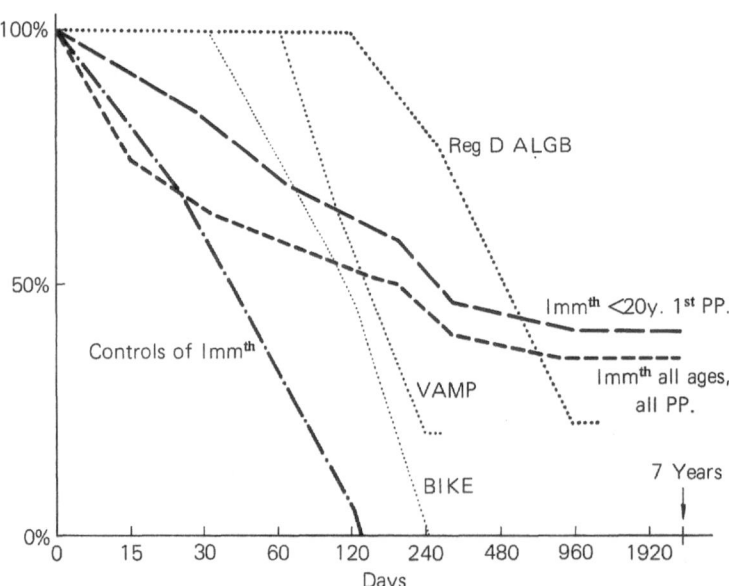

Fig. 14-5. Actuarial curve of duration of complete remissions after termination of chemotherapy in patients submitted to active immunotherapy compared to the control patients not receiving immunotherapy. The results of immunotherapy are compared with the unmaintained remissions after BIKE, VAMP, and the ALGB regimen D (see p. 254). Note that the time scale is geometric —— Immunotherapy in patients under 20 years of age treated in the initial phase of their disease,- - - - Immunotherapy in all patients, irrespective of age or phase of their disease

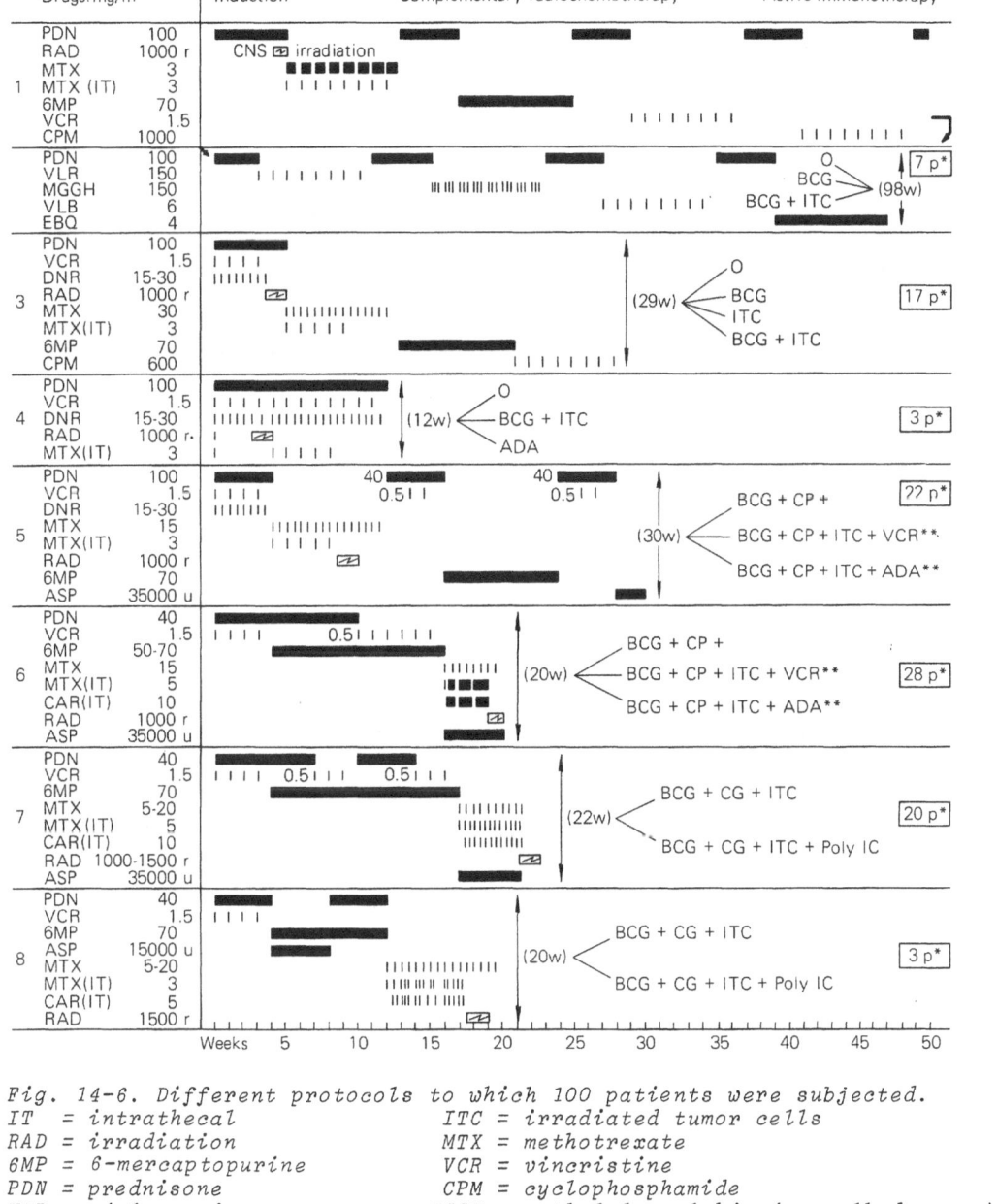

Fig. 14-6. Different protocols to which 100 patients were subjected.
IT = intrathecal   ITC = irradiated tumor cells
RAD = irradiation   MTX = methotrexate
6MP = 6-mercaptopurine   VCR = vincristine
PDN = prednisone   CPM = cyclophosphamide
VLR = vinleurosine   MGGH = methylglyoxal-bis (guanylhydrazone)
VLB = vinblastine   EBQ = ethylene-imino-benzo-quinone
DNR = daunorubicine   ASP = L-asparaginase
CAR = cytosine arabinoside   ADA = adamantadine
CP = Corynebacterium parvum   CG = C. granulosum
 * = Number of patients for whom diagnostic bone marrow smears were
      available to be reviewed. (From MATHE et al. (45))

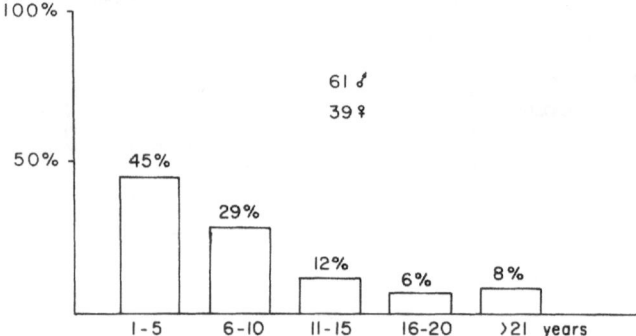

Fig. 14-7. Distribution of 100 patients with ALL according to age and sex (From MATHE et al. (111))

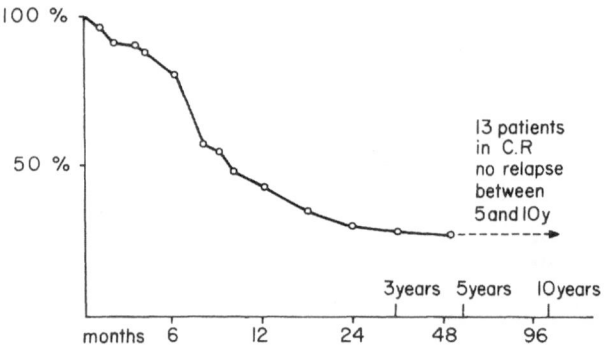

Fig. 14-8. Acute lymphoid leukemia (ALL). Cumulative duration of first complete remission after active immunotherapy (BCG + cells) is started (100 patients). Note that the time scale is geometric (From MATHE et al. (111))

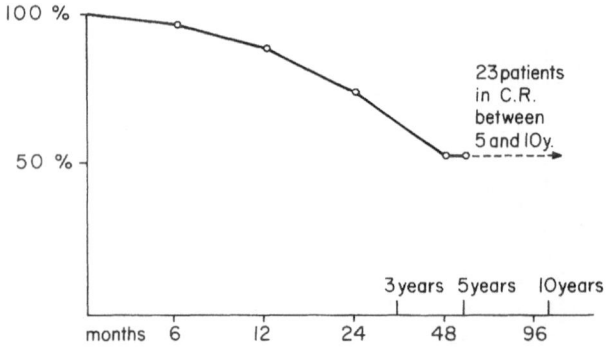

Fig. 14-9. Acute lymphoid leukemia. Cumulative duration of survival of 100 patients after active immunotherapy is started. Note that time scale is geometric (From MATHE et al. (111))

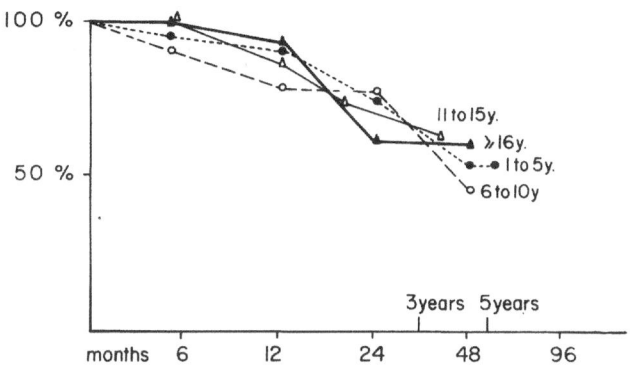

Fig. 14-10. Acute lymphoid leukemia. Cumulative duration of survival of 100 patients (submitted to active immunotherapy) according to age (From MATHE et al. (111))

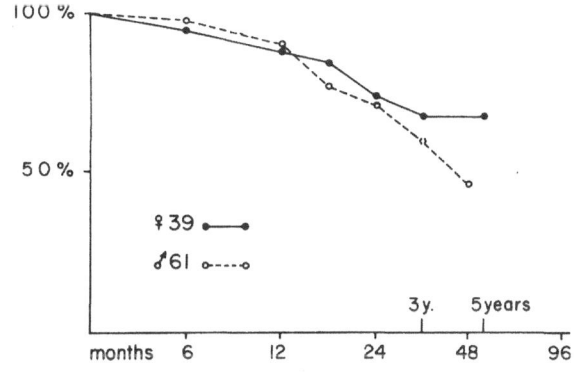

Fig. 14-11. Survival according to sex of 100 patients with ALL treated with immunotherapy (From MATHE et al. (111))

Table 14-6. Distribution of 100 patients with ALL according to their cytological types (From MATHE et al. (111))

	Number of patients
Prolymphocytic	42
Microlymphoblastic	27
Macrolymphoblastic	20
Prolymphoblastic	11
Total	100

Figure 14-14 shows the survival of patients submitted to active immunotherapy according to cytological typing. The survival at 5 years is
considerably higher for the microlymphoblastic type than for the others.
Between 3 and 5 years a plateau is reached representing 85% of the
patients. The prolymphoblastic (or undifferentiated) type has the worst
prognosis, while it is intermediate for the macrolymphoblastic and the
prolymphocytic types (between 40 and 50% of the patients are alive at
5 years and their survival curve forms a plateau).

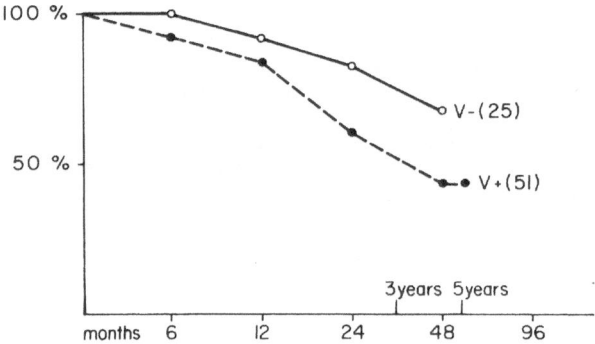

*Fig. 14-12. Acute lymphoid leukemia. Cumulative duration of survival
of 76 patients (submitted to active immunotherapy) according to volume
of neoplasia (From MATHE et al. (111))*

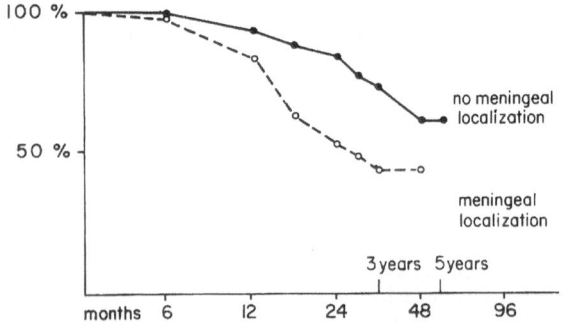

*Fig. 14-13. Acute lymphoid leukemia. Cumulative duration of survival
of patients submitted to active immunotherapy, according to presence
or absence of detectable meningeal localization at first presentation
of the disease or at first relapse (From MATHE et al. (111))*

In another computerized study, HAUSS (117) found that only the cytological type is related to all the other prognostic factors; of all these
factors taken as a constant, the cytological type alone maintains its
prognostic value; on the other hand, in case of a constant cytological
type, the other factors loose their prognostic value.

It is interesting to note in Figure 14-14 that the prognostic value of
this cytological typing is only found by J. BERNARD's group (115) for

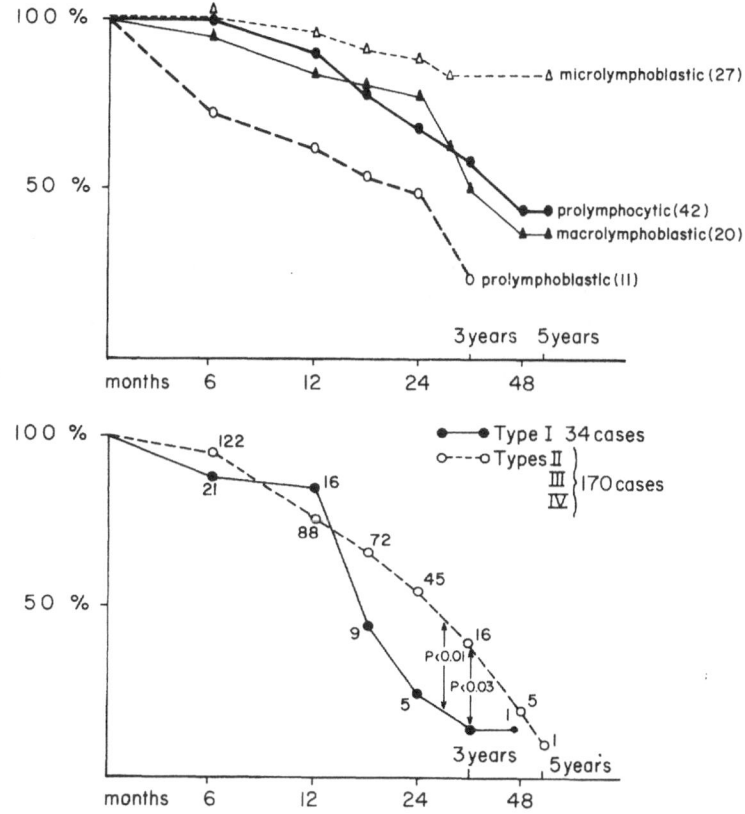

Fig. 14-14. (a) Acute lymphoid leukemia. Cumulative duration of survival of 100 patients submitted to active immunotherapy according to cytological types. Note that time scale is geometric (b) Acute lymphoid leukemia. Cumulative duration of survival of Jean Bernard's patients submitted to maintenance chemotherapy according to cytological types (From BERNARD et al. (115)). Type I: prolymphoblastic; type II: macrolymphoblastic; type III: microlymphoblastic; type IV: prolymphocytic (From MATHE et al. (111))

the prolymphoblastic (or undifferentiated) variety. This may be due to differences between immunotherapy and chemotherapy sensitivities; hence the high cure rate (85%) of the microlymphoblastic type seems to be due to active immunotherapy.

Since the cytological type determines the sensitivity to immunotherapy it should help to select the proper therapy. In our current treatment program (protocol 12, Fig. 14-15) patients with the microlymphoblastic variety are submitted to a safe chemotherapy preceding the immunotherapy while a more intensive and longer chemotherapy is used for the less immunosensitive varieties. Immunotherapy is maintained during 5 years as it is only after 48 months that no more relapses occurs.

BCG immunotherapy is well tolerated. Its toxicity is negligible compared to that of the maintenance chemotherapies which are responsible for 5-30% deaths of patients in remission (111)

Protocol 12 α

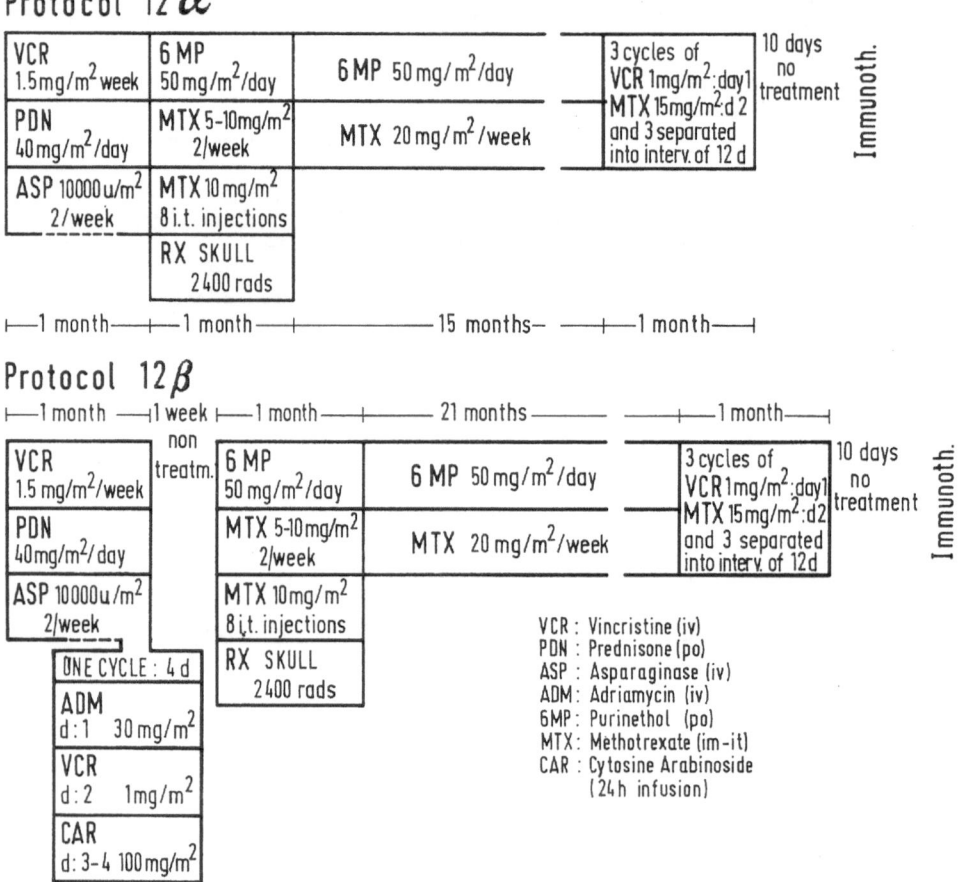

Protocol 12 β

Fig. 14-15. Protocol 12: induction and complementary cell-reducing chemotherapy prior to immunotherapy (currently in progress at ICIG, Villejuif)

The importance of the type of immunoadjuvant and the technique used to stimulate the immune response is stressed in several reports. Bordetella pertussis vaccine given intramuscularly delayed the occurrence of relapse but did not result in long-term remissions (84). BCG obtained from Glaxo and administered by means of a Heaf gun rather than by linear scarifications failed to show any beneficial effect over control patients (85).

The effect of immunotherapy in ALL was confirmed by the EORTC Hemopathies Working Party (118) which found that active immunotherapy (with living fresh Brussels Pasteur Institute BCG) is more, or at least as

efficacious in maintaining the remission of patients after 2 years (62%)
than 6MP and MTX chemotherapy (55%) (this difference is not significant), and that its lethal cost is nil (0 death out of 21 patients)
compared to that of chemotherapy (3 death/17 patients). Preliminary
results of ECKERT and JOSE also indicate that BCG interspersed with
chemotherapy is more efficacious in maintaining remission of ALL than
chemotherapy alone (119).

2. Surgery and Radiotherapy

We have already referred to the limited role of surgery in ALL (86).
Radiotherapy, on the other hand, is an integral part of the management
of CNS leukemia. Leukemic localizations in other "sanctuaries", for
example in testes, occasionally require radiotherapy (102-104).

C. DISCUSSION

There is one conclusion upon which all investigators concerned with
the treatment of ALL agree: therapy should be aimed from the start at
cure and not just palliation. The total eradication of the leukemic
cell population requires carefully planned, sophisticated, potentially
toxic (109) treatment extended over a long period. Although the results
of our current protocol, as discussed above, are encouraging, the cure
rate for ALL is still too uncertain and too low for complacency. For
these reasons we believe, like most experts in the field, that acute
leukemia should not be left to the general practice of pediatrics or
medicine (16, 87). We strongly encourage the practicing physician to
refer his patient promptly, before giving any therapy, to a leukemia
center for inclusion in protocol studies. He will be doing a service
to his patient, himself, and science, while still actively participating in the care of his patient.

Two treatment philosophies have emerged from years of organized studies
designed to eradicate the leukemic cells in ALL. The first, which is the
one we practice, employs chemotherapy of moderate intensity and moderate
duration, followed by immunotherapy. The other depends on intensive,
long-term chemotherapy (HOLLAND, PINKEL, DOWLING, SPIERS, BERNARD, and
others). The proponents of either approach feel that the value of their
method has been established while that of the other remains to be proven.
Each side is so convinced of the benefits and effectiveness of their
method, that they are not prepared to undertake comparative trials. In
this state of affairs, it is difficult to be objective in recommending
a particular approach. On the basis of our refined cytological subclassification, we have formulated specific, objective criteria for selecting the best type of treatment. We re-emphasize that it is important
to look not only at the reported results of studies but also at the
cost in toxicity.

REFERENCES

1. SPIERS. A.S.: Cure as the aim in therapy for the acute leukaemias. Lancet 2, 473 (1972).
2. EDITORIAL: Radical treatment of acute leukaemia in childhood. Lancet 2, 910 (1972).
3. MATHE, G., WEINER, R.: Criteria for short-term results in the treatment of acute leukemia. In: Nomenclature, Methodology and Results of Clinical Trials in Acute Leukemia (eds. G. Mathé, P. Pouillart, L. Schwarzenberg). Recent Results in Cancer Research, Vol. 43, Berlin-Heidelberg-New York: Springer-Verlag 1973.
4. MATHE, G., POUILLART, P., WEINER, R., HAYAT, M., STERESCO, M., LA-FLEUR, M.: Classification and subclassification of acute leukemias correlated with clinical expression, therapeutic sensitivity and prognosis. In: Nomenclature, Methodology and Results of Clinical Trials in Acute Leukemias, p. 7 (eds. G. Mathé, P. Pouillart, L. Schwarzenberg). Recent Results in Cancer Research, Vol. 43. Berlin-Heidelberg-New York: Springer-Verlag 1973.
5. MATHE, G., POUILLART, P., STERESCO, M., AMIEL, J.L., SCHWARZENBERG, L., SCHNEIDER, M., HAYAT, M., DE VASSAL, F., JASMIN, C., LAFLEUR, M.: Subdivision of classical varieties of acute leukemia: correlation with prognosis and cure expectancy. Europ. J. Clin. biol. Res. 16, 554 (1971).
6. MATHE, G., RAPPAPORT, H.: Histological and cytological typing of neoplastic diseases of the haematopoietic and lymphoid tissues, Vol. 1. Geneva: W.H.O. 1976.
7. FARBER, S., DIAMOND, L.K., MERCER, R.D., SYLVESTER, Jr., R.E., WOLFF, J.A.: Temporary remission in acute leukemia in children produced by folic antagonist 4-aminopteroylglutamic acid (aminopterin). New Engl. J. Med. 238, 787 (1948).
8. MATHE, G.: La chimiothérapie des cancers (leucémies, hématosarcomes, tumeurs solides), Vol. 1. Paris: Expansion Scient. Franc. 1966.
9. MATHE, G.: Strategy for the treatment of acute lymphoblastic leukemia, p. 21. In 13th Intern. Congress Pediatrics. Vienna: Wiener Med. Akad. 1971.
10. HENDERSON, E.S.: Treatment of acute leukemia. In: Leukemias and lymphosarcomas, Vol. 1, p. 47 (eds. J.F. Holland, P.A. Miescher, R.A. Jaffé). New York: Grune and Stratton 1969.
11. GOLDIN, A., SANDBERG, J.S., HENDERSON, E.S., NEWMAN, J.S.: The chemotherapy of human and animal acute leukemia. Cancer Chemother. Rep. 55, 309 (1971).
12. SPIERS, A.S.D.: Chemotherapy of acute leukemias. Clinics in Haematology 1, 127 (1972).
13. SCHWARZENBERG, L., MATHE, G., HAYAT, M., DE VASSAL, F., AMIEL, J.L., CATTAN, A., SCHNEIDER, M., SCHLUMBERGER, J.R., ROSENFELD, C., JASMIN, C., NGO MINH MAN: Une nouvelle combinaison de méthotrexate-acide folinique pour le traitement des cancers: Presse méd. 77, 385 (1969).
14. MATHE, G., HAYAT, M., SCHWARZENBERG, L., AMIEL, J.L., SCHNEIDER, M., CATTAN, A., SCHLUMBERGER, J.R., JASMIN, C.: Acute lymphoblastic leukemia treated with a combination of prednisone, vincristine and rubidomycin. Lancet 2, 380 (1967).
15. HOLLAND, J.F.: Therapy of acute leukemia. In: Cancer chemotherapy, Vol. 1, p. 279 (ed. F. Elkerbout). Leiden: Leiden Univ. Press 1971.
16. HOLLAND, J.F., GLIDEWELL, O.: Chemotherapy of acute lymphocytic leukemia of childhood. Cancer 30, 1480 (1972).
17. PINKEL, D., HERNANDEZ, K., BORELLA, L., HOLTEN, C., AUR, R., SAMOY, G., PRATT, C.: Drug dosage and remission duration in childhood lymphocytic leukemia. Cancer 27, 247 (1971).

18. BERRY, D.H., PULLEN, J., GEORGE, S., VIETTI, T.J., SULLIVAN, M.P., FERNBACH, D.: Comparison of prednisolone, vincristine, methotrexate, and 6-mercaptopurine vs. vincristine and prednisone induction therapy in childhood acute leukemia. Cancer 36, 98 (1975).
19. KOMP, D.M., GEORGE, S.L., FALLETTA, J., LAND, V.J., STARLING, K.A., HUMPHREY, G.B., LOWMAN, J.: Cyclophosphamide-asparaginase-vincristine-prednisone induction therapy in childhood acute lymphocytic and nonlymphocytic leukemia. Cancer 37, 1243 (1976).
20. MATHE, G., AMIEL, J.L., HAYAT, M., DE VASSAL, F., SCHWARZENBERG, L., SCHNEIDER, M., JASMIN, C., ROSENFELD, C.: Adriamycin in the treatment of acute leukemias. In: International Symposium Adriamycin. Vol. 1. Berlin-Heidelberg-New York: Springer 1972
21. MATHE, G., SCHWARZENBERG, L., MERY, A.M., CATTAN, A., SCHNEIDER, M., AMIEL, J.L., SCHLUMBERGER, J.R., POISSON, J., WAJCNER, G.: An extensive histological survey of patients with acute leukaemia in complete remission. Brit. Med. J., 1, 640 (1966).
22. FREI, E.III, FREIREICH, E.J.: Progress and perspectives in the chemotherapy of acute leukaemia. Adv. Chemother. 2, 269 (1965).
23. ELLISON, R.R., MURPHEY, M.L.: "Apparent doubling time" of leukemic cells in marrow. Clin. Res. 12, 284 (1964).
24. SKIPPER, H.E., SCHABEL, F.M., WILCOX, W.S.: Experimental evaluation of potential anticancer agents. XIII. On the criteria and kinetics associated with "curability" of experimental leukemia. Cancer Chemother. Rep. 35, 1 (1964).
25. SKIPPER, H.E., SCHABEL, F.M., WILCOX, W.S.: Experimental evaluation of potential anticancer agents. XIV. Further study of certain basic concepts underlying chemotherapy of leukemia. Cancer Chemother. Rep. 45, 5 (1965).
26. SKIPPER, H.E., SCHABEL, F.M., WILCOX, W.: XXI. Scheduling of arabinosylcytosine to take advantage of its S-phase specificity against leukemia cells. Cancer Chemother. Rep. 51, 125 (1967).
27. HYMAN, C.B., BORDA, F., BRUBAKER, C., HAMMOND, D., STURGEON, P.: Prednisone in childhood leukemia: comparison of interrupted with continuous therapy. Pediatrics 24, 1005 (1959).
28. KARON, M., FREIREICH, E.J., FREI, E.III, TAYLOR, R., WOLMAN, I.J., DJERASSI, I., LEE, S.L., SAWITSKY, A., HANANIAN, J., SELAWRY, O., JAMES, Jr., D., GEORGE, P., PATTERSON, R.B., BURGERT, Jr., O., HAURANI, F.I., OBERFIELD, R.A., MACY, C.T., HOOGSTRATEN, B., BLOM, J.: The role of vincristine in the treatment of childhood acute leukemia. Clin. Pharmacol. Ther. 7, 332 (1966).
29. FREIREICH, E.J., GEHAN, E., FREI, E.III, SCHROEDER, L.R., WOLMAN, I.J., AMBARI, R., BARGERT, E.E., MILLS, S.D., PINKEL, D., SELAWRY, O.S., MOON, J.H., GENDEL, B.R., SPURR, C.L., STORRS, R., HAURANI, F., HOOGSTRATEN, B., LEE, S.: The effect of 6-mercaptopurine on the duration of steroid-induced remission in acute leukemia: A model for evaluation of other potentially useful therapy. Blood 21, 699 (1963).
30. SELAWRY, O.S., HANANIAN, J., WOLMAN, I.J., ALBIR, R., CHEVALIER, L., GOURDEAU, R., DENTON, R., GUSSOFF, B., LEVY, R., BURGERT, O., MILLS, S.D., BLOM, J., JONES, B., PATTERSON, R.B., McINTYRE, O.R., HAURANI, F.I., MOON, J.H., HOOGSTRATEN, B., KUNG, F.H., SHECHE, P., FREI, E.III, HOLLAND, J.F.: New treatment schedule with improved sur survival in childhood leukemia (ALGB) J. Amer. Med. Ass. 154, 75 (1965).
31. WOLFF, J.A., BRUBAKER, C.A., MURPHY, M.L., PIERCE, M.I., SEVERO, I.: Prednisone therapy of acute childhood leukemia: Prognosis and duration of response in 330 patients. J. Pediat. 70, 626 (1967).
32. HOLLAND, J.F., GLIDEWELL, O.: Complementary chemotherapy in acute leukemia. Recent Results in Cancer Research, Vol. 30, p. 95. Berlin-Heidelberg-New York: Springer-Verlag 1970.
33. HOLLAND, J.F.: E pluribus unum. Cancer Res. 31, 1319 (1971).

34. DOWLING, M.D., HAGHBIN, M., GEE, T.S., CUNNINGHAM, B., TAN, C.T.C., CLARKSON, B.D., BURCHENAL, J.H.: Comparative results obtained in the treatment of acute leukemia. In: Nomenclature, Methodology and Results of Clinical Trials in Acute Leukemias. (eds. G. Mathé, P. Pouillart, L., Schwarzenberg). Recent Results in Cancer Research, Vol. 43, p. 133. Berlin-Heidelberg-New York: Springer-Verlag 1973.
35. GEORGE, P., HERNANDEZ, K., BORELLA, L., PINKEL, D.: "Total therapy" of acute lymphocytic leukemia in children. (abstr.) Proc. Amer. Ass. Cancer Res. 7, 23 (1966).
36. FREIREICH, E.J., KARON, M., FREI, E.III: Quadruple combination therapy (VAMP) for acute lymphocytic leukemia of childhood. Proc. Amer. Ass. Cancer Res. 5, 20 (1964).
37. FREIREICH, E.J., KARON, M., FLATOW, F., FREI, E.III: Effect of intensive cyclic chemotherapy (BIKE) in remission duration in acute lymphoblastic leukemia (abstr.). Proc. Amer. Ass. Cancer Res. 6, 20 (1965).
38. HENDERSON, E.S., FREIREICH, E.J., KARON, M., ROSSE, W.: High-dose combination chemotherapy in acute lymphocytic leukemia of childhood. (abstr.) Proc. Amer. Ass. Cancer Res. 7, 30 (1966).
39. SAUNDERS, E.F., KAUDER, E., MAUER, A.M.: Sequential therapy of acute leukemia in childhood. J. Pediat. 70, 632 (1967).
40. WOLFF, J.A., BRUBAKER, C.A., MURPHY, M.L., PIERCE, M.I., SEVERO, N.: Prednisone therapy of acute childhood leukemia: Prognosis and duration of response in 330 treated patients. J. Pediat. 70, 626 (1967).
41. ZUELZER, W.W.: Implications of long-term survival in acute stem cell leukemia of childhood treated with composite cyclic therapy. Blood 24, 477 (1964).
42. BRUBAKER, C.A., GILCHRIST, G.S., HAMMOND, D., HYMAN, C.B., SHORE, N.A., WILLIAMS, K.O.: Induction of remission in acute leukemia with prednisone and intravenous methotrexate. J. Pediat. 73, 623 (1968).
43. BERNARD, J.: Traitement des leucémies aiguës lymphoblastiques. Effets de la méthode de réinduction. Nouveaux médicaments (rubidomycine). Sem. Hôp. Thérapeutique 44, 308 (1968).
44. SIMONE, J., AUR, J.A., HUSTU, H.O., PINKEL, D.: "Total therapy" studies of acute lymphocytic leukemia in children. Current results and prospects for cure. Cancer 30, 1488 (1972).
45. MATHE, G., POUILLART, P., SCHWARZENBERG, L., AMIEL, J.L., SCHNEIDER, M., HAYAT, M., DE VASSAL, F., JASMIN, C., ROSENFELD, C., WEINER, R., RAPPAPORT, H.: Attempts at immunotherapy of 100 acute lymphoid leukemia patients. Some factors influencing results. Nat. Cancer Inst. Monogr. 35, 361 (1972).
46. AUR, R.J.A., SIMONE, J.V., HUSTU, H.O., VERZOSA, M.: A comparative study of central nervous system irradiation and intensive chemotherapy early in remission of childhood acute lymphocytic leukemia. Cancer 29, 381 (1972).
47. HUSTU, H.O., AUR, R.J.A., VERZOSA, M.S., SIMONE, J.V., PINKEL, D.: Prevention of central nervous system leukemia by irradiation. Cancer 32, 585 (1973).
48. REPORT TO THE MEDICAL RESEARCH COUNCIL BY THE LEUKAEMIA COMMITTEE AND THE WORKING PARTY ON LEUKAEMIA IN CHILDHOOD: Treatment of acute lymphoblastic leukaemia: Effect of "prophylactic" therapy against central nervous system leukaemia. Brit. med. J. 2, 381 (1973).
49. EDITORIAL: Irradiation of C.N.S. in leukaemia. Brit. med. J. 2, 377 (1973).
50. POUILLART, P., SCHWARZENBERG, L., SCHNEIDER, M., AMIEL, J.L., MATHE, G.: Les méningites lymphoblastiques. Fréquence, prévention et traitement. Nouv. Press méd. 1, 387 (1972).

51. GEISER, C.F., BISHOP, Y., FREI, E.III.: Toxic effects of intra-
    thecal methotrexate in central nervous system prophylaxis of leu-
    kemic children: clinical and morphologic studies. Proc. Amer.
    Ass. Cancer Res. 15, 77 (1974).
52. SAIKI, J.H., THOMPSON, S., SMITH, F., ATKINSON, R.: Paraplegia fol-
    lowing intrathecal chemotherapy. Cancer 29, 370 (1972).
53. PROBERT, J.C., PARKER, B.R., KAPLAN, H.S.: Growth retardation in
    children after megavoltage irradiation of the spine. Cancer 32,
    634 (1973).
54. HENDIN, B., DE VIVO, D.C., TORACK, R., LELL, M.-E., RAGAB, A.H.,
    VIETTI, T.: Parenchymatous degeneration of the central nervous
    system in childhood leukemia. Cancer 33, 468 (1974).
55. VERZOSA, M., AUR, R., HUSTU, O., SIMONE, J., PINKEL, D.: Central
    nervous system status 5 years after preventive CNS therapy for
    childhood acute lymphocytie leukemia (ALL). Proc. Amer. Ass. Cancer
    Res. 15, 98 (1974).
56. SITARZ, A.L., ALBO, V., MOVASSACHI, M.K., HAMMOND, D., WEINER, J.,
    REED, A.: Dibromodulcitol (NSC-104800) compared with cyclophospha-
    mide (NSC-26271) as remission maintenance therapy in previously
    treated children with acute lymphoblastic leukemia or acute un-
    differentiated leukemia: possible effectiveness in reducing the
    incidence of central nervous system leukemia. Cancer Chemother.
    Rep. Part 1, 59, 989 (1975).
57. SULLIVAN, M.P., VIETTI, T.J., HAGGARD, M.E., DONALDSON, M.H., CRALL,
    J.M., GEHAN, E.A.: Remission maintenance therapy for meningeal
    leukemia: Intrathecal methotrexate vs. intravenous bis-Nitrosourea.
    Blood, 38, 680 (1971).
58. YOUNG, D.F., SHAPIRO, W.R., MEHTA, B., HUTCHISON, D.J.: Cerebro-
    spinal fluid distribution of methotrexate (MTX) in patients with
    meningeal leukemia and carcinomatosis. Proc. Amer. Ass. Cancer Res.
    15, 140 (1974).
59. SPIERS, A.S., BOOTH, A.E. Reservoirs for intraventricular chemo-
    therapy. Lancet 1, 1263 (1973).
60. NIES, B.A., BODNEY, G.P., THOMAS, L.B., BRECHER, G., FREIREICH,
    E.J.: The persistence of extramedullary leukemic infiltrates
    during bone marrow remission of acute leukemia. Blood 26, 133
    (1965).
61. SIMONE, J.V., HOLLAND, E., JOHNSON, W.: Fatalities during remissions
    of childhood leukemia. Blood 39, 759 (1972).
62. BERNARD, J., BOIRON, M., JACQUILLAT, Cl., WEIL, M.: Recent results
    in acute leukemias at the Hospital Saint Louis. In: Nomenclature,
    Methodology and Results of Clinical Trials in Acute Leukemias.
    (eds. G. Mathé, P. Pouillart, L. Schwarzenberg). Recent Results
    in Cancer Research, Vol. 43, Berlin-Heidelberg-New York: Springer-
    Verlag 1973.
63. MATHE, G.: Immunological approaches to the treatment of acute leu-
    kemia. Clinics in Haematology 1, 165 (1972).
64. MATHE, G.: La dernière cellule. Presse méd. 75, 2591 (1967).
65. MATHE, G., POUILLART, P., LAPEYRAQUE, F.: Active immunotherapy of
    L 1210 leukaemia applied after the graft of tumour cells. Brit.
    J. Cancer 23, 814 (1969).
66. SKIPPER, H.E., SCHABEL, F.M., TRADER, M.W., RUSSEL LASTER, W.: Res-
    ponse to therapy of spontaneous, first passage, and long passage
    lines of AKR leukemia. Cancer Chemother. Rep. 53, 345 (1969).
67. POLLARD, M., SHARON, N.: Prevention and treatment of spontaneous leu-
    kemia in germ-free AKR mice. Soc. exp. Biol. Med. 137, 1494 (1971).
68. THOMAS, E.D., BUCKNER, C.D., FEFER, A., NEIMAN, P., BRYANT, J.I.,
    CLIFT, R.A., JOHNSON, F.L., RAMBERG, R.E., STORB, A.: Leukemic
    transformation of engrafted human marrow cells in vivo. Lancet 1,
    1310 (1972).

69. MATHE, G., POUILLART, P., LAPEYRAQUE, F.: Active immunotherapy of
    L1210 leukaemia applied after the graft of tumour cells. Br. J.
    Cancer 23, 814 (1969).
70. MATHE, G., POUILLART, P., LAPEYRAQUE, F.: Active immunotherapy of
    mouse RC 19 and E $_2$ K$_1$ leukaemias applied after intravenous trans-
    plantation of the tumour cells. Experientia (Basel) 27, 446 (1971).
71. MATHE, G., HALLE-PANNENKO, O., BOURUT, Ch.: Active immunotherapy
    of AKR mice spontaneous leukemia. Exp. Haemat. 1, 110 (1973).
72. MATHE, G., POUILLART, P.: Unpublished data.
73. DORE, J.F., MOTTA, R., MARHOLEV, L., HRSAK, Y., COLAS DE LA NOUE,
    H., SEMAN, G., DE VASSAL, F., MATHE, G.: New antigens in human
    leukaemic cells and antibody in the serum of leukaemic patients.
    Lancet 2, 1396 (1967).
74. YOSHIDA, T.O., IMAI, K.: Auto-antibody to human leukemic cell mem-
    brane as detected by immune adherence. Eur. J. clin. biol. Res.
    15, 61 (1970).
75. FRIDMAN, W.H., KOURILSKY, F.M.: Stimulation of lymphocytes by auto-
    logous leukaemic cells in acute leukaemia. Nature 224, 277 (1969).
76. LEVENTHAL, R.G., HALTERMAN, R.H., HEBERMANN, R.B.: In vitro and
    in vivo immunologic reactivity against autochtonous leukemic cells.
    (Abstr. 203). Proc. Amer. Ass. Cancer Res. 12, 51 (1971).
77. MATHE, G.: Unpublished data.
78. MATHE, G., AMIEL, J.L., SCHWARZENBERG, L., SCHNEIDER, M., CATTAN,
    A., SCHLUMBERGER, J.R., HAYAT, M., DE VASSAL, F.: Active immuno-
    therapy for acute lymphoid leukemia. Lancet 1, 697 (1969).
79. MATHE, G., AMIEL, J.L., SCHWARZENBERG, L., SCHNEIDER, M., HAYAT,
    M., DE VASSAL, F., JASMIN, C., ROSENFELD, C., POUILLART, P.: Pre-
    liminary results of a new protocol for the active immunotherapy
    of acute leukemia: inhibition of the immunotherapeutic effect by
    vincristine or adamantadine. Europ. J. clin. biol. Res. 16, 216
    (1971).
80. BORELLA, L., GREEN, A.A., WEBSTER, R.G.: Immunological rebound
    after cessation of long-term chemotherapy in acute leukemia. Blood
    40, 42 (1972).
81. BORELLA, L., GREEN, A.A., AUR, R.J.A., SIMONE, J.V., PINKEL, D.:
    Clinical and immunological recovery of children with acute leukemia
    admitted to "Total Therapy" studies. In: Nomenclature, Methodology,
    and Results of Clinical Trials in Acute Leukemias. (eds. G. Mathé,
    P. Pouillart, L. Schwarzenberg). Recent Results in Cancer Research,
    Vol. 43, p. 145. Berlin-Heidelberg-New York: Springer-Verlag 1973.
82. SCHNEIDER, M., MATHE, G., SCHWARZENBERG, L., POUILLART, P., WEINER,
    R., AMIEL, J.L., HAYAT, M., JASMIN, C., DE VASSAL, F.: Non-specific
    immune responses in hematosarcomas and acute leukemias. In: Investi-
    gations and stimulation of immunity in cancer patients (eds. G.
    Mathé, R. Weiner). Heidelberg: Springer-Verlag 1974.
83. CURRIE, G.A., BAGSHAWE, K.D.: Active immunotherapy with Coryne-
    bacterium parvum and chemotherapy in murine fibrosarcomas. Brit.
    med. J. 1, 541 (1970).
84. GUYER, R.J., CROWTHER, D.: Active immunotherapy in treatment of
    acute leukaemia. Brit. med. J. 4, 406 (1969).
85. MEDICAL RESEARCH COUNCIL: Treatment of acute lymphoblastic leukemia.
    Comparison of immunotherapy (BCG), intermittent methotrexate, and
    no therapy after a five-month intensive cytotoxic regimen (Concord
    trial). Brit. med. J. 4, 189 (1971).
86. SPIERS, A.S.: Surgery in management of patients with leukemia. Brit.
    med. J. 3, 528 (1973).
87. HOLLAND, J.F.: Who should treat acute leukemia? J. amer. Med. Ass.
    209, 1511 (1969).
88. LEVENTHAL, B.G.: New looks in leukemia. Cancer 35, 1015 (1975).
89. MATHE, G., BELPOMME, D., DANTCHEV, D., POUILLART, L., et al.:
    Search for correlations between cytological types and therapeutic
    sensitivity of acute leukemias. Blood Cells 1, 37 (1975).

90. MATHE, G., BELPOMME, D., DANCHEV, D., POUILLART, P., JASMIN, C. et al.: Immunoblastic acute lymphoid leukaemia: an undescribed type. Biomedicine. 20, 333 (1974).
91. JOHNSTON, P.G.B., HARDISTY, R.M., KAY, H.E.M., SMITH, P.G.: Myelo-suppressive effect of colaspace (L-asparaginase) in initial treatment of acute lymphoblastic leukaemia. Brit. Med. J. 3, 81 (1974).
92. MURIEL, F.S., PAVLOVSKY, S., PENALVER, J.A., HIDALGO, G., BONESANA, A.C. et al.: Evaluation of induction of remission, intensification, and central nervous system prophylactic treatment in acute lympho-blastic leukemia. Cancer 34, 418 (1974).
93. MATHE, G., POUILLART, P., SCHWARZENBERG, L.: Meningeal localisation of acute leukemia. Acta Neuropath. Suppl. VI, 235 (1975).
94. BAND, P.R., HOLLAND, J.F., BERNARD, J., WEIL, M., WALKER, M., RALL, D.: Treatment of central nervous system leukemia with intra-thecal cytosine arabinoside. Cancer 32, 744 (1973).
95. HITTLE, R., ORTEGA, J., DONALDSON, M., KARON, M., NESBIT, M.: Effectivenss of presymptomatic treatment on the occurrence of central nervous system disease in childhood lymphoblastic leukemia. Proc. Am. Soc. Clin. Oncol. 16, 256 (1975).
96. KOMP, D., FALLETTA, J., RAGAB, A., HUMPHREY, G.B.: Is cranial ra-diation necessary for CNS prophylaxis in ALL of childhood? Proc. Am. Soc. Clin. Oncol. 16, 232 (1975).
97. RUBINSTEIN, L.J., HERMAN, M.M., LONG, T.F., WILBUR, J.R.: Dis-seminated necrotizing leukoencephalopathy: a complication of treated central nervous system leukemia and lymphoma. Cancer 35, 291 (1975).
98. FLAMENT-DURAND, J., KETELBANT-BALASSE, P., MAURUS, R., REGNIER, R., SPEHL, M.: Intracerebral calcification appearing during the course of acute lymphocytic leukemia treated with methotrexate and X-rays. Cancer 35, 319 (1975).
99. PRICE, R.A., JAMIESON, P.A.: The central nervous system in child-hood leukemia-II. Subacute leukoencephalopathy. Cancer, 35 306 (1975).
100. AUR, R., VERZOSA, M., HUSTU, O., SIMONE, J., BARKER, L.: Leuko-encephalopathy during initial complete remission in children with acute lymphocytic leukemia receiving methotrexate. Proc. Am. Ass. Cancer Res. 16, 92 (1975).
101. SULLIVAN, M.P., HUMPHREY, G.B., VIETTI, T.J., HAGGARD, M.E., LEE, E.: Superiority of conventional intrathecal methotrexate therapy with maintenance over intensive intrathecal methotrexate therapy, unmaintained, or radiotherapy (200-2500 rads tumor dose) in treat-ment for meningeal leukemia. Cancer 35, 1066 (1975).
102. STOFFEL, T.J., NESBIT, M.E., LEVITT, S.H.: Extramedullary involve-ment of the testes in childhood leukemia. Cancer 35, 1203 (1975).
103. PRIETO, C., HUSTU, O., AUR, R., SIMONE, J.: Testicular involve-ment in childhood acute lymphocytic leukemia. Proc. Am. Ass. Can-cer Res. 16, 178 (1975).
104. SULLIVAN, M.P., FERNANDEZ, C., PEREZ, C., DYMENT, P.: Radiotherapy for testicular leukemia, 2500 rads: local control and relation-ship to subsequent disease. Proc. Am. Soc. Clin. Oncol. 16, 226 (1975).
105. HAGHBIN, M., TAN, C.C., CLARKSON, B.D., MIKE, V., BURCHENAL, J.H.: Intensive chemotherapy in children with acute lymphoblastic leukemia (L-2 protocol). Cancer 33, 1491 (1974).
106. SIMONE, J.V., AUR, R.J.A., HUSTU, H.O., VERZOSA, M., PINKEL, D.: Combined modality therapy of acute lymphocytic leukemia. Cancer 35, 25 (1975).
107. MATHE, G., AMIEL, J.L., SCHWARZENBERG, L., HAYAT, M., POUILLART, P. et al.: Immunotherapie active des leucémies aigues et des lympho-sarcomes leucémiques. Bilan de 10 ans-etude de 200 cas. Nouv. Presse Med. 4, 1337 (1975).

108. MATHE, G., SCHWARZENBERG, L., AMIEL, J.L., POUILLART, P., HAYAT, M., et al.: Immunotherapy of leukaemia. Proc. roy. Soc. Med. <u>68</u>, 211 (1975).
109. VIETTI, T.J., RAGAB, A.H.: Complications and total care of a child with acute leukemia. Cancer <u>35</u>, 1007 (1975).
110. RAGAB, A.H., SUTOW, W.W., KOMP, D.H., STARLING, K.A., LYON, G.M., GEORGE, S.: Adriamycin in the treatment of childhood acute leukemia. Cancer <u>36</u>, 1223 (1975).
111. MATHE, G., DE VASSAL, F., DELGADO, M., POUILLART, P., BELPOMME, D., JOSEPH, R., SCHWARZENBERG, L., AMIEL, J.L., SCHNEIDER, M., CATTAN, A., MISSET, J.L., JASMIN, C.: 1975 Current results of the first 100 cytologically typed acute lymphoid leukemias submitted to BCG active immunotherapy. Cancer Immunol. Immunother. <u>1</u>, 77 (1976).
112. MATHE, G.: Cancer active immunotherapy, immunoprophylaxis and immunorestoration. Berlin-Heidelberg-New York. Springer-Verlag 1976.
113. MAUER, A.M., SIMONE, J.V.: The current status of the treatment of childhood acute lymphoblastic keukemia. Cancer Treat. Rev. <u>3</u>, 17 (1976).
114. DRITSCHILO, A., CASSADY, J.R., CAMITTA, B., JAFFE, N., FURMAN, L., TRAGGIS, D.: The role of irradiation in central nervous system treatment and prophylaxis for acute lymphoblastic leukemia. Cancer <u>37</u>, 2729 (1976).
115. BERNARD, J., WEIL, M., JACQUILLAT, C.: Prognostic factors in human acute leukemias. In: Workshop on prognostic factors in human acute leukemia. Oxford: Pergamon Press, 1975, Vol. I, p. 97.
116. RIVERA, G., PRATT, C.B., AUR, R.J.A., VERZOZA, M., HUSTU, H.O.: Recurrent childhood lymphocytic leukemia following cessation of therapy. Cancer <u>37</u>, 1679 (1976).
117. HAUSS, G.: Aplication des méthodes statistiques à l'étude pronostique rétrospective de 161 cas de leucémies aigues lymphoides. Thèse de Doctorat en Médecine, Université Paris-Sud, Faculté de Médecine Paris-Sud, 1975.
118. EORTC Hemopathies Working Party. Immunotherapy versus chemotherapy during complete remission of acute lymphoblastic leukemia. Third Meeting of the International Society of Haematology. European and African Division, London, 24-28, August 1975 (abstract 21:06).
119. EKERT, H., JOSE, D.G.: Chemotherapy and BCG in acute lymphoblastic leukemia. Lancet <u>2</u>, 713 (1975).

Chapter 15
Acute Myeloid Leukemia

Many of the concepts discussed in Chapter 14 on acute lymphoid leukemia are pertinent to this discussion and will not be repeated in detail.

Acute myeloid leukemia (AML) can occur at any age and is the predominant form of acute leukemia in adults. It generally presents as a disseminated malignancy of the hematopoietic system, but a localized tumor, better known as a chloroma, or myeloid sarcoma, may in rare cases precede the classic phase of the disease (1). The malignant cells, which are incapable of complete differentiation, belong to the granulocytic series and are produced by the proliferation of their stem cells in the bone marrow.

A major question which remains to be answered is whether there are two relatively independently regulated cell populations, one leukemic and the other normal, or whether the hematopoietic tissues are completely populated by leukemic cells (2). In the latter case, it is postulated that the leukemic stem cells retain the capacity to differentiate, but do not do so because of one or more defects in the mechanisms that ordinarily regulate differentiation. When remission is induced, conditions are established that permit regulatory function and hence the production of apparently normal, functional, mature blood cells from leukemic stem cells. The answer to this question is not merely of academic interest; our approach to therapy depends on it. If the two-population theory is correct, it is reasonable to try to eradicate the entire leukemic population. If, instead, we are dealing with one population, therapy should be designed to provide conditions that would be compatible with the differentiation of leukemic cells. Neither model is at present firmly established. There are arguments in favor of either hypothesis, but treatment programs have thus far been directed toward the total eradication of the leukemic cell population.

AML, like ALL, presents two clinical syndromes. One is the infiltration of the marrow by leukemic cells and, less consistently, of the peripheral blood, spleen, lymph nodes, and other organs. The other problem is marrow insufficiency, generally more marked, more dangerous and more resistant to correction than in ALL.

Three subtypes of acute myeloid leukemia (AML) have been distinguished morphologically according to their degree of differentiation, or lack of it: promyeloblastic, myeloblastic, and promyelocytic leukemia (see plates 1 and 2) (1, 3). The last variety is often clinically associated with bleeding manifestations and a syndrome of intravascular coagulation.

In ALL, only the lymphoid cells appear to be qualitatively affected by the neoplastic process while the marrow elements, although decreased in number, appear normal. In contrast, in AML, not only do the leukemic

cells present morphologic abnormalities but frequently also the monocytic, normoblastic, and megakaryocytic series. The entire myeloid
tissue seems to be affected, except in truly mixed forms such as erythroleukemia or the much more common myelomonocytoid leukemia (AMMoL)
Two variants of the latter are recognized: one in which the leukemic
cells appear unique and homogeneous, for each cell one hesitates between its granulocytic or monocytoid nature; in the other variety described by NAEGELI (4), two distinct cell populations seem to coexist,
a granulocytic and a monocytoid. It is interesting that, in bone marrow cultures in agar, granulocytes and monocytes are derived from the
same precursor cell, which yields mixed cultures (5, 6).

Finally, there is a variety in which enough leukemic cells seem to belong to the granulocytic series for it to be classified as AML, yet
a considerable percentage of cells, sometimes up to 50 percent have
no distinctive features or may resemble immature cells of the lymphoid
series (1, 3). It is arguable whether the unidentifiable cells are:
(a) precursor cells of the myeloblast, (b) cells in which granule formation is defective, or (c) blast cells of a different origin, perhaps
lymphoid. This last possibility would imply the existence of acute leukemias with mixed cellular populations (myeloid and lymphoid). This
type of acute leukemia is called by some "AML with many lymphoblast-
like cells" (3). Cytochemical procedures and electron microscopy may
help to give answers (3, 6, 7, 92).

Acute monocytoid leukemia (AMoL) does not differ from the other variant
in its clinical manifestations except for more frequent involvement of
the gums and skin. Monoblasts, promonocytes, or promonoblasts may predominate. There is some evidence that prognosis and response to therapy
depend to some extent on these morphologic features.

Progress in the treatment of AML has proceeded at a much slower pace
than for ALL. While, for the latter, treatment objectives have advanced
over the years from palliation to remission induction, remission maintenance, and finally cure, with AML we are still trying to induce remissions in the majority of patients, or to maintain them in those who have
obtained one. Though it is known that children respond better to therapy,
the poorer results in AML cannot be explained on the basis of age alone,
since the response to chemotherapy of children with AML is much less
than that of those with ALL. Chemotherapy remains the major and almost
exclusive treatment modality. Immunotherapy has rarely been evaluated
since there are few patients in whom the leukemic cell population can
be reduced to a number low enough to be handled by immune stimulation.
Therapy is directed at the destruction of the leukemic population and
the protection of the patient during the period required to correct the
hematopoietic insufficiency. Techniques for the prevention and treatment of infection and bleeding, the major causes of death during the
initial phase of therapy, are discussed in Chapter 11.

A. CHEMOTHERAPY

1. Induction of Remission

AML has proven to be much less sensitive to a number of agents than ALL
(2, 8-16, 92, 93). The reason for this is not always clear and cannot
be explained on the basis of cell kinetics alone, as there are no characteristic differences in the cell-cycle parameters (17, 18). The first
drug that promised some activity in AML was 6-MP, introduced in 1953
(19). Many textbooks continued to recommend it as the drug "of choice"
until the mid- or even late 1960's not because of its effectiveness

(CR 11.5 percent) (13), but rather because it was the least ineffective of the agents available at that time. The response rates are no better for cyclophosphamide (1.3 percent CR) (13), MTX (17.5 percent CR) (13), 6-thioguanine (20), 6-MMPR (O percent CR) (15), prednisone (11.7 percent CR) (13), vincristine (inadequate data in adults) (13), and L-asparaginase (13 percent CR + PR) (21). We mention these drugs not because of their effectiveness but because they are still used in combination programs. Table 15-1 lists the drugs for which a 25 percent or better response rate has been reported, at least in some studies. Results from both screening and operational research are tabulated. Response rates vary widely for the same drug, for a number of reasons. When screening studies are made, the best mode of administration for a given drug is often unknown. The patient population selected for the different trials may not be comparable. The criteria whereby responses are evaluated are not uniform. We have already discussed the importance of making a distinction between regressions and remissions (see p. 192) (22). Some reports are based on small numbers of patients. Not all participants have intensive hematologic care units. Of the drugs listed, only four can be seriously considered: cytosine arabinoside (CAR), daunorubicin (DRB), adriamycin (ADM) and possibly methyl-GAG (MGGH). DRB and ADM, being chemically closely related, would be expected to be cross-resistant; this assumption has been confirmed by those who have evaluated it (40, 41). Daunorubicin is the most effective single agent (depending on the aggressiveness of treatment) but also the most toxic drug for AML. It is difficult to handle, since the range of doses and and schedules that will induce destruction of leukemic cells, while sparing hematopoietic stem cells, is narrow. It should not be used in hospitals not equipped to support a patient in marrow aplasia. The optimum schedule for induction was recently investigated by the ALGB (37). They obtained 34 percent CR with 5 daily doses of 60 mg/m^2, 20 percent for the same dose twice weekly, and 16 percent once weekly. The cumulative dose should not exceed 600 mg/m^2 (42). Because of the toxicity of DRB, many hematologists and oncologists consider CAR as the drug of choice (43). Note that the effectiveness of CAR and of DRB is schedule-dependent (see comparative trials, Table 15-1) (32, 44). Methyl-GAG has been used less frequently because of its toxicity and narrow therapeutic index (13, 23-26, 37). Making allowance for patient selection, elimination of inadequate trials, and differences in response evaluation, it would be fair to say that the best agent currently available, given in its most effective schedule, yields at best 25-30 percent of complete remissions.

The four drugs named are not only less effective than the remission-induction agents (PDN, VCR) available for ALL, but also much more myelosuppressive. If we add the cardiac toxicity of DRB and ADM, the severe marrow insufficiency, and the older age of the patients affected with AML, it is not surprising that the cost in toxicity is high. Preliminary reports suggest that 5-azacytidine is active in refractory AML (94, 95).

The results of single-agent therapy being rather poor, many investigators have resorted to combinations. Here we remind the reader of a general principle of combination chemotherapy: not much can be expected from the combination of agents that are not very effective individually. Furthermore, combination of agents in AML does not follow the formula of FREI and FREIREICH, illustrated in Table 6-2, page 123. In the example cited by these authors (the combination of 6-MP and PDN) only one agent is myelosuppressive, so that both drugs can be given in full dosage in combination. All drugs have some activity in AML are myelotoxic; their dosage must therefore be reduced in combinations.

It·is a difficult task to evaluate the results and even more difficult to make recommendations on the basis of the plethora of studies available

Table 15-1. Single agents for induction of remission in acute myeloid leukemia

Drug schedule	Personal experience or EORTC	Literature
Methyl-GAG	26% MATHE el al. (1963) (23) SCHWARZENBERG et al. (1966) (24)	0% REGELSON and HOLLAND (1963) (25) 69% FREIREICH et al. (1962) (26)
Cytosine arabinoside (CAR)		
50 mg/m², i.v., q 3h x 8; repeat: every 3 days	26% SCHWARZENBERG et al. (1969) (27)	
75-100 mg/m², 4h infusion, qd x 4, repeat: after 5-10 days	17.5% EORTC (1973) (28, 29)	44% HENDERSON et al. (1968) (30)
100 mg/m², q 12h, x 7-10 days repeat: after 10 days	25% EORTC (90)	
200 mg/m², continuous infusion, qd x 5; repeat every 2 weeks		31% FREIREICH et al. (1970) (31)
800 mg/m² over 48h infusion 1000 mg/m² over 120h infusion repeat: every 2 weeks		20% SWCCG (32) 38% SWCCG (1974)
200 mg/m² in divided doses, rapid i.v. injection every 8h, qd x 5; repeat: every 2 weeks		31% SWCCG (1974) (33)
Daunorubicin (DRB)		
70-80 mg/m², i.v. qd x 5	25% MATHE et al. (1967) (34) 25% EORTC (1969) (35)	
2 mg/kg, i.v. qd, until toxicity or CR		55% BOIRON et al. (36)
60 mg/m², i.v., qd x 5		34% ALGB (37)
60 mg/m², i.v., twice weekly		20% ALGB (37)
60 mg/m², i.v., once weekly		16% ALGB (37)
DRB-benzoyl-hydrazone chlorhydrate		
3-5 mg/kg, i.v., qd x 4-7		45% JACQUILLAT et al. (38)
Adriamycin (ADM)		
0.4 mg/kg, i.v. qd x 4; repeat after 3-day rest period	30% MATHE et al. (39)	

in the literature, since these studies are often not in agreement and sometimes contradictory. Combinations of two agents have the advantage that their effects can be easily compared, using 3 groups of patients, with that of each agent separately. Unfortunately, as with single-agent trials, the results of combination studies are not always in agreement.

Cytosine arabinoside and daunorubicin, the two most effective agents, have been combined with each other or with various other agents in an attempt to improve remission induction.

The combination of DRB with CAR, the two most effective single agents, seems logical. CROWTHER (45) reported a 60 percent CR rate for this combination, a result not confirmed by the EORTC LEUKEMIA HEMATOSAR-COMA GROUP (21 percent CR (28, 29)) or the earlier studies of the ALGB (36 percent CR + PR (46)) (Table 15-2). In a more recent study, the ALGB obtained their highest remission rate (77 percent) with CAR for 7 days and DRB for 3 days (56). GLUCKMAN et al. used these two agents in close sequence in AML and in combination in promyelocytic leukemia and reported respectively 12/22 and 4/8 CR (47).

The combination of DRB and PDN (CR = 27 percent) was no more effective than DRB alone (48). This is not too surprising, since neither the cyto-toxic effect of PDN in AML nor its capacity to modify the hematologic toxicity of chemotherapy have been properly documented. GEE et al. chose to combine 6-TG with CAR because this combination was synergistic in experimental studies (49). Since the metabolism of 6-TG does not in-volve the enzyme xanthine oxidase, its dosage must not be altered if allopurinol is administered concomitantly. GEE et al. obtained 50 per-cent CR plus PR. Their results were confirmed by CLARKSON et al. (65 percent CR) (2), who administered both drugs every 12 hours rather than once a day, and LEVI et al. (41 percent CR + 27 percent PR) (50). Hy-droxyurea was given prior to the CAR+6-TG combination in LEVI's proto-col as a "priming" agent in an attempt to induce cell synchrony. These results could not be confirmed by the EORTC LEUKEMIA HEMATOSARCOMA GROUP when CAR + 6-TG (15 percent CR) was compared with CAR alone (16 percent CR), and CAR + DRB (21 percent CR) (28, 29, 90).

The ALGB recently reported 23 percent CR + 22 percent PR for the CAR+ 6-TG combination (51). This same group has also evaluated CAR + 6-MP, obtaining 21 percent CR + 17 percent PR (52). A group from New Zealand reported 8 CR and 4 PR in 25 patients with the same two drug combina-tion (53).

CAR combined with cyclophosphamide was evaluated in adults on the basis of a synergism noted in L 1210 leukemia, and a CR was obtained in 9/19 patients entered in the study (54). Synergism was also noted for the combination of CAR + BCNU in L 1210 leukemia. However, results in one clinical study failed to confirm a synergistc action (response rate 7/29 PR + CR = 24 percent) (55). The ALGB had more success with CAR + CCNU: 30 percent CR and 8 percent PR (51) in a randomized trial com-paring this combination with CAR-6-TG (see above).

Another combination of two drugs to show synergism in experimental systems is 6-MP + 6-MMPR, giving 24 percent CR in adult AML whereas the single agents are ineffective (6-MP: 9 percent CR; 6-MMPR: 0%). However, this combination has since been abandoned by its proponents (15).

Various triple and quadruple combinations have been thought up and evaluated, with response rates varying from 22 percent to 67 percent (Table 15-3) (73).

Table 15-2. Two-drug combinations for induction of remission in acute myeloid leukemia

Drug schedule		Repeat	No. of patients	% complete remission	Reference
Cytosine arabinoside (CAR)	Daunorubicin				
100 mg/m², continuous infusion, qd x 7 idem qd x 5	45 mg/m², i.v., qd x 3 idem qd x 2		43 43	77% 53%	RAI et al. (56)
2 mg/kg, i.v., qd x 5 (+/- ASP)	1.5 mg/kg, i.v., day 1	5d	23	60%	CROWTHER et al. (45)
100 mg/m², continuous infusion, qd x 5	100 mg/m², i.v., day 6, 7, 8		22	55%	GLUCKMAN et al. (47)
100 mg/m², 1 h infusion,	45 mg/m², i.v., day 1, 2, 10 & 11			36% (CR+PR)	ALGB (46)
100 mg/m², i.v., q 12 h, for 7-10 days	60 mg/m², i.v., day 1	19-26d	61	31%	EORTC (90)
75-100 mg/m², 4 h infusion, qd x 4	60 mg/m², 4 h infusion, qd x 4	5-10d	58	21%	EORTC (28, 29)
Cytosine arabinoside	6-Thioguanine				
100 mg/m², i.v., q 12 h x 7-10 days	80 mg/m², p.o., q 12 h until CR or hypoplasia	+21d	43 (un-treated) 41 (prev. treated)	65% 41%	CLARKSON (2)
(initially Gee's schedule; later in study: Clarkson's)			64 (>50yr)	44%	GRANN et al. (57)
3 mg/kg, i.v. (8-10 h after 6-TG), qd until hypoplasia	2.5 mg/kg, p.o., qd until hypoplasia	1-5 weeks	36	41%	GEE et al. (49)
150 mg/m², s.c. (8 h after 6-TG), qd for 3-11 days	2 mg/kg, p.o., for 3-11 days	10d	22	41%	LEVI et al. (50)
100 mg/m², contin. infusion qd x 5	100 mg/m², p.o., q 12 h x 5d	14d	69	23%	ALGB (51)
100 mg/m², i.v., q 12 h, for 7-10 days	80 mg/m², p.o., q 12 h, for 7-10 days. First dose given 6 h before CAR	19-26d	70	30%	EORTC (90)
75-100 mg/m², 4 h infusion, qd x 4	75-100 mg/m², qd x 5	5-10d	53	15%	EORTC (28, 29)

Table 15-2. (continued)

Drug schedule	Repeat	No. of patients	% complete remission	Reference
Cytosine arabinoside				
2.5 mg/kg, 30 min infusion, q 12 h, x 8			21%	ALGB (52)
6-Mercaptopurine				
2.5 mg/kg, p.o., qd x 4	7-10d	25	32%	BUCHANAN et al. (53)
Cytosine arabinoside				
150 mg/m^2, in divided doses q 8 h, rapid infusion, qd x 4				
Cyclophosphamide				
150 mg/m^2, in divided doses q 8 h, rapid infusion, qd x 4	14d	29	40%	BODEY et al. (54)
Cytosine arabinoside				
30 mg/m^2, infusion, qd x 3 or 5				
BCNU				
100 mg/m^2, i.v., day 1	CAR, 3 weeks; BCNU, 6 weeks	29	24%(CR+PR)	VOGLER (55)
CCNU				
100 mg/m^2, contin. infusion, qd x 5				
6-Mercaptopurine				
100 mg/m^2, p.o., on day 1 (of 1st cycle only)	14d	60	30%	ALGB (51)
6MMPR				
		22	24%	FREIREICH (15)

Table 15-3. Multiple-drug combinations for induction of remission in acute myeloid leukemia

Drug schedule	No. of patients	% complete remission	Reference
PDN, DRB, MGGH		41%	MATHE, 1966 (58)
6-MP, MTX, MGGH		35%	BERNARD, 1967 (59)
PDN, 6-MP, MGGH, CAR	24	43%	BERNARD, 1967 (59)
PDN, VCR, 6-MP, MTX	23	22%	THOMPSON et al., 1965 (60)
POMP			
PDN 150-1000 mg/m^2, qd x 5		67%	KARON et al., 1965 (61)
VCR 2 mg/m^2, day 1 MTX 5-7.5 mg/m^2, qd x 5	83	29%	HENDERSON and SERPICK, 1967 (62)
6-MP 500 mg/m^2, qd x 5 repeat after 9 days	51	45% (adults) 70% (children)	HENDERSON and SAMAHA, 1969 (9)
	21	28%	WIERNIK and SERPICK, 1972 (64)
	51	25%	RODRIGUEZ et al., 1973 (63)
CAV			
CPM 40 mg/m^2, i.v. push, q 8 h x 12 CAR 40 mg/m^2, i.v. push, q 8 h x 12	20	45%	ABU-ZAHRA et al., 1972 (65)
VCR 2.0 mg, day 1 repeat at 2-week intervals			
DRB 1 mg/kg, i.v. push, qd x 3-6$^+$			
CAR 2 mg/kg, i.v. push, qd x 3-6$^+$	23	55%	ROSENTHAL and MOLONEY, 1972 (66)
VCR 1.5 mg, day 1 (and 4$^+$)			
$^+$if blasts still present in BM on day 4			
VCR 2 mg, i.v., day 1			
CAR 100 mg/m^2, qd x 10 d (continuous infusion)	111	51%	HEWLETT et al., 1975 (97)
PDN 100 mg, p.o. x 5 d			
COAP			
CPM 100 mg/m^2 qd (i.v.,3 divided doses q 8 h) x 5 days VCR 2 mg, i.v., day 1	19	53% 46 %	FREIREICH et al., 1970 (31) FREI et al., 1970 (10)
CAR 100 mg/m^2 (i.v., 3 divided doses q 8 h) x 5 days	39	44%	WHITECAR et al., 1972 (67)

286

Table 15-3. (continued)

Drug schedule	No. of patients	% complete remission	Reference
PDN 25 mg, p.o., q.i.d x 5d	66	48%	BODEY et al., 1974 (33)
repeat at 2-weeks interval	40	15%	STOUTENBOROUGH and MEYERS, 1975 (98)
A-OAP			
ADM 40 mg/m^2, i.v., followed on day 5 by: CAR 100 mg/m^2 qd x 5d (continuous infusion)			
VCR 2 mg, i.v., on day 1	33	70%	McCREDIE et al., 1974 (72)
PDN 100 mg qd x 5d repeat on day 19			
VCR 1-2 mg/m^2, i.v., weekly			
DRB 1-2 mg/kg, i.v., weekly	103	30%	PAVLOVSKY et al., 1973 (68)
PDN-alone 100 mg/m^2, p.o., qd until CR			
VCR 1-2 mg/m^2, i.v., d 1, 7, and 14			
DRB 1 mg/kg, i.v., d 1, 7, and 14			
PDN 40 mg/m^2, p.o., qd x 21d			
CAR 100 mg/m^2, qd, rapid i.v. injection 6-MP, 2.5 mg/kg, qd, p.o. days: 20-24 and 30-34	114	42%	EPPINGER-HELFT et al., 1975 (99)
Maintenance: MTX + 6-MP with reinforcements with DRB + VCR + PDN, alternating with CAR.			
Hammersmith Protocol (M) **TRAP (for induction)**			
6-TG 100 mg/m^2, p.o., qd x 5			
DRB 40 mg/m^2, i.v., day 1 CAR 100 mg/m^2, i.v. or i.m., qd x 5 PDN 30 mg/m^2, p.o., qd x 5 repeat at 2-week intervals x 6	27	48%	PAOLINO et al., 1973 (69)
Maintenance: alternating cycles of COAP, TRAP, and POMP			
CAM			
CPM 1.0 g/m^2, i.v., h 0-0.5			
CAR 300 mg/m^2, i.v., h 0.5-1	14	50%	SKEEL et al., 1973 (70)

Table 15-3. (continued)

Drug schedule	No. of patients	% complete remission	Reference

MTX 80 mg/m^2, i.v., h 0-24
   repeat once weekly
   until hypoplasia or CR.			

CAP
  CPM 50 mg/m^2, i.v., twice qd
  CAR 50 mg/m^2, i.v., twice qd
  PDN-olone 40 mg/m^2, i.v., twice qd
 	
  days: 1-4
  repeat on day 15
	25	28%	GAHRTON, et al. 1974 (100)

CAPA idem as CAP, followed by L-ASP 1000 i.u./kg i.v., qd, d 5-35	27	33%	GAHRTON et al., 1974 (100)
DRB 1.5 mg/kg, i.v., day 1 CAR 2 mg/kg, i.v. q 12 h x 7d 6-TG 2 mg/kg, p.o., q 12 h x 7 d VCR 1.0 mg, i.v., day 1 and 7 PDN 1 mg/kg, p.o., qd x 5d repeat on day 15	23	78%	GLUCKSBERG et al., 1975 (71)

2. Maintenance Therapy

Not only is it much more difficult to obtain a complete remission in AML than in ALL, but maintaining the remission is also more of a problem. Maintenance of remission has been attempted in three different ways: (1) employing the same agents that were used to induce remission, (2) switching to different agents for maintenance, (3) relying on immunotherapy or chemo-immunotherapy. In ALL we distinguish between inducing agents, the non-myelotoxic PDN, VCR, L-ASP, and maintenance agents, such as 6-MP and MTX, whose myelosuppressive effect is not very dangerous when given in remission. Switching to different agents during maintenance decreases the risk of selecting resistant cell lines, and allows the cell number to be further reduced. In AML, we are generally forced to use the same drugs or combinations for maintenance that were used to obtain a remission because there are not enough really effective agents to allow us to design a variety of complementary cell-reducing or reinforcement regimens. Most of the combinations described above consist of intensive courses of chemotherapy, given at 2 to 3-week intervals. They are generally continued, but often at slightly prolonged intervals in remission (31, 50, 54, 67, 71). In a few protocols, a switch was made to different agents for maintenance (2, 37, 48, 65, 101).

Some protocols have been designed to incorporate efforts directed against the fraction of resting cells during the maintenance phase (74, 75, 96) (Figs. 15-1 and 15-2). SPIERS is evaluating a protocol of three four-drug combinations (COAP, POMP, TRAP) in sequence (14). Preliminary results of a similar protocol have been reported (69). Some other protocols under study were reviewed by CARTER (73). CNS leukemia is seldom a problem in AML, at least at the present time, so that prophylactic measures are not part of current programs (92).

The results obtained with various combinations suggest that the response rate is slightly improved (CR = 35-50 percent) over that of single-agent therapy (CR = 25-35 percent). No particular protocol has emerged as clearly superior, and results are often not confirmed by subsequent studies.

In selecting a drug or a combination for AML, it is important to consider not only the response rate but also its toxicity, and the quality of life of the subjects treated. Our major aim during remission induction therapy should be to keep the patient alive while trying to kill leukemic cells, in that order! This may seem obvious but the delicate nature of the balance between these two objectives is illustrated by a recent report (64) of 52 percent mortality during induction therapy with POMP for a response rate of 28 percent CR. This is much too high a price to pay.

Most proponents of a particular combination claim certain advantages for their cocktail. ROSENTHAL et al. stress the rapidity with which induction is obtained, thereby shortening the period at risk for infection and bleeding (66). WHITECAR et al. claim for COAP the longest duration of remission and survival on record (33, 67). More recently MANASTER et al. (101) have made similar claims. The combination of 6-TG + CAR, currently favored in the US, has an advantage in employing only 2 drugs rather than 3 or 4; unfortunately, its efficacy is in dispute (28, 29, 90). The reasons for the failure of EORTC to confirm the results of some American groups is not clear. It could not be related to age differences in the patient population, the modalities of administration, or the availability of intensive hematologic care.

Some of the factors that influence the outcome of therapy have already been mentioned. In all evaluations it is confirmed that older patients respond much less frequently. GRANN, however, did obtain a 44 percent CR rate in patients over 50 years with CAR + 6-TG (57). One observation which needs confirmation is that women over 40 years old respond significantly better than men over 40, at least to DRB (48). The prognostic value of initial WBC or platelet counts is insignificant for individual patients. In a study using intermittent courses of CAR, CPM, and VCR, one of us (AC) noted that, in patients who subsequently responded to treatment, the first course of therapy usually cleared the peripheral blood of blast cells (65).

The influence of prior therapy is quite variable (37). Some studies report better results in previously treated subjects, either because these patients are under close observation and hence treated early in relapse by a new regimen, or because they represent a previously selected group of chemotherapy-sensitive patients, or a cohort that was strong enough to survive the high death rate early in the course of clinical disease (67). Other studies report that previously treated patients do worse (2) or no differently from untreated ones (49, 50). The "response" to prior therapy is important. A patient who had a 2-year remission on 6-MP can be expected to do better than a patient who failed to respond to DRB and CAR. Both the level of immunocompetence and changes in this level help in predicting the probability of remission and impending

289

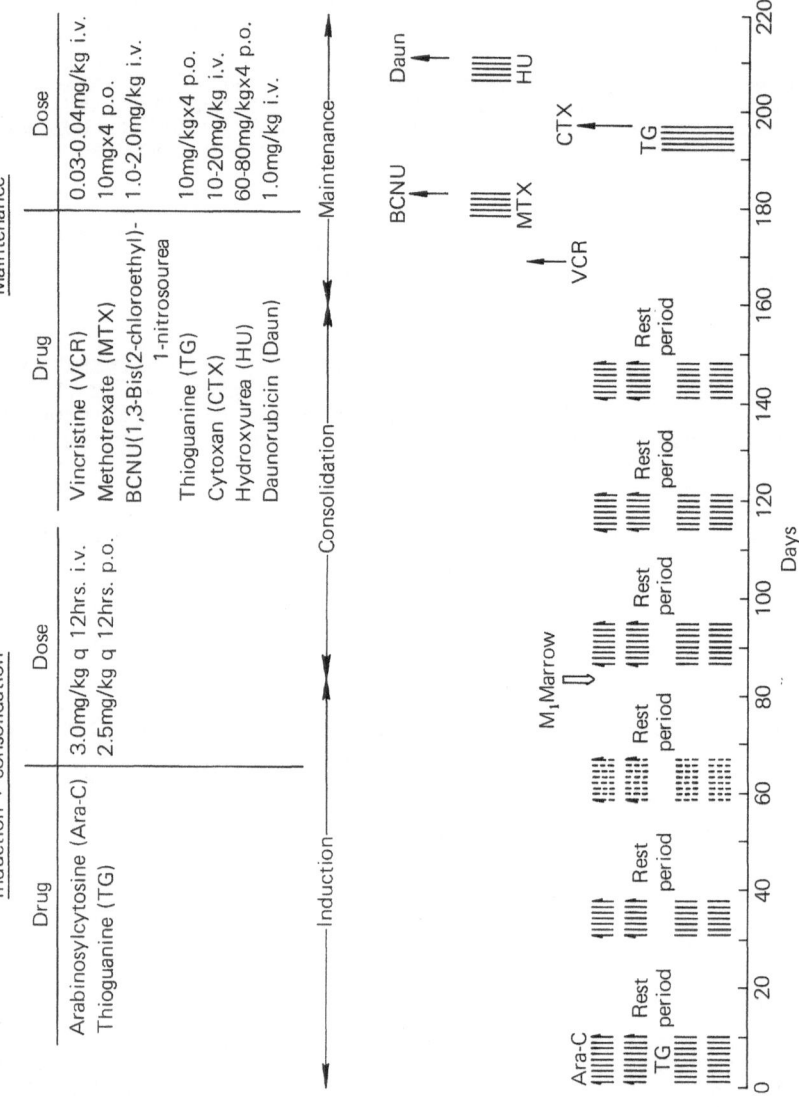

INTENSIVE "L-6" TREATMENT PROTOCOL FOR ACUTE MYELOBLASTIC LEUKEMIA
(Revised 1972)

Induction + consolidation

Drug	Dose
Arabinosylcytosine (Ara-C)	3.0mg/kg q 12hrs. i.v.
Thioguanine (TG)	2.5mg/kg q 12hrs. p.o.

Maintenance

Drug	Dose
Vincristine (VCR)	0.03-0.04mg/kg i.v.
Methotrexate (MTX)	10mgx4 p.o.
BCNU(1,3-Bis(2-chloroethyl)-1-nitrosourea	1.0-2.0mg/kg i.v.
Thioguanine (TG)	10mg/kgx4 p.o.
Cytoxan (CTX)	10-20mg/kg i.v.
Hydroxyurea (HU)	60-80mg/kgx4 p.o.
Daunorubicin (Daun)	1.0mg/kg i.v.

Fig. 15-1. The L-6 protocol for acute myeloid leukemia. (From DOWLING et al. (25))

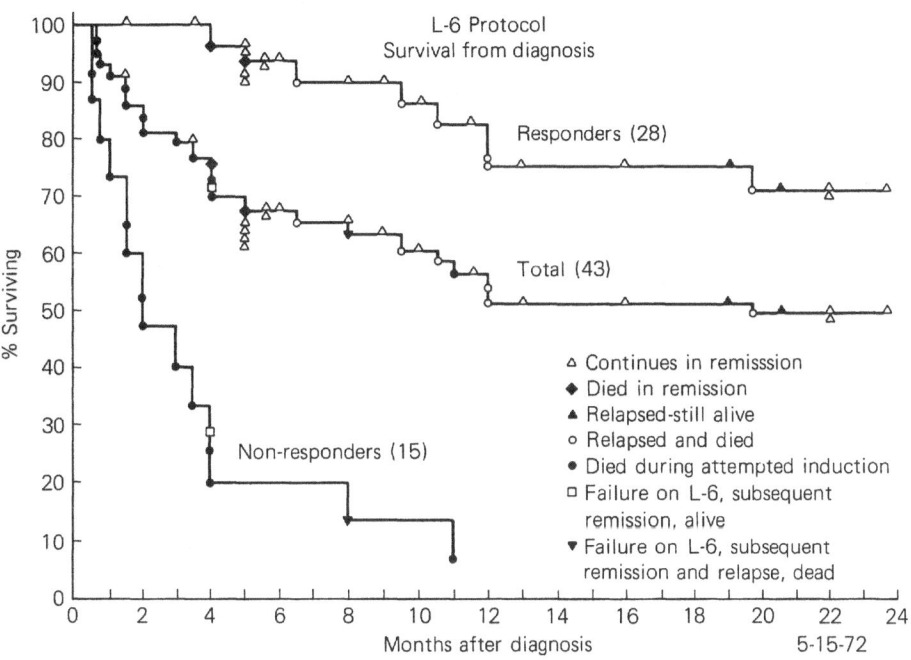

Fig. 15-2. Survival from diagnosis with the L-6 protocol. (From DOWLING et al. (75))

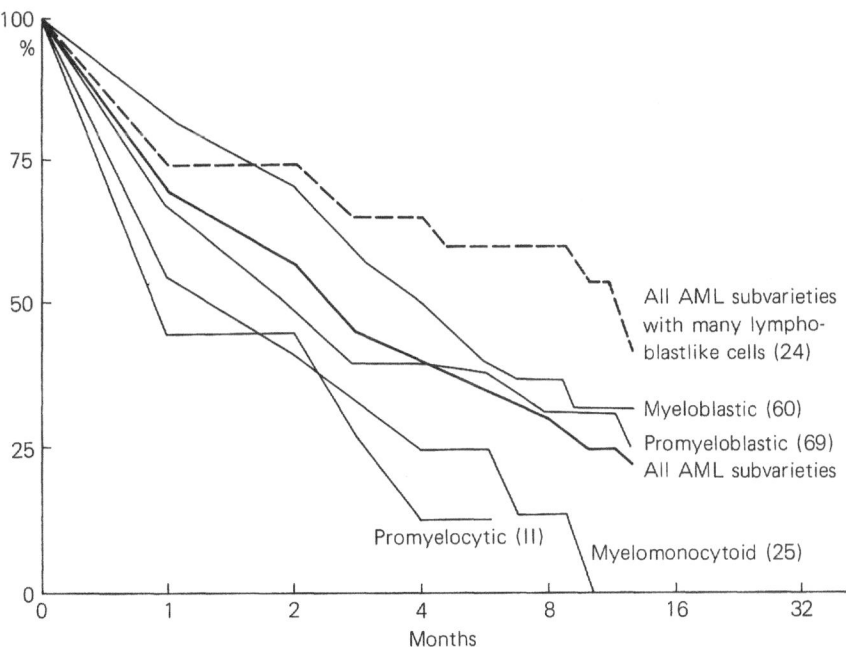

Fig. 15-3. Actuarial curve of cumulative survival of all AML patients submitted to trial AML[1] (1970-1971) (CAR or CAR + 6-TG or CAR + DRB) (EORTC, Leukemia and Hematosarcoma Group), according to the different cytological varieties. (From MATHE et al. (3))

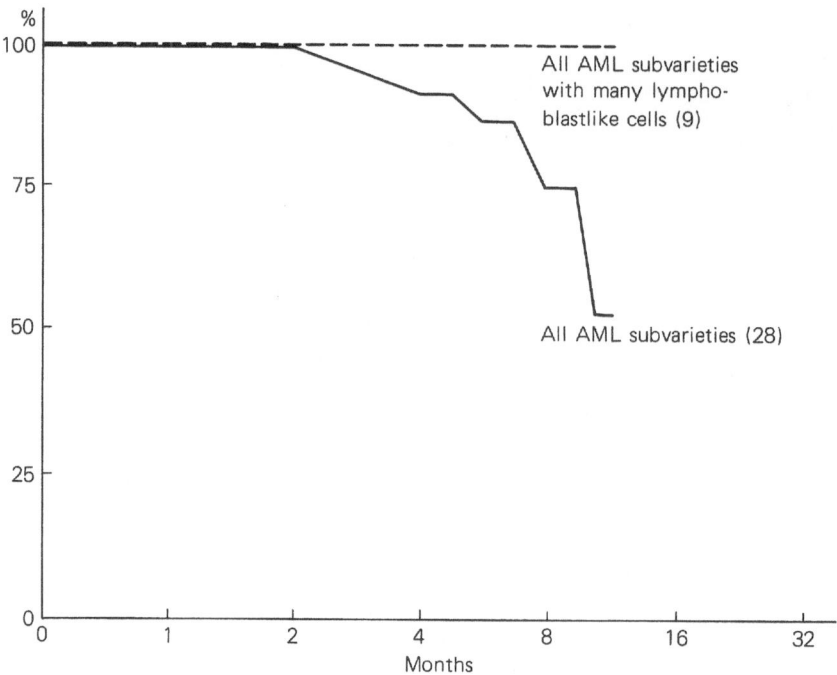

%

Fig. 15-4. Actuarial curves of cumulative duration of "complete" remissions of AML patients submitted to trial AML[1] (1970-1971) (CAR or CAR
+ 6-TG or CAR + DRB) (EORTC, Leukemia and Hematosarcoma Group), according to the abundant presence of "lymphoblast-like" cells on the first
smear. (From MATHE et al. (3))

relapse in patients with acute leukemia (76). SAKURAI and SANDBERG have
stressed the prognostic and therapeutic value of chromosomal findings
(102).

Better results are obtained in trials conducted in centers equipped
with the facilities for intensive hematologic care (90). The ade-
quacy of the latter is reflected by the percentage of patients who receive an "adequate trial" (variably defined in different studies but
generally meaning a minimum of 6 weeks of remission induction chemotherapy at full dose). Currently, 80 percent of AML patients should be
able to receive an adequate trial. It is also not uncommon for the proponent of a regimen to have better results than subsequent users. This
probably illustrates the importance of the experience, confidence and
faith of the therapist in the treatment's potential value, since these
factors determine the intensity with which he treats leukemia and its
complications. For this raison, we would advise individual physicians
who do not participate in cooperative trials to familiarize themselves
with one particular regimen rather than to switch with each new publication that claims a 5 percent higher response rate than the previous
one. There is no doubt that patients who respond do benefit from therapy and that they enjoy longer survival periods than non-responders (2,
33, 49, 54, 57, 63, 65, 68). Increased survival depends on the induction
of remission. Patial remission are of much less value and should be
reported separately from complete remissions.

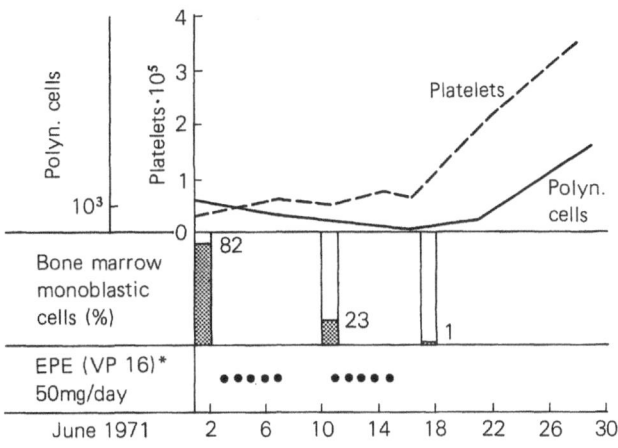

*4'-Demethyl-epipodophyllotoxine-β-D-ethylidene glucoside

*Fig. 15-5. Complete regression with complete remission obtained in
a woman aged 80 with acute momocytoid leukemia treated with VP 16213.
(From SCHWARZENBERG et al. (91))*

There have been no great differences in the response rates for the various morphologic subclasses of acute nonlymphoid leukemia in adults.
Most reports place them together. However, there may be some value in
considering some variants separately. Several investigators have observed that promyelocytic leukemia responds better to DRB than do other
variants of AML (37, 42), and possibly also erythroleukemia (48, 77).
The EORTC LEUKEMIA HEMATOSARCOMA GROUP obtained significantly more
complete remissions in a comparative trial with CAR, CAR + 6-TG or
CAR + DRB, in the subvariety AML "with many lymphoblast-like cells" (3)
than in the other cytological variants (Figs. 15-3 and 15-4), however,

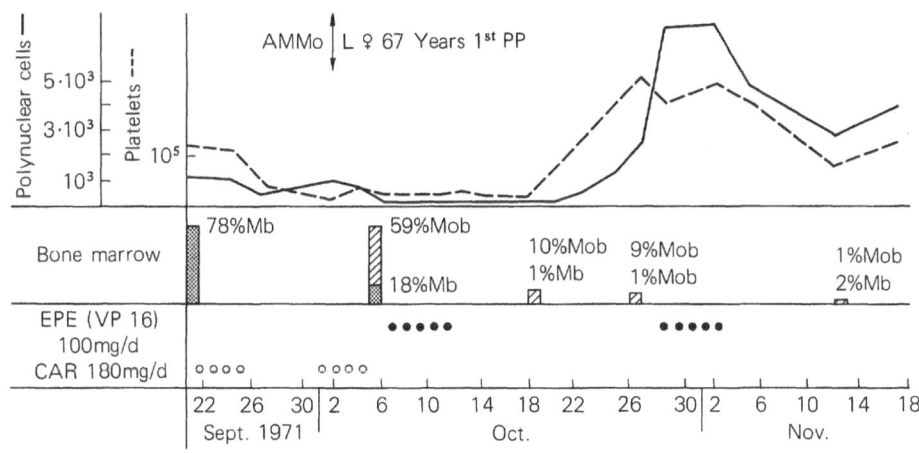

*Fig. 15-6. Acute myelomonocytoid leukemia: the myeloblasts were much
reduced after a course of CAR while the monoblasts increased but disappeared after a course of VP 16213. (From MATHE et al. (3))*

this was not confirmed by a second trial (29). The same group obtained
2/5 CR with VP 16213 or EPE, a podophyllotoxin derivative, in the otherwise poorly responsive acute monoblastoid leukemia (78) (Figs. 15-5 and
15-6). They also reported that in acute myelomonoblastic leukemias
(AMMoL) the myeloid leukemic cells may disappear after administration
of CAR, CAR + DRB, or CAR + 6-TG, while the monocytoid cells persist
(33). In several patients, the remission could be completed by VP 16213,
to which monocytoid cells seem to be most sensitive (103). VM 26, though
closely related, does not seem to have this selective effect. Hence,
they suggest the combination of CAR + VP 16213 for acute myelomonoblastic leukemia. VP 16213 had no effect in pure AML while CAR is ineffective in pure AMoL (3). Remissions have also been induced in acute monoblastic leukemia with vinblastine (104) and with daunorubicin (105)

B. STRATEGY

1. Immunotherapy

Preliminary results of trials in progress are encouraging and seem to
confirm MATHE's observations of the value of active immunotherapy in
acute leukemia, when used to treat residual disease (79-82, 92, 106);
others use a combination of chemotherapy and immunotherapy for maintenance and some for induction of remission as well (107-111).

2. Bone Marrow Transplantation

A few research centers are investigating the role of bone marrow transplantation in the treatment of AML. Though still a highly experimental
procedure, it has been proposed on the assumption that the disease
affects all hematopoietic cell lines. It would thus be logical to eradicate and replace them (83-89).

REFERENCES

1. MATHE, G., RAPPAPORT, H.: Histological and cytological typing of the
   neoplastic diseases of the haematopoietic and lymphoid tissues.
   Geneva: W.H.O. 1973.
2. CLARKSON, B.D.: Acute myelocytic leukemia in adults. Cancer 30, 1572
   (1972).
3. MATHE, G., POUILLART, P., WEINER, R., HAYAT, M., STERESCO, M., LA-
   FLEUR, M.: Classification and subclassification of acute leukemias
   correlated with clinical expression, therapeutic sensitivity and
   prognosis. In: Nomenclature, Methodology and Results of Clinical
   Trials in Acute Leukemias, (eds. G. Mathé, P. Pouillart, L. Schwarzenberg). Recent Results in Cancer Research, Vol. 43, p. 7. Berlin-
   Heidelberg-New York: Springer-Verlag 1973.
4. NAEGELI, O.: Blutkrankheiten und Blutdiagnostik. Berlin: Springer-
   Verlag 1931.
5. CLARYSSE, A.M.: unpublished observations.
6. POUILLART, P.: Contribution of cultures in agar to the classification
   of acute leukemias: preliminary results. In: Nomenclature, Methodology and Results of Clinical Trials in Acute Leukemias, p. 88 (eds.
   G. Mathé, P. Pouillart, L. Schwarzenberg). Berlin-Heidelberg-New
   York: Springer-Verlag 1973

7. BESSIS, M.: Cytologic diagnosis of leukemias by electron microscopy. In: Nomenclature, Methodology, and Results of Clinical Trials in Acute Leukemias, p. 63 (eds. G. Mathé, P. Pouillart, L. Schwarzenberg). Berlin-Heidelberg-New York: Springer 1973.

8. HENDERSON, E.S.: Treatment of acute leukemia. Seminars in Hematology, 6, 271-319 (1969).

9. HENDERSON, E.S., SAMAHA, R.J.: Evidence that drugs in multiple combination have materially advanced the treatment of human malignancies. Cancer Res. 29, 2272 (1969).

10. FREI, E.III, BODEY, G.P., WHITECAR, J., HART, J., FREIREICH, E.J.: Advances in the chemotherapy of acute leukemia. In: Comparative leukemia research, Vol. 1, p. 690 (ed. R.M. Dutcher). Basle: Karger 1970.

11. WEIL, M., JACQUILLAT, C., BERNARD, J.: Traitement des leucémies aigues myéloblastiques. Rev. Méd. 11, 261 (1970).

12. GOLDIN, A., SANDBERG, J.S., HENDERSON, E.S., NEWMAN, J.W., FREI, E. III, HOLLAND, J.F.: The chemotherapy of human and animal leukemia. Cancer Chemother. Rep. 55, 309 (1971).

13. LIVINGSTON, R.B., CARTER, S.K.: Single agents in cancer chemotherapy. New York: IFI/Plenum 1970.

14. SPIERS, A.S.D.: Chemotherapy of acute leukaemia. Clinics in Haematology 1, 127 (1972).

15. FREI, E. III: Chemotherapy of acute leukemia. In: Cancer Chemotheapy II, p. 315 (eds. I. Brodsky, S.B. Kahn, J.H. Moyer). New York: Grune and Stratton 1972.

16. RODRIGUEZ, V., BODEY, G.P., FREIREICH, E.J.: Combination chemotherapy for lymphomas and leukemias. Disease-A-Month (Chic.) April 1973.

17. GREENBERG, M.L., CHANANA, A.D., CRONKITE, E.P., GIACOMELLI, G., RAI, K.R., SCHIFFER, L.M., STRYCKMANS, P.A., VINCENT, P.C.: The generation time of human leukemic myeloblasts. Lab. Invest. 26, 245 (1972).

18. STRYCKMANS, P., MANASTER, J.: Kinetic aspects of leukaemia therapy. In: The Design of Clinical Trials in Cancer Therapy, p. 132 (ed. M. Staquet). Brussels: Editions Scientifiques Européennes 1972.

19. BURCHENAL, J.H., MURPHY, M.L., ELLISON, R.R., SVKES, M.P., TAN, T.C., LEONE, L.A., KARNOFSKY, D.A., CRAVER, L.F., DARGEON, H.W., RHOADS, C.P.: Clinical evaluation of a new antimetabolite, 6-mercaptopurine, in the treatment of leukemia and allied disease. Blood 8, 965 (1953).

20. MURPHY, M.D., TAN, T.C., ELLISON, R.R., KARNOFSKY, D.A., BURCHENAL, J.H.: Clinical evaluation of chloropurine and thioguanine. Proc. Amer. Ass. Cancer Res. 2, 36 (1966).

21. TAN, C.: L-Asparaginase in leukemia. Hospital Practice 99, July 1972.

22. MATHE, G., WEINER, R.: Criteria for short term results in the treatment of acute leukemia. In: Nomenclature, Methodology and Results of Clinical Trials in Acute Leukemias, Vol 1 (eds. G. Mathé, P. Pouillart, L. Schwarzenberg). Berlin-Heidelberg-New York: Springer-Verlag 1973.

23. MATHE, G., AMIEL, J.L., SCHNEIDER, M., CATTAN, A, SCHWARZENBERG, L., COUDIERE, M.: Essai de traitement des leucémies aigues par la méthylglyoxal bis (guanylhydrazone). Rev. franc. Etudes clin. biol. 8, 1035 (1963).

24. SCHWARZENBERG, L., SCHNEIDER, M., CATTAN, A., AMIEL, J.R., SCHLUMBERGER, J.R., MATHE, G.: Le traitement des leucémies aigues par la méthylglyoxal bis(guanylhydrazone) et son association à la hydroxystilbamidine. Sem. Hôp. Paris 42, 2955 (1966).

25. REGELSON, W., HOLLAND, J.F.: Clinical experience with methylglyoxal bis(guanylhydrazone) dihydrochloride: a new agent with clinical activity in acute myelocytic leukemias and lymphomas. Cancer Chemother. Rep. 27, 15 (1963).

26. FREIREICH, E.J., FREI, E.III, KARON, M.: Methylglyoxal bis(guanyl-hydrazone): a new agent active against acute myelocytic leukemia. Cancer Chemother. Rep. 16, 183 (1962).
27. SCHWARZENBERG, L., MATHE, G., HAYAT, M., DE VASSAL, F., AMIEL, J.L., CATTAN, A., SCHNEIDER, M., SCHLUMBERGER, J.R., ROSENFELD, C., JAS-MIN, C.: Essai de traitement des leucémies aigues par la cytosine arabinoside selon la méthode de Skipper. Nouv. Rev. franc. Hématol. 9, 199 (1969).
28. EORTC, Leukemia and Haematosarcoma Cooperative Group: A comparative trial of remission induction (by cytosine arabinoside, or CAR and thioguanine, or CAR and daunorubicin) and maintenance therapy (by CAR or methylgag) in acute myeloid leukemia. Biomedicine 18, 192 (1973).
29. EORTC, Leukemia and Haematosarcoma: Preliminary result of a trial on acute myeloid leukemia comparing the effects of cytosine arabino-side, the combination of cytosine arabinoside and thioguanine, and the combination of cytosine arabinoside and daunorubicin. In: No-menclature, Methodology and Results of Clinical Trials in Acute Leukemias. (eds. G. Mathé, P. Pouillart, L. Schwarzenberg). Berlin-Heidelberg-New York: Springer-Verlag 1973.
30. HENDERSON, E., SERPICK, A., LEVENTHAL, B., HENRY, P.: Cytosine arabinoside infusions in adult and childhodd acute myelocytic leu-kemia. Proc. Amer. Ass. Cancer Res. 9, 29 (1968).
31. FREIREICH, E.J., BODEY, G.P., HART, S., RODRIGUEZ, V., WHITECAR, J.P., FREI, E. III,: Remission induction in adults with acute mye-logenous leukemia. In: Advances in treatment of acute blastic leu-kemias, p. 85. (ed. G. Mathé). Paris: C.N.R.S. 1970.
32. SOUTHWEST ONCOLOGY GROUP: Cytarabine for acute leukemia in adults. Effect of schedule on therapeutic response. Arch. intern. Med. 133, 251 (1974).
33. BODEY, G.P., COLTMAN, C.A., FREIREICH, E.J., BONNET, J.D., GEHAN, E.A., HAUT, A.B., HEWLETT, J.S., McCREDIE, K.B., SAIKI, J.H., WILSON, H.E.: Chemotherapy of acute leukemia. Comparison of cytara-bine alone and in combination with vincristine, prednisone, and cyclophosphamide. Arch. intern. Med. 133, 260 (1974).
34. MATHE, G., HAYAT, M., SCHWARZENBERG, L., SCHNEIDER, M., CATTAN, A., SCHLUMBERGER, J.R., AMIEL, J.L.: Essai de traitement des leucémies aigues par la rubidomycine (ou daunomycine) seule ou en association. Path. et Biol. 15, 933 (1967).
35. EORTC, Groupe Coopérateur des Leucémies et Hématosarcomes: Essai de traitement des leucémies aigues granulocytaires par la dauno-rubicine. Europ. J. Cancer 5, 339 (1969).
36. BOIRON, M., JACQUILLAT, C., WEIL, M., TANZER, J., LEVY, J., SULTAN, C., BERNARD, J.: Daunorubicin in the treatment of acute myelocytic leukaemia. Lancet 1, 330 (1969).
37. WEIL, M., GLIDEWELL, O.J., JACQUILLAT, C., LEVY, R., SERPICK, A.A., WIERNIK, P.H., CUTTNER, J., HOOGSTRATEN, B., WASSERMAN, L., ELLISON, R.R., GAILANI, S., BRUNNER, K., SILVER, R.T., REGE, V.B., COOPER, M.R., LOWENSTEIN, L., NISSEN, N.I., HAURANI, F., BLOM, J., BOIRON, M., BERNARD, J., HOLLAND, J.F.: Daunorubicin in the therapy of acute granulocytic leukemia. Cancer Res. 33, 921 (1973).
38. JACQUILLAT, C., WEIL, M., GEMON, M.F., IZRAEL, V., BOIRON, M., BERNARD, J.: A new agent active in the treatment of acute myelo-blastic leukemia: 22050 RP. In: Nomenclature, Methodology and Re-sults of Clinical Trials in Acute Leukemias, p. 155 (eds. G. Mathé, P. Pouillart, L. Schwarzenberg). Berlin-Heidelberg-New York: Springer-Verlag 1973.
39. MATHE, G., AMIEL, J.L., HAYAT, M., DE VASSAL, F., SCHWARZENBERG, L., SCHNEIDER, M., JASMIN, C., ROSENFELD, C.: Adriamycin in the treatment of acute leukemias. In: International Symposium Adriamycin. Berlin-Heidelberg-New York: Springer-Verlag 1972.

40. CARTER, S.K., DI MARCO, A., GHIONE, M., KRAKOFF, I.H., MATHE, G.: International Symposium on Adriamycin. Heidelberg: Springer Verlag 1972.
41. WHITEHOUSE, J.M.A., CROWTHER, D., BATEMAN, C.J.T., BEARD, M.E., MALPAS, J.S.: Adriamycin in the treatment of acute leukaemia. Brit. med. J. 1, 482 (1972).
42. BERNARD, J., WEIL, M., BOIRON, M., JACQUILLAT, C., FLANDRIN, G., GEMON, M.F.: Acute promyelocytic leukemia: results of treatment by daunorubicin. Blood 41, 489 (1973).
43. FREI, E. III.: Acute granulocytic leukemia in adults. New Engl. J. Med. 286, 1211 (1972).
44. ELLISON, R.R., HOLLAND, J.F., WEIL, M., JACQUILLAT, C., BOIRON, M., BERNARD, J., SAVITSKY, A., ROSNER, F., GUSSOFF, B., SILVER, R.T., KARANAS, A., CUTTNER, J., SPURR,-HAYES, D.M., BLOM, J., LEONE, L.A., HAURANI, F., KYLE, R., HUTCHISON, J.L., FORCIER, R.J., MOON, J.H.: Arabinosyl cytosine: a useful agent in the treatment of acute leukemias in adults. Blood 32, 507 (1968).
45. CROWTHER, D., BATEMAN, C.J.T., VARTAN, C.P., WHITEHOUSE, J.M.A., MALPAS, J.S., HAMILTON-FAIRLEY, G., BODLEY SCOTT, R.: Combination chemotherapy using L-asparaginase, daunorubicin and cytosine arabinoside in the treatment of acute myelogenous leukemia. Brit. med. J., 4, 513 (1970).
46. CAREY, R.W. (ALGB): Comparative study of cytosine arabinoside therapy alone and combined with thioguanine or mercaptopurine and daunorubicin in acute myelocytic leukemia. Proc. Amer. Ass. Cancer Res. 11, 15 (1970).
47. GLUCKMAN, E., BASCH, A., VARET, B., DREYFUS, B.: Combination chemotherapy with cytosine arabinoside and rubidomycin in 30 cases of acute granulocytic leukemia. Cancer 31, 487 (1973).
48. BLOOMFIELD, C.D., BRUNNING, R.D., THEOLOGIDES, A., KENNEDY, B.J.: Daunorubicin-prednisone remission induction with hydroxyurea maintenance in acute non-lymphocytic leukemia. Cancer 31, 931 (1973).
49. GEE, T.S., YU, K.P., CLARKSON, B.D.: Treatment of adult acute leukemia with arabinosylcytosine and thioguanine. Cancer 23, 1019 (1969).
50. LEVI, J.A., VINCENT, P.C., GUNZ, F.W.: Combination chemotherapy of adult acute nonlymphoblastic leukemia. Ann. intern. Med. 76, 397 (1972).
51. WALLACE, Jr., H.J., HOAGLAND, H.C., ELLISON, R.R., GLIDEWELL, O., HOLLAND, J.F.: CCNU plus cytosine arabinoside in the treatment of acute myelocytic leukemia compared with thioguanine plus ARA-C. Proc. Amer. Ass. Cancer Res. 14, 100 (1973).
52. HOLLAND, J.F.: Acute leukemia chemotherapy. In: Oncology 1970, Vol. 4, p. 433 (eds. R.L. Clark, R.M. Cumley, McCay) Chicago: Yearbook Medical Publishers 1971.
53. BUCHANAN, J.G., MATTHEWS, J.R.D., DAVIDSON, J.G., GRIGOR, R.R., CASEY, T.P.: Treatment of acute myeloid leukemia of adults with cytosine arabinoside in combination with 6-mercaptopurine. Cancer 32, 789 (1973).
54. BODEY, G.P., RODRIGUEZ, V., HART, J., FREIREICH, E.J.: Therapy of acute leukemia with the combination of cytosine arabinoside (NSC-63878) and cyclophosphamide (NSC-26271). Cancer Chemother. Rep. 54, 255 (1970).
55. VOGLER, W.R.: BCNU and cytosine arabinoside combination in acute leukemia. Proc. Amer. Ass. Cancer Res. 9, 74 (1968).
56. RAI, K.R., HOLLAND, J.F., GLIDEWELL, O.: Improvement of remission induction therapy of acute myelocytic leukemia. Proc. Am. Soc. Clin. Oncol. 16, 265 (1975).
57. GRANN, V., ERICHSON, R., FLANNERY, J., FINCH, S., CLARKSON, B.: The therapy of acute granulocytic leukemia in patients more than 50 years old. Ann. intern. Med. 80, 15 (1974).

58. MATHE, G.: La chimiothérapie des cancers (leucémies, hématosarcomas, tumeurs solides), 2e éd. Paris: L'Expansion Scient. Franc. (1966).
59. BERNARD, J.: Acute leukemia treatment. Cancer Res. <u>27</u>, 2567 (1967).
60. THOMPSON, I., HALL, T.C., MOLONEY, W.C.: Combination therapy of acute myelogenous leukemia experience with the simultaneous use of vincristine, amethopterine, 6-mercaptopurine and prednisone. New Engl. J. Med. <u>273</u>, 1302 (1965).
61. KARON, M., FREIREICH, E.J., CARBONE, P.P.: Effective combination therapy of adult acute leukemia. Proc. Amer. Ass. Cancer Res. <u>6</u>, 34 (1965).
62. HENDERSON, E.S., SERPICK, A.: The effect of combination drug therapy and prophylactic oral antibiotic treatment in adult acute leukemia. Clin. Res. <u>15</u>, 336 (1967).
63. RODRIGUEZ, V., HART, J.S., FREIREICH, E., BODEY, G.P., McCREDIE, K.B., WHITECAR, J.P., COLTMAN, Jr., C.A.: POMP combination chemotherapy of adult acute leukemia. Cancer <u>32</u>, 69 (1973).
64. WIERNIK, P.H., SERPICK, A.A.: A randomized clinical trial of daunorubicin and a combination of prednisone, vincristine, 6-mercaptopurine, and methotrexate in adult acute nonlymphocytic leukemia. Cancer Res. <u>32</u>, 2023 (1972).
65. ABU-ZAHRA, H., CLARYSSE, A., COWAN, D.H., HASSELBACK, R., BERGSAGEL, D.E.: Treatment of acute myeloblastic leukemia in adults: remission induction with a combination of cyclophosphamide, cytarabine and vincristine. Canad. med. Ass. J. <u>107</u>, 1073 (1972).
66. ROSENTHAL, D.S., MOLONEY, W.C.: The treatment of acute granulocytic leukemia in adults. New Engl. J. Med. <u>286</u>, 1176 (1972).
67. WHITECAR, J.P., Jr., BODEY, G.P., FREIREICH, E.J., McCREDIE, K.B., HART, J.S.: Cyclophosphamide (NSC-26271), vincristine (NSC-67574), cytosine arabinoside (NSC-63878), and prednisone (NSC-10023) (COAP) combination chemotherapy for acute leukemia in adults. Cancer Chemother. Rep. <u>56</u>, 543 (1972).
68. PAVLOVSKY, S., PENALVER, J., EPPINGER-HELFT, M., SACKMANN, F., BERGNA, L., SUAREZ, A., VILASECA, G., PAVLOVSKY, A.A., PAVLOVSKY, A.: Induction and maintenance of remission in acute leukemia. Effectiveness of combination therapy in 227 patients. Cancer <u>31</u>, 274 (1973).
69. PAOLINO, W., RESEGOTTI, L., ROSSI, M., INFELISE, V.: Treatment of acute myeloid leukaemia according to the Hammersmith protocol: Preliminary report. Brit. med. J. <u>3</u>, 567 (1973).
70. SKEEL, R.T., MARSH, J.C., DECONTI, R.C., MITCHELL, M.S., HUBBARD, S., BERTINO, J.R.: Development of a combination chemotherapy program for adult acute leukemia. CAM and CAM-L. Cancer <u>32</u>, 76 (1973).
71. GLUCKSBERG, H., COLEMAN, D., RUDOLPH, R., FASS, L., FEFER, A., THOMAS, E.D.: Combination chemotherapy in adult non-lymphocytic acute leukemia. Proc. Am. Ass. Cancer Res. <u>16</u>, 120 (1975).
72. McCREDIE, K.B., BODEY, G.P., GUTTERMAN, J.U., RODRIGUEZ, V., FREIREICH, E.J.: Sequential adriamycin-cytosine arabinoside (A-OAP) for remission induction of adult acute leukemia. Proc. Amer. Ass. Cancer Res. <u>15</u>, 62 (1974).
73. CARTER, S.K.: Clinical trials and combination chemotherapy. Cancer Chemother. Rep. Part 3, <u>2</u>, 81 (1971).
74. CLARKSON, B.D., FRIED, J.: Changing concepts of treatment in acute leukemia. Medical Clinics of North America <u>55</u>, 561 (1971).
75. DOWLING, M.D., HAGHBIN, M., GEE, T.S., CUNNINGHAM, B., TAN, C.T.C., CLARKSON, B.D., BURCHENAL, J.H.: Comparative results obtained in the treatment of acute leukemia. In: Nomenclature, Methodology and Results of Clinical Trials in Acute Leukemias, p. 133 (ed.s G. Mathé, P. Pouillart, L. Schwarzenberg). Recent Results in Cancer Research, Vol. 43. Berlin-Heidelberg-New York: Springer-Verlag 1973
76. HERSH, E.M.: Serial studies of immunocompetence in patients undergoing chemotherapy for acute leukemia. Proc. Amer. Ass. Clin. Oncol. <u>15</u>, 166 (1974).

77. BLOOMFIELD, C.D., BRUNNING, R., KENNEDY, B.J.: Daunorubicin treatment of erythroleukemia. Proc. Amer. Ass. Cancer Res. <u>15</u>, 17 (1974).
78. E.O.R.T.C., Clinical Screening Group: Epipodophyllotoxin VP 16213 in the treatment of acute leukaemias, heamatosarcomas and solid tumours. Brit. Med. J. <u>3</u>, 199 (1973).
79. CROWTHER, D., BATEMAN, C.J.T., VARTAN, C.P., WHITEHOUSE, J.M.A., MALPAS, J.S., HAMILTON-FAIRLEY, G., BODLEY SCOTT, R.: Combination chemotherapy using L-asparaginase, daunorubicin and cytosine arabinoside in adults with acute myelogenous leukaemia. Brit. med. J. <u>4</u>, 513 (1970).
80. POWLES, R.: Immunotherapy for acute myelogenous leukaemia. Brit. J. Cancer <u>28</u>, 262 (1973).
81. HAMILTON-FAIRLEY, G., POWLES, R., CROWTHER, D.: Active immunotherapy of acute myeloid leukemias. In: Investigation and Stimulation of Immunity in Cancer Patients. (eds. G. Mathé, R. Weiner). Paris-Heidelberg: CNRS and Springer 1973.
82. VOGLER, W.R., CHAN, Y-K.: Effect of BCG in prolongation of remissions in acute myeloblastic leukemia. Proc. Amer. Ass. Cancer Res. <u>15</u>, 164 (1974).
83. MATHE, G., AMIEL, J.L., SCHWARZENBERG, L., SCHNEIDER, M., CATTAN, A., SCHLUMBERGER, J.R., HAYAT, M., DE VASSAL, F.: Démonstration de l'efficacité de l'immunothérapie active dans la leucémie aiguë lymphoblastique humaine. Rev. franc. Etudes clin. biol. <u>13</u>, 454 (1968).
84. SANTOS, G.W., OWENS, Jr., A.H.: Syngeneic and allogeneic marrow transplants in the cyclophosphamide pretreated rat. In: Advances in Transplantation, Proc. 1st Intern. Congress Transplant. Soc., p. 431. Copenhagen: Munkspaard 1968.
85. MATHE, G., AMIEL, J.L., SCHWARZENBERG, L., CHOAY, J., TROLARD, P., SCHNEIDER, M., HAYAT, M., SCHLUMBERGER, J.R., JASMIN, C.: Bone marrow graft in man after condioning by antilymphocytic serum. Brit. med. J. <u>2</u>, 131 (1970).
86. GRAW, Jr., R.H., ROGENTINE, Jr., G.N., LEVENTHAL, B.G., HALTERMAN, R.H., BERARD, C., HERZIG, G.P., YANKEE, R.A., WHANG PENG, J., KRUGER, G., HENDERSON, E.S.: Graft-versus-host reaction complicating HL-A-matched bone marrow transplantation. Lancet <u>2</u>, 1053 (1970).
87. MATHE, G., AMIEL, J.L., SCHWARZENBERG, L.: Bone marrow transplantation and leucocyte transfusions. Springfield, Ill.: Charles C Thomas 1971.
88. THOMAS, E.D., BRYANT, J.I., BUCKNER, C.D., CLIFT, R.A., FEFER, A., JOHNSON, F.L., NEIMAN, P., RAMBERG, R., STORB, R.: Leukemic transformation of engrafted human marrow cells in vivo. Lancet <u>1</u>, 1310 (1972).
89. ABU-ZAHRA, H., AMATO, D., AYE, M.T., BERGSAGEL, D.L., CLARYSSE, A.M., COWAN, D.H., FORNASIER, V.L., HASSELBACK, R., ISCOVE, N.N., McCULLOCH, E.A., MESSNER, H., MILLER, R.G., PHILLIPS, R.A., RAGAB, A.H., RIDER, W.D., SENN, J.S.: Bone marrow transplantation in patients with acute leukemia. Ser. Haematol. <u>5</u>, 189 (1972).
90. EORTC, Leukemia and Heamatosarcoma Cooperative Group: A second comparative trial of remission induction (by cytosine arabinoside given every 12 hours, or CAR and thioguanine, or CAR and daunotubicin) and maintenance therapy (by CAR or methylgag) in acute myeloid leukemia. Europ. J. Cancer <u>10</u>, 413 (1974).
91. SCHWARZENBERG, L., MATHE, G., POUILLART, P., WEINER, R., HAYAT, M., AMIEL, J.L., JASMIN, C., ROSENFELD, C., DE VASSAL, F., SCHNEIDER, M., CATTAN, A.: Comparative results obtained in the treatment of acute lymphoid leukemia and acute monocytoid leukemia. In: Nomenclature, Methodology and Results of Clinical Trials in Acute Leukemias, p. 160 (eds. G. Mathé, P. Pouillart, L. Schwarzenberg). Berlin-Heidelberg-New York: Springer 1973.

92. BEARD, M.E.J., HAMILTON-FAIRLEY, G.: Acute leukemia in adults. Semin. Hematol. 11, 5 (1974).
93. WILLOUGHBY, M.L.N.: Acute myeloblastic leukemia. Brit. med. J. 4, 337 (1974).
94. LEVI, J.A., WIERNIK, P.H., EGAN, J.J., SUTHERLAND, J.C.: Comparative study of 5-azacytidine and guanazole in previously treated adult non-lymphocytic leukemia. Proc. Am. Ass. Cancer Res. 16, 83 (1975).
95. VOGLER, W.R., MILLER, D., KELLER, J.W.: Remission induction in refractory myeloblastic leukemia with continuous infusion of 5-azacytidine. Proc. Am. Ass. Cancer Res. 16, 155 (1975).
96. CLARKSON, B.D., DOWLING, M.D., GEE. T.S., CUNNINGHAM, I.B., BURCHENAL, J.H.: Treatment of acute leukemia in adults. Cancer 36, 775 (1975)
97. HEWLETT, J.S., BALCERZAK, S., GUTTERMAN, J., FREIREICH, E.J.: Remission induction in adult acute leukemia by 10-day continuous intravenous infusion of ara-C, plus oncovin and prednisone. Maintenance with and without BCG. Proc. Am. Soc. Clin. Oncol. 16, 234 (1975).
98. STOUTENBOROUGH, K.A., MEYERS, M.C.: Cytosine arabinoside versus cyclophosphamide, vincristine, cytosine arabinoside and prednisone in the treatment of acute nonlymphocytic leukemia in adults. Proc. Am. Soc. Clin. Oncol. 16, 258 (1975).
99. EPPINGER-HELFT, M., PAVLOVSKY, S., SUAREZ, A., MURIEL, F.S., HIDALGO, G., et al.: Sequential therapy for induction and maintenance of remission in acute myeloblastic leukemia. Cancer 35, 347 (1975).
100. GAHRTON, G., ENGSTEDT, L., FRANZEN, S., GULLBRING, B., HOLM, G. et al.: Induction of remission with L-asparaginase, cyclophosphamide, cytosine arabinoside, and prednisolone in adult patients with acute leukemia. Cancer 34, 472 (1974).
101. MANASTER, J., COWAN, D.H., CURTIS, J.E., HASSELBACK, R., BERGSAGEL, D.E.: Remission maintenance of acute nonlymphoblastic leukemia with BCNU(NSC-409962) and cyclophosphamide (NSC-26271). Cancer Chemother. Rep. Part 1, 59, 537 (1975).
102. SAKURAI, M., SANDBERG, A.A.: Chromosomes and causation of human cancer and leukemia. 33, 1548 (1974).
103. MATHE, G., SCHWARZENBERG, L., POUILLART, P., OLDHAM, R., WEINER, R. et al.: Two epipodophyllotoxin derivatives, VM 26 and VP 16213, in the treatment of leukemias,hematosarcomas, and lymphomas. Cancer 34, 985 (1974).
104. GEISER, C.F., MITUS, J.W.: Acute monocytic leukemia in children and its response to vinblastine. Cancer Chemother. Rep. Part 1, 59, 385 (1975).
105. BERNARD, J., WEIL, M., FLANDRIN, G., SEBAOUN, G., DANIEL, M.T., JACQUILLAT, C.: Clinical study of acute monoblastic leukemia. Proc. Am. Ass. Cancer Res. 16, 201 1975.
106. VOGLER, W.R., CHAN, Y.K.: Prolonging remission in myeloblastic leukaemia by Tice-strain bacillus Calmette-Guerin. Lancet 2, 128 (1974).
107. GUTTERMAN, J.U., RODRIGUEZ, V., MAVLIGIT, G., BURGESS, M.A., GEHAN, E. et al.: Chemo-immunotherapy of adult acute leukemia: prolongation of remission in myeloblastic leukemia with BCG. Lancet 2, 1405 (1974).
108. GUTTERMAN, J.U., HERSH, E.M., McCREDIE, K.B., RODRIGUEZ, V., BODEY, G.P., FREIREICH, E.J.: BCG immunotherapy in remission maintenance of adult acute leukemia: a 3 year study. Proc. Am. Ass. Cancer Res. 16, 127 (1975).
109. McCREDIE, K.B., HESTER, J.P., GUTTERMAN, J.U., GEHAN, E.A., FREIREICH, E.J.: Survival of adults with acute leukemia. Proc. Am. Ass. Cancer Res. 16, 141 (1975).

110. BEKESI, J.G., HOLLAND, J., CUTTNER, J., SILVER, R., COLEMAN, M., JAROWSKI, C., VINCEGUERRA, V.: Immunotherapy in acute myelocytic leukemia with neuraminidase treated allogeneic myeloblasts with or without MER. Proc. Amer. Ass. Cancer Res. 17, 184 (1976)

111. RUSSELL, J.A., CHAPUIS, B., POWLES, R.L.: Various uses of BCG and allogeneic acute leukemia cells to treat patients with acute myelogenous leukemia. Cancer Immunol. Immunother. 1, 87 (1976)

Chapter 16
Chronic Myeloid Leukemia

Chronic myeloid leukemia (CML) is a disseminated, progressive proliferation of the cells of the granulocytic series at all stages of maturation (1). The increase (10 to 150 times the normal) in the total
granulocyte mass (TGM) is the main feature. The bone marrow is hyper-
cellular with a preponderance of the granulocytic cell series at all
stages of maturation. The peripheral blood shows increased numbers of
mature and immature polymorphonuclear cells (predominantly myelocytes
and metamyelocytes), basophils and eosinophils. Splenomegaly and sternal
tenderness are the most frequent physical findings.

The Philadelphia chromosome (Ph') is found in 85 percent of cases; this
is an abnormal G chromosome, recently identified as number 22 (2, 3).
New evidence suggests that it represents a translocation between the
long arm of 22 and the long arm of 9 (4). Ph' is found in the myeloid
precursors, erythroblasts, and megakaryocytes (5), which indicates that
they are all derived from the same abnormal stem cell. Though stem cell
proliferation tends toward granulopoiesis, other cell lines, especially the megakaryocytic series, may be similarly affected. Some authors
consider CML as a variant with granulocytic predominance of the so-
called "myeloproliferative diseases" (6). Ph'-negative cases tend to
be different from the typical Ph'-positive CML (7-9). They are older,
present with low platelet and leukocyte levels, and have more myeloblasts in the bone marrow and peripheral blood. They respond less well
to chemotherapy,enter blastic crisis earlier (54) and have a shorter
median survival (8 months compared to 40 months for Ph'-positive CML).

CML typically runs a chronic course for months or years before changing,
in the majority of cases, into an acute blastic crisis.

Chemotherapy, splenic irradiation or radioactive isotopes can reduce
the expanded TGM; however, these treatments seem unable to eradicate
the abnormal population, since Ph' persists during such remissions.
"Total cell kill" cannot be attempted until we have determined whether
or not a normal hematopoietic stem cell is present beside the abnormal
one (Ph') (see p. 281). If there is none, a successful technique of
bone marrow transplantation would have to be available before total
cell kill can be attempted.

CML is one of the most responsive malignancies. Remissions can be obtained in approximately 90 percent. Induction of remission does not
result in significant prolongation of survival as is the case for acute
leukemias, but gives a striking improvement in the quality of life.

A. CHEMOTHERAPY

1. Remission Induction with Busulfan

Therapy with busulfan (BSF) is the treatment of choice in CML (10-14).
It occupies the place once held by radiotherapy or radioactive ^{32}P (15).
It was found to be superior to splenic irradiation, although neither
can prevent the occurence of blastic transformation (16). Busulfan is
given initially in relatively large doses, 0.075 to 0.1 mg/kg, or 3 to
4 mg/m^2 with a maximal dose of 6 mg/d. As a rule, the dose is halved
when the WBC drops by half, and then titrated until the WBC reaches
10,000 to 15,000/mm^3 when therapy is stopped. If it is not, irreversible
bone marrow aplasia may be the result. The WBC will often continue to
drop after therapy has been discontinued. One can also use a constant
dose of BSF and plot serial WBC's on a semilogarithmic scale. The leucocyte count falls exponentially and, by extrapolation, it can be estimated how long treatment would have to be continued to bring the WBC to
between 5,000 and 10,000/mm^3 (17). Subsequent remissions last longer
if this level is achieved (11). Platelets are sometimes more sensitive
than granulocytes and therapy must be discontinued if they drop below
100,000, regardless of the WBC count.

2. Maintenance Therapy with Busulfan

Once the TGM is reduced, which is reflected in a return of the peripheral counts and the enlarged spleen to normal, the cells can be kept
under control by either continuous or intermittent maintenance therapy
with BSF. In the former method, BSF is given in smaller doses, daily,
every other day, or twice weekly, to maintain the blood counts approximately within the normal range. The proponents of this method argue
that it is undesirable to allow overt relapse with its potential complications, or the possible development of irreversible manifestations.
With intermittent therapy, BSF is withheld once a remission is obtained
and is not restarted until the WBC reaches an arbitraty figure of 35,000
to 50.000/mm^3 (11). This ensures that the total duration of exposure
to BSF is considerably shorter, so protecting the patient against the
toxicity of long-term therapy. Another advantage of the intermittent
method is that the leukocyte doubling time can be calculated during
the first unmaintained remission. This parameter correlates with subsequent survival, patients with long DT's surviving longer (17). The
period of control may last for months up to several years. It has been
noted that with successive relapses the DT becomes progressively shorter
(12, 18) (Fig. 16-1). STRYCKMANS et al. predict that blastic crisis
will occur within 12 months once the DT of the leukocyte population
falls below 12 days (18).

Among the side-effects of BSF, we mention skin pigmentation (19), amenorrhea, pulmonary fibrosis (20-23), and a Addison-like syndrome (24, 25).
However, the most serious one is bone marrow aplasia. BSF is one of the
most frequent causes of fatal aplasia in patients referred to the hematologic intensive care unit of the ICIG.

3. Other Agents Effective in CML

Chlorambucil (26), uracil mustard (27), 6-MP (28), pipobroman (29),
piposulfan (30), mitomycin C (31), and demecolcine (32) have occasionally been used in treating CML, but none of these proved superior to
BSF. Two of the newer agents deserve discussion: hydroxyurea (HUR)
(33, 34) and dibromomannitol (DBM) (35-39). In a randomized trial DBM

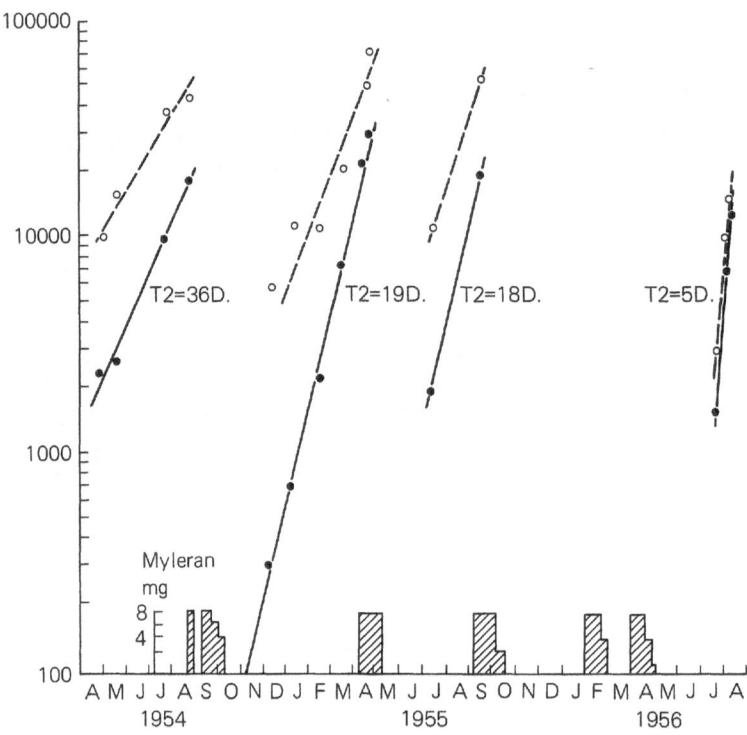

Fig. 16-1. Measurement of the doubling time of mature and immature myeloid cells in the peripheral blood during 4 successive·exacerbations in a patient with chronic myeloid leukemia.○ Circulating mature and immature myeloid cells/mm³. ● Circulating immature myeloid cells/mm³. (From STRYCKMANS et al. (18))

and BSF were equivalent as far as the rate of remission induction, duration of remission, the frequency of blastic transformation, and survival (39). Dibromomannitol was not particularly effective in busulfan-resistant CML (35). Hydroxyurea can induce remissions but, when treatment is stopped, the leukocyte count rises much faster than after a BSF induction. Continuous therapy is thus required. Hydroyurea and DBM are unlikely to replace BSF as the primary agent for CML but they can be tried in cases that have developed resistance to BSF. Table 16-1 tabulates the results obtained at the ICIG with different agents.

Hydroxyurea is often used at the ICIG precisely because it causes rapid remissions, of short duration if therapy is stopped. This ensures the availability of a pool of CML patients with elevated leucocyte counts who can be used as donors for white-cell transfusions (40). These have proven very useful in the prevention and control of infections in granulocytopenic patients (see Table 11-1). The survival of patients treated with intermittent HUR and repeated leucaphoresis is no different from that of patients treated more conventionally with BSF, DBM, ^{32}P and splenic irradiation (Fig. 16-2) (11, 16, 38, 41, 42).

Dibromodulcitol (DBD), and 3,3'-iminodi-1-1propanol, dimethanesulfonate (ester), p-toluenesulfonate (43) are new agents under investigation.

Table 16-1. Single agents for induction or remission in chronic myeloid leukemia

Drug	Number of courses	Complete remissions	Incomplete remissions	Failures	Fatal toxicity
Busulfan (1)	41	18	12	7	1[a]
Hydroxyurea (2)	43	1	39	2	1[a]
Dibromomannitol (3)	12	3	6	2	1[a]
Desacetyl-methyl-colchicine (4)	7	2	3	2	
Piposulfan (5)	10	3	4	2	1[a]

(1) 4-6 mg/d until remission
(2) 1,500-2,500 mg/d until remission, then 500 mg/d
(3) 250-500 mg/d for 7 days, every 15 days
(4) 1-3 mg/d until remission
(5) 25-50 mg/d for 20-30 days

[a] Bone marrow aplasia.

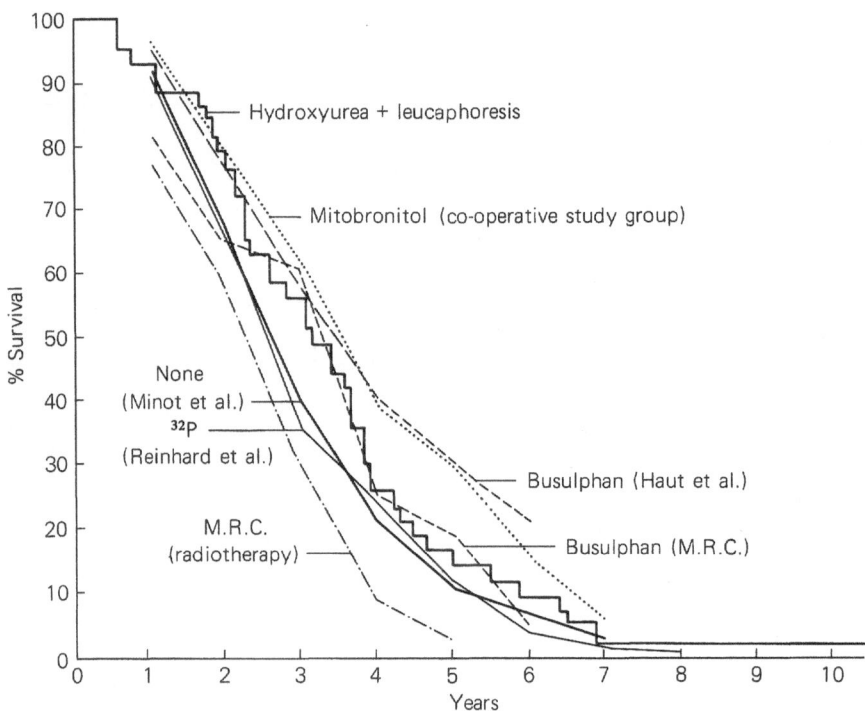

Fig. 16-2. *Cumulative survival time of patients subjected to hydroxy-urea + leucaphoresis compared with survival of patients submitted to other protocols. (From SCHWARZENBERG et al. (40))*

B. STRATEGY

Surgery and Radiotherapy

Radiotherapy was for half a century the preferred treatment for CML; it is now only occasionally used, for instance, for persistent spleno-megaly in cases where chemotherapy has controlled the leukocytosis.

It has been suggested that splenectomy early in the disease be recon-sidered to remove a large pool of granulocytes (44). Splenectomy per-formed during the first remission does not significantly prolong survi-val (Fig. 16-3) (40).

C. TREATMENT OF ACUTE BLASTIC TRANSFORMATION

The majority of patients with CML die in so-called "blastic crisis" (50-80 percent). Many consider it as part of the natural history of CML, the end phase for those who have not died as a result of a thera-peutic accident or an intercurrent complication. It is characterized by an increasing proportion of blast cells in the bone marrow and peri-pheral blood with progressive marrow failure (worsening of anemia, throm-bocytopenia), which is no longer responsive to previously effective therapy. The transition into blast crisis must be differentiated from

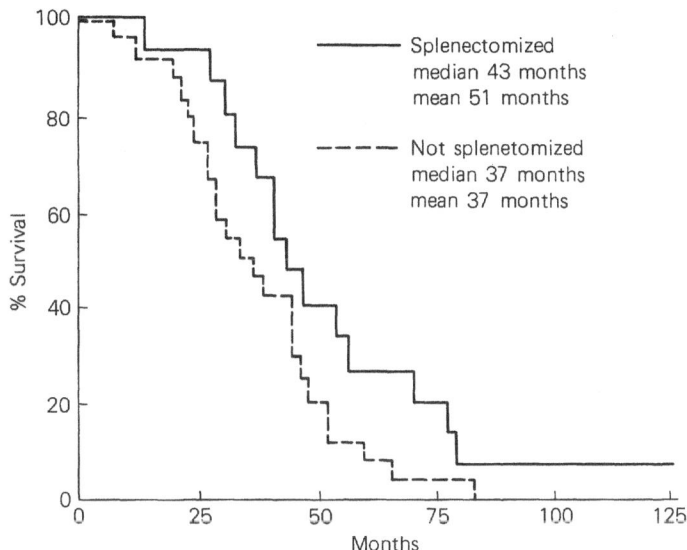

Fig. 16-3. Cumulative survival times of splenectomized and non-splenectomized patients with chronic myeloid leukemia. (From SCHWARZENBERG et al. (40))

the development of myelofibrosis. Chromosome studies indicate that blastic transformation represents a progression in a malignant process that has arisen by mutation. Many of the cytotoxic drugs used in AML are capable of reducing the number of blast cells but these reductions are short-lived, usually incomplete, and not accompanied by a regeneration of the normal hematopoietic elements (45, 46). FOLEY et al. obtained one CR and two PR in 13 patients with blastic crisis using a combination of VCR, PDN, MTX, and 6-MP (45). This combination was very toxic and resulted in four drug-related deaths. CANELLOS et al. obtained 6 CR (mean duration 5 months, range 1-9 months) and 3 PR in 30 patients treated with a combination of vincristine and prednisone (47, 48). This combination was selected in the hope that it might spare platelet and granulocyte reserves, while still having a cytotoxic effect on blast-cell proliferation. Our group (1) observed that the blasts either resemble lymphoblasts, in which case they are sensitive to VCR (Fig. 16-4), monoblasts, or, most frequently, myeloblasts. In the last case, we have tried cytosine arabinoside, but the results have been unsatisfactory. Table 16-2 shows the results obtained at the ICIG (49) and by CARBONE et al. (50) with various drugs and combinations. Most remissions are of short duration.

The ALGB has evaluated intravenous 6-MP, 6-TG plus azaserine, and a combination of CAR plus BCNU and CAR, BCNU, VCR plus PDN (56). None of the treatments were successful enough to warrant recommendation for general use against blastic crisis of CML. SPIERS et al. tried several combinations in 43 patients, most of them without impressive results (57). However, the use of seven or eight drugs (TRAMPCO or TRAMPCOL, i.e., 6-TG, DRB, CAR, MTX, PDN, CPM, VCR without or with L-asparaginase) in nine patients produced four satisfactory responses with a mean survival of more than nine months. Several single agents and various combinations did not appear to be satisfactory to VALLEJOS et al. at the M.D. Anderson hospital (54). COAP (CPM, VCR, CAR, PDN) produced the best

Table 16-2. Results of single agents and combination chemotherapy for induction of remission in blastic transformation of chronic myeloid leukemia (From CATTAN et al. (49), CARBONE et al. (50) and MATHE et al. unpubl.)

Drugs	Number of courses evaluated	Number of CR
Methotrexate	3	0
Cytosine arabinoside	10	1
BCNU	4	0
Methyl-GAG	16	2
L-asparaginase	1	0
Vincristine	10	3
Prednisone	4	1
CAR, PDN	1	0
MGGH, PDN	4	1
ASP, PDN	4	0
VCR, PDN	30	6
CAR, BCNU	13	1
DRB, VCR, PDN	1	0
MTX, 6-MP, VCR, PDN	13	1
CAR, MGGH, DRB, PDN	1	0

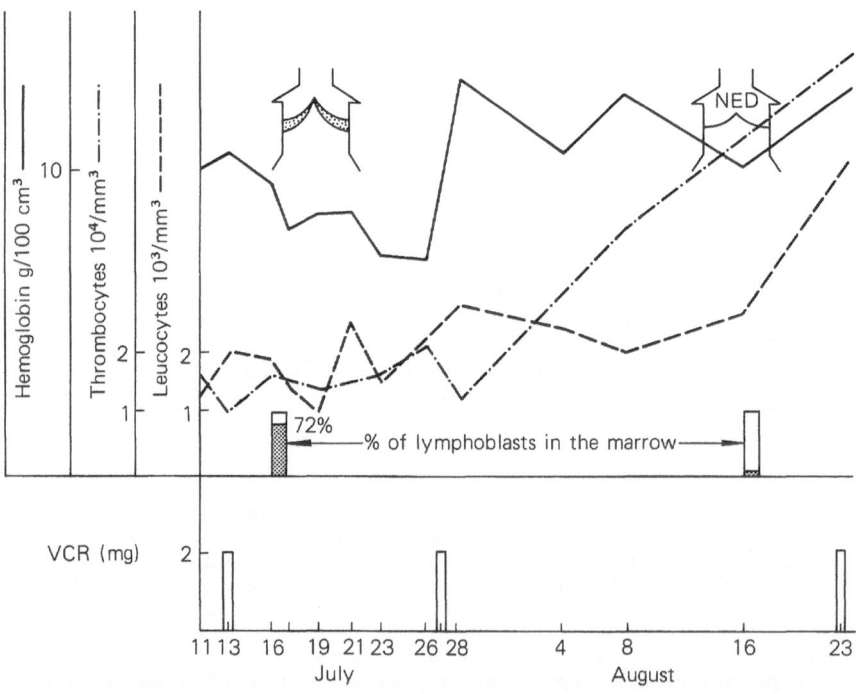

Fig. 16-4. Blastic transformation of chronic myeloid leukemia with blasts resembling lymphoblasts; induction of complete remission with vincristine

308

response with five remissions and one hematologic improvement in 11 patients.

CANELLOS et al., in a randomized trial, obtained 7 responses (2 CR) in 19 patients treated with vincristine plus prednisone and 4 responses (1 CR) in 12 patients receiving CAR plus 6-TG (58).

We were unable to observe any beneficial effect of splenectomy on the subsequent incidence and responsiveness of blastic crisis (Table 16-3) (40).

Table 16-3. Effect of splenectomy on course of blastic crisis (From SCHWARZENBERG et al. (40))

	Splenectomy	No Splenectomy
Blastic crisis	13/15	19/24
Complete remission obtained	2/13	3/19
Median survival time from onset of blastic crisis	2 months	1 month
Mean survival time from onset of blastic crisis	3.3 months	2.1 months

D. DISCUSSION

It appears that the survival of CML patients will not improve until we have learned to prevent or treat the blastic crisis. Some investigators are evaluating prophylactic antiblastic therapy with periodic administration of phase-dependent agents to eliminate possible developing clones of cells capable of causing a blastic transformation. The EORTC LEUKEMIA AND HEMATOSARCOMA GROUP is evaluating the effect of intermittent administration of VCR plus CAR. CLARKSON proposes more aggressive therapy at the time of diagnosis to eliminate the neoplastic population early in the disease, but assumes that a normal population of hematopoietic stem cells remains (51). The protocol consists of (1) splenic irradiation; (2) splenectomy; (3) three or more courses of CAR, 120 mg/m^2, i.v., and 6-thioguanine 100 mg/m^2, p.o., every 12 h; (4) L-asparaginase 8,000 u/m^2, i.v., for 14 days with vincristine 1.5 mg/m^2, i.v., on days 7 and 14; and (5) maintenance treatment with hydroxyurea (51). It is too soon to know whether survival will be affected. SOKAL et al. attack developing clones by immunologic stimulation (BCG plus leukemic cells) in an attempt to prevent blastic transformation (52).

Another potential new development is the use of maturation regulators. Indeed, leukemic myeloblasts that fail to mature into granulocytes in patients in the terminal phase may do so in vitro cultures.

Arguments in favor of further exploration of the role of leucaphoresis in the treament of CML were advanced by GATTI et al. (53).

REFERENCES

1. MATHE, G., RAPPAPORT, H.: Histological and cytological typing of
   the neoplastic diseases of the hematopoietic and lymphoid tissues.
   Geneva: W.H.O. (1973).
2. NOWELL, P.C., HUNGERFORD, D.A.: Chromosome studies in human leukemia. II. Chronic granulocytic leukemia. J. nat. Cancer Inst. 27,
   1013 (1961).
3. CASPERSSON, T., GAHRTON, G., LINDSTEN, J., ZECH, L.: Identification
   of the Philadelphia chromosome as a number 22 by quinacrine mustard
   fluorescence analysis. Exp. Cell Res. 63, 238 (1970).
4. ROWLEY, J.: A new consistent chromosomal abnormality in chronic
   myelogenous leukemia identified by quinacrine fluorescence and
   Giemsa staining. Nature 243, 290 (1973).
5. TRUJILLO, O.A., OHNO, S.: Chromosomal alteration of erythropoietic
   cells in chronic myeloid leukemia. Acta Hematol. 29, 311 (1963).
6. GILBERT, H.S., DAMESHEK, W.: The myeloproliferative disorders.
   Disease-a-Month, October (1970).
7. EZDINLI, E.Z., SOKAL, J.E., CROSSWHITE, L., SANDBERG, A.A.: Phila-
   delphia-chromosome-positive and -negative chronic myelocytic leukemia. Ann. intern. Med. 72, 175 (1970).
8. THEOLOGIDES, A.: Unfavorable signs in patients with chronic myelocytic leukemia. Ann. intern. Med. 76, 95 (1972).
9. BASERGA, I., CASTOLDI, G.I.: The Philadelphia chromosome. Europ.
   J. clin. Biol. Res. 18, 89 (1973).
10. GALTON, D.A.: Myleran in chronic myeloid leukemia. Lancet 1, 208
    (1953).
11. HAUT, A., ABBOTT, W.S., WINTROBE, M.M., CARTWRIGHT, G.E.: Busulfan
    in the treatment of chronic myelocytic leukemia. The effect of
    long-term intermittent chemotherapy. Blood 17, 1 (1961)
12. GALTON, D.A.G.: Chemotherapy of chronic myelocytic leukemia. Semi-
    nars Hematol. 6, 323 (1969).
13. HUGULEY, Jr., C.M.: Chronic myelocytic and chronic lymphocytic
    leukemia. Cancer 30, 1583 (1972).
14. SOKAL, J.E.: Current concepts in the treatment of chronic myelo-
    genous leukemia. Ann. Rev. Med. 24, 281 (1973).
15. OSGOOD, E.E.: Treatment of chronic leukemia. J. nucl. Med. 5, 139
    (1964).
16. Medical Research Council's Working Party for Therapeutic Trials in
    Leukaemia: Chronic granulocytic leukaemia: comparison of radio-
    therapy and busulphan therapy. Brit. med. J. 1, 201 (1968).
17. BERGSAGEL, D.E.: The chronic leukemias: A review of disease mani-
    festations and the aims of therapy. Canad. med. Ass. J. 96, 1615
    (1967).
18. STRYCKMANS, P.A., MANASTER, J., PELTZER, T., SOQUET, M., VAMECQ,
    G.: Cell proliferation in chronic myeloid leukemia under discon-
    tinuous treatment from diagnosis to blastic crisis. In: Advances
    in the treatment of acute (blastic) leukemias, p. 156 (ed. G. Mathé)
    Recent Results in Cancer Research, Vol. 30. Berlin-Heidelberg-New
    York: Springer-Verlag 1970.
19. MATHE, G., BRULE, G., DEBRAY, J., LAUFER, J.: Mélanodermies appa-
    rues après une longue administration de myleran chez trois patients
    atteints de leucémie myéloide chronique. Nouv. Rev. franc. Hématol.
    1, 624 (1961).
20. OLINER, H., SCHWARTZ, R., RUBIO, Jr., F., DAMESHEK, W.G.: Intersti-
    tial pulmonary fibrosis following busulfan therapy. Amer. J. Med.
    31, 134 (1961).
21. FEINGOLD, M.L., KOSS, L.G.: Effects of long-term administration of
    busulfan. Report of a patient with generalized nuclear abnormali-
    ties, carcinoma of vulva, and pulmonary fibrosis. Arch. intern.
    Med. 124, 66 (1969).

22. KIRSCHNER, R.H., ESTERLY, Y.R.: Pulmonary lesions associated with busulfan therapy of chronic myelogenous leukemia. Cancer 27, 1074 (1971).
23. MIN, K.W., GYORKEY, F.: Interstitial pulmonary fibrosis, atypical epithelial changes and bronchiolar cell carcinoma following busulfan therapy. Cancer 22, 1027 (1968).
24. KYLE, R.A., SCHWARTZ, R.S., OLINER, H.L., DAMESHEK, W.: A syndrome resembling adrenal cortical insufficiency associated with long-term busulfan therapy. Blood 18, 497 (1961).
25. VIVACQUA, R.J., HAURANI, F.I., ERSLEY, A.: Selective pituitary insufficiency secondary to busulfan. Ann. intern. Med. 67, 380 (1967).
26. RUNDLES, R.W., GRIZZLE, Y., BELL, W.N., CORBEY, C.D., PROMMEYER, Jr., W.B., GREENBERG, B.G., HUGULEY, Jr., C.M., JAMES, C.W., JONES, Jr., R., LARSEN, W.E., LOEB, V., LEONE, L.A., PALMER, J.G., RISER, Jr., W.H., WILSON, S.J.: Comparison of chlorambucil and myleran in chronic lymphocytic and granulocytic leukemia. Amer. J. Med. 27, 424 (1959).
27. ROBERTSON, J.H.: Uracil mustard in the treatment of thrombocythemia. Blood 35, 288 (1970).
28. HUGULEY, Jr., C.M., GRIZZLE, J., RUNDLES, R.W., BELL, W.N., CORLEY, C.C., FROMMEYER, W.B., GREENBERG, B.G., HAMMACK, W., HERION, J.C., JAMES, G.W., LARSEN, W.E., LOEB, V., LEONE, L.A., PALMER, J.G., WILSON, S.J.: Comparison of 6-mercaptopurine and busulfan in chronic granulocytic leukemia. Blood 21, 89 (1963).
29. BOND, W.H., ROHN, R.J., HODES, M.E., YARDLEY, J.M.: Clinical evaluation of compound 8103-Abbott. Cancer Chemother. Rep. 16, 209 (1962).
30. KENIS, Y.: Effect of piposulfan on malignant lymphomas and solid tumors. Cancer Chemother. Rep. 52, 433 (1968).
31. HOSHINO, A.: Mitomycin C in the treatment of chronic myelogenous leukemia. Nagoya J. med. Sci. 29, 317 (1967).
32. MOESCHLIN, S., MEYER, H., LICHTMAN, A.: Ein neues Colchicum Nebenalkaloid (Demecolcin Ciba) als Cytostaticum myeloischer Leukämine. Schweiz. Med. Wschr. 83, 990 (1953).
33. FISHBEIN, W.N., CARBONE, P.P., FREIREICH, E.J., MSRA, D., FREI, E. III,: Clinical trials of hydroxyurea in patients with cancer and leukemia. Clin. Pharmacol. Ther. 5, 574 (1964).
34. KENNEDY, B.J.: Hydroxyurea therapy in chronic myelogenous leukemia. Cancer 29, 1052 (1972).
35. ECKHARDT, S., SELLEI, C., HOKVATH, I.P., INSTITORISZ, L.: Effect of 1,6 dibromo-1-6 deoxy d-mannitol on chronic granulocytic leukemia. Cancer Chemother. Rep. 33, 57 (1963).
36. MATHE, G., SCHNEIDER, M., CATTAN, A., SCHWARZENBERG, L., AMIEL, J.L.: Essai de traitement de la leucémie myéloide chronique par le dibromomannitol. Presse méd. 72, 2185 (1964).
37. CASAZZA, A.R., CAHN, E.L., CARBONE, P.P.: Preliminary studies with dibromomannitol (NSC-94100) in patients with chronic myelogenous leukemia. Cancer Chemother. Rep. 51, 91 (1967).
38. DIBROMOMANNITOL COOPERATIVE STUDY GROUP: Survival of chronic myeloid leukaemia patients treated by dibromomannitol. Europ. J. Cancer 9, 583 (1973).
39. CANELLOS, G.P., YOUNG, R.C., NIEMAN, P., DEVITA, V.T.: Dibromomannitol (DBM) in the treatment of chronic granulocytic leukemia: a randomized comparison with busulfan (B). Cancer Chemother. Rep. 57, 97 (1973).
40. SCHWARZENBERG, L., MATHE, G., POUILLART, P., SCHNEIDER, M., DE VASSAL, F., HAYAT, M., AMIEL, J.L., SCHLUMBERGER, J.R., JASMIN, C., ROSENFELD, C.: Chemotherapy with hydroxyurea, leucaphoresis and splenectomy in the treatment of chronic myeloid leukemia at the problastic phase. Brit. med. J., 1, 700 (1973).

41. MINOT, G.R., BUCKMAN, T.E., ISAACS, R.: Chronic myelogenous leukemia, age, incidence, duration and benefit derived from irradiation. J. Amer. Med. Ass. 82, 1489 (1924).
42. REINHARDT, E.H., NEEZLY, C.L., SAMPLES, D.M.: Radioactive phosphorus in the treatment of chronic leukemias. Long-term results over a period of 15 years. Ann. intern. Med. 50, 942 (1959).
43. HIRANO, M., MIURA, M., KAKIZAWA, H., MORITA, A., UETANI, T., OHNO, R., KAWASHIMA, K., NISHIWAKI, H., YAMADA, K.: Treatment of chronic myelogenous leukemia with 3,3'-iminodi-1-propanol, dimethanesulfonate (ester), p-toluenesulfonate (NSC-140117) given orally. Cancer Chemother. Rep. 56, 335 (1972).
44. SPIERS, A.S.: Surgery in management of patients with leukemia. Brit. med. J. 3, 528 (1973).
45. FOLEY, H.T., BENNETT, J.M., CARBONE, P.P.: Combination chemotherapy in accelerated phase of chronic granulocytic leukemia. Arch. intern. Med. 123, 166 (1969).
46. BRIERE, J., REYES, F., BILSKI-PASQUIER, G.: Les épisodes aigus terminaux des leucémies chroniques. Rev. Méd. (Paris) 313 (1970)
47. CANELLOS, G.P., DEVITA, V.T., WHANG-PENG, J., CARBONE, P.P.: Hematologic and cytogenetic remission of blastic transformation in chronic granulocytic leukemia. Blood 38, 671 (1971).
48. CANELLOS, G.P., WHANG-PENG, J., SCHNIPPER, L., BROWN, C.H. III.: Prolonged cytogenetic and hematologic remission of blastic transformation in chronic granulocytic leukemia. Cancer 30, 288 (1972).
49. CATTAN, A., MATHE, G., AMIEL, J.L., SCHLUMBERGER, J.R., SCHWARZENBERG, L., SCHNEIDER, M., BERUMEN, L.: Treatment of blastic crisis in chronic myeloid leukemia. In: Advances in the Treatment of Acute Blastic Leukemias, p. 152 (ed. G. Mathé). Berlin-Heidelberg-New York: Springer 1970.
50. CARBONE, P.P., CANELLOS, G.P., DE VITA, V.T.: Therapy of the blastic phase of chronic granulocytic leukemia. In: Advances in the Treatment of Acute Blastic Leukemias, p. 142 (ed. G. Mathé). Berlin-Heidelberg-New York: Springer 1970.
51. DOWLING, M.D., HOPFAN, S., KNAPPER, W.H., VAARTAJA, T., GEE, T., HAGHBIN, M., CLARKSON, B.D.: Attempt to induce true remission in chronic myelogenous leukemia (CML). Proc. Amer. Ass. Cancer Res. 15, 189 (1974).
52. SOKAL, J.E., AUNGST, C.W., GRACE, J.T.: Immunotherapy of myeloid leukemia. Ann. intern. Med. 76, 878 (1972).
53. GATTI, R.A., ROBINSON, W.A., DEINARD, A.S., NESBIT, M., McCULLOUGH, J.J., BALLOW, M., GOOD, R.A.: Cyclic leukocytosis in chronic myelogenous leukemia: New perspectives on pathogenesis and therapy. Blood 41, 771 (1973).
54. VALLEJOS, C.S., TRUJILLO, J.M., CORK, A., BODEY, G.P., McCREDIE, K.B., FREIREICH, E.J.: Blastic crisis in chronic granulocytic leukemia: experience in 39 patients. Cancer 34, 1806 (1974).
55. LEVIN, W.C., MIMS, C.H., HAUT, A.: Dibromomannitol: a clinical study of previously treated patients with refractory chronic myelocytic leukemia and blastic transformation. Cancer Chemother. Rep. Part 1, 58, 223 (1974).
56. HAYES, D.M., ELLISON, R.R., GLIDEWELL, O., HOLLAND, J.F., SILVER, R.T.: Chemotherapy for the terminal phase of chronic myelocytic leukemia. Cancer Chemother. Rep. Part 1, 233 (1974).
57. SPIERS, A.D.S., COSTELLO, C., CATOVSKY, D., GALTON, D.A.G., HOLDMAN, G.M.: Chronic granulocytic leukemia: multiple drug chemotherapy for acute transformation. Brit. Med. J. 3, 77 (1974).
58. CANELLOS, G.P., YOUNG, R.C., CHABNER, B.A., SCHEIN, P.S., WHANG-PENG, J., DEVITA, V.T.: Chemotherapy of the blastic phase of chronic granulocytic leukemia: Prospective comparison of vincristine/prednisone with cytosine arabinoside/6-thioguanine and effect of prior splenectomy. Proc. Am. Soc. Clin. Oncol. 16, 252 (1975).

Chapter 17

Polycythemia Vera (Vaquez-Osler) and Myelosclerosis with Myeloid Metaplasia

POLYCYTHEMIA VERA

Polycythemia vera (PV) is defined as a slowly progressive panmyelosis
(mean survival 13 years), characterized by persistent erythrocytosis,
leukocytosis, thrombocytosis, increased total red cell mass, hypervolemia, and severe irreversible hyperplasia of the bone marrow, involving
the cells of the normoblastic, granulocytic, and megakaryocytic series.
PV may often progress to myelosclerosis with myeloid metaplasia, at
times to "acute leukemia" or "blastic crisis", and occasionally to erythroleukemia or acute erythremia (1). Splenomegaly is usually present.
The leukocyte alkaline phosphatase is elevated. Most of the symptoms
are related to the expanded red cell mass. This increase must be documented by a direct measurement of the RBC mass. Thrombosis, embolism
and/or hemorrhage are common complications and should be prevented.
It is essential to differentiate polycythemia vera from stress polycythemia and secondary erythrocytosis caused by inappropriate or compensatory erythropoietin elaboration (2, 3).

Therapy can be either symptomatic, through removal of the endproduct
of proliferation by phlebotomy, or seek to correct the panmyelosis by
means of myelosuppressive agents. Both methods are often used, in combination or sequentially. Since PV runs a relatively benign and prolonged course, therapy must not be aggressive and should be such as to
be given over extended periods.

A. CHEMOTHERAPY

Alkylating agents are the cytotoxic drugs most commonly used in PV.
Chlorambucil (CLB) (6-10 mg, qd), cyclophosphamide (CPM) (100-150 mg,
qd), busulfan (BSF) (4-6 mg, qd) (4, 5) and melphalan (MPH) (4-6 mg,
qd) (6) have replaced nitrogen mustard, TEM and thioTEPA (7). There
are no randomized trials comparing the relative merits of these four
alkylating agents in PV. All control the excessive proliferation of the
three hematopoietic cell lines in 80-90 percent of cases. A decrease
in WBC and platelet count precedes the effect on the hematocrit (Hct),
which reaches its maximum in 3-4 months. The effect on splenomegaly is
more variable. The spleen disappears in 40-76 percent of patients, chlorambucil being most effective in this regard. Unmaintained remissions
last twice as long for BSF (15 months) as for CPM and CLB (6 months)
(Fig. 17-1) (5). BSF, the most effective agent, is also the most dangerous one because of the high risk of severe and prolonged thrombocytopenia (8). Cyclophosphamide is relatively platelet-sparing, but causes more side-effects (GI distress, dysuria, hematuria) than the other
alkylating agents. One the Hct has been stabilized at near normal

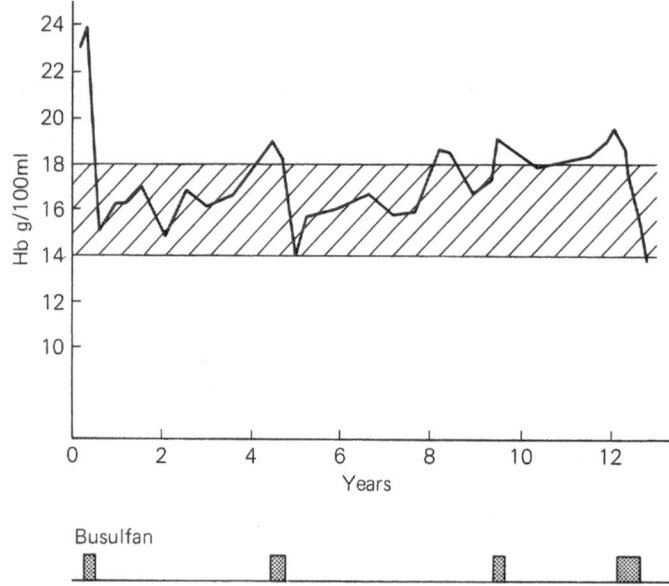

Fig. 17-1. Effect of busulfan (4 courses over 12 years) on the hemo-globin level in a patient with polycythemia vera

levels, maintenance therapy, starting with approximately one-half of the induction therapy, may be indicated in cases with rapid proliferation.

Prolonged BSF therapy is best avoided because of the side-effects associated with long-term therapy and the risk of thrombocytopenia and delayed aplasia.

Antimetabolites such as CAR (9), MTX (9), azauridine (10) and 6-MP (11) are inferior to alkylating agents (9). Neither hydroxyurea (9), dibromomannitol (12, 13), pipobroman (14-16), nor piposulfan (17) have replaced the oral alkylating agents in the primary therapy of PV.

B. STRATEGY

1. Phlebotomy

Some form of therapy is often indicated when the diagnosis of PV is made, especially to prevent the frequent episodes of thrombosis, embolism and/or hemorrhage (50 percent mortality in the first 18 months in untreated patients).

Phlebotomy is the preferred immediate therapy to relieve symptoms and reduce the total RBC mass. Any form of myelosuppressive therapy requires several months to reach its maximum effect. DAMESHEK (18) advocated that the majority of patients could be treated by phlebotomies alone. Following an initial series of venesections, the degree of erythroid activity is monitored by serial Hct determinations. In patients with relatively indolent erythroid activity, 4-6 phlebotomies a year may suffice to maintain a normal Hct. It may be continued, often for years, as long as no bothersome manifestations or complications of panmyelosis are present or imminent.

2. Myelosuppressive Therapy

The advocates of myelosuppressive therapy for PV argue that it has an effect, not only on the erythroid mass, but also on splenomegaly and increased granulocyte, platelet, and uric acid production.

Myelosuppressive therapy is indicated when phlebotomy is required rather frequently to control the expanded RBC mass, or when other manifestations of panmyelosis demand correction. Cytotoxic drugs and radioactive ^{32}P are equally effective and can produce long remissions, even without maintenance therapy. The long-term results of the EORTC Leukemia Hematosarcoma Group trial (BSF vs. ^{32}P) and the Polycythemia Vera Study Group (phlebotomy vs. CLB vs. ^{32}P) (19) will have to be known before a definitive position can be taken up with regard to their relative merits. ^{32}P is easy to use, its effect is predictable in most cases, its side-effects are few, and many fewer patient visits are required than for chemotherapy (20). A major concern of its opponents is the definite risk of a leukemogenic action of ionizing irradiation (7). The advocates object that the benefits conferred on the patient in terms of reduced morbidity and prolonged survival outweigh the possible risk of acute leukemia. Furthermore, uncertainty continues as to whether the increased frequency of acute leukemia is the result of prolonged survival thanks to radioisotopic therapy, (21, 22) or of the leukemogenic effect of radiation in a condition already predisposed to leukemic transformation (7).

Hyperuricemia and hyperuricaciduria can be effectively controlled with allopurinol. Androgens may be useful to stimulate erythropoiesis in the stage of myelosclerosis with myeloid metaplasia.

Splenectomy may be indicated in selected cases of severe hemolysis and "hypersplenism," provided that the spleen is not the major site of erythropoietic activity (8).

The leukemic transformation should be treated like classic AML or like a blastic crisis in CML.

MYELOSCLEROSIS WITH MYELOID METAPLASIA

This condition is defined as a progressive panmyelosis characterized by intramedullary fibrosis, atypical megakaryocytic proliferation, and myeloid metaplasia in which all three types of myeloid cells are represented. The metaplasia is usually limited to the spleen, liver, and lymph nodes, but may occasionally involve other sites. The disease is frequently associated with osteosclerosis. A blastic crisis may occur terminally (1). Primary myelofibrosis must be differentiated from forms secondary to the effects of chemicals, physical agents, infection, and malignancy (3).

Symptoms and findings are related to massive splenomegaly and progressive marrow failure with anemia, but leukocyte and platelet counts may be variable (2, 3, 23).

STRATEGY

The management of myelofibrosis with myeloid metaplasia is difficult and controversial, reflecting the lack of a uniformly effective therapy (23). Many asymptomatic patients are better off if left untreated.

Splenic irradiation, ^{32}P and alkylating agents (e.g., BSF) (24, 25) can reduce spleen size and the peripheral WBC and platelet count (if they are elevated), but this is rarely associated with clinical improvement or any prolongation of survival. These therapeutic measures have a very small margin of safety in the presence of an already compromised bone marrow and may precipitate severe cytopenia. A limited dosage schedule often makes it difficult to obtain splenic shrinkage.

Androgens and steroids are rarely very effective. However, they remain the most popular form of therapy because they are the least dangerous, though not devoid of serious side-effects; anemia may improve with their prolonged administration (26, 27).

Splenectomy has both its proponents and opponents. It may be indicated in selected cases where it can be demonstrated that the spleen is more harmful than beneficial in maintaining a normal blood count (3). In some cases, an acceleration of the extramedullary hematopoiesis occurs post-splenectomy in the liver, lymph nodes, and other sites, with increasing leukocyte and platelet counts.

REFERENCES

1. MATHE, G., RAPPAPORT, H.: Histological and cytological typing of the neoplastic diseases of the hematopoietic and lymphoid tissues, Geneva: W.H.O. 1973.
2. GILBERT, H.S., DAMESHEK, W.: The myeloproliferative disorders. Disease-a-Month October (1970).
3. GILBERT, H.S.: The spectrum of myeloproliferative disorders. Med. Clin. N. Amer. 57, 355 (1973).
4. ISRAELS, M.C.G.: Treatment and prognosis of polycythaemia managed by non-radioactive methods. Proc. Roy. Soc. Med. 59, 1100 (1966).
5. GILBERT, H.S.: Problems relating to control of polycythemia vera: the use of alkylating agents. Blood 32, 500 (1968).
6. LOGUE, G.L., GUTTERMAN, J.U., McGINN, T.G., LASZIO, J., RUNDLES, R.W.: Melphalan therapy of polycythemia vera. Blood 36, 70 (1970).
7. MODAN, B.: The polycythemic disorders. Springfield Ill.: Charles C. Thomas 1971.
8. WASSERMAN, L.R., GILBERT, H.S.: The treatment of polycythemia vera. Med. Clin. N. Amer. 50, 1051 (1966).
9. NAJEAN, Y., DRESCH, C., RAIN, J.D., DELOBEL, J., PECKING, A.: Les élements du choix thérapeutique dans les polyglobulies vraies. 1. L'efficacité de la chimiothérapie. Nouv. Press. Méd. 2, 1431 (1973).
10. DECONTI, R.C., CALABRESI, P.: Treatment of polycythemia vera with azauridine and azaribine. Ann. intern. Med. 73, 575 (1970).
11. SHULLENBERGER, C.C.: Long-range treatment of polycythemia vera with 6-mercaptopurine. Cancer Chemother. Rep. 16, 251 (1962).
12. SZENTKLARAY, J.: Evaluation of the therapeutic effect of myelobromol on polycythemia vera based on five years' observation. Orv. Hetil, 110, 651 (1969).
13. TURA, S., BACCARANI, M.: The management of polycythaemia vera with dibromomannitol. Haematologia. 4, 67 (1970).
14. MONTO, R.W., TENPAS, A., BATTLE, Jr., J.D., ROHN, R.J., LOUIS, J., LOUIS, N.B.: A-8103 in polycythemia. J. Amer. med. Ass. 190, 833 (1964).
15. BILSKI-PASQUIER, G., BLANC, C.M., BOUSSER, J.: Traitement de la polycythémie de Vaquez par le 1-4-bis(3 bromopropionyl-pipérazine). Etude de 36 cas, Presse méd. 76, 1953 (1968).
16. COUNCIL ON DRUGS: Evaluation of two antineoplastic agents, pipo-broman (vercyte) and thioguanine. J. Amer. med. Ass. 200, 619 (1967).

17. NELSON, N.A., TALLEY, R.W., REED, M.L., EVANS, A.M., ISAACS, B.L., HUFFMAN, P., LOUIS, J.: Midwest cooperative group evaluation of piposulfan (A-20968) in cancer. Clin. Pharmacol. Ther. $\underline{8}$, 385 (1967).
18. DAMESHEK, W.: The case for phlebotomy in polycythemia vera. Blood 32, 488 (1968).
19. WASSERMAN, L.R.: The treatment of polycythemia. A panel discussion. Introduction. Blood $\underline{32}$, 483 (1968).
20. OSGOOD, E.E.: The case for ^{32}P in treatment of polycythemia vera. Blood $\underline{32}$, 492 (1968).
21. LAWRENCE, J.H., WINCHELL, H.S., DONALD, W.G.: Leukemia in polycythemia vera. Relationship to splenic myeloid metaplasia and therapeutic radiation dose. Ann. intern. Med. $\underline{70}$, 763 (1969).
22. OSGOOD, E.E.: Contrasting incidence of acute monocytic and granulocytic leukemias in P^{32}-treated patients with polycythemia vera and chronic lymphocytic leukemia. J. Lab. clin. Med. $\underline{64}$, 560 (1964).
23. WARD, H.P., BLOCK, M.H.: The natural history of agnogenic myeloid metaplasia (AMM) and a critical evaluation of its relationship with the myeloproliferative syndrome. Medicine $\underline{50}$, 357 (1971).
24. BOURONCLE, B.A., DOAN, C.A.: Myelofibrosis: clinical, hematologic and pathologic study of 110 patients. Amer. J. med. Sci. $\underline{243}$, 697 (1962).
25. SILVER, R.T., JENKINS, Jr., D.E., ENGLE, Jr., R.L.: Use of testosterone and busulfan in the treatment of myelofibrosis with myeloid metaplasia. Blood $\underline{23}$, 341 (1964).
26. KENNEDY, B.J.: Effect of androgenic hormone in myelofibrosis. J. Amer. med. Ass. $\underline{182}$, 116 (1962).
27. GARDNER, F.H., NATHAN, D.G.: Androgens and erythropoiesis. III. Further evaluation of testosterone treatment of myelofibrosis. New. Engl. J. Med. $\underline{274}$, 420 (1966).

Chapter 18
Chronic Lymphoid Leukemia

Chronic lymphoid leukemia (CLL) is a disseminated neoplastic proliferation of cells with the morphological characteristics of mature lymphocytes (1). Bone marrow, lymphoid tissues, and eventually other tissues
are infiltrated by lymphoid cells. For some time it was thought that
these cells, which resemble morphologically mature lymphocytes, were
physiologically immature, since phytohemagglutinin (PHA) transforms
only the same absolute number of lymphocytes in CLL patients as in normal individuals (2). Now we know that PHA stimulates only T lymphocytes
(3). Recent studies suggest that the excessive lymphocytes in CLL are
B lymphocytes (2, 46). The presence of immunoglobulins on their surface
supports this hypothesis (4, 5).

It is not clearly known to what degree the increase in lymphoid mass
results from excessive production or from accumulation of lymphocytes
due to a defect in their removal mechanism, in other words a prolongation of survival (47). DAMESHEK (6) was among those who believe that the
disease is due to accumulation of a clone of immunologically incompetent
lymphocytes, which do not function but survive for a long time and gradually accumulate.

CLL runs a chronic course. The median survival of untreated cases is
slightly over 3 years but ranges from a few weeks to over 20 years. Two
types of CLL, or two phases in its course, can be recognized clinically.
The first phase, referred to as "indolent" disease, is relatively asymptomatic (7). The lymphocyte count rises very slowly or remains stable
for prolonged periods; neither lymphadenopathy nor splenomegaly are impressive. Systemic symptoms are absent and there is no evidence of marrow failure. The second, active phase is characterized by a steadily increasing lymphoid mass, systemic symptoms (fever, night sweats, weight
loss, decreased performance status), immunoincompetence, and bone marrow
insufficiency. Anemia, bleeding, and susceptibility to infections, especially viral (Herpes zoster, generalized vaccinia as a result of small
pox vaccination), are common complications. Blastic transformation, as
seen in AML, does not occur. The patient may be at either clinical stage
at the time of diagnosis. The need for and type of therapy differs with
this clinical stage.

A variety of complications are seen in the later stages. Anemia is a
common problem. An autoimmune hemolytic anemia occurs in approximately
15 percent of patients; in others anemia is associated with the "packed-
marrow syndrome." The pathogenesis of the suppression of erythropoiesis
is unknown, but it is unlikely to be just a problem of space (8).

Hypo-γ-globulinemia and impairment of both humoral and cellular immunity tend to become more severe as the disease progresses. Anergy is associated with more aggressive disease and poorer prognosis (48).

A. CHEMOTHERAPY

1. Remission Induction

Chemotherapy is the treatment modality used most frequently in the management of CLL. However, complete remissions as seen in acute leukemias are rare (9, 10). Tumor regressions (decrease in size of lymph nodes and spleen, and a fall in the number of lymphocytes in the blood and marrow) are rarely complete and not always accompanied by complete restoration of the hematopoietic function (or remission).

Chlorambucil (CLB) is the drug most commonly used for CLL. It appears as effective as any other drug, and is relatively nontoxic and easy to use. The induction dose is 4 to 8 mg/m² or 0.1 to 0.2 mg/kg, p.o. daily. It is customary to halve the dose once the WBC falls by half. The response rate is 50 to 80 percent, depending on the criteria (11-14). The rate of fall of the WBC is dose-related, and it may take 1 to 3 months to reach 10,000 to 15,000. Despite the WBC reduction, lymphocytosis often persists. Hematocrit (Hct), neutrophil, and platelet counts may improve or deteriorate.

A number of other drugs are capable of inducing response rates probably not unlike those obtained with CLB. However, they have never displaced CLB as the primary agent for CLL because they are more myelotoxic. Among these are HN2 (15), cyclophosphamide (16), melphalan, triethylene-melamine (17), streptonigrin (18), and mitoclomine (19, 50) (Fig. 18-1). They may be useful in cases of primary (30 percent of CLL) or secondary resistance to CLB. Because of the kinetic characteristics of the malignant cells in CLL, one would not except significant responses to phase-dependent agents for induction.

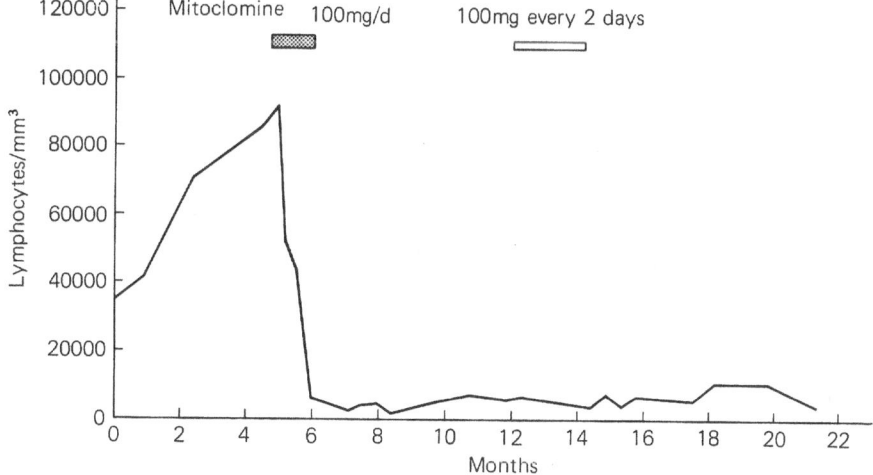

Fig. 18-1. Effect of mitoclomine on the peripheral blood lymphocytes in a patient with chronic lymphoid leukemia

Prednisone (PDN) has been used in CLL, either for its lympholytic effect or for symptomatic therapy. Regressions in the size of lymph nodes, and

319

less often of the spleen, may be dramatic but temporary (20, 21). The initial effect on the lymphocyte count is often a paradoxical increase, while the lymphoid organs melt away. It is thought to be a result of flooding of the blood by the lymphocytes discharged from the rapidly shrinking lymphoid tissues. An improvement in the Hct and platelet count may be noted. The major advantage of PDN is that it is not myelotoxic. It can therefore be used as part of the initial therapy in patients that present severe marrow insufficiency (anemia, thrombocytopenia) which precludes the use of alkylating agents (8). However, they should be tapered and discontinued as soon as possible, since their effect is only temporary and obtained at the cost of serious side-effects. A recent comparative trial reports the superiority of CLB + PDN over CLB alone in a small number of patients (22). Few other reports of combination chemotherapy in CLL can be found (51, 52). Four complete remissions were reported in 8 patients treated with CAR + CPM given in a 4-day course every 3 weeks (23).

2. Maintenance Therapy

Once a tumor response has been obtained, the disease can be kept under control either by continuous low-dose maintenance therapy or by inter-mittent courses of CLB, prescribed each time the disease tends to become worse. Two studies comparing both methods showed no difference in survival (24, 25). The proponents of intermittent therapy argue that there is less risk of cytopenia (14). If maintenance therapy is indicated, it may be logical (on the basis of the treatment principles discussed in Chapter 6) to try a high-dose intermittent schedule (25, 26). We are evaluating a program of treatment cycles, lasting 2 to 3 weeks, at the dose level mentioned above, with intervals off therapy. The latter are determined by the clinical condition and the urgency for control of certain disease manifestations. However, they should last for a minimum of 2 to 3 weeks to permit recovery of the hematopoietic and immune systems. The SECSG is currently studying the effectiveness of CLB administered in single high doses every 2 weeks (27, 28).

B. STRATEGY

1. Radiotherapy and Radioactive Isotopes

Other treatment modalities besides cytotoxic agents can reduce the expanded mass and may thus be useful at some stage. Local radiotherapy may be indicated for symptomatic local disease caused by enlarged spleen or lymph nodes, for example, bronchial obstruction caused by mediastinal adenopathy, disfigurement from cervical or submandibular glands, interference with movement of an extremity due to axillary or inguinal adenopathy. Irradiation of the spleen with small doses can result in a significant volume reduction (49). It can be considered as a method to influence lymphocytes as they pass through the spleen without affecting the normal hematopoietic tissue (29). Furthermore, the spleen is one of the organs, most rich in B lymphocytes. In spite of a beneficial effect in individual cases with correction of anemia, the overall results are unsatisfactory. Anemia and/or thrombocytopenia are sometimes aggravated.

Fractionated whole-body irradiation has been reported to induce a high rate of "complete" remissions (8/17) (30, 31).

Extracorporeal irradiation (32) of the blood with a cesium-137, cobalt-60, or strontium-90 source, or with ultraviolet light (33) can reduce lymphocytosis and the volume of lymphoid organs. However, this method does not offer any advantage over other methods of irradiation and is technically complicated and impractical.

Internal irradiation with radiophosphorus is as effective as other methods of irradiation in reducing the lymphoid mass (34, 35). No special equipment is required but oncologists continue to prefer cytotoxic agents with which they have more experience. Indeed, the superiority of ^{32}P over CLB remains to be shown in a randomized trial. The risks of aplasia, and more remotely of induction of leukemia, are greater with the isotope than with CLB (34).

2. Antilymphocyte Serum and Lymphocytophoresis

Lymphocytosis and adenopathy can also be reduced for a brief period with antilymphocyte serum (36, 37). This method could theoretically be used to destroy cells remaining after intensive chemotherapy.

Finally, lymphocytes can be removed by lymphocytophoresis with a blood cell separator (38), a method without advantage over the others, except possibly for a case of extreme lymphocytosis with marrow failure.

3. Indications for Therapy

We have been thus far describing conventional and more exotic methods for treating CLL, but we have not yet discussed the indication to treat in the first place. The "total-cell-kill-oriented" oncologist may not have noted this omission. Should not all malignancies be treated intensively, as soon as they are diagnosed? A less aggressive oncologist will interject that he has followed many a patient with CLL for years, doing well without any therapy. There are even those who feel that therapy in this disease may trigger autoimmune complications (39). No-one will deny that symptoms or complications related to organ size or marrow failure constitute indications to treat. The argument in CLL centers around the advisability of initiating therapy in patients diagnosed in the asymptomatic, stable, or slowly progressive (indolent) phase of the disease. Should an attempt be made at all times to rid the patient of all evidence of disease, as in acute leukemia?

Studies that have compared patients treated only when the disease became aggressive or symptomatic, and then long enough to achieve control, with patients (at other centers) treated irrespective of the presence or absence of symptoms, yielded the same survival results. It is even questioned whether therapy in CLL has improved survival at all (8). More recent data indicate that survival is improving, especially in the minority of patients in whom complete remission can be obtained (9). GRAY et al. have shown that the prognosis of CLL correlated with the degree of blood and marrow lymphocytosis (40). Thus more aggressive, rather than symptomatic therapy may be indicated. We cannot take a formal stand on this debate until the results of study of the EORTC LEUKEMIA AND HEMATOSARCOMA GROUP are known. Patients with small lymph nodes and a lymphocyte count of less than 50,000/mm³ are randomized. In the meantime, it is not unreasonable for the practicing oncologist to continue with the traditional approach that consists in reducing symptoms, improving the performance status, and delaying marrow failure rather than aggravating it, since most patients die as a result of its complications. Special centers and study groups can investigate the value of more agressive treatment. If the guidelines for protocol studies are followed, results from different studies can be compared (7).

4. Treatment of Refractory Cases and Complications

Some special management problems remain to be discussed. CLB-resistant
CLL may respond to some of the second-line cytotoxic agents listed
above. For those resistant to all chemotherapy, some form of radiotherapy, external or other, may be indicated. Local radiotherapy may
be useful in cases with massive adenopathies or splenomegaly but discrete blood and marrow lymphocytosis. The most difficult patients to
treat are those showing marrow failure with marked lymphocytosis. As
initial therapy, we recommend prednisone, to be followed by chemotherapy
as soon as improvement in the blood picture is noted (especially platelet and neutrophil counts). If PDN fails to produce the desired effect,
one may be forced to use chemotherapy under coverage of packed red
cells, platelet and/or leukocyte transfusions. For those adequately
equipped, preliminary leukaphoresis is a third possibility.

Controlling some of the complications of CLL may be equally challenging,
especially autoimmune hemolytic anemia. This type of anemia may respond to steroid therapy (Fig. 18-2). If no improvement is obtained following an adequate trial of steroids, splenectomy should be considered
(14, 41-43). A favorable result can be expected if there is a gamma
type of direct Coombs reaction, significant splenic sequestration, or
other signs of hypersplenism. Relative contraindications to splenectomy are a bone marrow packed with lymphocytes and devoid of megakaryocytes, normoblasts and granulocyte precursors, a non-gamma direct Coombs
test, or lack of evidence of splenic sequestration. Androgens and/or
prednisone can be tried to stimulate erythropoiesis in the packed-mar-
row syndome (44, 45).

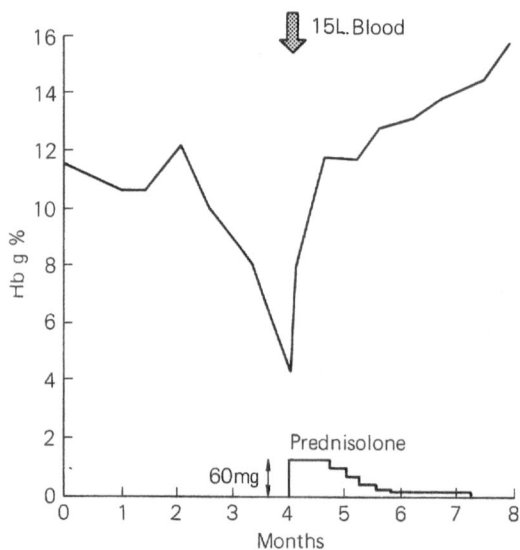

Fig. 18-2. Effect of prednisolone on autoimmune hemolytic
anemia in a patient with
chronic lymphoid leukemia

REFERENCES

1. MATHE, G., RAPPAPORT, H.: Histological and cytological typing of the
   neoplastic diseases of the haematopoietic and lymphoid tissues.
   Geneva: W.H.O. 1973.

2. RUBIN, A.D., JOHNSON, L.I., BROWN, S.M.: Lymphocyte proliferation and lymphoproliferative disorders. Prog. exp. Tumor Res. 13, 135 (1970).
3. JANOSSY, G., GREAVES, M.F.: Lymphocyte activation. I. Response of T and B lymphocytes to phytomitogens. Clin. exp. Immunol. 9, 483 (1971).
4. AISENBERG, A.C., BLOCK, K.J.: Immunoglobins on the surface of neoplastic lymphocytes. New Engl. J. Med. 287, 272 (1972).
5. SELIGMANN, M., PREUD'HOMME, J.L.: Cell surface bound immunoglobulins as markers in lymphoproliferative diseases. In: 14th Hematological Congress, p. 94. Sao-Paulo 1972.
6. DAMESHEK, W.: Chronic lymphocytic leukemia. An accumulative disease of immunologically incompetent lymphocytes. Blood 29, 566 (1967).
7. COMMITTEE OF THE CHRONIC LEUKEMIA-MYELOMA TASK FORCE, NATIONAL CANCER INSTITUTE: Proposed guidelines for protocol studies. III. Chronic lymphocytic leukemia. Cancer Chemother. Rep. Part 3, 4, 159 (1973).
8. BERGSAGEL, D.E.: The chronic leukemias: A review of disease manifestations and the aims of therapy. Canad. med. Ass. J. 96, 1615 (1967).
9. HUGULEY, Jr., C.M.: Chronic myelocytic and chronic lymphocytic leukemia. Cancer 30, 1583 (1972).
10. KNOSPE, W.H., GREGORY, S.A., TROBAUGH, Jr., F.E., SCHREK, R.: Complete remission in chronic lymphocytic leukemia: Clinical, cytological and electron-microscopic studies. Proc. Amer. Soc. Clin. Oncol. 15, 192 (1974).
11. BERNARD, J., MATHE, G., WEIL, M.: Essai de traitement par l'acide p-di-2-chloroéthylamine-phénylbutyrique, de la maladie de Hodgkin, de la leucémie lymphoide chronique et de divers hématosarcomes et leucémies. Rev. franc. Etudes clin. Biol. 1, 1121 (1956).
12. RUNDLES, R.W., GRIZZLE, Y., BELL, W.N., CORBEY, C.D., FROMMEYER. Jr., W.B., GREENBERG, B.G., HUGULEY, Jr., C.M., JAMES, G.W., JONES, Jr., R., LARSEN, W.E., LOEB, V., LEONE, L.A., PALMER, J.G., RISER, Jr., W.H., WILSON, S.J.: Comparison of chlorambucil and myleran in chronic lymphocytic and granulocytic leukaemia. Amer. J. Med. 27, 424 (1959).
13. GALTON, D.A.G., WHITSHAW, E., SZUR, L., DACIE, J.V.: The use of chlorambucil and steroids in the treatment of chronic lymphatic leukemia. Brit. J. Haematol. 7, 73 (1967).
14. SILVER, R.T.: The treatment of chronic lymphocytic leukemia. Seminars in Hematol. 6, 344 (1969).
15. LIVINGSTON, R.B., CARTER, S.K.: Single Agents in Cancer Chemotherapy. New York: IFI/Plenum 1970.
16. MOLONEY, W.C.: Treatment of chronic leukemia. In: Proc. Intern. Conf. on leukemia and lymphomas. (ed. C. Zarafondis), Philadelphia: Lea and Febiger 1968.
17. BIGLEY, R.H.: Treatment of chronic lymphocytic leukemia with triethylene melamine and chlorambucil. Cancer Chemother. Rep. 30, 2 (1963).
18. KAUNG, D.T., WHITTINGTON, R.M., SPENCER, H.T., PATNO, M.E.: Comparison of chlorambucil and streptonigrin in the treatment of chronic lymphocytic leukemia. Cancer 23, 597 (1969).
19. KENIS, Y., DE MEUTER, R., MANASTER, J., STRYCKMANS, P., VERRIEST, M.: Etude préliminaire d'un agent alkylant ayant une action prédominante sur les lymphocytes: la mitoclomine. Session Plénière de l' O.E.R.T.C. Paris, 20-21 juin 1969.
20. KYLE, R.A., McFARLAND, C.E., DAMESHEK, W.: Large doses of prednisone and prednisolone in the treatment of malignant lympho-proliferative disorders. Ann. intern. Med. 57, 717 (1962).
21. EZDINLI, E.Z., STUTZMAN, L.: Corticosteroid therapy for lymphomas and chronic lymphocytic leukemia. Cancer 23, 900 (1969).

22. HAN, T., EZDINLI, E.Z., SHIMAOKA, K., DESAI, D.V.: Chlorambucil vs. combined chlorambucil-corticosteroids therapy in chronic lympho-cytic leukemia. Cancer 31, 502 (1973).

23. GUTTERMAN, J.U., CURTIS, J.E., FREIREICH, E.J.: Combination chemo-therapy with cytosine arabinoside (Ara-C) and cyclophosphamide (CTX) of chronic lymphocytic leukemias (abstr.). Proc. Amer. Ass. Clin. Oncol. (1972).

24. EZDINLI, E.Z., STUTZMAN, L.: Chlorambucil therapy for lymphomas and chronic lymphocytic leukemia. J. amer. Med. Ass. 191, 444 (1965).

25. HUGULEY, C.M.: Long-term study of chronic lymphocytic leukemia - Interim report after 45 months. Cancer Chemotherapy Rep. 16, 241 (1962).

26. SPECK, B.: The treatment of chronic lymphocytic leukemia and myelo-proliferative syndromes. In: Cancer chemotherapy, p. 241 (ed. F. Elkerbout). Leiden: Leiden Univ. Press 1971.

27. KNOSPE, W.H., LOEB, Jr., V., HUGULEY, Jr., C.M.: Bi-weekly chlor-ambucil treatment of chronic lymphocytic leukemia. Cancer 33, 555 (1974).

28. KNOSPE, W.H., LOEB, V., HUGULEY, C.M.(for Southeastern Cancer Study Group): Intermittent chlorambucil in the therapy of chronic lympho-cytic leukemia. Proc. Amer. Ass. clin. Oncol. Abstract 44 (1973).

29. SCHLIENGER, M., PARMENTIER, C., LAUGIER, A., SCHLUMBERGER, J.R., BOK, B., MATHE, G., TUBIANA, M.: La radiothérapie splénique dans le traitement des leucémies lymphoïdes chroniques. Ses analogies avec l'irradiation extracorporelle. Nouv. Rev. Franc. Hématol. 8, 719 (1968).

30. JOHNSON, R.E., KAGAN, A.R., GRALNICK, H.R., FASS, L.: Radiation-induced remissions in chronic lymphocytic leukemia. Cancer 20, 1382 (1967).

31. JOHNSON, R.E.: Total body irradiation of chronic lymphocytic leu-kemia: incidence and duration of remission. Cancer 25, 523 (1970).

32. THOMAS, E.D., EPSTEIN, R.B., ESCHBACH, J.W., PRAYER, D., BUCHNER, L.D., MARSAGLIA, G.: Treatment of leukemia by extracorporal irra-diation. New Engl. J. Med. 273, 6 (1965).

33. BINET, J.L., VILLENEUVE, B., VAN RAPPENBUSCH, R., MIGNON, F., BECA, R., VAUGIER, G., BERNARD, J.: Irradiation extracorporelle du sang par les rayons ultra-violets. Nouv. Rev. Franc. Hématol. 8, 733 (1968).

34. OSGOOD, E.E.: Contrasting incidence of acute monocytic and granulo-cytic leukemia in P32-treated patients with polycythemia vera and chronic lymphocytic leukemia. Blood 22, 820 (1963).

35. STEINKAMP, R.C., LAWRENCE, J.H., BORN, J.L.: Long-term experience with use of P32 in treatment of chronic lymphocytic leukemia. J. nucl. Med. 4, 92 (1963).

36. MATHE, G., SCHWARZENBERG, L., AMIEL, L.: Approches immunologiques du traitement des leucémies. Premiers résultats chez l'homme. Nouv. Rev. Franc. Hématol. 7, 721 (1967).

37. LASZLO, J., BUCKLEY, C.E. III, AMOS, D.B.: Infusion of isologous immune plasma in chronic lymphocytic leukemia. Blood 31, 104 (1968).

38. CURTIS, J.E., HERSH, E.M., FREIREICH, E.J.: Leukophoresis therapy of chronic lymphocytic leukemia. Blood 39, 163 (1972).

39. LEWIS, F.B., SCHWARTZ, R.S., DAMESHEK, W.: X-radiation and alkylating agents as possible trigger mechanisms in the autoimmune complica-tions of malignant lymphoproliferative disease. Clin. exp. immun. 1, 3 (1966).

40. GRAY, J.L., JACOBS, A., BLOCK, M.: Prognosis of chronic lymphatic leukemia. In: Abstr. 14th Hematological Congress, Abstr. 54, Sao Paulo.

41. EBBE, S., WITTELL, J.B., DAMESHEK, W.: Auto-immune thrombocytopenic purpura (ITP-Type) with chronic lymphocytic leukemia. Blood 19, 23 (1962).

42. SCHUBOTHE, H.: The cold agglutinin disease. Seminars in Hematol. 3, 27 (1966).
43. YAM, L.T., CROSBY, W.H.: Early splenectomy in lymphoproliferative disorders. Arch. intern. Med. 133, 270 (1974).
44. SPIERS, A.S.: Surgery in the management of patients with leukemia. Brit. med. J. 3, 528 (1973).
45. KENNEDY, B.J.: Androgenic hormone therapy in lymphatic leukemia. J. Amer. med. Ass. 190, 1130 (1964).
46. ROWLANDS, D.T., DANIELE, R.P., NOWELL, P.C., WURZEL, H.A.: Characterization of lymphocyte subpopulations in chronic leukemia. Cancer 34, 1962 (1974).
47. MANASTER, J., FRUHLING, P., STRYCKMANS, P.: Kinetics of lymphocytes in chronic lymphocytic leukemia. I. Equilibrium between blood and a "readily accessible pool". Blood 41, 425 (1973).
48. MOAYERI, H., HAN, T., SOKAL, J.E.: Delayed hypersensitivity responses, palpable disease and survival in chronic lymphocytic leukemia. Proc. Am. Soc. Clin. Oncol. 16, 239 (1975).
49. BYHARDT, R.W., KIRKLAND, C.B., WIERNIK, P.H.: The role of splenic irradiation in chronic lymphocytic leukemia. Cancer 35, 1621 (1975).
50. LONGEVAL, E., GANGJI, D., STRYCKMANS, P., KENIS, Y.: Phase I-II clinical trial with mitoclomine (NSC-114575) in chronic lymphocytic leukemia. Cancer Chemother. Rep. Part 1, 59, 1173 (1975)
51. KELLER, J.W., KNOSPE, W.H., HUGULEY, C.M.: Biweekly chlorambucil and prednisone in chronic lymphocytic leukemia consolidating remissions with same or cycle-active therapy. Proc. Amer. Soc. Clin. Oncol. 17, 280 (1976).
52. KEMPIN, S., GEE, T., LEE, B., DOWLING, M., CLARKSON, B.: Combination chemotherapy (M-2) treatment of chronic lymphocytic leukemia. Proc. Amer. Soc. Clin. Oncol. 17, 297 (1976).

Chapter 19
Multiple Myeloma and Primary Macroglobulinemia (Waldenström)

MULTIPLE MYELOMA

Multiple myeloma is a plasma cell neoplasm. Myeloma cells generally maintain the morphologic characteristics of plasma cells, but may have lymphoid features. Thus, the malignant transformation affects cells which are normally destined to produce immunoglobulins. Most myeloma cells continue to produce immunoglobulins or fragments thereof, which may or may not be secreted. These appear on electrophoresis of serum or concentrated urine as a narrow band of homogeneous immunoglobulin or subunits, referred to as M components (M for monoclonal). In some patients, heavy- and light-chain synthesis is "balanced" and only an intact immunoglobulin is secreted; in others, light chain is excessive and synthesis unbalanced, leading to Bence Jones proteinuria. In some cases, the only abnormality that can be detected is the excretion of light chain in the urine (Bence Jones proteinuria). The normal immunoglobulins and serum albumin are usually reduced.

Multiple myeloma, as the name infers, is most often a disseminated malignancy. However, truly solitary plasmocytomas, often extraskeletal, do occur. The spectrum of plasma cell neoplasms includes beside multiple myeloma (1) the macroglobulinemias and heavy-chain (α, γ and μ) diseases (2).

The symptoms and manifestations of the disease are related to the presence of M protein in the serum and/or urine and the infiltration of bones, bone marrow, and to a lesser extent of other tissues by myeloma cells (59). Much of the morbidity and most of the mortality are caused by disease complications: infections, various combinations of cytopenia, renal failure, bone fractures, hyperuricemia, and hypercalcemia (Table 19-1). Hypercalcemia is thought to be due to the secretion of a soluble factor by myeloma cells that in turn stimulates osteoclastic activity in adjacent bone (60).

The quantity of M protein synthesized in a given patient reflects the size of his tumor burden. SALMON et al. (3, 4, 5) have calculated the total body myeloma cell number at various stages of the disease and therapy from the total-body M-component synthetic rate (in vivo) and the cellular M-component sythetic rate (determined in vitro). The M-component synthetic rates range from 2.5 pg to 35 pg per myeloma cell per day (most patients fall in the 10-20 pg range). In molecular terms, 5,200 to 87,500 molecules of immunoglobulin are secreted per cell per minute. Their studies indicate that the growth of myeloma is Gompertzian. At early diagnosis, at least 0.2×10^{12} myeloma cells are present in the body; only 4 doublings are required to bring the tumor mass to 3×10^{12}, the number present at death. This lethal number is similar to the lethal cell number in acute leukemia. The doubling time during the clinical phase of disease (plateau phase) is 4 to 6 months.

Table 19-1. Clinical manifestations and complications of multiple myeloma

---

1. Manifestations related to M components

    - Hypervolemia: spurious fall in Hgb concentration
                    pseudohyponatremia
                    congestive heart failure
    - Shortened RBC and platelet survival
    - Hyperviscosity syndrome (12)
    - Bleeding diathesis: defective function of platelets
                          interaction with coagulation factors (13)
    - Proteinuria ⟶ renal insufficiency
    - Rouleaux formation, accelerated ESR
    - Cold sensitivity if M component is cold-precipitable

2. Manifestations related to myeloma cell infiltration of

    Bones   - pain
                            - lytic lesions, diffuse osteoporosis,
                              rarely osteoblastic lesions
                            - pathologic fractures
                            - cord compression
                            - hypercalcemia due to increased resorption
                              of bone salts

    Bone marrow   - plasmocytosis: 10-95%
                            - anemia; additional contributing factors:
                                  - decreased erythropoiesis
                                  - renal insufficiency
                                  - hemolysis
                                  - therapy (cytotoxic, radiation)
                            - leukopenia
                            - thrombocytopenia

    Other organs, tissues   - plasmacytomas
                            - organomegaly
                            - organ dysfunction

3. Additional disease complications

    Renal Failure due to

    - Bence Jones proteinuria ⟶ protein precipitates ⟶ tubular ob-
                 obstruction and degeneration "Myeloma kidney"
    - Hyaline bodies, probably BJ protein in tubular cells ⟶ defects
                 in tubular resorption "adult Fanconi syndrome"
    - Hypercalcemia, hypercalciuria ⟶ impaired tubular re-absorption,
                 dehydration, nephrocalcinosis
    - Pyelonephritis
    - Amyloidosis
    - Myeloma cell infiltration of kidneys
    - Hyperuricemia ⟶ crystallization of uric acid in tubules

    Infections, due to
    - decrease of normal immunoglobulins and deficient antibody
      response
    - cell-mediated immune responses may also be impaired
    - disease- or therapy-related neutropenia
    - steroid therapy
    - immobilization, paraplegia ⟶ decubitus ulcers, urinary reten-
      tion, pneumonia

    Amyloidosis
    macroglossia, carpal-tunnel syndrome, hepatosplenomegaly, peri-
    pheral neuropathy, nephritic syndrome, cardiac decompensation (14)

A number of factors influence the outcome of the disease. Heavy Bence Jones proteinuria, uremia, low serum albumin, hypercalcemia refractory to therapy, plasma-cell leukemia, a rapid response to chemotherapy, poorly differentiated tumor, and a large myeloma cell mass are unfavorable prognostic features (4-7, 63). The low response rate from melphalan therapy in myeloma producing only lambda Bence Jones proteins (8) was not confirmed in subsequent studies (9-11). There has been no consistent correlation between the specific type of M component and response to alkylating agents.

A. SUPPORTIVE THERAPY

Vigorous therapy of complications or, better, prophylactic measures to prevent their occurrence are an essential aspect of the management of multiple myeloma (10, 15).

Infections must be dealt with promptly (see Chapt. 11). Gram-negative organisms, rather than gram-positive ones, are isolated most frequently from myeloma patients (16). Prophylactic antibiotics are generally contraindicated. In a controlled, double-blind study, prophylactic γ-globulin administration failed to prevent infection (17).

Many of the complications of skeletal involvement can be prevented by maintaining adequate ambulation. A regular program of exercise (walking, swimming, and other mild sports) should be encouraged. However, excessive straining and heavy lifting must be avoided. To permit this program of active ambulation, relief of bone pain must be provided with analgesics or localized radiotherapy for the most painful areas of the skeleton. A palliative dose of 1200-1500 rads is usually adequate for relief of pain. Excessive radiation doses and field sizes should be avoided to limit damage to the bone marrow reserve, which would compromise further cytotoxic therapy.

Chemotherapy will often relieve bone pain in previously untreated patients. Corsets, spine braces, walkers, and other orthopedic supports may be helpful in alleviating pain. Sodium fluoride produces skeletal fluorosis (18) and increases bone density on roentgenograms; however, a controlled study failed to show any clinical benefit (19). More encouraging results have been obtained with the combination of sodium fluoride and calcium carbonate (68).

Adequate hydration (with a urine output of 1500-2500 ml) should be maintained to avoid hypercalcemia, hyperuricemia, and azotemia. Allopurinol effectively reduces uric acid production. Hypercalcemia must be treated as a medical emergency (see p. 205).

Effective chemotherapy ameliorates the anemia, which is often present at the time of diagnosis. Transfusions of packed red cells may be required until chemotherapy takes effect. Androgens will often raise the hemoglobin concentration in patients whose anemia is mainly due to reduced erythropoiesis and who do not respond to chemotherapy.

Repeated plasmaphoresis may be lifesaving during the acute stage of the hyperviscosity syndrome and in hypervolemia due to increased plasma volume (with dilutional anemia) (12, 20-22).

B. CHEMOTHERAPY

1. Single Agents

The median survival of patients with untreated myeloma is approximately
7-11 months (23, 24). Since the introduction of effective chemotherapy
in the early 1960's, survival times have been increased three- to seven-
fold (24-50 months) (10). This improvement has been largely due to alkylating agents. ^{32}P, urethane, stilbamide, antimetabolites, and mitotic
poisons have not proved of practical value in this disease (7, 24, 25).

Melphalan (MPH), and to a lesser extent cyclophosphamide (CPM), have
been used most often in myeloma (Table 19-2). They appear to be equally
effective in producing objective improvement (30-50 percent) and in
prolonging survival (10, 26). This effect has been documented by a
comparative trial of both drugs administered continuously (6, 27) but
high-dose intermittent CPM versus MPH has not been compared. There is a
a significant difference in survival from onset of therapy between responders (median survival: 41 months) and nonresponders (9 months) (28).
The question of the best mode of administration of MPH and CPM remains
unsettled. Melphalan has been administered in low-dose, daily therapy,
4 mg qd without interruption adjusted on basis of WBC and platelet
counts (29); a loading dose of 0.15 mg/kg qd for 7 days followed promptly (10) of after a rest period (30) by continuous low-dose maintenance
therapy; high-dose intermittent therapy, 0.25 mg/kg, qd, for 4 days every
6 weeks (31), or 0.15 mg/kg, qd, for 7 days every 5 weeks (32). In a
comparative trial of the SWCCG, intermittent high-dose therapy proved
superior to long-term low-dose therapy (32 percent versus 19 percent
response rate) (31) while in a study by the ALGB, intermittent MPH
(0.15 mg/kg, qd for 7 days every 5 weeks) was inferior to a regimen
using continuous MPH maintenance therapy (32). McARTHUR concluded that
experienced investigators achieve a similar proportion of objective
responses and the same prolongation of survival with all three dosage
schedules (29).

Intermittent therapy has the advantage that blood counts are required
only at 6-week intervals, once the pattern of hematologic toxicity has
been determined for a particular patient.

Most trials with CPM have used low-dose continuous therapy (33-35).
BERGSAGEL and HUMPHREY have used intermittent high-dose CPM with good
results (36, 37). The problem of cross-resistance between CPM and MPH
in myeloma requires further investigation. Preliminary data indicate
that patients who are resistant to MPH (primary or secondary) may bene-
benefit from subsequent CPM therapy (36, 65) (not confirmed by KYLE
et al. (66))

A beneficial effect of steroid therapy in myeloma was first reported
by THORN (38), who noted a correction of the protein abnormality and
the anemia and a decrease of the marrow infiltrate following ACTH. Similar types of response have been observed in subsequent studies (25,
39, 40) but there has been no improvement in survival (39). This indicates that prednisone by itself has at best a minimal direct antineoplastic effect (36). The lowering of the serum concentration and urinary
excretion of M proteins while on steroid therapy could result from increased catabolism rather than from a direct lethal effect on myeloma
cells. The possibility of a synergistic effect of steroids in combination therapy is discussed later in this chapter.

Procarbazine (PCZ) yields a 15 percent response rate (26, 41), adriamycin 13 percent (42, 67). The nitrosoureas appear promising new agents
(43).

Table 19-2. Effectiveness of single agents in multiple myeloma

	No. evaluated	% response	Reference
6-Mercaptopurine	19	10 %	LIVINGSTON and CARTER (26)
Hydroxyurea	12	O	LIVINGSTON and CARTER (26)
BCNU	31	39 %	CARTER (43)
Procarbazine	33	15 %	LIVINGSTON and CARTER (26)
Nitrogen mustard	9	11 %	LIVINGSTON and CARTER (26)
Chlorambucil	15	33 %	LIVINGSTON and CARTER (26)
Cyclophosphamide	413	29 %	LIVINGSTON and CARTER (26)
Melphalan	499	42 %	LIVINGSTON and CARTER (26)
Mitomycin C	15	O	LIVINGSTON and CARTER (26)
Adriamycin	23	13 %	O'BRYAN et al. (42)
Bleomycin	14	O	BLUM et al. (58)
Prednisone	39	49 %	LIVINGSTON and CARTER (26)

2. Combinations

Combination therapy has been not evaluated as extensively in multiple myeloma as in some of the other hematologic malignancies, since the choice of effective drugs is limited (Table 19-3). Until recently prednisone and either MPH or CPM were the only active drugs.

Table 19-3. Response rates to combinations in multiple myeloma

Combination	No. evaluated	% response	Reference
MPH, PDN	205	48 %	ALEXANIAN et al. (9)
PCZ, MPH, PDN	139	59 %	ALEXANIAN et al. (9)
BCNU, CPM, MPH, PDN	19	100 %	HARLEY et al. (44)
BCNU, CPM, MPH, VCR, PDN	32	60-90 %	LEE et al. (46)
BCNU, CPM, PDN	in progress	-	SECSG, ECOG (43)
BCNU, MPH, PDN	in progress	-	ALGB (43)

ALEXANIAN (31) reported better results with the combination of prednisone and MPH (48 percent) than with MPH alone (24 percent). Adding PCZ to the MPH-PDN combination further improved the response rate (59 percent) but without evident prolongation in either median survival or remission duration (9). BCNU together with PDN is more effective than either drug alone and is equivalent to MPH plus PDN (ALGB quoted by CARTER (43)). The addition of prednisone (for 10 weeks in the dosage

used) to a loading dose of MPH, followed by long-term maintenance therapy with MPH, considerably improved the response rate and the survival
in "good risk" patients but had an adverse effect in "poor risk" patients (11).

The combinations MPH + BCNU + PDN (ALGB) and CPM + BCNU + PDN (SECCG,
ECOG) are being compared with MPH + PDN (43, 64). HARLEY, at the University of West Virginia, has combined all 3 alkylating agents (BCNU +
MPH + CPM + PDN) and reported a 100 percent response rate in 19 patients
(43, 44). A protocol combining the same 4 drugs, with VCR in addition,
resulted in an 86 percent response (45, 46). Part of the rationale for
the simultaneous use of several alkylating agents with different cellular uptake mechanisms is that it may increase tumor cell kill and at
the same time retard the development of resistance to alkylating agents.
It remains to be determined whether it is better to treat myeloma with
one alkylating agent until resistance develops before changing to another, or whether two or more alkylators should be administered alternatively or concurrently. The conbination of BCNU + ADM has been effective for myeloma relapsing on alkylating agents (69).

The kinetic studies of SALMON (4) and DREWINKO et al. (61) indicate
that recruitment occurs following a good response to alkylating agents.
As a result of such therapy (which is associated with a considerable
clinical benefit) tumor load is reduced by only 1-2 logs and then remains at a plateau. However, while only 3 percent of myeloma cells are
in DNA synthesis prior to therapy, the growth fraction progressively
rises to 30 percent after repetitive cycles of chemotherapy. It would,
therefore, be logical to try, during the plateau phase of myeloma, phase-
dependent agents which are ineffective in advanced disease. Treatment
with VCR at this stage, indeed, induces further significant reductions
in the total-body myeloma cell number (47).

For the practicing oncologist, we recommend the combination of MPH +
PDN. Personally, we prefer the intermittent high-dose method of administration. CPM + PDN may be preferable in patients with impaired marrow
reserve (leukopenia, thrombocytopenia). Since the doubling time of
myeloma at the clinical stage is very long (48) (4-6 months), prolonged
therapy is necessary. The newer developments described in the preceding
paragraphs await verification by further clinical trials.

Most oncologists feel that the benefits of alkylating-agent therapy
far outweigh the potential risk of inducing acute myelomonoblastic leukemia (49). Sideroblastic anemia may precede the leukemic transformation (50).

C. STRATEGY

Radiotherapy and Surgery

Since myeloma is generally a disseminated malignancy, chemotherapy is
the principal treatment modality. Radiotherapy is mainly used for palliation of bone pain, pathologic fractures, and cord compression.

Truly localized plasmocytomas should be treated with radiotherapy with
curative intent, surgical excision depending on the localization, or a
combination of both treatment modalities. Subsequent dissemination is
not uncommon and these patients must be followed up for a long time
(62).

Macroglobulinemia, first described by WALDENSTRÖM, represents a malignancy of the cell population normally responsible for the synthesis of
IgM globulins. The involved organs are infiltrated with cells that have
the morphologic appearance of lymphocytes, plasma cells or intermediate
cells, so-called "lymphocytoid plasma cells". Abnormal quantities of
IgM globulin are produced. The clinical picture may resemble that of
a lymphoma with lymphadenopathy and hepatosplenomegaly rather than that
of multiple myeloma. Lytic bone lesions occur in only 10 percent of
cases and bone pains are unusual. The majority of symptoms are related
to the presence of cryoglobulins, hyperviscosity, and protein-protein
interactions with bleeding manifestations. Anemia is common.

A. STRATEGY

Plasmaphoresis and Chemotherapy

The need for therapy depends to a great extent on the clinical status
of the patient. A long asymptomatic period often precedes the manifest
disease phase. Significant anemia, bleeding, and symptoms related to
hyperviscosity or cryoglobulinemia are indications for therapy. The
latter can be rapidly and usually effectively controlled by repeated
plasmaphoresis (51). Long-term control of excessive IgM production and
organ infiltration is effected by chemotherapy. Chlorambucil (CLB) has
been used most often, administered as in CLL (52-55).

Since no comparative trials are available, it cannot be stated whether
CLB is indeed superior to other alkylating agents such as cyclophosphamide (52, 55, 56) TEM (53) or melphalan (55), which have also been
used successfully in this disease. MACKENZIE et al. (55) noted that
their patients responded to much lower doses of alkylating agents than
are usually recommended and warned that the customary doses of CLB carries a severe risk of inducing aplastic anemias.

Steroids have mainly a palliative effect: possible improvement of the
general condition, anemia, bleeding tendency and, in some cases, dimi-
nution of organomegaly and the IgM peak. (57).

REFERENCES

1. SNAPPER, I., KAHN, A.I.: Myelomatosis: Fundamentals and clinical
   features. Baltimore: University Park Press 1971.
2. FRANGIONE, B., FRANKLIN, E.G.: Heavy chain diseases: clinical features and molecular significance of the disordered immunoglobulin
   structure. Seminars in Haematol. 10, 53 (1973).
3. SALMON, S.E., SMITH, B.A.: Immunoglobulin synthesis and total body
   tumor cell number in IgG multiple myeloma. J. Clin. Invest. 49, 1114
   (1970).
4. SALMON, S.E.: Immunoglobulin synthesis and tumor kinetics of multiple
   myeloma. Seminars in Haematol. 10, 145 (1973).
5. DURIE, B.G., SALMON, S.E.: A clinical staging system for multiple
   myeloma. Correlation of measured myeloma cell mass with presenting
   clinical features, response to treatment, and survival. Cancer 36,
   842 (1975).

6. REPORT OF THE MEDICAL RESEARCH COUNCIL's WORKING PARTY FOR THERA-
PEUTIC TRIALS IN LEUKAEMIA. Myelomatosis: Comparison of melphalan
and cyclophosphamide therapy. Brit. med. J. 1, 640 (1971).
7. LEE, B.J., PINSKY, C., MILLER, D.G.: The management of plasma cell
neoplasms. Med. Clin. N. Amer. 55, 603 (1971).
8. BERGSAGEL, D.E., MIGLIORE, P.J., GRIFFITH, K.M.: Myeloma proteins
and the clinical response to melphalan therapy. Science 148, 376
(1965).
9. ALEXANIAN, R., BONNET, J., GEHAN, E., HAUT, A., HEWLETT, J., LANE,
M., MONTO, R., WILSON, H.: Combination chemotherapy for multiple
myeloma. Cancer 30, 382 (1972).
10. FARHANGI, M., OSSERMAN, E.F.: The treatment of multiple myeloma.
Seminars in Hematol. 10, 149 (1973).
11. COSTA, G., ENGLE, Jr., R.L., SCHILLING, A., CARBONE, P.P., KOCHWA,
S., NACHMAN, R.L., GLIDEWELL, O.: Melphalan and prednisone: an effective combination for the treatment of multiple myeloma. Amer.
J. Med. 54, 589 (1973).
12. BLOCH, K.J., MAKI, D.G.: Hyperviscosity syndrome associated with
immunoglobulin abnormalities. Seminars in Haematol. 10, 113
(1973).
13. LACKNER, H.: Haemostatic abnormalities associated with dysprotein-
emia. Ser. Haematol. 10, 125 (1973).
14. GLENNER, G.G., PERRY, W.D., ISERSKY, C.: Amyloidosis: its nature
and pathogenesis. Seminars in Haematol. 10, 65 (1973).
15. ALEXANIAN, R.: Multiple myeloma II. Treatment for complications.
Cancer Bull. 25, 15 (1973).
16. MEYERS, B.R., HIRSCHMAN, S.Z., AXELROD, J.A.: Current patterns of
infection in multiple myeloma. Amer. J. Med. 52, 87 (1972).
17. SALMON, S.E., SAMAL, B.A., HAYES, D.M., HOSLEY, H., MILLER, S.P.,
SCHILLING, A.: Role of gammaglobulin for immunoprophylaxis in multiple myeloma. New Engl. J. Med. 277, 1336 (1967).
18. CARBONE, P.P., ZIPKIN, I., SOKOLOFF, L., FRAZIER, P., COOK, P.,
MULLINS, F.: Fluoride effect on bone in plasma cell myeloma. Arch.
intern. Med. 121, 130 (1968).
19. HARLEY, J.B., SCHILLING, A., GLIDEWELL, O.: Ineffectiveness of
fluoride therapy in multiple myeloma. New Engl. J. Med. 24, 1283
(1972).
20. WOLF, R.E., ALPERIN, J.B., RITZMANN, S.E., LEVIN, W.C.: IgG-K multiple myeloma with hyperviscosity syndrome - response to plasmapheresis. Arch. intern. Med. 129, 114 (1972).
21. MacKENZIE, M.R., FUDENBERG, H.H., O'REILLY, R.A.: The hyperviscosity
syndrome. I. In IgG myeloma. The role of protein concentration and
molecular shape. J. clin. Invest. 49, 15 (1970).
22. PRUZANSKI, W., WATT, J.G.: Serum viscosity and hyperviscosity syndrome in IgG multiple myeloma. Ann. intern. Med. 77, 853 (1972).
23. OSGOOD, E.E.: The survival time of patients with plasmacytic myeloma. Cancer Chemother. Rep. 9, 1 (1960).
24. HOLLAND, J.F., HOSLEY, H., SCHARLAU, C., CARBONE, P.P., FREI, E.,
III, BRINDLEY, C.O., HALL, T.C., SHNIDER, B.I., GOLD, G.L., LASAGNA,
L., OWENS, Jr., A.H., MILLER, S.P.: A controlled trial of urethane
treatment in multiple myeloma. Blood 27, 328 (1966).
25. BERGSAGEL, D.E., GRIFFITH, K.M., HAUT, A., STUCKEY, Jr., W.J.: The
treatment of plasma cell myeloma. In: Advances in Cancer Research,
Vol. 10, p. 31 (eds. A. Haddow, S. Weinhouse). London: Academic
Press 1967.
26. LIVINGSTON, R.B., CARTER, S.K.: Single Agents in Cancer Chemotherapy.
New York: IFI/Plenum 1970.
27. RIVERS, S.L., PATNO, M.E.: Cyclophosphamide vs. melphalan in treatment of plasma cell myeloma. J. Amer. med. Ass. 207, 1328 (1969).
28. ALEXANIAN, R., BERGSAGEL, D.E., MIGLIORE, G.J., VAUGHN, W.K., HOWE,
C.D.: Melphalan therapy for plasma cell myeloma. Blood, 31, 1 (1968).

29. McARTHUR, J.R., ATHENS, J.W., WINTROBE, M.M., CARTWRIGHT, G.E.: Melphalan and myeloma. Experience with a low-dose continuous regimen. Ann. intern. Med. 72, 665 (1970).
30. HOOGSTRATEN, B., SHEEHE, P.R., CUTTNER, J., COOPER, T., KYLE, R.A., OBERFIELD, R.A., TOWNSEND, S.R., HARLEY, J.B., HAYES, D.M., COSTA, G., HOLLAND, J.F.: Melphalan in multiple myeloma. Blood 30, 74 (1967).
31. ALEXANIAN, R., HAUT, A.U., LANE, M., McKELVEY, E.M., MIGLIORE, P.J., STUCKEY, Jr., W.J., WILSON, H.E.: Treatment of multiple myeloma. Combination chemotherapy with different melphalan dose regimens. J. Amer. med. Ass. 208, 1680 (1969).
32. HOOGSTRATEN, B., COSTA, J., CUTTNER, J., FORCIER, J., LEONE, L.A., HARLEY, J.B., GLIDEWELL, O.L.: Intermittent melphalan therapy in multiple myeloma. J. Amer. med. Ass. 209, 251 (1969).
33. KORST, D.R., CLIFFORD, G.O., FOWLER, W.M., LOUIS, J., WILL, J., WILSON, H.E.: Multiple myeloma. II. Analysis of cyclophosphamide therapy in 165 patients. J. Amer. med. Ass. 189, 758 (1964).
34. TOURTELLOTTE, C.R., CALL, M.K.: Prolonged remission of myeloma with cyclophosphamide. Arch. intern. Med. 113, 758 (1964).
35. SKOOG, W.A., ADAMS, W.S.: Clinical and metabolic investigations of eight cases of multiple myeloma during prolonged cyclophosphamide administration. Amer. J. Med. 41, 76 (1966).
36. BERGSAGEL, D.E.: Plasma cell myeloma. An interpretative review. Cancer 30, 1588 (1972).
37. HUMPHREY, R.L., KVOLS, L.K., BRAINE, H.G., ABELOFF, M.D.: High-dose cytoxan therapy of poor risk myeloma and Waldenström's macroglobulinemia. Proc. Amer. Ass. Cancer Res. 14, 54 (1973).
38. THORN, G.W., FORSHAM, P.H., FRAWLEY, T.F., RICHARDSON HILL, Jr., S., ROCHE, M., STAEHELIN, D., LAURENCE WILSON, D.: The clinical usefulness of ACTH and cortisone (continued). New Engl. J. Med. 242, 824 (1950).
39. MASS, R.E.: A comparison of the effect of prednisone and a placebo in the treatment of multiple myeloma. Cancer Chemother. Rep. 16, 257 (1962).
40. SALMON, S.E., SHADDUCK, R.K., SCHILLING, A.: Intermittent high-dose prednisone (NSC-10023) therapy for multiple myeloma. Cancer Chemother. Rep. 51, 179 (1967).
41. ORGANISATION EUROPEENNE DE RECHERCHE SUR LE TRAITEMENT DU CANCER.: Essai de traitement du myélome multiple par une méthylhydrazine. Europ. J. Cancer 3, 437 (1967).
42. O'BRYAN, R.M., LUCE, J.K., TALLEY, R.W., GOTTLIEB, J.A., BAKER, L.H., BONADONNA, G.: Phase II evaluation of adriamycin in human neoplasia. Cancer 32, 1 (1973).
43. CARTER, S.K.: An overview of the status of the nitrosoureas in other tumors. Cancer Chemother. Rep. Part 3, 4, 35 (1973).
44. HARLEY, J.B., RAMANAN, S.V., KIM, I. et al.: The cyclic use of multiple alkylating agents in multiple myeloma. W.Va. Med. J. 68, 1 (1972).
45. LEE, B.J., CLARKSON, B., KRAKOFF, I.: Combination chemotherapy in multiple myeloma. Proc. amer. Soc. Clin. Oncol., abstract No. 30 (1973).
46. LEE, B.J., SAHAKIAN, G., CLARKSON, B.D., KRAKOFF, I.H.: Combination chemotherapy of multiple myeloma with alkeran, cytoxan, vincristine, prednisone, and BCNU. Cancer 33, 533 (1974).
47. SALMON, S.E., SMITH, B.A.: Induction of tumor sensitivity to cyclic agents in IgG multiple myeloma. Clin. Res. 20, 570 (1972) (abstr.)
48. HOBBS, J.R.: Paraproteins, benign or malignant? Brit. med. J. 3, 699 (1967).
49. KYLE, R.A., PIERRE, R.V., BAYRD, E.D.: Multiple myeloma and acute myelomonocytic leukemia. Report of four cases possibly related to melphalan. New Engl. J. Med. 283, 1121 (1970).

50. KHALEELI, M., KEANE, W.M., LEE, G.R.: Sideroblastic anemia in multiple myeloma: a preleukemic change. Blood, 41, 17 (1973).
51. SOLOMON, A., FAHEY, J.L.: Plasmapheresis therapy in macroglobulinemia. Ann. intern. Med. 58, 789 (1963).
52. BUCKLE, R.M., JENKINS, G.C., MILLS, G.L.: Waldenström's , macroglobulinaemia treated with cyclophosphamide and chlorambucil. J. Clin. Path. 19, 55 (1966).
53. COHEN, R.J., BOHANNON, R.A., WALLENSTEIN, R.O.: Waldenström's macroglobulinemia. A study of ten cases. Amer. J. Med. 41, 274 (1966).
54. McALLISTER, B.D., BAYRD, E.D., HARRISON, E.G., McGUCKIN, W.F.: Primary macroglobulinemia. Review with a report on 31 cases and notes on the value of continuous chlorambucil therapy. Amer. J. Med. 43, 394 (1967).
55. MACKENZIE, M.R., FUDENBERG, H.H.: Macroglobulinemia: An analysis of forty patients. Blood 39, 874 (1972).
56. BOURONCLE, B.A., DATTA, P., FRAJOLA, W.J.: Waldenström's macroglobulinemia. Report of three patients treated with cyclophosphamide. J. Amer. med. Ass. 189, 729 (1964).
57. O'REILLY, R.A., MacKENZIE, M.R.: Primary macroglobulinemia. Remission with adrenal corticosteriod therapy. Arch. intern. Med. 120, 234 (1967).
58. BLUM, R.H., CARTER, S.K., AGRE, K.: A clinical review of bleomycin - a new antineoplastic agent. Cancer 31, 903 (1973).
59. KYLE, R.A.: Multiple myeloma. Review of 869 cases. Mayo Clin. Proc. 50, 29 (1975).
60. MUNDY, G.R., RAISZ, K.G., COOPER, R.A., SCHECHTER, G.P., SALMON, S.E.: Evidence for the secretion of an osteoclast stimulating factor in myeloma. New Engl. J. Med. 291, 1041 (1974).
61. DREWINKO, B., BROWN, B.W., HUMPHREY, R., ALEXANIAN, R.: Effect of chemotherapy on the labelling index of myeloma cells. Cancer 34, 526 (1974).
62. MEYER, J.E., SCHULZ, M.D.: "Solitary" myeloma of the bone. A review of 12 cases. Cancer 34, 438 (1975).
63. ALEXANIAN, R., BALCERAK, S., BONNET, J.D., GEHAN, E.A., HAUT, A., HEWLETT, J.S., MONTO, R.W.: Prognostic factors in multiple myeloma. Cancer 36, 1192 (1975).
64. COHEN, H.J., ABRAMSON, N., BARTOLUCCI, A., BAILOR, J.: BCNU, cyclophosphamide, and prednisone versus melphalan and prednisone in myeloma. Proc. Amer. Soc. Clin. Oncol. 17, 280 (1976)
65. BERGSAGEL, D.E., COWAN, D.H., HASSELBACK, R.: Plasma cell myeloma: response of melphalan-resistant patients to high-dose intermittent cyclophosphamide. Can. Med. Assoc. J. 107, 851 (1972).
66. KYLE, R.A., SELIGMAN, B.R., WALLACE, H.J., SILVER, R.T., GLIDEWELL, O., HOLLAND, J.F.: Multiple myeloma resistant to melphalan (NSC-8806) treated with cyclophosphamide (NSC-26271), prednisone (NSC-10023), and chloroquine (NSC-187208). Cancer Chemother. Rep. Part 1, 59, 557 (1975).
67. ALBERTS, D.S., SALMON, S.E.: Adriamycin (NSC-123127) in the treatment of alkylator-resistant multiple myeloma. Cancer Chemother. Rep. Part 1, 59, 345 (1975).
68. KYLE, R.A., JOWSEY, J., KELLY, P.J., TAWES, D.R.: Multiple myeloma: Effect of sodium fluoride and calcium carbonate or placebo. New Engl. Med. 293, 1329 (1975).
69. ALBERTS, D.S., SALMON, S.E.: Adriamycin-BCNU:Effective therapy for myeloma relapsing on alkylating agents. Proc. Amer. Ass. Cancer Res. 17, 123 (1976).

Chapter 20
Hodgkin's Disease

Tremendous progress has been made in the past two decades in the treatment of Hodgkin's disease, thanks to a better understanding of the disease (1-3) and to advances in both radiotherapy and chemotherapy.

Hodgkin's disease is a neoplastic disease in which typical Sternberg-Reed cells and mononuclear cells with corresponding nuclear features represent the neoplastic elements and in which a variety of inflammatory cells are intimately associated with the malignant cellular proliferations. The inflammatory components of the lesion often form the bulk of the tumor (4).

LUKES et al. (5) proposed a new histological classification to replace that of JACKSON and PARKER (6), which distinguished Hodgin's granuloma, paragranuloma, and sarcoma as three prognostically different types. The new classification was based on the proposal that the histologic variations reflect differences in host reactivity, number of lymphocytes, and characteristic types of fibrosis, while the basic process involves principally the Sternberg-Reed cells. At the Rye conference, a modification (7, 8) was generally accepted which recognizes four main histological subtypes (4, 9) (Table 20-1). There is a definite relationship between histologic type, clinical stage, and survival (9, 10). Lymphocyte predominance (LP) has the best prognosis and is strongly associated with clinical stages I and II (see below). Nodular sclerosis (NS) enjoys the second prognosis; it is seen most often as stage II and has a strong propensity to involve lower cervical lymph nodes, the mediastinum, and contiguous structures. Mixed cellularity (MC) is next and occurs in all clinical stages without any strong associations. Lymphocyte depletion (LD) has the worst prognosis and is seen primarily as stages III and IV. RAPPAPORT et al.(11, 12) and others (131-133) have stressed the importance of vascular invasion as a histologic parameter influencing prognosis; it occurs in 10 percent of lymph-node biopsies, and is more likely to be found in the more malignant variants of HD (in 50 percent of LD). Some authors question its value as an indicator of biologic behavior (13, 132).

The prognostic and therapeutic importance of the extent of the disease (stage) was first recognized by radiotherapists (14). The new Ann Arbor staging classification (15) (Table 20-2) replaces the Rye system (16). The recommendations of the Committee on HD Staging Procedures (Ann Arbor) are shown in Table 20-3 (17), and are reviewed by DRESSER et al. (18).

The clinical stage (CS) (physical examination, laboratory tests, roentgenograms, including lymphangiography, scans, and the initial biopsy to establish the diagnosis) is distinguished from the pathologic staging (PS) (findings of exploratory laparotomy; cytological studies of the liver, bone-marrow biopsy, mediastinoscopy, laparoscopy; any cytological studies in addition to the first biopsy, and pathological

Table 20-1. Histologic types of Hodgkin's
disease. (Rye classification) (7, 8)

Lymphocytic predominance	LP
Nodular sclerosis	NS
Mixed cellularity	MC
Lymphocytic depletion	LD

studies). A clear distinction is also made between extranodal (E) involvement in continuity with lymph-node disease (per continuitatem) and by dissemination (per disseminationem) to other more distant organs and tissues (19). The former can be included to its full extent in the curative radiation treatment. The local or regional character of the disease is thus maintained. This form of extranodal disease has the same prognosis as lymph-node involvement of a similar extent and is therefore transferred from stage IV (Rye classification) to the relevant lower stage in the Ann Arbor classification. The presence of one or more of the following symptoms will place a patient in group B: (1) unexplained weight loss of more than 10 percent during the 6 months previous to diagnosis; (2) unexplained fever (more than 38°C) and night sweats (15). Pruritus alone no longer qualifies patients for B classification. A method for classification of relapses was recently proposed (20).

The question of a unifocal versus a multifocal origin of HD and of its mode of spread, especially of hematogenous dissemination relatively early in the disease, remains unanswered (3, 11, 12, 21-25, 134).

The answer to this question is not merely of academic interest. Extended-field radical therapy has been based on the premise that the disease arises at a single focus and spreads in a predictable manner to adjacent lymph-nodes (25).

Other factors besides histological type, vascular invasion, and stage (extent of disease and presence or absence of constitutional symptoms) influence the prognosis and the selection of and reponse to the therapy (20, 26). Recent clinical studies have emphasized the importance of the clinical presentation, that is the lymph-node areas that are invaded.

Table 20-2. Hodgkin's disease. Ann Arbor staging Classification (17)

Stage I. Involvement of a single lymph node region (I) or of a single extralymphatic organ or site (I_E).

Stage II. Involvement of two or more lymph node regions on the same side of the diaphragm (II) or localized involvement of extralymphatic organ or site and of 1 or more lymph node regions on the same side of the diaphragm (II_E). An optional recommendation is that the numbers of node regions involved be indicated by a subscript (e.g., II_3).

Stage III. Involvement of lymph node regions on both sides of the diaphragm (III), which may also be accompanied by localized involvement of the extralymphatic organ or site (III_E) or by involvement of the spleen (III_S), or both (III_{SE}).

Stage IV. Diffuse or disseminated involvement of 1 or more extralymphatic organs or tissues with or without associated lymph node enlargement . The reason for classifying the patient as Stage IV should be identified further by defining site by symbols.

Table 20-3. Recommendations of the Committee on Staging Procedures for Hodgkin's Disease, Ann Arbor (17)

A. Required Evaluation Procedures

1. Adequate surgical biopsy, reviewed by a hematopathologist
2. Detailed history (fever, sweating, pruritus, and weight loss)
3. Complete physical examination with attention to lymphadenopathy, Waldeyer's ring, liver, spleen, and bone tenderness
4. Laboratory studies:
   Complete blood count, platelet count, erythrocyte sedimentation rate, serum alkaline phosphatase level. Evaluation of renal function and liver function
5. Radiologic studies:
   a) Chest roentgenogram (postero-anterior and lateral views)
   b) Intravenous pyelogram
   c) Bilateral lower extremity lymphogram
   d) Skeletal survey, especially thoraco-lumbar vertebrae, pelvis, proximal extremities, and areas of bone tenderness and/or pain.

B. Required Evaluation Procedures under Certain Conditions

1. Whole chest tomography, if abnormality on chest roentgenogram
2. Inferior cavography for equivocal lymphogram or pyelogram
3. Bone marrow biopsy, by a needle or open surgical technique if:
   a) Serum alkaline phosphatase elevated
   b) Unexplained anemia or other blood count depression
   c) Roentgenographic or scintigraphic evidence of osseous disease
   d) Generalized disease of Stage III category or greater
4. Exploratory laparotomy and splenectomy, if management decisions will depend on the identification of abdominal disease.

C. Useful Ancillary Procedures, not Definitive for Diagnosis

1. Skeletal scintigrams
2. Hepatic and spleen scintigrams
3. Serum chemistries, including calcium and uric acid
4. Estimate of patients' delayed hypersensitivity.

D. Procedures and Tests Promising for Clinical Study at Selected Centers but Experimental at this Time

1. Whole body gallium and selenium scintigrams
2. Determinations of: Serum iron and iron binding capacity, copper and ceruloplasmin, zinc, haptoglobin, fibrinogen, alpha-2-globulin: as well as, urinary hydroxyproline, leukocyte alkaline phosphatase, absolute lymphocyte count, antibodies to Epstein-Barr virus, human lymphocyte antibody typing

---

(26, 28). Involvement of the spleen is associated with a poor prognosis, even in stage II. According to KAPLAN (not confirmed by FERGUSON et al. (29) and SHIPLEY et al. (135)), it constitutes presumptive evidence of concomitant microscopic involvement of the liver, even in patients with an apparently normal liver at laparotomy and a negative liver biopsy (23, 30). It is not certain whether the spleen becomes involved through lymphatic spread (retrogradely from the para-aortic nodes) or whether it reflects hematogenous dissemination (24, 31). Involvement of the spleen can no longer be viewed as merely equivalent to that of another lymph node. Age and sex are of prognostic significance. Younger patients and females do better than older patients and males (32).

Several studies have demonstrated impairment of immune competence in HD, especially of cell-mediated immunity (33-35). This defect is progressive and is more extensive in stages III and IV and in the MC and LD varieties (34, 35). SOKAL (36) observed that patients who have a negative reaction to a tuberculin test but who convert after BCG vaccination have a distinctly better survival rate than those who do not. While one would expect individuals with normal immunity to have better prognosis, YOUNG et al. (33) failed to demonstrate that initial delayed hypersensitivity and lymphocyte transformation influence prognosis and survival in HD. Thus, it is not clear to what extent knowledge of immune status will improve prognostication over that based only on clinical stage and histologic type (154). The blood lymphocyte count is correlated with histological type and has a small independent prognostic value (32, 33).

The adverse effect of prior therapy, especially chemotherapy, has been noted in most drug trials. On the other hand, the disease-free interval following prior therapy is important. Patients with HD who remain relapse-free for 5 years after radiotherapy have at least a 95 percent chance of being permanently cured (37). Since all the factors described in the preceding paragraphs influence prognosis and response to therapy, it is important that they be recorded and reported in clinical trials.

A. CHEMOTHERAPY

1. Single Agents

Hodgkin's disease, like childhood ALL, is sensitive to a variety of cytotoxic agents (38-40). Alkylating agents, the Vinca alkaloids, and procarbazine (PCZ) are the most effective agents (Table 20-4). Nitrogen mustard (HN2) is probably the most active of the alkylating agents and is especially useful when a rapid effect is desired. Vinblastine (VLB) seems to induce longer remission than vincristine (VCR) but no studies are available that compare the two Vinca alkaloids. PCZ induces the highest percentage of complete remissions (41). It is probably the most active of all agents, especially since it has often been evaluated as a drug of last resort. Corticosteroids have a mainly palliative effect, lysis of fever, improved appetite, and a feeling of well-being, but sustained, objective responses are uncommon (38, 42, 43). Any decrease in tumor volume is due to reduction of the granulomatous reaction rather than of the malignant cells themselves. Steroids are also useful in progressive disease, while the marrow is suppressed, and in secondary hemolytic anemias. Antimetabolites and the older antibiotics have rarely been evaluated (38).

A number of promising experimental agents are still under study. BCNU is effective in far-advanced HD that is resistant to both alkylating agents and Vinca alkaloids (44, 45, 136). CCNU is even more active (46). The ALGB recently initiated a study comparing CCNU with Me-CCNU (47). At least one third of patients respond to adriamycin (48, 49, 137). A similar response rate is reported for bleomycin (50-52) but to date most of the patients treated had far-advanced disease, often refractory to conventional agents. Its lack of bone marrow toxicity makes it especially useful in patients with impaired marrow reserve and for inclusion in combination chemotherapy. Because of its concentration in lung tissue, bleomycin may be indicated for pulmonary lesions provided its pulmonary toxicity is not prohibitive (50).

Table 20-4. Effectiveness of single agents in Hodgkin's disease

Drug	No. evaluated	Response rate	Complete remission	Reference
Methotrexate	44	30 %	–	GOLDSMITH and CARTER (40)
6-Mercaptopurine	34	35 %	–	–
Imidazole carboxamide	18	56 %	5 %	FREI et al. (57)
5-Fluorouracil	23	26 %	–	GOLDSMITH and CARTER (40)
BCNU	149	50 %	5 %	–
CCNU	19	74 %	21 %	SELAWRY and HANSEN (46)
MeCCNU	16	56 %	–	TRANUM and HAUT (127)
Streptozotocin	16	44 %	6 %	SCHEIN et al. (139)
Procarbazine	366	69 %	38 %	GOLDSMITH and CARTER (40)
Nitrogen mustard	796	64 %	13 %	–
Chlorambucil	305	60 %	16 %	–
Cyclophosphamide	469	54 %	12 %	–
ThioTEPA	64	41 %	–	–
Actinomycin D	18	50 %	–	–
Adriamycin	64	36 %	–	BLUM and CARTER (137)
Bleomycin	122	37 %	6 %	BLUM et al. (52)
Vincristine	115	58 %	36 %	GOLDSMITH and CARTER (40)
Vinblastine	682	68 %	30 %	–
VM-26	22	31 %	O	MATHE et al. (138)
Prednisone	105	61 %	O	GOLDSMITH and CARTER (40)

Preliminary reports indicate some activity of the semisynthetic podo-phyllotoxin derivatives, VM26 and VP 16213 (53-56, 138). Imidazole car-boxamide (57), streptonigrin (39, 58, 59), piposulfan (60), dibromo-dulcitol (39), streptozotocin (139), and 1-methyl-1-nitrosourea (140) are also effective.

Although different classes of agents have considerable activity (50-70 percent response rate) in HD, the rate of complete remissions is rela-tively low (10-30 percent) (see Table 20-4). Furthermore, remissions induced by single-agent therapy are of short duration. As active agents were marketed, it became standard practice to use each one until primary or secondary resistance developed. The patient thus became successively resistant to alkylating agents, Vinca alkaloids, procarbazine, and cor-ticosteroids.

In the early '60s, some investigators began to evaluate combination chemotherapy in advanced HD, first low-dose continuous (61), and later high-dose intermittent therapy (62, 63). Gradually, a similar approach has evolved as in ALL. Applying the same principles (see Chap. 14), one can now distinguish induction, consolidation and maintenance chemotherapy programs (64-67).

2. Combinations

(i) Remission Induction

Most combinations for induction of advanced HD include an alkylating agent, a Vinca alkaloid, procarbazine and prednisone. MOPP, a combination of nitrogen mustard, vincristine, procarbazine and prednisone, given over 14 days, every 28 days (Fig. 20-1) for 6 cycles has been the most effective and therefore the most popular combination (40, 63, 65, 68, 141). Of 43 previously untreated patients with advanced HD, 81 percent achieved complete remission with a median duration of 36 months determined from the time of termination of treatment. Fifteen (43 percent) of these have remained continuously free of disease for at least 5 and up to 7 years with no further therapy beyond the initial 6 cycles (66). Twenty of the 35 (58 percent) who had a CR relapsed in a median time of 11 months. The median survival point has not yet been reached, but will exceed 60 months in the group with CR. To date, there have been no relapses in any patient who after the initial 6 cycles of MOPP remained free of disease for longer than 42 months (65, 157). These results have been confirmed by several other investigators. The Cancer Therapy Evaluation Branch of the National Cancer Institute has data on file for 709 patients treated with MOPP with a complete response rate of 60 percent (40). This response rate has been improved by substituting cyclophosphamide or BCNU for HN2 or VLB for VCR (40, 69-71) (Table 20-5). Several three-drug combinations have not been as effective as MOPP (40, 47, 72-74). New active agents are being added to MOPP in an attempt to improve the remission induction rate. Table 20-6 lists some of the protocols under study.

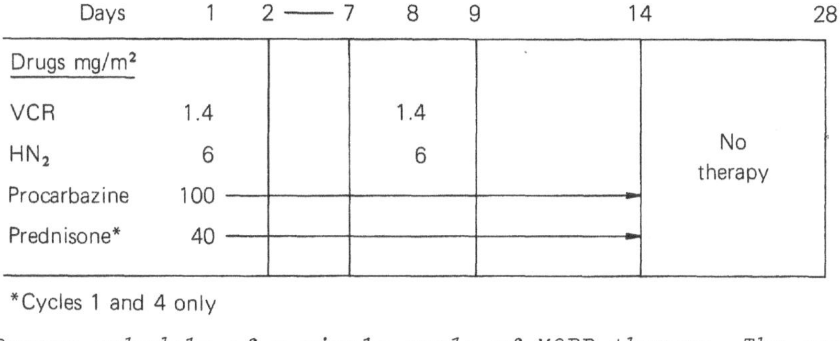

Days	1	2 ——— 7	8	9	14	28
Drugs mg/m²						
VCR	1.4		1.4			
HN₂	6		6		No therapy	
Procarbazine	100					
Prednisone*	40					

*Cycles 1 and 4 only

Fig. 20-1. Dosage schedule of a single cycle of MOPP therapy. The cycle is repeated on day 29. (From DE VITA et al. (63))

Combination chemotherapy is clearly superior to single-agent therapy by historical comparison (38, 40) and in one controlled study (MOPP vs. HN2: CR of 50 percent vs. 19 percent) (75). This superiority applies to percentage of complete remissions, duration of unmaintained remissions, and survival. Few trials have compared the MOPP regimen with the same agents administered sequentially (76). The ALGB compared

Table 20-5. Results of combination chemotherapy in Hodgkin's disease

Combinations	Number evaluated	% CR	Reference
TEM VLB PCZ PDN	29	41%	AMIEL et al. (1966) (128)
M HN2 – 6 mg/m², i.v., days 1 and 8 O VCR – 1.4 mg/m², i.v., days 1 and 8 P PCZ – 100 mg/m², p.o., days 1-14 P PDN – 40 mg/m², p.o., days 1-14 (cycles 1 and 4 only) Total of six 2-week cycles, 14 days on and 14 days off.	43	81%	DEVITA et al. (1970) (63)
MOPP	709	60%	GOLDSMITH and CARTER (1974) (40)
M HN2 – 6 mg/m², i.v., days 1 and 8 V VLB – 10 mg/d, i.v., days 1, 8, and 14 P PCZ – 100 mg/m²/d, p.o., x 14 days P PDN – olone – 40 mg/d, p.o., x 14 days (courses 1 and 4 only)	52	58%	NICHOLSON et al. (1970) (69)
6 courses; 4 wks between each Maintenance: induction regimen q 3 mos x 1 yr and q 4 mos in 2nd yr.	148	51%	FAIRLEY (1973) (70)
C CPM – 1000 mg/m², i.v., day 1 V VLB – 0.1 mg/kg, i.v., days 1 and 8 P PCZ – 100 mg/m², p.o., days 1-7 P PDN – 40 mg/m², p.o., days 1-7 repeat on day 21	20 previously treated 17 previously untreated	55% 65%	KVOLS et al. (154)
C CPM – 600 mg/m², i.v., days 1 and 8 O VCR – 1.4 mg/m², i.v., days 1 and 8 P PCZ – 100 mg/m²/d, p.o., x 10 days P PDN – 40 mg/m²/d, p.o., x 14 days (courses 1 and 4 only) Every month for 6 courses	138	66%	MORGENFIELD et al. (1975) (129)

Table 20-5. (continued)

Combinations	Number evaluated	% CR	Reference
C CPM – 800 mg/m², i.v., day 1 (impairment marrow – 400 mg/m²)	107	36%	LUCE et al. (1971) (74)
O VCR – 2 mg, i.v., day 1 P PDN – 60 mg/m²/d, p.o., x 5 days, taper over 3 days 6 courses at 14-day intervals			

CPM – 10 mg/kg, i.v., weekly
   VLB – 0.2 mg/kg, i.v., weekly
   PDN – 1 mg/kg, p.o., daily
	32	34%	LENHARD (1970) (72)

A ADM – 25 mg/m², i.v. days B BLM – 10 mg/m², i.v. 1 and 14 repeat on day 28 V VLB – 6 mg/m², i.v. D DIC – 150 mg/m², i.v. days 1 to 5 6 cycles	20	75%	BONADONNA et al. (1975) (130)

Table 20-6. Combination chemotherapy for Hodgkin's disease. Studies in progressa

BOP	BCNU, VCR, PDN	ALGB
BOPP	BCNU, VCR, PCZ, PDN	ALGB
	CCNU, VCR, PCZ, PDN	ALGB
	CCNU, VLB, PCZ, PDN	ALGB
MOPP-B	MOPP + BLM	SWCCG
BCVPP	BCNU, CPM, VLB, PCZ, PDN	SEG
BVVPP	BCNU, VCR, VLB, PCZ, PDN	SEG
MABOP	HN2, ADM, BLM, VCR, PDM	BONADONNA

aFor dosage schedules, see references 40 and 47.

MOPP to a five-drug combination (VCR, PCZ, VLB, CLB, and PDN) and to
each of these drugs used singly in sequence. The complete remission
rate and the median duration of remission achieved with each combination
proved superior to the same drugs used in sequence (64, 65, 71).

The long duration of unmaintained remissions with MOPP, in almost half
of the patients suggests that it is capable of reducing the tumor cell
population to low levels. In contrast, one would expect single-agent
sequential therapy to provide only palliation of symptoms or control
of disease progression. High response rates have also been obtained
with MOPP in patients who have received prior radiotherapy (74-76 percent CR) (66, 77, 141, 142) but not in patients with prior exposure to
chemotherapy (40 percent CR) (77), or to both (35 percent CR) (69, 77,
78). All histologic types respond to MOPP. Advanced age, the presence
of constitutional symptoms, or bone marrow involvement adversely affect
the results of MOPP therapy (141-142).

MOPP is generally tolerated by most patients. The dosage of all drugs
except prednisone must often be reduced with each cycle because of progressive myelosuppression (63); 75 to 92 percent of the total projected
dose of the agents can be administered. Nausea and vomiting frequently
occur with injections of HN2. Vincristine neurotoxicity is also common.
The long-term effects of MOPP are not yet known. Prolonged aspermia,
possibly permanent, is an important consideration in young males. The
incidence of cancer and leukemia is not yet known.

In the context of our studies on intermittent cyclic sequential chemotherapy we are evaluating a protocol (CISC III) that uses most of the
agents active in Hodgkin's disease (ADM, VM 26, CPM, PDN, VLB, CLB, and
PCZ). Several other combinations containing mainly of drugs not included
in the MOPP combination are also effective (133, 155-161).

(ii) Maintenance Therapy
About half the patients with MOPP-induced complete remissions will relapse within 2 years if no further therapy is given. Therefore maintenance programs were introduced, with either further courses of MOPP at
2- or 3-monthly intervals or single conventional or experimental agents.
The NCI group in a controlled trial noted no beneficial effect for maintenance therapy with either BCNU every 3 months for 15 months or two
consecutive monthly cycles of MOPP every 3 months for 15 months (79).

The SWCCG found no benefit from maintenance therapy with a series of
injections of actinomycin D or methotrexate every 2 months for 18 months
(80). VLB every 2 weeks for 18 months, however, was better than no maintenance therapy. The same group reported significantly fewer relapses
in patients on maintenance therapy with MOPP every 2 months (77, 198).
Thus, 75 percent of the maintained patients were in CR 3 years later
compared with 46 percent for the unmaintained controls. There was no
difference in overall survival at 4 years between the maintained and
unmaintained patients in complete remission. This was due largely to
more effective secondary treatment in patients receiving only 6 courses
of MOPP (77 percent chance of reentering CR with MOPP). According to
the ALGB, maintenance therapy with VLB (weekly or every 2 weeks), or
with chlorambucil plus monthly reinforcement doses of VCR + PDN, is
superior to maintenance with CLB alone (71). The Stanford group initiated a randomized trial of maintenance using drugs (CCNU versus VLB
plus CLB) not included in the MOPP combination (142). Although the data
are not fully in agreement (especially the difference between the NCI
and the SWCCG with respect to maintenance therapy with MOPP), it would
seem that maintenance therapy is beneficial. The best regimen, however,
remains to be determined.

B. STRATEGY

1. Surgery

Surgery has had no place in the treatment of HD since the advent of
radiotherapy (81-83). Its role was limited to initial biopsy for diagnosis and treatment of certain complications, for example hypersplenism
(143) and obstruction by tumor masses. In an attempt to determine more
accurately the extent of disease in the abdomen and to plan therapy
more appropriately, exploratory laparotomy and splenectomy have become
popular in recent years (81, 84-88, 144). A great deal has been learned
through this procedure about the progression of HD and its clinical
behavior. It offers the opportunity to check the accuracy of the various
staging procedures (lymphangiography, scans, liver function tests, etc.).
Staging changes in 25-50 percent of patients after laparotomy, which
may affect therapy in a considerable percentage of these. In addition,
splenectomized patients are more tolerant of subsequent radiotherapy
(89) and chemotherapy (90, 91, 143) (according to IHDE et al. (145) only
in patients with hypersplenism); in female patients an oophoropexy can
be carried out to shield the ovaries (30, 92) from excessive radiation.
Splenectomy simplifies subsequent irradiation of the abdomen. The debate about the subsequent increased risk of bacterial infections, especially in younger patients (146) and viral infections (93) continues
(94-98, 143). The effect of early splenectomy on the course of HD is
not yet known. Preliminary data suggest that it does not prolong survival (147).

It is beyond the scope of this text to discuss in detail the indications for exploratory laparotomy and splenectomy (29, 81, 86, 87, 99-
102, 143). To summarize: in practice, surgery should be used selectively in those cases in which the findings will alter therapy. Unsuspected
HD in the spleen is especially important because of its possible association with liver involvement (23, 30).

2. Radiotherapy

The radiotherapeutic principles for HD have undergone considerable
changes in the past 30 years (103, 104). First, it was learned that
a dose of 4000 rads is required to sterilize HD and to prevent local
recurrences. The fact that relapses were frequently noted at the margin
of treated fields led to the concept of prophylactic "extended-field"
irradiation, to include contiguous lymph-node areas. The availability of
high-energy sources permitted this concept to be expended to all lymph-
node areas (total nodal irradiation: mantle, inverted Y, and spleen),
both prophylactically (Stages I and II) and with curative intent (Stage
III). The superiority of total nodal irradiation over extended-field
therapy for localized disease was demonstrated by a prospective clinical trial (105). This aggressive therapy, however, does not exclude
subsequent relapse, especially extranodal, in all patients thus treated.
Exploratory laparotomy and splenectomy were therefore introduced to
allow the true extent of the disease to be determined in order to avoid
such failures. It was also hoped to identify certain patient groups that
do not require total nodal irradiation for localized disease (Stages
I and II). Finally, laparotomy indicates certain groups of patients
with a high risk of unsuspected extranodal dissemination at the time
of diagnosis. These include patients with "B" symptoms, vascular invasion, splenic involvement, or the lymphocytic-depletion type (even in
Stages I and II) HD (11, 12, 23, 106-107). Some of the newer radiotherapeutic techniques permit treatment of some of these extranodal sites:
entire abdomen (108), liver (109, 148), or lungs (110). The acute and

late reactions to extensive irradiation in HD patients must be familiar to those who care for them (104, 111, 149, 150).

3. Combined Chemotherapy-Radiotherapy

As long as radiotherapy was the only treatment modality with a curative potential in HD, the selection of therapy was relatively easy. In recent years all cases with disease limited to the lymph nodes (Stage I to III) have been treated with radiotherapy. Chemotherapy was reserved for patients with extranodal involvement (Stage IV per dissemination) and radiation failures (107). Since the introduction of drug combinations, however, the curative potential of chemotherapy may be becoming a reality. Its role in the overall management of HD therefore needs to be reassessed. Several trials in progress are studying the value of chemotherapy (1) as an adjuvant to radiotherapy in localized disease (Stages I and II) and (2) as an integral part (together with radiotherapy) in the intermediate stages (IIB, IIIA + B) and for the high-risk groups described in the preceding section (26, 112, 113, 151, 156).

For Stages I and II, the EORTC has reported a beneficial effect from weekly vinblastine injections following extended-field radiotherapy for the mixed cellularity type, and to a lesser extent for the lymphocytic-depletion variants (see Fig. 13-6) (26, 114). This trial demonstrated that chemotherapy is capable of sterilizing some subclinical lesions in the non-irradiated areas (26). A study is in progress at Stanford to assess the value of six courses of MOPP as adjuvant to radiotherapy, (strictly local to subtotal nodal, depending on favorable or unfavorable clinical features in Stages IA and IIA). Preliminary results of a randomized study of Stages I(A and B), II(A and B), and IIIA HD indicate fewer relapses in patients treated with involved-field radiotherapy, followed by adjuvant MOPP, than in patients receiving extended-field radiation without MOPP (112). Since localized radiotherapy results in 40-50 percent survival rates in Stages I and II, it must be concluded that many patients in these stages are now being overtreated. It is hoped that with better techniques for evaluating the extent of the disease and better appreciation of prognositc factors and of the natural history of the different variants of HD, it will be possible to be more selective in determining the intensity of therapy (radiotherapy, with or without chemotherapy) and its extent for certain subgroups in each of these stages. This approach should reduce the number of overtreated patients without decreasing the proportion of long-term survivors (26, 115).

4. Immunotherapy

Some trials are now beginning to incorporate BCG vaccination in the treatment of patients in remission following chemotherapy (47, 73).

5. Treatment Plan for Stages I and II

For those not participating in cooperative studies, we recommend the following therapy in Stages I and II (Table 20-7). Radiotherapy is the primary treatment modality. It should, for the time being, include, for supradiaphragmatic localizations, mantle therapy and irradiation of the upper abdominal lymph nodes and spleen. Some radiotherapists think that for certain favorable localizations less extensive radiotherapy suffices (103, 108, 118). Laparotomy and splenectomy are indicated in high-risk patients (B symptoms, mixed cellularity, or lymphocytic

Table 20-7. Treatment plan for Hodgkin's disease (for physicians not participating in cooperative studies)

Stages I and II	Supra-diaphragmatic (without high-risk factors)	1. Radiotherapy: mantle + upper abdominal lymph nodes
	Infra-diaphragmatic (without high-risk factors)	1. Laparotomy + splenectomy 2. Radiotherapy: inverted Y
	If high-risk factors: 1. B symptoms 2. Lymphocytic depletion 3. Vascular invasion	1. Laparotomy + splenectomy 2. Total nodal radiation (TNR) 3. Adjuvant chemotherapy

Stage III	Options:
	1. TNR
	2. Combination chemotherapy
	3. Combination: chemotherapy → radiotherapy[a] radiotherapy → chemotherapy chemotherapy → radiotherapy → → chemotherapy
	Recommended:
	In absence of high-risk[b] factors: TNR
	In presence of high-risk factors: chemotherapy → radiotherapy (to pretreatment involved areas) → chemotherapy

Stage IV	Combination chemotherapy (MOPP)

[a] = 1) TNR or
2) radiotherapy to areas involved prior to therapy
[b] (same as above plus splenic involvement)

depletion (107). For those, total nodal radiotherapy is recommended and it is resonable to supplement it with adjuvant chemotherapy. Experienced physicians can use MOPP in the knowledge that the bone marrow reserve may be diminished (117). Preliminary results of this combination are encouraging. The disease-free survival is significantly improved compared to controls treated with radiotherapy alone (112, 118, 119, 151, 156). Longer follow-up is required to determine whether survival is also improved. Less experienced physicians could use VLB. Better drug selections will certainly be developed in the future for adjuvant therapy in HD. The EORTC is currently investigating VLB + PCZ for this purpose. For Stage-I and -II localizations below the diaphragm, laparotomy and splenectomy are recommended, followed by radiotherapy (inverted Y). Adjuvant chemotherapy is given in high-risk patients as for supradiaphragmatic disease.

Incidentally, chemotherapy alone cannot at this time be recommended
for localized disease. However, the outcome of an ongoing study of
chemotherapy in a country where radiation therapy is not available deserves our attention (120).

6. Treatment Plan for Stage III

For Stage-III disease (involvement on both sides of the diaphragm) a
new approach is under study: the combination of radiotherapy and chemotherapy as primary therapy. This approach is justified by the difference in the modes of action of the two agents and by the fact that their
limiting factors are not the same (26). Radiotherapy exerts a local
action but presents local risks. Chemotherapy can reach a malignant
cell wherever it is located, but the total dose is limited by the risk
of hematologic aplasia. Radiotherapy is not very effective against
cells in S phase (121) but it does act on resting cells. Chemotherapy,
on the other hand, is effective against cells in the proliferative cycle
but has little effect on resting cells. Chemotherapy preceding radiotherapy has several advantages. It may permit completion of scheduled
radiotherapy in patients with severe constitutional symptoms, who otherwise tolerate nodal radiotherapy only with difficulty (113). Subsequent
radiation fields can be considerably reduced in patients who present
with large tumor masses. Effective chemotherapy may have a curative potential in treating occult foci of extranodal disease (26), which are a
frequent source of relapse after total nodal irradiation, while subsequent radiotherapy is used for curative therapy of gross disease. Relapses after chemotherapy with MOPP tend to occur in areas of most involvement before treatment (77). Relapses occur rarely in sites not previously involved (152). This is consistent with the hypothesis that relapses result from persisting tumor cells. The larger the tumor mass,
the more likely it is that kinetic and pharmacologic conditions will
favor the persistence of clonogenic cells. This concept strongly suggests that, after patients on chemotherapy enter CR, it is a rational
approach to irradiate sites of major pretreatment involvement (156).

Many radiotherapists, however, are concerned about the myelosuppressive
effect of chemotherapy prior to radiotherapy and prefer to reverse the
sequence, beginning with radiotherapy. Chemotherapy following radiotherapy may be more effective because of recruitment resulting form
tumor cell reduction effected by radiation (see Chap. 13). In one study
comparing both modalities, the ALGB reported that fewer technical problems were experienced when total nodal radiation therapy preceded sequential chemotherapy with VLB and HN2 (122). The reserved sequence had
a pronounced effect on platelet count and hemoglobin level. The SWCCG
has managed to give three courses of MOPP preceding radiotherapy (123).
The Stanford Group has been able to give six cycles of MOPP therapy
after total nodal irradiation in Stage III A and B (118, 119).

If chemotherapy is to be used as an integral part of the treatment plan
in Stage III, the question of the extent of radiotherapy will have to
be investigated in a comparative prospective trial. Is total nodal
therapy necessary, or is therapy to sites of major pretreatment involvement sufficient? The problem of their most effective sequence also needs
to be studied.

Thus, for Stage III disease, three modalities are possible: (1) total
nodal irradiation (124, 125), (2) combination chemotherapy (63), (3)
combination of chemotherapy plus radiotherapy (total nodal (113, 118,
119) or limited to pretreatment of involved areas (113)). In the latter
situation, one can start with either chemotherapy or radiotherapy (118,
119). Another option is to begin with chemotherapy (126) for remission

Table 20-8. Treatment scheme for Hodgkin's disease integrating EORTC protocols

Histologic classification[a] / Stage	1 and 2	3 and 4
I and Supra-diaphragmatic, Protocol H2 EORTC	Randomized → Laparotomy + splenectomy / Irradiation (splenic hilar area) followed by:	Laparotomy + splenectomy / Irradiation (splenic hilar area) followed by:
II	irradiation (mantle + lumbo-aort.)	irradiation (mantle + lumbo-aort.) followed by (randomized) → VLB / VLB + procarbazine
A and B Infra-diaphragmatic	Laparotomy + splenectomy followed by: irradiation (inverted Y)	Laparotomy + splenectomy followed by: irradiation (inverted Y) followed by: VLB or VLB + procarbazine
IIIA	Laparotomy + splenectomy followed by: irradiation (total nodal) followed or not followed by chemotherapy or	(VLB or combination)
IIIB Protocol H3B EORTC	Laparotomy + splenectomy followed by: Randomized → MOPP / Irradiation followed by VLB + procarbazine	
IV A and B	MOPP or phase-II trial	

a 1 = lymphocytic predominance; 2 = nodular sclerosis;
  3 = mixed cellularity; 4 = lymphocytic depletion.

induction, followed by radiotherapy for consolidation, and to end with short-term (153) or prolonged maintenance chemotherapy (67, 26). Appropriate studies are still needed to demonstrate which of these approaches is the most effective, and for which patient subgroups (115). The current treatment scheme of the EORTC Group tries to answer some of these questions (Table 20-8).

In Stage III without high-risk features, extranodal lesions are rare and it seems logical to treat these like Stage II, thus primarily by radiotherapy (total nodal). In Stage III with high-risk factors (B symptoms, splenic involvement, vascular invasion, MC or LD histology) the risk of extranodal dissemination is high and chemotherapy is required. The sequence of moderately intensive chemotherapy (e.g., 2-3 x MOPP), followed by complementary radiotherapy to pretreatment-involved areas, terminating with long-term maintenance therapy (e.g., MOPP q 2 months for 18 months) is a reasonable program for the time being.

7. Treatment Plan for Stage IV

Stage IV patients (per dissemination) are treated primarily by combination chemotherapy.

Patients who have become refractory to MOPP can be treated with one of the newer agents: the nitrosoureas, bleomycin, adriamycin, DIC, or VM 26. They are listed more or less in decreasing order of effectiveness. Preliminary reports suggest that several new combinations (ABVD, CAVe) are useful in MOPP-failures (130, 155, 156).

REFERENCES

1. KAPLAN, H.S.: Hodgin's disease. Cambridge: Harvard University Press. 1972.
2. ULTMANN, J.E., MORAN, E.M.: Clinical course and complications in Hodgkin's disease. Arch. intern. Med. 131, 332 (1973).
3. STRUM, S.B.: The natural history, histopathology, staging and mode of spread of Hodgkin's disease. Ser. Haematol. 6, 20 (1973).
4. MATHE, G., RAPPAPORT, H.: Histological and cytological typing of the neoplastic diseases of the haematopoietic and lymphoid tissues. Geneva: W.H.O. 1973.
5. LUKES, R.J., BUTLER, J.J., HICKS, E.B.: Natural history of Hodgkin's disease as related to its pathologic picture. Cancer 19, 317 (1966).
6. JACKSON, Jr., H., PARKER, F.: Hodgkin's disease. II. Pathology. New Engl. J. Med. 231, 35 (1944).
7. LUKES, R.J., BUTLER, J.J.: The pathology and nomenclature of Hodgkin's disease. Cancer Res. 26, 1063 (1966).
8. LUKES, R.J., CRAVER, L.F., HALL, T.C., RAPPAPORT, H., RUBIN, P.: Report of the nomenclature committee. Cancer Res. 26, 1131 (1966).
9. BUTLER, J.J.: Relationship of histological findings to survival in Hodgkin's disease. Cancer Res. 31, 1770 (1971).
10. BERARD, C.W., THOMAS, L.B., AXTELL, L.M., KRUSE, M., NEWELL, G., KAGAN, R.: The relationship of histopathological subtype to clinical stage of Hodgkin's disease at diagnosis. Cancer Res. 31, 1776 (1971).
11. RAPPAPORT, H., STRUM, S.B.: Vascular invasion in Hodgkin's disease: its incidence and relationship to the spread of the disease. Cancer 25, 1304 (1970).
12. RAPPAPORT, H., STRUM, S.B., HUTCHISON, G., ALLEN, L.W.: Clinical and biological significance of vascular invasion in Hodgkin's disease. Cancer Res. 31, 1794 (1971).

13. KIRSCHNER, R.H., ABT, A.B., O'CONNELL, M.J., SKLANSKY, B.D., GREENE, W.H., WIERNIK, P.H.: Vascular invasion and hematogenous dissemination of Hodgkin's disease. Cancer 34, 1159 (1974).

14. PETERS, V.: A study of survivals in Hodgkin's disease treated radiologically. Amer. J. Roentgenol. 63, 299 (1950).

15. CARBONE, P.P., KAPLAN, H.S., MUSSHOFF, K., SMITHERS, D.W., TUBIANA, M.: Report of the Committee on Hodgkin's disease staging classification. Cancer Res. 31, 1860 (1971).

16. ROSENBERG, S.A.: Report of the committee on the staging of Hodgkin's disease. Cancer Res. 26, 1310 (1966).

17. ROSENBERG, S.A., BOIRON, M., DE VITA, V.T., JOHNSON, R.E., LEE, B.J., ULTMANN, J.E.: VIAMANTE, M.: Report of the committee on Hodgkin's disease staging procedures. Cancer Res. 31, 1862 (1971).

18. DRESSER, R.K., MORAN, E.M., ULTMANN, J.E.: Staging of Hodgkin's disease and lymphoma. Diagnostic procedures including staging laparotomy and splenectomy. Med. Clin. N. Amer. 57, 479 (1973).

19. MUSSHOFF, K.: Prognostic and therapeutic implications of staging in extranodal Hodgkin's disease. Cancer Res. 31, 1814 (1971).

20. MATHE, G., TUBIANA, M.: The development of ideas on the natural history and the therapy of Hodgkin's disease. Ser. Haematol. 6, 5 (1973).

21. RAPPAPORT, H.: The clinical and biologic significance of recent observations concerning the spread of Hodgkin's disease. Rev. franc. Etud. clin. biol. 14, 449 (1969).

22. SMITHERS, D.W.: Spread of Hodgkin's disease. Lancet 1, 1262 (1970).

23. KAPLAN, H.S.: Contiguity and progression in Hodgkin's disease. Cancer Res. 31, 1811 (1971).

24. AISENBERG, A.C.: Hematogenous dissemination of Hodgkin's disease. Ann. intern. Med. 77, 810 (1972).

25. ROSENBERG, A., KAPLAN, H.S.: Evidence for an orderly progression in the spread of Hodgkin's disease. Cancer Res. 26, 1225 (1966).

26. TUBIANA, M., MATHE, G.: Combined radiotherapy and chemotherapy in the treatment of Hodgkin's disease. Ser. Haematol. 6, 202 (1973).

27. FULLER, L.M., GAMBLE, J.F., SCHULLENBERGER, C.C., BUTLER, J.J., GEHAN, E.A.: Prognostic factors in localized Hodgkin's disease treated with regional radiation. Radiology 98, 641 (1971).

28. PETERS, V.: The need for a new clinical classification in Hodgkin's disease. Cancer Res. 31, 1713 (1971).

29. FERGUSON, D.J., ALLEN, L.W., GRIEM, M.L., MORAN, M.E., RAPPAPORT, H., ULTMANN, J.E.: Surgical experience with staging laparotomy in 125 patients with lymphoma. Arch. intern. Med. 131, 356 (1973).

30. BAGLEY, Jr., C.M., ROTH, J.A., THOMAS, L.B., DE VITA, Jr., V.T.: Liver biopsy in Hodgkin's disease. Clinicopathologic correlations in 127 patients. Ann. intern. Med. 76, 219 (1972).

31. HALIE, M.R., SELDENRATH, J.J., STAM, H.C., NIEWEG, H.O.: Curative radiotherapy in Hodgkin's disease: significance of hematogenous dissemination established by examination of peripheral blood and spleen. Brit. med. J. 2, 611 (1972).

32. TUBIANA, M., ATTIE, E., FLAMANT, R., GERARD-MARCHANT, R., HAYAT, M.: Prognosis factors in 454 cases of Hodgkin's disease. Cancer Res. 31, 1801 (1971).

33. YOUNG, R.C., CORDER, M.P., BERARD, C.W., DeVITA, V.T.: Immune alterations in Hodgkin's disease. Arch. intern. Med. 131, 446 (1973).

34. AISENBERG, A.C.: Value of immunologic testing. J. amer. Med. Ass. 222, 1301 (1972).

35. SCHNEIDER, M., MATHE, G., SCHWARZENBERG, L., POUILLART, P., WEINER, R., AMIEL, J.L., HAYAT, M., JASMIN, C., DE VASSAL, F.: Nonspecific immune responses in hematosarcomas and acute leukemias. In: Investigations and Stimulation of Immunity in Cancer Patients. Recent Results in Cancer Research, Vol. 47, p. 42. (eds. G. Mathé, R. Weiner). Heidelberg: Springer-Verlag 1974.

36. SOKAL, J.E., AUNGST, C.W.: Response to BCG vaccination and survival in advanced Hodgkin's disease. Cancer 24, 128 (1969).
37. KAPLAN, H.S.: Prognostic significance of the relapse-free interval after radiotherapy in Hodgkin's disease. Cancer 22, 1131 (1968).
38. CARTER, S.K., LIVINGSTON, R.B.: Single-agent therapy for Hodgkin's disease. Arch. intern. Med. 131, 377 (1973).
39. DRESSER, R.J., ULTMANN, J.E.: The sensitivity of Hodgkin's disease to chemotherapeutic agents administered singly. Ser. Haematol. 6, 152 (1973).
40. GOLDSMITH, M.A., CARTER. S.K.: Combination chemotherapy of advanced Hodgkin's disease. Cancer 33, 1 (1974).
41. MATHE, G., BERUMEN, L., SCHWEIGUTH, O., BRULE, G., SCHNEIDER, M., AMIEL, J.L., CATTAN, Z., SCHWARZENBERG, L.: Methyl-hydrazine in treatment of Hodgkin's disease and various forms of haematosarcoma and leukemia. Lancet 2, 1077 (1963).
42. KOFMAN, S., PERLIA, C.P., BOESEN, E., EISENSTEIN, R., TAYLOR, S.G., III: The role of corticosteroids in the treatment of malignant lymphomas. Cancer 15, 338 (1962).
43. HALL, T.C., ABADI, A., KRANT, M.J.: High-dose corticoid therapy in Hodgkin's disease and other lymphomas. Ann. intern. Med. 66, 1144 (1967).
44. YOUNG, R.C., DE VITA, V.T., SERPICK, A.A., CANELLOS, G.R.: Treatment of advanced Hodgkin's disease with (1,3 bis (2 chloroethyl)-1-nitrosourea) BCNU. New Engl. J. Med. 285, 475 (1971).
45. LESSNER, H.: BCNU (1,3bis(2-chloroethyl)-1-nitrosourea) effects on advanced Hodgkin's disease and other neoplasia. Cancer 22, 451 (1968).
46. SELAWRY, O., HANSEN, H.: Superiority of CCNU over BCNU in the treatment of advanced Hodgkin's disease. Proc. Am. Ass. Cancer Res. 13, 46 (1972) (abstr.).
47. CARTER, S.K.: An overview of the status of the nitrosoureas in other tumors. Cancer Chemother. Rep. Part 3, 4, 35 (1973).
48. CARTER, S.K.: Current status of new agents. Cancer Chemother. Rep. Part 3, 3, 33 (1972).
49. O'BRYAN, R.M., LUCE, J.K., TALLEY. R.W., GOTTLIEB, J.A., BAKER, L.H., BONADONNA, G.: Phase II evaluation of adriamycin in human neoplasia. Cancer 32, 1 (1973).
50. E.O.R.T.C. Co-operative Group for Leukaemia and Haematosarcomas: Bleomycin in the reticuloses. Brit. med. J. 1, 285 (1972).
51. YAGODA, A., MUKHERJI, B., YOUNG, C., ETCUBANAS, E., LAMONTE, C., SMITH, J.R., TAN, C.T.C., KRAKOFF, I.H.: Bleomycin, an antitumor antibiotic. Ann. intern. Med. 77, 861 (1972).
52. BLUM, R.H., CARTER, S.K., AGRE, K.: A clinical review of bleomycin - a new antineoplastic agent. Cancer 31, 903 (1973).
53. DOMBERNOWSKY, P., NISSEN, N.I., LARSEN, V.: Clinical investigation of a new podophyllum derivative epipodophyllotoxin 4'-demethyl-9-(4,6-O-2.thenylidene-ß-D-glucopyranoside) (NSC-122819), in patients with malignant lymphomas and solid tumors. Cancer Chemother. Rep. 56, 71 (1972).
54. E.O.R.T.C. Co-operative Group for Leukaemia and Haematosarcomas: Clinical screening of epipodophyllotoxin VM 26 in malignant lymphomas and solid tumours. Brit. med. J. 2, 744 (1972).
55. GOLDSMITH, M.A., CARTER, S.K.: 4'-demethyl-epipodophyllotoxin-ß-D-thenylidene glucoside (VM-26). A brief review. Europ. J. Cancer 9, 477 (1973).
56. E.O.R.T.C. Clinical Screening Group. Epipodophyllotoxin VP 16213 in the treatment of acute leukaemias, haematosarcomas and solid tumours. Brit. Med. J. 3, 199 (1973).
57. FREI, E. III, LUCE, J.K., TALLEY, R.W., VAITKEVICIUS, V.K., WILSON, H.E.: 5-(3,3-dimethyl-1-triazeno) imidazole-4-carboxamide (NSC-45388) in the treatment of lymphoma. Cancer Chemother. Rep. 56, 667 (1972).

58. HUMPHREY, E.W., DIETRICH, F.S.: Clinical experience with the methyl ester of streptonigrin (NCS-45384). Cancer Chemother. Rep. 33, 21 (1963).
59. KAUNG, D.T., WITTINGTON, R.M., SPENCER, H., PATNO, M.E.: Comparison of chlorambucil and streptonigrin (NSC-45383) in the treatment of malignant lymphomas. Cancer 23, 1280 (1969).
60. KENIS, Y.: Effect of piposulfan (NSC-47774) on malignant lymphomas and solid tumors. Cancer Chemother. Rep. 52, 433 (1968).
61. LACHER, M.J., DURANT, J.R.: Combined vinblastine and chlorambucil therapy of Hodgkin's disease. Ann. intern. Med. 62, 468 (1965).
62. FREI, E., DE VITA, V., MOXLEY, J., CARBONE, P.: Approaches to improving the chemotherapy of Hodgkin's disease. Cancer Res. 26, 1284 (1966).
63. DE VITA, Jr., V.T., SERPICK, A.A., CARBONE, P.P.: Combination chemotherapy in the treatment of advanced Hodgkin's disease. Ann. intern. Med. 73, 881 (1970).
64. CARTER, S.K.: Clinical trials and combination chemotherapy. Cancer Chemother. Rep. Part 3, 2, 81 (1971).
65. DE VITA, V.T., CARBONE, P.P.: Current chemotherapeutic combinations. Ser. Haematol. 6, 182 (1973).
66. CANELLOS, G.P., YOUNG, R.C., BERARD, C.W., DE VITA, V.T.: Combination chemotherapy and survival in advanced Hodgkin's disease. Arch. intern. Med. 131, 388 (1973).
67. RODRIGUEZ, V., BODEY, G.P., FREIREICH, E.J.: Combination chemotherapy for lymphomas and leukemias. Disease-A-Month, (Chic.) April 1973.
68. DE VITA, V.T., CARBONE, P.P.: Chemotherapeutic implications of staging in Hodgkin's disease. Cancer Res. 31, 1838 (1971).
69. NICHOLSON, W.M., BEARD, M.E.J., CROWTHER, D., STANSFELD, A.G., VARTAN, C.P., MALPAL, J.S., HAMILTON FAIRLEY, G., SIR RONALD BODLEY SCOTT: Combination chemotherapy in generalized Hodgkin's disease. Brit. med. J. 3, 7 (1970).
70. HAMILTON-FAIRLEY, G.: The use of different drugs and combinations in the treatment of Hodgkin's disease. Ser. Haematol. 6, 196 (1973).
71. NISSEN, N.I., STRUTZMAN, L., HOLLAND, J.F., GLIDEWELL, O.J.: Chemotherapy of Hodgkin's disease in studies by Acute Leukemia Group B. Arch. intern. Med. 131, 396 (1973).
72. LENHARD, Jr., R.E.: Combination chemotherapy of Hodgkin's disease. Proc. Amer. Ass. Cancer Res. 11, 48 (1970).
73. LENHARD, Jr., R.E.: Eastern Cooperative Oncology Group studies. Arch. intern. Med. 131, 418 (1973).
74. LUCE, J.K., GAMBLE, J.F., WILSON, H.E., MONTO, R.W., ISAACS, B.L., PALMER, R.L., COLTMAN, Jr., C.A., HEWLETT, J.S., GEHAN, E.A., FREI, E.: Combined cyclophosphamide, vincristine, and prednisone therapy of malignant lymphoma. Cancer 28, 306 (1971).
75. HUGULEY, C.M., DURANT, J.R., MOORES, R.R., YICK-KWONG CHAN, DORFMAN, R.F., JOHNSON, L.: A comparison of nitrogen mustard, vincristine, procarbazine, and prednisone (MOPP) vs nitrogen mustard in advanced Hodgkin's disease. Cancer 36, 1227 (1975).
76. BROOK, J., GOCKA, E.: Comparison of single agent with combination therapy in Hodgkin's disease. Proc. Amer. Ass. Cancer Res. 12, 12 (1971).
77. FREI, E., III., LUCE, J.K., GAMBLE, Jr., C.A., CONSTANZI, J.J., TALLEY, R.W., MONTO, R.W., WILSON, H.E., HEWLETT, J.S., DELANEY, F.C., GEHAN, E.A.: Combination chemotherapy in advanced Hodgkin's disease. Induction and maintenance of remission. Ann. intern. Med. 79, 376 (1973).
78. LOWENBRAUN, S., DE VITA, V.T., SERPICK, A.A.: Combination chemotherapy with nitrogen mustard, vincristine, procarbazine and prednisone in previously treated patients with Hodgkin's disease. Blood 36, 704 (1970).
79. YOUNG, R.C., CANELLOS, G.P., CHABNER, B.A., SCHEIN, P.S.: Maintenance chemotherapy for advanced Hodgkin's disease in remission. Lancet 1, 1339 (1973).

80. COLTMAN, C., FREI, E., DELANEY, F.: Effectiveness of actinomycin D, methotrexate, and vinblastine in prolonging the duration of combination chemotherapy (MOPP) induced remission in advanced Hodgkin's disease. Proc. Amer. Soc. Clin. Oncol. 1973 (abstr. 78).

81. TRUEBLOOD, H.W., GUERNSEY, J.M., COHN, R.: Hodgkin's disease and non-Hodgkin's lymphoma. The surgeon's role in therapy. Current Problems in Surgery. Aug. (1972).

82. LEE, Y.N., SAY, C., HORI, J.M., SPRATT, Jr., J.S.: Major surgery in Hodgkin's disease and other malignant lymphomas. J. Surg. Oncol. 465 (1973).

83. YAM, L.T., CROSBY, W.H.: Early splenectomy in lymphoproliferative disorders. Arch. intern. Med. 133, 270 (1974).

84. GLATSTEIN, E., GUERNSEY, J.M., ROSENBERG, S.A., KAPLAN, H.S.: The value of laparotomy and splenectomy in the staging of Hodgkin's disease. Cancer 24, 709 (1969).

85. LOWENBRAUN, S., RAMSEY, H., SUTHERLAND, J., SERPICK, A.A.: Diagnostic laparotomy and splenectomy for staging Hodgkin's disease. Ann. intern. Med. 72, 655 (1970).

86. LACHER, M.J.: Laparotomy and splenectomy in Hodgkin's disease. Hosp. Practice, Aug. 87, (1971).

87. JOHNSON, R.E.: Is staging laparotomy routinely indicated in Hodgkin's disease? Ann. intern. Med. 75, 459 (1971).

88. PIRO, A.J., HELLMAN, S., MOLONEY, W.C.: The influence of laparotomy on management decisions in Hodgkin's disease. Arch. intern. Med. 130, 844 (1972).

89. SALZMAN, J.R., KAPLAN, H.S.: Effect of splenectomy on hematological tolerance during total lymphoid radiotherapy of patients with Hodgkin's disease. Cancer 27, 471 (1971).

90. LOWENBRAUN, S., RAMSEY, H.E., SERPICK, A.A.: Splenectomy in Hodgkin's disease for splenomegaly, cytopenias and intolerance to myelosuppressive chemotherapy. Amer. J. Med. 50, 49 (1971).

91. PANETTIERE, F., COLTMAN, Jr., C.A.: Splenectomy effects on chemotherapy in Hodgkin's disease. Arch. Intern. Med. 131, 362 (1973).

92. BAKER, J.W., MORGAN, R.L., RECKHAM, M.J., SMITHERS, D.W.: Preservation of ovarian function in patients requiring radiotherapy for paraaortic and pelvic Hodgkin's disease. Lancet 1, 1307 (1972).

93. GOFFINET, D.R., GLADSTEIN, E.J., MERIGAN, T.C.: Herpes zoster-Varicella infections and lymphoma. Ann. intern. Med. 76, 235 (1971).

94. STIVER, G., SHARRAR, R., KENDRICK, M., EICKHOFF, T.: Bacterial risk in staging splenectomy. Ann. intern. Med. 76, 670 (1972).

95. RAVRY, M., MALDONADO, N., VELEZ-GARCIA, E., MONTALVO, J., SANTIAGO, P.J.: Serious infection after splenectomy for the staging of Hodgkin's disease. Ann. intern. Med. 77, 11 (1972).

96. NIXON, D.W., AISENBERG, A.C.: Fatal Hemophilus influenzae sepsis in an asymptomatic splenectomized Hodgkin's disease patient. Ann. intern. Med. 77, 69 (1972).

97. DRESSER, R.K., ULTMANN, J.E.: Risk of severe infection in patients with Hodgin's disease or lymphoma after diagnostic laparotomy and splenectomy. Ann. intern. Med. 77, 143 (1972).

98. CORMIA, Jr., F.E., CAMPOS, L.T.: Infections after splenectomy. Ann. intern. Med. 78, 149 (1973).

99. ULTMANN, J.E.: Hodgkin's disease: Laparotomy or not? Ann. intern. Med. 76, 330 (1972).

100. LOKICH, J.J.: Staging laparotomy. Ann. intern. Med. 76, 143 (1972).

101. AISENBERG, A.C., GOLDMANN, J.M., BAKER, J.W., WANG, C.C.: Spleen involvement at the onset of Hodgkin's disease. Ann. intern. Med. 74, 544 (1971).

102. ROSENBERG, S.A.: A critic of the value of laparotomy and splenectomy in the evaluation of patients with Hodgkin's disease. Cancer Res. 31, 1737 (1971).

103. PETERS, M.V.: The evolution of the radiotherapeutic concept in Hodgin's disease. Ser. Haematol. 6, 117 (1973).

104. KAPLAN, H.S.: Hodgkin's disease. Modern radiotherapy techniques and their results. Ser. Haematol. 6, 139 (1973).

105. JOHNSON, R.E., THOMAS, L.B., SCHNEIDERMAN, M., GLENN, D.W., FAW, F., HAFERMANN, M.D.: Preliminary experience with total nodal irradiation in Hodgkin's disease. Radiology 96, 603 (1970).

106. JOHNSON, R.E., THOMAS, L.B., CHRETIEN, P.: Correlation between clinicohistologic staging and extranodal relapse in Hodgkin's disease. Cancer 25, 1071 (1970).

107. DURANT, J.R.: Treatment of Hodgkin's disease: With what and by whom? Ann. intern. Med. 73, 1033 (1970).

108. FULLER, L.M., SULLIVAN, M.P., BUTLER, J.J.: Results of regional radiotherapy in localized Hodgkin's disease in children. Cancer 32, 640 (1973).

109. KRAUT, J.W., KAPLAN, H.S., BAGSHAW, M.A.: Combined fractionated isotopic and external irradiation of the liver in Hodgkin's disease. A study of 21 patients. Cancer 30, 39 (1972).

110. PALOS, B.A., KAPLAN, H.S., KARZMARK, C.J.: The use of thin shields to deliver limited whole-lung irradiation during mantlefield treatment of Hodgkin's disease. Radiology 101, 441 (1971).

111. GLICKSMAN, A.S., NICKSON, J.J.: Acute and late reactions to irradiation in the treatment of Hodgkin's disease. Arch. intern. Med. 131, 369 (1973).

112. O'CONNELL, M.J., WIERNIK, P.H., BRACE, K.C., BYHARDT, R.W., GREENE, W.H.: A combined modality approach to the treatment of Hodgkin's disease. Cancer 35, 1055 (1975).

113. HOOGSTRATEN, B., GLIDEWELL, O.: Chemotherapy-radiotherapy for stage III Hodgkin's disease. Proc. Amer. Ass. Clin. Oncol. 160 (1974).

114. E.O.R.T.C. Radiotherapy Co-operative Group: A randomized study of irradiation and vinblastine in stages I and II of Hodgkin's disease (Preliminary results). Europ. J. Cancer 8, 353 (1972).

115. MATHE, G., TUBIANA, M.: Hodgkin's disease: considerable progress and more to be achieved. Ser. Haematol. 6, 244 (1973).

116. IBRAHIM, E., FULLER, L.M., GAMBLE, J.F.: Stage I Hodgkin's disease: Changing concepts. Cancer. Bull. (Tex.) 24, 109 (1972).

117. CURRAN, R.E., JOHNSON, R.E.: Tolerance to chemotherapy after prior irradiation for Hodgkin's disease. Ann. intern. Med. 72, 505 (1970).

118. MOORE, M.R., BULL, J.M., JONES, S.E., ROSENBERG, S.A., KAPLAN, H.S.: Sequential radiotherapy and chemotherapy in the treatment of Hodgkin's disease. A progress report. Ann. intern. Med. 77, 1 (1972).

119. ROSENBERG, S.A., MOORE, M.R., BULL, J.M., JONES, S.E., KAPLAN, H.S.: Combination chemotherapy and radiotherapy for Hodgkin's disease. Cancer 30, 1505 (1972).

120. ZIEGLER, J.L., BLUMING, A.Z., FASS, L., MAGRATH, I.T., TEMPLETON, A.C.: Chemotherapy of childhood Hodgkin's disease in Uganda. Lancet 2, 679 (1972).

121. SINCLAIR, W.K.: Cyclic X-ray responses in mammalian cells in vitro. Radiat. Res. 33, 620 (1968).

122. HOOGSTRATEN, B., HOLLAND, J.F., KRAMER, S., GLIDEWELL, O.J.: Combination chemotherapy-radiotherapy for Stage III Hodgkin's disease. Arch. intern. Med. 131, 424 (1973).

123. GAMBLE, J.F., FULLER, L.M., IBRAHIM, E., BUTLER, J.J., SCHULLENBERGER, C.C.: Combined chemotherapy. Arch. intern. Med. 131, 435 (1973).

124. JOHNSON, R.E.: Modern approaches to the radiotherapy of lymphoma. Seminars Hematol. 6, 357 (1969).

125. KAPLAN, H.S.: Clinical evaluation and radiotherapeutic management of Hodgkin's disease and the malignant lymphomas. New Engl. J. Med. 278, 892 (1968).

126. FREI, E.III: Status and perspectives in chemotherapy of Hodgkin's disease. Arch. intern. Med. 131, 439 (1973).

127. TRANUM, B.L., HAUT, A.: Methyl CCNU in Hodgkin's disease and other tumors. Proc. Amer. Ass. Cancer Res. 15, 171 (1974).
128. AMIEL, J.L., BERUMEN, L., SCHWARZENBERG, L., SCHNEIDER, M., CATTAN, A., SCHLUMBERGER, J.R., MATHE, G.: Essai de traitement de la maladie de Hodgkin généralisée par une chimiothérapie multiple. Sem. Hôp. Paris 42, 2970 (1966).
129. MORGENFIELD. M.C., PAVLOVSKY, A., SUAREZ, A., SOMOZA, N., PAV-LOVSKY, S., PALAU, M., BARROS, C.A.: Combined cyclophosphamide, vincristine, procarbazine, and prednisone (COPP) therapy of maligant lymphoma. Cancer 36, 1241 (1975).
130. BONADONNA, G., ZUCALI, R., MONFARDINI, S., DE LENA, M., USLENGHI, C.: Combination chemotherapy of Hodgkin's disease with adriamycin, bleomycin, vinblastine, and imidazole carboxamide versus MOPP. Cancer 36, 252 (1975).
131. NAEIM, F., WAISMAN, J., COULSON, W.F.: Hodgkin's disease: The significance of vascular invasion. Cancer 34, 655 (1974).
132. LAMOUREUX, K.B., JAFFE, E.S., BERARD, C.W., JOHNSON, R.E.: lack of identifiable vascular invasion in patients with extra-nodal dissemination of Hodgkin's disease. Cancer 31, 824 (1974).
133. TEILLET, F., WEISGERBER, C., DNA, M., FEINGOLD, N., CHELLOUL, et al.: Maladie de Hodgkin. Traitement des formes localisées I et II par association de radiothérapie et chimiothérapie. Presse med. 3, 1925 (1974).
134. SMITHERS, D.W., LILLICRAP, S.C., BARNES, A.: Patterns of lymph node involvement in relation to hypotheses about the modes of spread of Hodgkin's disease. Cancer 34, 1779 (1974).
135. SHIPLEY, W.U., PIRO, A.J., HELLMAN, S.: Radiation therapy of Hodgkin's disease: significance of splenic involvement. Cancer 34, 223 (1974).
136. REGE, V.B., OWENS, A.H.: BCNU in the treatment of advanced Hodg-kin's disease, lymphosarcoma, and reticulum cell sarcoma. Cancer Chemother. Rep. Part 1, 58, 383 (1974).
137. BLUM, R.H., CARTER, S.K.: Adriamycin. Ann. intern. Med. 80, 249 (1974).
138. MATHE, G., SCHWARZENBERG, L., POUILLART, R., WEINER, R. et al.: Two epipodophyllotoxin derivatives, VM 26 and VP 16213, in the treatment of leukemias, hematosarcomas, and lymphomas. Cancer 34, 985 (1974).
139. SCHEIN, P.S., O'CONNELL, M.J., BLOM, J., HUBBARD, S., MAGRATH, I.T. et al.: Clinical antitumor activity and toxicity of strepto-zotocin. Cancer 34, 993 (1974).
140. EMMANUEL, N.M., BERMEL, E.M., OSTROVSKAYA, L.A., KORMAN, N.P.: Ex-perimental and clinical studies of the antitumor activity of 1-methyl-1-nitrosourea. Cancer Chemother. Rep. Part 1, 58, 135 (1974).
141. NIXON, D.W., AISENBERG, A.C.: Combination therapy of Hodgkin's disease. Cancer 33, 1499 (1974).
142. MOORE, M.R., JONES, S.E., BULL, J.M., WILLIAM, L.A., ROSENBERG, S.A.: MOPP chemotherapy for advanced Hodgkin's disease. Prognostic factors in 81 patients. Cancer 32, 52 (1973).
143. COOPER, I.A., IRONSIDE, P.N.J., MADIGAN, J.P., MORRIS, P.J., EWING, M.R.: The role of splenectomy in the management of advanced Hodgkin's disease. Cancer 34, 408 (1974).
144. HELLMAN, S.: Current studies in Hodgkin's disease: What laparotomy has brought. New Engl. J. Med. 1290, 894 (1974).
145. IHDE, D.C., DE VITA, V.T., CANELLOS, G.P., CHABNER, B.A., YOUNG, R.C.: Effect of splenectomy on tolerance to combination chemothera-py in patients with lymphoma. Proc. Am. Soc. Clin. Oncol. 16, 230 (1975).

146. CHILCOTE, R.R., BAEHNER, R.L.: The incidence of overwhelming infection in children staged for Hodgkin's disease. Proc. Am. Soc. Clin. Oncol. 16, 224 (1975).
147. PANETTIERE, F.J., COLTMAN, C.A., DELANEY, F.C.: Splenectomy and survival in Hodgkin's disease. Proc. Am. Soc. Clin. Oncol. 16, 243 (1975).
148. NISCE, L.Z., GELLER, W., D'ANGIO, G.J.: Total nodal and hepatic irradiation for bad risk stage III Hodgkin's disease. Am. Soc. Clin. Oncol. 16, 251 (1975).
149. RUCKDESCHEL, J.C., MARTIN, R.G., BRYHARDT, R.W.: Non-radiotherapeutic factors in the development of radiation-related pericardial effusions in patients treated for Hodgkin's disease. Proc. Am. Soc. Clin. Oncol. 16, 238 (1975).
150. BYHARDT, R., BRACE, K., RUCKDESCHEL, J., CHANG, P., MARTIN, R., WIERNICK, P.: Dose and treatment factors in radiation-related pericardial effusion associated with the mantle technique for Hodgkin's disease. Cancer 35, 795 (1975).
151. ROSENBERG, S.A., KAPLAN, H.S.: The management of stages I, II and III Hodgkin's disease with combined radiotherapy and chemotherapy. Cancer 35, 55 (1975).
152. YOUNG, R.C., CANELLOS, G.P., CHABNER, B.A., DE VITA, V.T.: Patterns of relapse after complete remission in Hodgkin's disease treated with MOPP chemotherapy. Proc. Am. Soc. Clin. Oncol. 16, 249 (1975).
153. FARBER, L.R., PROSNITZ, L.R., DeCONTI, R.C., BERTINO, J.R., FISCHER, J.J.: Combination chemotherapy-low dose radiotherapy for stage III-B and IV Hodgkin's disease. Proc. Am. Soc. Clin. Oncol. 16, 266 (1975).
154. TSE-CHIANG CHANG, STUTZMAN, L., SOKAL, J.E.: Correlation of delayed hypersensitivity responses with chemotherapeutic results in advanced Hodgkin's disease. Cancer 36, 950 (1975).
155. KAPLAN, H.S., ROSENBERG, S.A.: The management of Hodgkin's disease. Cancer 36, 796 (1975).
156. BONADONNA, G., USLENGHI, C., ZUCALI, R.: Resent trends in the medical treatment of Hodgkin's disease. Eur. J. Cancer 11, 251 (1975).
157. DeVITA, V., CANELLOS, G., HUBBARD, S., CHABNER, B., YOUNG, R.: Chemotherapy of Hodgkin's disease with MOPP: a 10 year progress report. Proc. Amer. Soc. Clin. Oncol. 17, 269 (1976).
158. COLTMAN, C.A., HALL, W., FREI, E. III, MOON, T.E.: MOPP maintenance versus unmaintained remission for MOPP induced complete remission of advanced Hodgkin's disease: 7.2 year follow-up. Proc. Amer. Soc. Clin. Oncol. 17, 289 (1976).
159. BAKEMEIER, R.F., DeVITA, V.T., HORTON, J.: Chemotherapy and immunotherapy of Hodgkin's disease. Proc. Amer. Soc. Clin. Oncol. 17, 293 (1976).
160. VINCIGUERRA, V., COLEMAN, M., DEGNAN, T.J., JAROWSKI, C.I., SILVER, R.T.: BVDS-A polychemotherapy regimen for MOPP refractory Hodgkin's disease. Proc. Amer. Soc. Clin. Oncol. 17, 303 (1976).
161. HUM, G.J., SRIBOUR, L.M., BATEMAN, J.R.: A randomized phase III study for adult advanced Hodgkin's disease, MOPP versus CCNU, velban, prednisone. Proc. Amer. Soc. Clin. Oncol. 17, 310 (1976).

Chapter 21
Non-Hodgkin Lymphomas (Lymphosarcoma, Reticulosarcoma)

The treatment of non-Hodgkin lymphomas (NHL) has generally followed that of Hodgkin's disease. However, such conditions deserve a separate discussion because of certain peculiarities in their clinical behavior and relative sensitivity to cytotoxic drugs.

Several histologic variants are grouped together under the designation of non-Hodgkin lymphomas. The most popular classification in the USA in recent publications is that of RAPPAPORT (1) modified by BERARD (2), which considers cell type, degree of differentiation, and architectural pattern. The relationship between the older classification of lymphosarcoma (LS), and reticulum cell sarcoma (RCS) or reticulosarcoma (RS), the newer one, and the WHO classification (3) is outlined in Table 21-1. New classifications no longer based solely on histologic criteria but taking into consideration the functional capacity of the component cells may be expected in the near future (128).

Lymphosarcoma is either poorly differentiated or well differentiated. The latter form is composed of cells that may be morphologically indistinguishable from normal lymphocytes and in its histological appearance it is indistinguishable from chronic lymphoid leukemia (CLL). Unlike leukemias, lymphosarcomas seem to originate in lymphoid organs (lymph nodes, spleen, Waldeyer's ring, gastrointestinal tract) rather than in the bone marrow. They can also originate in extranodal sites, such as skin, testes, kidney, etc. Leukemic transformation may occur early or late in the course of poorly differentiated lymphosarcoma and can mimic acute lymphoid leukemia, especially in children, while such transformation in well-differentiated lymphosarcoma mimics CLL.

Reticulosarcomas are also classified as either poorly differentiated (immature-appearing cells with histiocytic features, so-called "histoblasts" or "prohistiocytes" with rare phagocytosis and sparse argyrophilic fibers) or well-differentiated (composed of histiocytes that show evidence of phagocytosis or production of argyrophilic fibers, or both) (3, 4). Leukemic transformation (5) can occur with poorly differentiated reticulosarcomas (in ± 20 percent) but is exceptional in the well-differentiated type.

Reticulolymphosarcoma (mixed histiocytic-lymphocytic lymphoma) is composed of a mixture of neoplastic (poorly and well-differentiated) histiocytes and lymphocytes in approximately equal proportions. It is very rare except in the nodular form.

The non-Hodgkin lymphomas tend to be more widespread at the time of diagnosis than Hodgkin's disease. Extranodular sites are often involved (RS 60 percent, LS 40 percent) and are commonly the primary site of disease. Bone marrow involvement is frequently seen, even in apparently localized stages (I and II) (6, 129). Constitutional symptoms ("B" symptoms) are less common than in HD.

Table 21-1. Classification of non-Hodgkin lymphomas

WHO Classification:	Classification of non-Hodgkin lymphomas	
	RAPPAPORT-BERARD[d]	Old terminology
1. Burkitts's tumor[a]	1. Malignant lymphoma, undifferen- tiated, Burkitt type	Burkitt's tumor
2. Reticulosarcoma, poorly differentiated	2. Malignant lymphoma, undifferen- tiated, pleiomorphic type	⎫ ⎬ Reticulum cell sarcoma
3. Reticulosarcoma, well differentiated	3. Malignant lymphoma, histiocytic type	⎭
4. Reticulolymphosarcoma	4. Malignant lymphoma mixed, histio- cytic-lymphocytic type	⎫
5. Lymphosarcoma, poorly differentiated	5. Malignant lymphoma, lymphocytic type, poorly differentiated	⎬ Lymphosarcoma
6. Lymphosarcoma, well differentiated	6. Malignant lymphoma, lymphocytic type, well differentiated	⎭
7. Follicular lymphoma[b]		
8. Unclassified tumors of lymphoid and histiocytoid cells[c]		

[a] For categories 1-5 and 8 the term "diffuse" or "nodular" should be added as indicated by the architectural pattern.
[b] This category is provided for those who regard the nodular forms of 1-5 and 8 as distinct entities.
[c] Cannot be clearly classified under way of the above headings.
[d] All forms may have nodular or diffuse pattern.

The same staging procedures can be used as for HD (see p. 340). Most, if not all, patients should have a bone marrow biopsy (6). Lymphangiograms are often positive in apparently early stages. The role of exploratory laparotomy in the workup of NHL is not yet well defined (7-11). Abdominal involvement is common (8, 9).

Most authors use the same staging system for NHL as for HD (see Table 20-2). However, lack of evidence of uniform sites of onset or predictable manner of progression to contiguous areas makes staging less valuable in NHL.

Several factors influence prognosis. Nodular lymphomas within each cell type are more favorable than the diffuse patterns (12-14, 130, 131). Histiocytic lymphomas (RS) have the worst prognosis, lymphocytic lymphomas the most favorable. Other prognostic features are the extent and the distribution of involvement, vascular invasion, and leukemic transformation and the immunologic state.

A. CHEMOTHERAPY

1. Single Agents

Most of the agents that are effective in HD are also effective in NHL, but the various types of NHL show differences in sensitivity, both among each other and compared to HD (Table 21-2), (12, 15-21, 132).

Alkylating agents are generally effective. Nitrogen mustard (HN2) seems to be less active in NHL than cyclophosphamide (CPM) while the reverse is true for HD. Cyclophosphamide (22-24) and chlorambucil (CLB) (25) tend to be more popular as alkylating agents in NHL. Both yield higher response rates in LS than in RS. Vincristine (VCR) (26, 27) is better for NHL than vinblastine (VLB) (28, 29). Response to prednisone (PDN) equals that to the alkylating agents and Vinca alkaloids (30). Although the overall response rates of the three most active agents (CPM, VCR, and PDN) are about 50-70 percent, complete remission occurs in less than 20 percent and responses to single-agent therapy are of short duration. Procarbazine, one of the best agents of the current drug armamentarium for HD, has been tested much less frequently in NHL (31-34).

No studies are available that compare the response rates for these agents in the new variants of LS and RS according to the RAPPAPORT-BERARD classification (see Table 21-1). In a retrospective study, JONES et al. (12) noted a higher percentage of complete remissions and a longer duration of response to alkylating agents in nodular lymphomas compared to diffuse lymphomas.

Several of the newer agents show promising activity in NHL. Among them are bleomycin (BLM) (35-38), adriamycin (ADM) (50 percent RR) (39, 40) (132, 133), rufochromomycin (41, 42), the nitrosoureas RR (43) BCNU: 28 percent; CCNU: 28 percent RR (134); MeCCNU: 26 percent RR (135), the podophyllotoxin derivative VM26 (44, 45), dimethyl triazeno imidazole carboxamide (46), and L-asparaginase (in lymphocytic lymphomas, particularly the poorly differentiated variant) (48-50). Adriamycin can already be classified among the most active agents for non-Hodgkin lympomas, while nitrosoureas are moderately effective. Bleomycin is especially useful in patients with severe myelosuppression.

Table 21-2. Effectiveness of single agents in non-Hodgkin lymphoma compared to Hodgkin's disease

Drug	Hodgkin's disease		Lymphosarcoma		Reticulosarcoma		Reference
	Number	%CR + PR	Number	% CR + PR	Number	% CR + PR	
Imidazole carboxamide	18	56 %	15	27 %	13	0	FREI et al. (46)
BCNU	149	50 %	107			28 %	CARTER (43)
Procarbazine	347	69 %	42	40.5 %	33	36 %	LIVINGSTON and CARTER (47)
Nitrogen mustard	432	63 %	154	49 %	17	18 %	-
Chlorambucil	282	61 %	90	68 %	46	39 %	-
Cyclophosphamide	452	54 %	276	65 %	219	56 %	-
Adriamycin	18	40 %	16	44 %	13	53 %	O'BRYAN et al. (40)
Bleomycin	122	37 %	34	44 %	42	40 %	BLUM et al. (38)
Vincristine	92	60 %	93	53 %	72	61 %	LIVINGSTON and CARTER (47)
Vinblastine	380	65 %	84			27 %	-
VM 26	22	27 %	19	30 % (all PR)	25	50 % (all PR)	EORTC
Prednisone	40	54 %	47	74 %			LIVINGSTON and CARTER (47)

2. Combinations

The various active agents can be used in sequence until primary or secondary resistance develops. As in HD, the current trend is toward the
use of high-dose intermittent combinations (Tables 21-3 and 21-4). The
majority of these have included the three most active agents: CPM, VCR,
and PDN. The ALGB and ECOG compared CPM alone with CPM + VCR + PDN at
two dose levels in six weekly cycles (51). In both LS and RS, the high-
dose combination was more effective than CPM alone. LENHARD et al. (52)
showed that PDN is essential in improving the response rate of the CPM
and VCR two-drug combination. However, the addition of VCR and BCNU
failed to improve the response rate over the combination of CPM plus
PDN (136).

A similar combination (COP at 2-week intervals) was studied by the SWCCG
(53) and again found to provide results superior to those of single
agents reported in the literature. The median duration of remission was
prolonged by maintenance (COP at 4-week intervals) in LS but not in RS.
BAGLEY et al. (54) used the same three drugs (CVP) at 3-week-intervals.
Two more cycles were given once complete remission was obtained. Of 35
patients with LS, 57 percent obtained CR and 34 percent had partial responses; median duration of CR was approximately 2 years. Thus, in all
three studies, the combination CPM + VCR + PDN significantly increased
both the percentage of complete remissions and the duration of remission. Survival of complete responders was significantly better than that
of partial responders (53, 54). SKARIN et al. using a modified COP regimen noted a 77 percent RR (10/13) for nodular lymphocytic lymphoma
compared to a 12 percent RR (2/17) for diffuse lymphocytic lymphoma
(130). Long-term remissions and possibly cures are registered with the
COP combination (137). Similar regression rates are obtained with a
combination of CPM + VCR + CCNU (13). Some investigators still question the superiority of combination chemotherapy over single-agent therapy (55, 139, 140).

Using the MOPP combination, LOWENBRAUN et al. (56) obtained 7/15 CR in
LS and 3/8 CR in RS with a mean duration of unmaintained CR of 11.7+
and 32+ months respectively. The same combination but with substitution of HN2 by CPM is under study at the NCI (19). HØST (57) substituted
CPM for HN2 and VLB for VCR, and obtained 61 percent and 42 percent
CR for LS and RS, respectively. The SWCCG is conducting a direct comparative study of MOPP, COP, and COAP (CPM, VCR, CAR, PDN). The same
group reported in abstract the results of a modified COP combination
plus bleomycin (BLM) (58). The CR of 61 percent compared favorably
with that of a previous study with COP. Even better response rates were
reported when ADM was added to CPM, VCR, and PDN (CHOP) or to the latter two drugs alone (HOP) (see Tables 21-3 and 21-4) (59, 142, 157)
Diffuse histiocytic lymphoma has been highly responsive to CHOP + BLM
(158) and a combination of CPM, VCR, CAR plus MTX-FA (C.O.M.A) (159).
DE LENA et al. (60, 132, 133) studied two schedules of an HN2, VCR, ADM,
BLM and PDN combination for induction of remission in advanced non-
Hodgkin lymphomas. CPM, VLB, PCZ, and MTX were used in a cyclic manner
for maintenance. The CR rate was 17 to 37 percent for LS and 42-62 percent for RS, depending on the schedule. BONADONNA et al. compared the
CVP combination to another three-drug regimen, ABP (ADM, BLM, and PDN)
(132, 133). Preliminary results show no difference, at least in lymphocytic lymphoma; CVP apparently produces a slightly higher number of CR's
in histiocytic lymphoma as compared to ABP (133). Impressive results
were obtained in RS by LEVITT et al. (61) using CPM and VCR pretreatment
to reduce the tumor masses and convert the remaining cell population to
logarithmic growth (recruitment), at which time the phase-specific antimetabolites, MTX and CAR, are used. MORGENFIELD et al. obtained 75% CR
in 52 patients with NHL treated with COPP combination (see Table 20-5)

(155). Our preliminary results with a cyclic combination (AVmCP) of
ADM, VM 26, CPM, and prednisone, based on pharmacokinetic considerations
of synchronization and potentiation are very encouraging (156).

Few investigators have reported their results in terms of the newer
classification of NHL (see Table 21-1) (14, 62) and comparison of the
results of different studies is often impossible because of differences
in terminology. Progress in NHL would be greatly benefited by more uniformity in methods of reporting. RS generally responds less well to
therapy, with either single agents or combinations. Many NHL's are initially very responsive to single-agent or combination chemotherapy;
however, with the exception of those with nodular and differentiated
histology, it is often difficult to maintain long-term remissions.

B. STRATEGY

1. Surgery

Radical surgery is rarely indicated in the management of NHL. In most
cases, the role of the surgeon is to obtain the biopsy required to establish the diagnosis. Some complications experienced in the course of
the disease may require surgery for their relief (65). The role of exploratory laparotomy and splenectomy is not yet well defined in NHL
(7-11).

2. Radiotherapy

It is well established that radiotherapy is capable of curing localized
NHL (21, 66, 67, 142). However, the selection of patients for primary
treatment by radiotherapy and the best radiotherapeutic techniques are
not well defined. Extended-field and total nodal radiotherapy have been
applied to NHL on the assumption that all sites of clinical or microscopic involvement must be exposed to adequate doses of radiotherapy.
What constitutes an adequate dose is also less well defined for NHL than
for HD. There may be a difference in the radiosensitivity of the different histologic variants and great variability within a subgroup
(66, 68). The results achieved with current radiotherapeutic approaches
do not equal those obtained in HD. The greater propensity of NHL to disseminate and to develop a leukemic transformation along with its more
unpredictable pattern of spread, rather than local recurrences have
been blamed for many of the failures. There are no studies that document the beneficial effect of extended field over involved-field radiotherapy. Relapses after radiotherapy for localized non-Hodgkin lymphoma
occur at sites outside treated fields. These sites were lymphatic rather
than extralymphatic in about half of the cases of diffuse histiocytic
(DH) and in about two thirds of the cases of nodular mixed (NM) and nodular lymphocytic poorly differentiated (NLPD) (69). KAPLAN (69) suggests that the high rate of lymphatic relapse in these histological
types might be prevented by initial total nodal therapy. PETERS (70)
recommends that radiation treatment should be extended beyond the major nodal sites, particularly in the abdomen. At Stanford NHL are currently treated with either involved-field or total nodal radiotherapy,
with or without combination chemotherapy, depending on the stage and
the histologic variant (69). JOHNSON (66, 67) has had considerable success in treating patients with Stage III and IV LS with bone marrow
involvement, and in some cases with visceral involvement, with low-dose,
spaced total-body irradiation. A comparative study of total-body radiotherapy versus CVP combination chemotherapy for advanced lymphocytic
lymphoma is in progress. Preliminary results are comparable in nodular
lymphoma; some advantage is noted for total-body radiotherapy in diffuse lymphoma (71). Palliative radiotherapy is useful for symptomatic
lesions and relief of certain complications.

Table 21-3. Results of combination chemotherapy in lymphosarcoma

Combination	Number of patients	% CR	% total response	Duration of remission (months)	Reference
CPM 15 mg/kg weekly x 6 VCR 0.025 mg/kg, i.v., weekly x 6 PDN 1.0 mg/kg, p.o., daily for 6 wks	16	31%	100%	3 (maint.) 1.5 (unmaint.)	HOOGSTRATEN et al 1969 (51)
C CPM 800 mg/m^2, i.v., q 14 d x 6 O VCR 2 mg, i.v., q 14 d x 6 P PDN 60 mg/m^2, p.o., 5 d; q 14 d x 6	74	50%	88%	12	LUCE et al. 1971 (53)
C CPM 400 mg/m^2, p.o., d 1-5 V VCR 1.4 mg/m^2, i.v., d 1 P PDN 100 mg/m^2, p.o., d 1-5 Repeat d 21	35	57%	91%	± 24	BAGLEY et al. 1972 (54)
CPM 10 mg/kg, i.v., weekly x 6 VCR 2 mg, i.v., weekly x 6 PDN 50 mg/daily for 21 days 25 mg " 7 " 12.5 mg " 7 " Repeat every 10 wks.	13 17	76% 22%	84% 58%	nodular lymphocytic diffuse lymphocytic	SKARIN et al. 1974 (62)
CVP	8	4/8	7/8		BONADONNA et al. 1975 (36)
A ADM 75 mg/m^2, i.v., d 1 B BLM 15 mg/m^2, i.v., d 1 and 8 P PDN 100 mg/m^2, p.o., i.m., d 1-5 Repeat d 21	9	4/9	8/9		BONADONNA et al. 1975 (36)

Table 21-3. (continued)

Combination	Number of patients	% CR	% total remission	Duration of remission (months)	Reference
MOPP					
(HN2, VCR, PCZ, PDN) (see Table 20-5)	15	47%	80%	11.7+	LOWENBRAUN et al., 1970 (56)
CPM 600 mg/m², i.v., d 1 and 8 VLB 6 mg/m², i.v., d 1 and 8 PCZ 100 mg/m², p.o., d 1 to 15 PDN 40 mg/m², p.o., qd, d 1 to 15 Repeat at 6-week intervals	23	61%	83%		HØST and ABRAHAMSEN 1973 (57)
HN2 6 mg/m² VCR 1.2 mg/m²) IV, d 1 and 8 ADM 25 mg/m²) BLM 30 mg/m²)	14	17% (6 cycles)			DE LENA et al., 1973 (60)
PDN 40 mg/m², i.m., d 1 to 14 (cycle 1, 3, 5,) or (1, 2) for 2 or 6 cycles		37% (2 cycles)			
Maintenance with sequential cyclic CPM, VLB, PCZ, MTX					
C CPM 750 mg/m², i.v., d 1 A ADM 50 mg/m², i.v., d 1 O VCR 1.4 mg/m² (Mx 2 mg) i.v., d 1 P PDN 25 mg, p.o., qid, d 1 to 5 Repeat at 2 to 3-week intervals		69%			McKELVEY et al., 1974 (59)

365

Table 21-3 (continued)

Combination	Number of patients	% CR	% total remission	Duration of remission (months)	Reference
A ADM 40 mg/m^2, i.v., d 1 VM VM 26 60 mg/m^2, i.v., d 2					
C CPM 300 mg/m^2, i.v. or i.m., d 3 and d 4	16	56%	80%		MISSET et al., 1975 (156)
P PDN 40 mg/m^2, d 3 to 7 Repeat d 15 to 21					
C CPM 1.0 g/m^2, i.v., d 1	78	22%	63%		EZDINLI et al, 1974 (63)
P PDN 100 mg/m^2 d 1 to 5 Repeat d 29					
B BCNU 120 mg/m^2, i.v., d 1	73	19%	64%		EZDINLI et al., 1974 (63)
P PDN 100 mg/m^2 d 1 to 5 Repeat d 29					

Table 21-4. Results of combination chemotherapy in reticulosarcoma

Combination	Number of patients	% CR	% total response	Duration of remission (months)	Reference
CPM, VCR, PDN (see Table 21-3)	13	30%	85%	3 (maint.) 1.5 (unmaint.)	HOOGSTRATEN et al., 1969 (51)
COP (see Table 21-3)	66	39%	78%	6	LUCE et al. 1971 (53)
CVP "	14	36%	71%	4+ (1-10.5+)	BONADONNA et al. (39)
ABP "	13	39%	85%	7+ (1+-10+)	BONADONNA et al. (39)
MOPP (see Table 20-5)	8	3/8	5/8	32+	LOWENBRAUN et al., 1970 (56)
CPM, VLB, PCZ, PDN (see Table 21-3)	36 (eval.)	42%	75%		HØST and ABRAHAMSEN 1973 (57)
CPM 1.5 g/m² i.v., day 1 VCR 1.4 mg/m² d 2, 9, 16 followed by (beginning day 23): MTX 120 mg/m², p.o., over 24 h; FA 25 mg/m², q 6 h x 4 beginning with last dose of MTX qw x8; CAR 300 mg/m², i.v., 16 h after starting MTX	15	60%	100%	10+	LEVITT et al., 1972 (61)
HN2, VCR, ADM, BLM, PDN (see Table 21-3) (Maintenance: sequential cyclic CPM, VLB, PCZ, and MTX)	43	62% (6 cycles) 52% (2 cycles)			DE LENA et al. 1973 (60)

Table 21-4. (continued)

Combination	Number of patients	% CR	% total response	Duration of remission (months)	Reference
CHOP (see Table 21-3)		69%			McKELVEY et al. 1974 (59)
HOP (same as CHOP minus CPM; ADM at 80 mg/m²)		70%			McKELVEY et al. 1974 (59)
MTX 30 mg/m², p.o., q 6 h x 4; then: CAR 150 mg/m², i.v., in 6 h FA 20 mg/m², i.m., q 6 h (24 h after first MTX injection) VCR 1 mg/m², i.v., d 15 and 22 CPM 1.5 mg/m², i.v., d 16 PDN 30 mg/m², p.o., d 15 to 29 Total of 6 cycles	8	7/8	100%		GOMEZ et al. 1974 (64)
AVmCP (see Table 21-3)	8	5/8	6/8		MISSET et al. 1975 (156)

3. Adjuvant Chemotherapy and Immunotherapy

Because of the high relapse rate following radiotherapy of apparently
localized lesions, adjuvant chemotherapy (single-agent or combination)
deserves a clinical trial (69, 132). A combination of radiotherapy and
chemotherapy is part of a prospective study at Stanford of unfavorable
histologic variants in all four clinical stages of NHL (69). A preliminary report (72) shows a statistically significant difference in relapse
rate in favor of Stage I and II lymphoma patients treated with adjuvant
immunotherapy (BCG) after radiotherapy as compared to untreated controls.

4. Treatment Plan for Localized NHL

The treatment of NHL is not very well standardized at the present time.
Many controlled studies are required to answer questions about the best
chemotherapy, the proper radiotherapy, or the most effective way to combine both modalities. Another essential requirement, if progress is to
be made, is that all investigators use the same staging and histological
classification and define their results in terms of these two parameters, so that the results of different studies can be properly compared.

Truly localized nodal and extranodal LS and RS can be cured by radiotherapy and this should, therefore, be the primary treatment modality
for localized disease. Presentations in the head and neck areas, skin,
gastrointestinal tract, and bone (144, 154) are among those most likely
to be localized. Trials in progress should determine the extent of the
field to be treated, whether involved areas only, or total nodal with
or without total abdomen. Extended-field has not improved on the result
of involved-field therapy. Involved-field therapy can be recommended
for the time being except for those participating in a protocol study
(145). The value of adjuvant chemotherapy in the early stages remains
to be established.

5. Treatment Plan for Disseminated NHL

Chemotherapy is reserved for advanced stages, or those where further
radiotherapy is undesirable. Studies in progress are designed to establish the role of radiotherapy, chemotherapy, or their combination in
different histologic subgroups of Stage III and IV NHL (69).

Many patients, especially older ones, with well-differentiated LS can
be easily managed with a single alkylating agent, for example intermittent chlorambucil (as for CLL). For more aggressive forms of lymphosarcomas, the CVP (CPM, VCR, PDN) possibly with ADM (CHOP, HOP) combination
is recommended. MOPP, CHOP, or HOP are for the time being recommended
for advanced RS.

If LEVITT's results (61) are confirmed, his protocol may be an alternative choice for RS or for those who fail on MOPP. Bleomycin, the nitrosoureas, VM 26, and L-asparaginase (for LS only) are second-line drugs,
useful in patients who have become resistant to CPM, VCR, PDN, and ADM.
At the ICIG we are currently investigating a combination of ADM, VM 26,
CPM, and PDN, based on the concept of selective tumor sensitivity, selective toxicity, synchronization, and potentiation (see Chapt. 7).

BURKITT'S TUMOR

Burkitt's tumor is recognized as a clinical syndrome and a histopathologic entity (73, 74). In the classification of non-Hodgkin lymphomas

proposed by RAPPAPORT et al. and modified by BERARD (see Table 21-1), it is listed among the undifferentiated lymphomas (1, 2). It is a malignant tumor composed of blast-like cells (like immunoblasts or transformed lymphocytes with intensive cytoplasmic basophilia (pyroninophilia) and many sudanophilic cytoplasmic inclusions. Macrophages are frequently interspersed among the tumor cells, forming a so-called "starry-sky" pattern. Although a prominent histological feature, this pattern is not specific to or pathognomonic of Burkitt's tumor (3).

Initially, Burkitt's tumor was thought to be endemic to tropical Africa, but cases occur world-wide (75-78), chiefly in children. The clinical presentation appeared to differ somewhat in African and American patients (73-75, 78); however, a recent study of the American Burkitt Lymphoma Registry observed clinical and epidemiological features in American patients closely resembling those in Africa. ZIEGLER (79) proposed a staging system based on the African syndrome; others have used a staging classification adapted to the syndrome seen in American children (75, 78). It is a rapidly progressing tumor; without therapy, most patients die within a few months.

Burkitt's tumor, in contrast to other lymphomas and solid tumors, is potentially "curable" by chemotherapy alone. Two factors are thought to contribute to this favorable outcome: (1) the tumor has an unusual sensitivity to chemotherapy, including single agents, which is assumed to be due to its favorable cell kinetics, that is rapid proliferation rate and high growth fraction (80, 81). Burkitt's tumor offers the closest human counterpart to the growth characteristics of the L 1210 mouse leukemia model; (2) there is much evidence that host immune defenses participate. Tumor regressions have been noted following smallpox vaccinations (82) and transfusions of serum of other patients in remission following chemotherapy (83) or spontaneously.

KLEIN (84) demonstrated the presence of a specific cell-surface antigen. A viral etiology has long been suspected, notably the Epstein-Barr-Virus (85, 86).

A. CHEMOTHERAPY

Tumor regressions and remissions have been reported with cyclophosphamide (CPM) (78, 79, 82, 88, 89), nitrogen mustard (82, 88) melphalan (82), orthomelphalan (88), methotrexate (MTX) (90), cytosine arabinoside (CAR) (88), actinomycin D (91), vincristine (VCR) (92), and BCNU (88). Cyclophosphamide and methotrexate appear to be the most effective agents, especially CPM in a high-dose intermittent schedule (79, 89). Complete and lasting remissions can be achieved with one or two doses of CPM (40 mg/kg) even in patients with Stage III disease. Intensive cytoreductive therapy early in the course of the disease is desirable, especially in patients with generalized tumors.

Sudden lysis of large volumes of tumor induced by effective chemotherapy may result in hyperkalemia, which can be fatal if unrecognized (93, 94). ZIEGLER (79, 89) achieved complete remissions in 95 percent of patients usually after a single dose of CPM; of these, 61 percent relapsed (39 percent of patients with localized disease, compared to 72 percent and 65 percent respectively with Stage III and IV disease).

Two patterns of relapse were noted: early relapse occurred within 10 weeks and late relapses after a median remission duration of 26 weeks from first treatment. Patients who have become unresponsive to cyclophosphamide may still respond to a combination of VCR, MTX, and CAR (79). Relapses after one year in CR are exceedingly rare. Such patients are presumably cured. It has been suggested that late relapses may result from reinduction of tumor (95). The prognosis is related to the clinical stage. Patients with localized disease have longer remissions, fewer relapses, and a higher incidence of long-term survivors (89, 94).

CNS involvement, as in childhood ALL, is a frequent problem (89). Intrathecal injections of MTX or CAR are effective initial therapy. Prophylaxis with intrathecal MTX in combination with CNS irradiation needs investigation.

B. STRATEGY

1. Surgery

Several studies have reported improved results in Stage III patients who underwent a surgical reduction of large tumor masses prior to chemotherapy (79, 96, 147).

2. Radiotherapy

Burkitt's tumor is radiosensitive. The role of radiotherapy has not been studied extensively (radiotherapy is not always available in areas of Africa where this tumor is most prevalent) and its role is not clearly defined (78, 97). A combined modality (chemotherapy and radiotherapy) trial is in progress in the USA (148).

3. Immunotherapy

Since host immune defenses may be important in this tumor, it is not surprising that immunotherapy is being evaluated (88, 89, 98).

4. Discussion

Chemotherapy, especially with high doses of CPM, is currently the favored mode of therapy for Burkitt's tumor. It remains to be determined by proper trials whether a combination of one or more of the four treatment modalities is superior to chemotherapy alone for some stages of Burkitt's tumor.

MYCOSIS FUNGOIDES

Mycosis fungoides is now generally thought of as a lymphoma arising within the skin. The cutaneous lesions progress slowly from eczematous patches through a plaque and tumor stage. Sooner or later, peripheral lymph nodes become involved and finally various internal organs, as in a systemic lymphoma (see Table 21-5).

The disease generally extends over years as long as there are no cutaneous tumors, cutaneous ulcers, or palpable nodes. Once these disease manifestations have appeared, the median survival is 2 to 2 1/2 years; after hepatosplenomegaly has developed it is only 3 months (99).

Table 21-5. Staging of Mycosis Fungoides. (From VAN SCOTT et al.(105))

Stage	Histologic diagnosis of cutaneous lesions	Clinical characteristics of skin lesions	Axillary, inguinal, or cervical lymphadenopathy	Internal lesions
0	0	0 or hyperpigmentation	0	0
I	Compatible with MF	Erythematous plaque or generalized erythema	0	0
II	MF	Indurated plaques or papules, with or without generalized erythema	0	0
III	MF	Tumors, with or without papules, plaques, or generalized erythema	0	0
IV	MF	Plaques, papules, or tumors with or without generalized erythema	+	0
V	MF	Any of the above	+	+

Extracutaneous dissemination is a clinicopathologically distinct aspect of the natural history of mycosis fungoides and is not due to the development of a different type of a malignant lymphoma (149, 150).

A. STRATEGY

Various local and systemic treatment modalities are more or less effective in this disease (100). Among the former are topical or intralesional cytotoxic agents or steroids, ultraviolet light, superficial X-irradiation, and electron beam therapy. Steroids and cytotoxic drugs can also be given systemically. The selection of therapy depends to a great extent on the disease stage.

1. Topical Therapy and Radiotherapy

The earlier stages of the cutaneous involvement may respond to topical (in high concentration with occlusive dressings) or intralesional steroid therapy (100-103). This may be a good choice as long as the diagnosis of mycosis fungoides is not firmly established or to reduce pruritus or erythema. Ultraviolet light can also be tried in early mildly infiltrative disease. Sustained complete remissions have been achieved with whole-body continuous topical applications of aqueous solutions of nitrogen mustard (HN2) and supplemental intralesional injections of heavily infiltrated plaques and tumors (104, 105). Approximately 55 percent of patients whose disease is still limited to the skin (Stages I-III) become free of evidence of disease. Many patients so treated develop hypersensitivity to HN2. Patients can then be desensitized by daily minute doses of HN2 given intravenously. Specific immune tolerance to HN2 can be achieved, prior to topical treatment, by a series of weekly i.v., injections of similarly minute doses of HN2 (105).

Remissions may also be achieved with adequate doses of electron therapy (106). Generalized cutaneous infiltrative tumors and plaques can be treated by total-body therapy, but lesions deeper than 1 cm beneath the skin will not be reached by the electron beam. Subsequent chemotherapy is indicated if such deep-seated lesions are present. Superficial "spot" X-irradiation is useful as long as the lesions are few in number.

A type of immunotherapy may be possible in this disease. It has been noted that delayed hypersensitivity reactions, for example to HN2 or other antigens, are sometimes associated with a distinct additional improvement (105, 107).

2. Chemotherapy

Systemic chemotherapy is indicated once lymph nodes (Stage IV) or internal organs (Stage V) are involved, or for cutaneous stages that have become refractory to local therapy. Laparotomies have been carried out to assist proper staging of the disease (151). Approximately 50 percent of patients respond to alkylating agents: nitrogen mustard (104), cyclophosphamide (99, 100, 108), or BCNU (99). Methotrexate, preferably in a weekly schedule, is equally effective (99, 100). Few other agents have been given adequate trial in this disease (99). Among the newer agents, bleomycin deserves further investigation (109, 110). It is active in lymphomas and high concentrations are attained in the skin. Systemic corticosteroids have mainly an unpredictable and temporary symptomatic effect (101).

Combination chemotherapy of the type used in lymphomas (MOPP, (100), COP + BLM (110), CPM + MTX (100)), BLM, VLB + PDN (112)) is currently under investigation.

In spite of sometimes remarkable results in terms of palliation, there is no evidence that therapy in recent years has improved survival (99). Infection is the most common cause of death.

HISTIOCYTOSIS-X

The discussion of the treatment of eosinophilic granuloma of bone, the Hand-Schüller-Christian syndrome, and the Letterer-Siwe syndrome is not simplified by lumping them together under the designation of histiocytosis-X, on the assumption that they are different expressions of a single disease of similar pathology. The debate between the "lumpers" (113, 114) and the "splitters" (115) continues. The relatively inexperienced physician might get the impression that the (more or less innocent) eosinophilic granuloma should be treated vigorously because it is said to be part of a disease spectrum that includes more fatal types of disorders. The problem is further compounded by the fact that the etiology remains unknown. The neoplastic nature of histiocytosis-X is not firmly established. Assuming an infectious etiology, several authors have used, sometimes successfully, antibiotic therapy (116).

A. STRATEGY

1. Localized Histiocytosis-X

Isolated eosinophilic granulomas are generally effectively treated with surgical excision or curettage, with or without postoperative radiotherapy. Radiotherapy (300-600 rads) can also be used as the primary therapy of single lesions or to eradicate a recurrence following surgery. Irradiation may be preferable for lesions occurring in vital areas (e.g., vertebral body), areas of stress (e.g., neck of femur), or where a good cosmetic effect is desirable (e.g., lateral orbital lesions) (115, 117).

2. Disseminated Histiocytosis-X

Disseminated forms require systemic therapy. Steroids often have a significant symptomatic effect (118). Active phases are suppressed and young patients are given a chance to reach an age where the disease loses most of its aggressiveness (119). Remissions initiated by steroids are sustained for 12 to 30 months.

A variety of cytotoxic agents have been used, often with considerable improvement of symptoms and abnormal physical findings in individual patients. No particular drug has established itself as the treatment of choice. Small numbers of patients have been treated with nitrogen mustard (120), cyclophosphamide (121, 122), procarbazine (152), 6-MP (120, 122), methotrexate (122-124), vinblastine (121, 122, 125), vincristine (121, 122), or daunorubicin (126), with or without concomitant steroid therapy. JONES obtained longer remissions with MTX than with VCR and maintenance therapy with MTX prolonged remission compared to an unmaintained control group (153).

Evaluation of combination therapy is in progress (122). One would expect combinations such as MOPP or CVP to be effective.

Small doses of radiotherapy or surgery may also be indicated in disseminated disease to treat hazardous sites with impending or actual complications (pathologic fractures, cord compression, etc.).

It is difficult to evaluate the effect of current treatment methods on morbidity and survival because of the variable and unpredictable course of the disease(s) under discussion. Several long-term remissions (up to 15 years without relapse) and apparent cures have from time to time been reported. DOEDE and RAPPAPORT (127) reviewed these cases and found that they had often been treated with steroids, with or without other treatment modalities.

REFERENCES

1. RAPPAPORT, H.: Tumors of the hematopoietic system. In: Atlas of Tumor Pathology, Section 3, Fasc. 8, p. 13. Washington. DC: Armed Forces Institute of Pathology 1966.
2. BERARD, C.W.: Histopathology of lymphoreticular disorders - conditions with malignant proliferative reponse-lymphoma. In: Principles of Hematology (eds. W. Williams, E. Beutler, A. Erslev, W. Rundles). New York: McGraw-Hill 1972.
3. MATHE, G., RAPPAPORT, H.: Histological and cytological typing of the neoplastic disease of the haematopoietic and lymphoid tissues. Geneva: WHO 1973.
4. MATHE, G., GERARD-MARCHANT, R., TEXIER, J.L., SCHLUMBERGER, J.R., BERUMEN, L., PAINTRAND, M.: The two varieties of lymphoid tissue "reticulo-sarcomas", histiocytic and histioblastic types. Brit. J. Cancer 24, 687 (1970).
5. SCHLUMBERGER, J.R., MATHE, G., TEXIER, J.L., AMIEL, J.L., CATTAN, A., SCHWARZENBERG, L., SCHNEIDER, M., BERUMEN, L.: Blastic leukemia complicating reticulo-sarcoma and lympho-sarcoma. In: Advances in the Treatment of Acute (Blastic) Leukemias. Recent Results in Cancer Research, Vol. 30, p. 162 (ed. G. Mathé). Berlin-Heidelberg-New York: Springer-Verlag 1970.
6. JONES, S.E., ROSENBERG, S.A., KAPLAN, H.S.: Non-Hodgkin's lymphomas I. Bone marrow involvement. Cancer 29, 954 (1972).
7. ALLEN, L.W.: Laparotomy and splenectomy in the staging of lymphomas other than Hodgin's disease. J. Lab. clin. Med. 76, 877 (1970).
8. MUGGIA, F.M., ULTMANN, J.E.: Exploratory laparotomy in reticulum cell sarcoma. Cancer 30, 454 (1972).
9. HANKS, G.E., TERRY, L.N., BRYAN, J.A., NEWSOME, J.F.: Contribution of diagnostic laparotomy to staging non-Hodgkin's lymphoma. Cancer 29, 41 (1972).
10. GOFFINET, D.R., CASTELLINO, R.A., KIM, H., DORFMAN, R.F., FUKS, Z., ROSENBERG, S.A., NELSEN, T., KAPLAN, H.S.: Staging laparotomies in unselected previously untreated patients with non-Hodgkin's lymphomas. Cancer 32, 672 (1973).
11. VERONESI, U., MUSUMECI, R., PIZZETTI, F., GENNARI, L., BONADONNA, G.: The value of staging laparotomy in non-Hodgkin's lymphomas (with emphasis on the histiocytic type). Cancer 33, 446 (1974).
12. JONES, S.E., ROSENBERG, S.A., KAPLAN, H.S., KADIN, M.E., DORFMAN, R.F.: Non-Hodgkin's lymphomas. II. Single-agent chemotherapy. Cancer 30, 31 (1971).
13. CARBONE, P.P.: Management of patients with non-Hodgin's lymphoma. Arch. intern. Med. 131, 455 (1973).

14. SCHEIN, P.S., CHABNER, B., CANELLOS, G., YOUNG, R.C., BERARD, C., DE VITA, V.T.: Potential for prolonged disease-free survival following combination chemotherapy of non-Hodgkin's lymphomas. Blood 43, 181 (1974).

15. ULTMANN, J.E., NIXON, D.D.: The therapy of lymphoma. Seminars Hematol. 6, 376 (1969).

16. ULTMANN, J.E.: Current status: The management of lymphoma. Seminars Hematol. 7, 441 (1970).

17. ULTMANN, J.E., GRIEM, M.L., KIRSTEN, W.H., WISSLER, R.W.: Current concepts in the management of lymphoma and leukemia. In: Recent Results in Cancer Research, Vol. 36. Berlin-Heidelberg-New York: Springer-Verlag 1971.

18. DE VITA, Jr., V.T., CANELLOS, G.P.: Treatment of the lymphomas. Seminars in Hematol. 9, 193 (1972).

19. CARBONE, P.P.: Non-Hodgkin's lymphoma: recent observations on natural history and intensive treatment. Cancer 30, 1511 (1972).

20. RUBIN, P.: Updated Hodgkin's disease: C. advanced disease and special problems. Comment: The non-Hodgkin's lymphomas. J. Amer. Med. Ass. 223, 175 (1973).

21. McELWAIN, T.J.: Chemotherapy of the lymphomas. Seminars Hematol. 11, 59 (1974).

22. HYMAN, G.A., CASSILETH, P.A.: Efficacy of cyclophosphamide in the management of reticulum cell sarcoma. Cancer 19, 1386 (1966).

23. JACOBS, E.M., PETERS, F.C., LUCE, J.K., ZIPPIN, C., WOOD, D.A.: Mechlorethamine HCl and cyclophosphamide in the treatment of Hodgkin's disease and the lymphomas. J. Amer. med. Ass. 203, 392 (1968).

24. MENDELSON, D., BLOCK, J.B., SERPICK, A.A.: Effect of large intermittent intravenous doses of cyclophosphamide in lymphoma. Cancer 25, 715 (1970).

25. EZDINLI, E.Z., STUTZMAN, L.: Chlorambucil therapy for lymphomas and chronic lymphocytic leukemia. J. Amer. med. Ass. 191, 444 (1965).

26. MATHE, G., SCHWEISHUTH, O., BRULE, G., BREZIN, C., AMIEL, J.L., SCHWARZENBERG, M., CATTAN, Cl., SMADJA, R.: Essai de traitement par la leurocristine de la leucémie aigue lymphoplastique et du lymphoblastosarcome. Presse méd. 71, 529 (1963).

27. DESAI, D.V., EZDINLI, E.Z., STUTZMAN, L.: Vincristine therapy of lymphomas and chronic lymphocytic leukemia. Cancer 26 352 (1970).

28. HILL, J.M., LOEB, E.: Treatment of leukemia, lymphoma, and other malignant neoplasms with vinblastine. Cancer Chemother. Rep. 15, 41 (1961).

29. WRIGHT, T.L., HURLEY, J., KORST, D.R., MONTO, R.W., ROHN, R.J., WILL, J.J., LOUIS, J.: Vinblastine in neoplastic disease. Cancer Res. 23, 169 (1963).

30. EZDINLI, E.Z., STUTZMAN, L., AUNGST, C.W., FIRAT, D.: Corticosteroid therapy for lymphoma and chronic lymphocytic leukemia. Cancer 32, 900 (1969).

31. MATHE, G., BERUMEN, L., SCHWEISGUTH, O., BRULE, G., SCHNEIDER, M., AMIEL, J.L., CATTAN, A., SCHWARZENBERG, L.: Methyl-hydrazine in treatment of Hodgkin's disease and various forms of heamatosarcoma and leukemia. Lancet 2, 1077 (1963).

32. MARTZ, G., D'ALESSANDRI, A., KEEL, H.J., BOLLAG, W.: Preliminary clinical results with a new antitumor agent RO 4-6467 (NSC-77213). Cancer Chemother. Rep. 33, 5 (1963).

33. KENIS, Y., WERLI, J., HILDENBRAND, J., TAGNON, H.J.: Action d'un dérivé de la méthylhydrazine, le RO4-6467, dans la maladie de Hodgkin, dans l'autres lymphomes malins et dans des leucémies. Europ. Cancer 1, 33 (1965).

34. STOLINSKY, D.C., SOLOMON, J., PUGH, R.P., STEVENS, A.R., JACOBS, E.M., IRWIN, L.E., WOOD, D.A., STEINFELD, J.L., BATEMAN, J.R.: Clinical experience with procarbazine in Hodgkin's disease, reticulum cell sarcoma, and lymphosarcoma. Cancer, 26, 984 (1970).

35. E.O.R.T.C. Co-operative Group for Leukemia and Haematosarcomas: Bleomycin in the reticuloses. Brit. med. J. 1, 285 (1972).
36. BONADONNA, G., DE LENA, M., MONFARDINI, S., BARTOLI, E., BAJETTA, E., BERETTA, G., FOSSATI-BELLANI, F. (1972). Clinical trials with bleomycin in lymphomas and in solid tumors. Europ. J. Cancer 8, 205 (1972).
37. RUDDERS, R.A.: Treatment of advanced malignant lymphomas with bleomycin. Blood 40, 317 (1972).
38. BLUM, R.H., CARTER, S.K., AGRE, K.: A clinical review of bleomycin - a new antineoplastic agent. Cancer 31, 903 (1973).
39. BONADONNA, G., MONFARDINI, S., DE LENA, M., FOSSATI-BELLANI, F., BERETTA, G.: Phase I and preliminary phase II evaluation of adriamycin (NSC 123127). Cancer Res. 30, 2572 (1970).
40. O'BRYAN, R.M., LUCE, J.K., TALLEY, R.W., GOTTLIEB, J.A., BAKER, L.H., BONADONNA, G.: Phase II evaluation of adriamycin in human neoplasia. Cancer 32, 1 (1973).
41 JACQUILLAT, C., BOIRON, M., WEILL, M., MAZELIER, A., BERNARD, J.: Résultat du traitement des hémopathies par la rufocromomycine (5278 R.P.) Presse méd. 73, 2003 (1965).
42. CHAUVERGNE, J., BIRABEN, J., LARGARDE, Cl.,HUGUES, A.: Etude clinique d'un antibiotique antimitotique: la rufocromomycine (5278 R.P.). Sur 166 observations. Intérêt dans les réticulopathies malignes. Bull. Cancer 53, 229 (1966).
43. CARTER, S.K.: An overview of the status of the nitrosoureas in other tumors. Cancer Chemother. Rep. Part 3, 4, 35 (1973).
44. E.O.R.T.C. Co-operative Group for Leukaemia and Haematocarcomas: Clinical screening of epipodophyllotoxin VM 26 in malignant lymphomas and solid tumors. Brit. med. J. 2, 744 (1972).
45. GOLDSMITH, M.A., CARTER, S.K.: 4'-demethyl-epipodophyllotoxin-B-D-thenylidene glucoside (VM-26). A brief review. Europ. J. Cancer 9, 477 (1973).
46. FREI, E., III, LUCE, J.K., TALLEY, R.W., VAITEVICIUS, V.K., WILSON, H.E.: 5-(3,3-dimethyl-1-triazeno) imidazole-4-carboxamide (NSC-45388) in the treatment of lymphoma. Cancer Chemother. Rep. 56, 667 (1972).
47. LIVINGSTON R.B., CARTER, S.K.: Single agents in cancer chemotherapy. New York: IFI/Plenum 1970.
48. HILL, J.M., ROBERTS, J., LOEB, E., KHAN, A., MACLELLAN, A., HILL, R.W.: L-Asparaginase therapy for leukemia and other malignant neoplasms. J. Amer. med. Ass. 202, 882 (1967).
49. BEARD, M.E.J., CROWTHER, D., GALTON, D.A.G., GUYER, R.J., HAMILTON FAIRLEY, G., KAY, H.E.M., KNAPTON, P.J., MALPAS, J.S., BODLEY SCOTT, R.: L-Asparaginase in treatment of acute leukemia and lymphosarcoma. Brit. med. J. 1, 191 (1970).
50. CLARKSON, B., KRAKOFF, I., BURCHENAL, J., KARNOFSKY, D., GOLBEY, R., DOWLING, M., OETTGEN, H., LIPTON, A.: Clinical results of treatment with E. coli L-asparaginase in adults with leukemia, lymphoma and solid tumors. Cancer 25, 279 (1970).
51. HOOGSTRATEN, B., OWENS, A.H., LENHARD, R.E., GLIDEWELL, O.J., LEONE, L.A., OLSON, K.B., HARLEY, J.B., TOWNSEND, S.R., MILLER, S.P., SPURR, C.L.: Combination chemotherapy in lymphosarcoma and reticulum cell sarcoma. Blood 33, 370 (1969).
52. LENHARD, R.E., OWENS, A.H.: Prednisone in combination chemotherapy of lymphoma. Proc. Amer. Ass. Cancer Res. 12, 35 (1971).
53. LUCE, J.K., GAMBLE, J.F., WILSON, H.E., MONTO, R.W., ISAACS, B.L., PALMER, R.L., COLTMAN, Jr., C.A., HEWLETT, J.S., GEHAN, E.A., FREI, E.: Combined cyclophosphamide, vincristine, and prednisone therapy of malignant lymphoma. Cancer 28, 306 (1971).
54. BAGLEY, Jr., C.M., DE VITA, V.T.: Advanced lymphosarcoma: intensive cyclical combination chemotherapy with cyclophosphamide, vincristine, and prednisone. Ann. intern. Med. 76, 227 (1972).

55. KAUFMAN, J.H., EZDINLI, E., AUNGST, W., STUTZMAN, L.: Combination chemotherapy vs. standard therapy in lymphosarcoma. Proc. Amer. Ass. Cancer Res. 14, 85 (1973).

56. LOWENBRAUN, S., DE VITA, V.T., SERPICK, A.A.: Combination chemotherapy with nitrogen mustard, vincristine, procarbazine and prednisone in lymphosarcoma and reticulum cell sarcoma. Cancer 25, 1018 (1970).

57. HØST, H., ABRAHAMSEN, A.F.: Combination chemotherapy with cyclophosphamide, vinblastine, procarbazine, and prednisone in the treatment of malignant lymphomas. Scand. J. Haemat. 10, 170 (1973).

58. LUCE, J.K., DELANEY, F.C., GEHAN, E.A.: Remission induction chemotherapy of disseminated malignant lymphoma with combination bleomycin, cyclophosphamide, vincristine and prednisone. Proc. Amer. Ass. Cancer Res. 14, 66 (1973).

59. McKELVEY, E.M., GOTTLIEB, J.A., COLTMAN, C.A., WILSON, H.E.: Treatment of non-Hodgkin's lymphoma with hydroxyldaunomycin (adriamycin) combination chemotherapy. Proc. Amer. Ass. Cancer Res. 15, 184 (1974).

60. DE LENA, M., MONFARDINI, S., BONADONNA, G., TANCINI, G., FOSSATI, F., VERONESI, U.: Combination chemotherapy in advanced non-Hodgkin's lymphomas. Proc. Amer. Ass. Cancer Res. 14, 55 (1973).

61. LEVITT, M., MARSH, J.C., DE CONTI, R.C., MITCHELL, M.S., SKEEL, R.T., FARBER, L.R., BERTINO, J.R.: Combination sequential chemotherapy in advanced reticulum cell sarcoma. Cancer 29, 630 (1972).

62. SKARIN, A., ROSENTHAL, D., MOLONEY, W., FREI, E.III: Treatment of advanced non-Hodgkin's lymphoma (NHL) with bleomycin, adriamycin cyclophosphamide, vincristine and prednisone (BACOP). Proc. Amer. Ass. Cancer Res. 15, 133 (1974).

63. EZDINLI, E.Z., POCOCK, S., BRUNK, S.F., AUNGST, C.W.: Intensive vs. moderate chemotherapy of lymphocytic lymphoma. Proc. Amer. Ass. Cancer Res. 15, 39 (1974).

64. GOMEZ, G.A., STUTZMAN, K.: Cell cycle agents and cyclophosphamide (CYP) in histiocytic (HL) and other lymphomas. Proc. Amer. Ass. Cancer Res. 15, 105 (1974).

65. LEE, Y.N., SAY, C., HORI, J.M., SPRATT, Jr., J.S.: Major surgery in Hodgkin's disease and other malignant lymphomas. J. Surg. Oncol. 465 (1973).

66. JOHNSON, R.E.: Modern approaches to the radiotherapy of lymphoma. Seminars Hematol. 6, 357 (1969).

67. JOHNSON, R.E., O'CONNOR, G.T., LEVIN, D.: Primary management of advanced lymphosarcoma with radiotherapy. Cancer 25, 787 (1970).

68. NEWALL, J., FRIEDMAN, M.: Reticulum-cell sarcoma. Part II. Radiation dosage for each type. Radiology 94, 643 (1970).

69. JONES, S.E., KAPLAN, H.S., ROSENBERG, S.A.: Non-Hodgkin's lymphomas. III. Preliminary results of radiotherapy and a proposal for new clinical trials. Radiology 103, 657 (1972).

70. PETERS, M.V.: Changing concepts in the radiotherapy for the lymphomas. In: Leukemia-Lymphoma, p. 261. Chicago: Year Book Medical Publishers 1970.

71. CANELLOS, G.P., DE VITA, V.T., YOUNG, R.C., CHABNER, B.A., SCHEIN, P.S., JOHNSON, R.E.: Intensive therapy for advanced lymphocytic lymphoma: a randomized trial between combination chemotherapy and total body radiotherapy. Proc. Amer. Ass. Cancer Res. 15, 172 (1974).

72. SOKAL, J.E., AUNGST, W., SNYDERMAN, M.: Prolongation of remission in Stage I and II lymphomas by BCG vaccination. Proc. Amer. Ass. Cancer Res. 15, 13 (1974).

73. BURKITT, D.: A sarcoma involving the jaws in African children. Brit. J. Surg. 46, 218 (1958).

74. BURKITT, D.P., WRIGHT, D.H.: Burkitt's lymphoma. Edinburgh-London: E. & S. Livingstone 1970.

75. DORFMAN, R.F.: Childhood lymphosarcoma in St. Louis, Missouri clinically and histologically resembling Burkitt's tumor. Cancer 18, 418 (1965).

76. O'CONNOR, G., RAPPAPORT, H., SMITH, E.B.: Childhood lymphoma resembling "Burkitt tumor" in the United States. Cancer 18, 411 (1965).
77. BRAS, G., MURRAY, S.M.: Sporadic occurrence in Jamaica of neoplasma resembling Burkitt's tumor. Lancet 2, 619 (1965).
78. COHEN, M.H., BENNETT, J.M., BERARD, C.W., ZIEGLER, J.L., VOGEL, C.L., SHEAGREN, J.N., CARBONE, P.P.: Burkitt's tumor in the United States. Cancer 23, 1259 (1969).
79. ZIEGLER, J.L., MORROW, Jr., R.H., FASS, L., KYALMAZI, S.K., CARBONE, P.P.: Treatment of Burkitt's tumor with cyclophosphamide. Cancer 26, 474 (1970).
80. COOPER, E.H., FRANK, G.L., WRIGHT, D.H.: Cell proliferation in Burkitt tumours. Europ. J. Cancer 2, 377 (1966).
81. IVERSEN, U., IVERSEN, O.H., BLUMING, A.Z., ZIEGLER, J.L., KYALWASI, S.: Cell kinetics of African cases of Burkitt lymphoma. A preliminary report- Europ. J. Cancer 8, 305 (1972).
82. CLIFFORD, P.: Further studies in the treatment of Burkitt's lymphoma. E. Afr. med. J. 43, 179 (1966).
83. NGU, V.A.: Clinical evidence of host defences in Burkitt tumour. In: Treatment of Burkitt's Tumour. U.I.C.C. Monograph 8, p. 204, (eds. J.H. Burchenal, D.P. Burkitt). Berlin-Heidelberg-New York: Springer-Verlag 1967.
84. KLEIN, G., CLIFFORD, P., KLEIN, E., STJERNSWARD, J.: Search for tumour specific immune reactions in Burkitt lymphoma patients by the membrane immunofluorescene reaction. In: Treatment of Burkitt's Tumour. U.I.C.C. Monograph 8, p. 209 (eds. J.H. Burchenal, D.P. Burkitt). Berlin-Heidelberg-New York: Springer-Verlag 1967.
85. EPSTEIN, M.A., HENLE, G., ACHONG, B.G.: Morphological and biological studies on a virus in cultured lymphoblasts from Burkitt's lymphoma. J. exp. Med. 121, 761 (1965).
86. SIMONS, P.H., ROSS, M.G.R.: The isolation of herpes virus from Burkitt tumours. Europ. J. Cancer 1, 135 (1965).
87. HENLE, W., DIEHL, V., KOHN, G., HAUSEN, H., HENLE, G.: Herpes-type virus and chromosome marker in normal leukocytes after growth with irradiated Burkitt cells. Science 157, 1064 (1967).
88. CLIFFORD, P., SINGH, S., STJERNSWÄRD, J., KLEIN, G.: Long-term survival of patients with Burkitt's lymphoma: an assessment of treatment and other factors which may relate to survival. Cancer Res. 27, 2578 (1967).
89. ZIEGLER, J.L.: Chemotherapy of Burkitt's lymphoma. Cancer 30, 1534 (1972).
90. OETTGEN, H.F., BURKITT, D., BURCHENAL, J.H.: Malignant lymphoma involving the jaw in African children: treatment with methotrexate. Cancer 16, 616 (1963).
91. OETTGEN, H.F., CLIFFORD, P., BURKITT, D.: Malignant lymphoma involving the jaw in African children: treatment with alkylating agents and actinomycin D. Cancer Chemother. Rep. 28, 25 (1963).
92. BURKITT, D.: African lymphoma. Observations on reponse to vincristine sulphate therapy. Cancer 19, 1131 (1966).
93. ARSENAU, J.C., BAGLEY, C.M., ANDERSON, T., CANELLOS, G.P.: Hyperkalaemia, a sequel to chemotherapy of Burkitt's lymphoma. Lancet 1, 10, (1973).
94. ANDERSON, T., MAGRATH, I., BRERETON, H., ZIEGLER, J., SCHEIN, P.: Burkitt's lymphoma: Prediction of early relapse and metabolic complications of therapy. Proc. Amer. Ass. clin. Oncol. 15, 169 (1974).
95. FIAKKOW, P.J., KLEIN, G., CLIFFORD, P.: Second malignant clone underlying a Burkitt-tumour exacerbation. Lancet 2, 629 (1972).
96. BURKITT's lymphoma. An assessment of treatment and other factors which may relate to survival. Cancer Res. 27, 2578 (1967).
97. STUTZ, A.J., GREENBERG, A.J., WILEY, A., GILBERT, E.F., OPPENHEIMER, J.: Burkitt's lymphoma: The role of radiotherapy. Radiology 104, 379 (1972).

98. MAGRATH, I.T., ZIEGLER, J.L.: BCG immunotherapy in Burkitt's lymphoma. Proc. Amer. Ass. clin. Oncol. Abstract no. 25 (1973).
99. EPSTEIN, Jr., E.H., LEVIN, D.L., CROFT, Jr., J.D., LUTZNER, M.A.: Mycosis fungoides. Survival, prognostic features, response to therapy and autopsy findings. Medicine 15, 61 (1972).
100. HAYNES, H.A., VAN SCOTT, E.J.: Therapy of mycosis fungoides. Prog. Dermatol. 3, 1 (1968).
101. CHAIMET, P.: Un cas d'eczéma prémycosique traité par la corticothérapie depuis 3 ans. Concours med. 85, 1879 (1963).
102. FARBER, E.M., COX, A.J., STEINBERG, J., McCLINTOCK, R.P.: Therapy of mycosis fungoides with topically applied fluocinolone acetonide under occlusive dressing. Cancer 19, 237 (1966).
103. MARMELZAT, W.L.: Mycosis fungoides; Local injection of triamcinolone. Calif. Med. 98, 139 (1963).
104. SIPOS, K.: Paintings with nitrogen mustard in mycosis fungoides. Dermatologica 130, 3 (1965).
105. VAN SCOTT, E.J., KALMANSON, J.D.: Complete remissions of mycosis fungoides lymphoma induced by topical nitrogen mustard (HN2). Control of delayed hypersensitivity to HN2 by desensitization and by induction of specific immunologic tolerance. Cancer 32, 18 (1973).
106. FUKS, Z., BAGSHAW, M.A.: Total-skin electron treatment of mycosis fungoides. Therapeut. Radiol. 100, 145 (1971).
107. WALDORF, D.S., HAYNES, H.A., VAN SCOTT, E.J.: Cutaneous hypersensitivity and desensitization to mechlorethamine in patients with mycosis fungoides lymphoma. Ann. intern. Med. 67, 282 (1967).
108. KREBS, J., LANDES, E.: Zur Endoxantherapie von malignen Wucherungen des reticulo-histiocytären Systems. (Mycosis Fungoides and Reticulosarkomatose). Hautarzt 16, 76 (1965).
109. DE BAST, C., MORIAME, N., WANET, J., LEDOUX, M., ACHTEN, G., KENIS, Y.: Bleomycin in mycosis fungoides and reticulum cell lymphoma. Arch. Derm. 104, 508 (1971).
110. SPIGEL, S.C., COLTMAN, Jr., C.A.: Therapy of mycosis fungoides with bleomycin. Cancer 32, 767 (1973).
111. UMEZAWA, H., ISHIZUKI, M., MAEDA, K., TAKEUCHI, T.: Studies on bleomycin. Cancer 20, 891 (1967).
112. DEBAST, C., KENIS, Y.: Unpublished data.
113. LICHTENSTEIN, L.: Histiocytosis X. Integration of eosinophilic granuloma of bone, "Letterer-Siwe disease", and "Schüller-Christian disease" as related manifestations of a single nosologic entity. Arch. Path. 56, 84 (1953).
114. GREEN, W.T., FARBER, S.:"Eosinophilic or solitary granuloma" of bone. J. Bone Joint Surg. 24, 499 (1942).
115. LIEBERMAN, P.H., JONES, C.R., DARGEON, H.W.K., BEGG, C.F.: A reappraisal of eosinophilic granuloma of bone, Hand-Schüller-Christian syndrome and Letterer-Siwe syndrome. Medicine (Balt.) 48, 375 (1969).
116. EIERMAN, H.R.: Apparent cure of Letterer-Siwe disease. Seventeen-year survival of identical twins with nonlipoid reticuloendotheliosis. J. Amer. med. Ass. 196, 156 (1966).
117. VOGEL, J.M., VOGEL, P.: Idiopathic histiocytosis: A discussion of eosinophilic granuloma, the Hand-Schüller-Christian syndrome, and the Letterer-Siwe syndrome. Seminars Hematol. 9, 349 (1972).
118. AVIOLI, L.V., LASERSOHN, J.T., LOPRESTI, J.M.: Histiocytosis X (Schüller-Christian disease): a clinico-pathological survey, review of ten patients and the results of prednisone therapy. Medicine 42, 119 (1963).
119. NEZELOF, Ch.: L'histiocytose X. Rev. franc. Etudes clin. biol. 11, 22 (1966)
120. DARGEON, H.W.: Considerations in the treatment of reticuloendotheliosis; the Janeway Lecture, 1964. Amer. Roentgen. 93, 521 (1965).

121. STARLING, K.A., DONALDSON, M.H., HAGGARD, M.E., VIETTI, T.J., SUTOW, W.W.: Therapy of histiocytosis X with vincristine, vinblastine, and cyclophosphamide. Amer. J. Dis. Child. 123, 105 (1972).

122. LEIKIN, S., FURUGANAN, G., FRANKEL, A., STEERMAN, R., CHANDRA, R.: Immunologic parameters in Histiocytosis X. Cancer 32, 796 (1973).

123. FREUD, P.: Treatment of reticuloendotheliosis. Use of corticosteroids and antifolic acid compounds. J. Amer. Med. Ass. 175, 82 (1961).

124. NEWTON, K.A., ANDERSON, I.M.: Long-term remission following methotrexate therapy in a case of Hand-Schüller-Christian disease. Postgrad. med. J. 41, 33 (1965).

125. SHARP, H., WHITE, J.G., KRIVIT, W.: Histiocytosis X treated with vinblastine sulfate. Cancer Chemother. Rep. 39, 53 (1964).

126. SEGNI, F., MASTRANGELO, R., TORTOROLO, G.: Daunomycin in Letterer-Siwe's disease. Lancet 2, 461 (1968).

127. DOEDE, K.G., RAPPAPORT, H.: Long-term survival of patients with acute differentiated histiocytosis (Letterer-Siwe disease). Cancer 20, 1783 (1967).

128. DORFMAN, R.F.: Classification of non-Hodgkin's lymphomas. Lancet 1, 1295 (1974).

129. DICK, F., BLOOMFIELD, C.D., BRUNNING, R.D.: Incidence, cytology, and histopathology on non-Hodgkin's lymphomas in the bone marrow. Cancer 33, 1382 (1974).

130. SKARIN, A.T., PINKUS, G.S., MYEROWITZ, R.L., BISHOP, Y.M., MOLONEY, W.C.: Combination chemotherapy of advanced lymphocytic lymphoma. Cancer 34, 1023 (1974).

131. PATCHEFSKY, A.S., BRODOVSKY, H.S., MENDUKE, H., SOUTHARD, M., BROOKS, J., NICKLAS, D., HOCH, W.S.: Non-Hodgkin's lymphomas: a clinicopathologic study of 293 cases. Cancer 34, 1173 (1974).

132. BONADONNA, G., MONFARDINI, S.: Chemotherapy of non-Hodgkin's lymphomas. Cancer Treat. Rev. 1, 167 (1974).

133. BONADONNA, G., DE LENA, M., MONFARDINI, S., BERETTA, G., VALAGUSSA, P.: Combination chemotherapy with adriamycin in malignant lymphomas. In: Adriamycin review. EORTC International Symposium, (eds, M. Staquet, H. Tagnon, Y. Kenis et al.) p. 200. Ghent: European Press Medikon 1975.

134. WASSERMAN, T.H., SLAVIK, M., CARTER, S.K.: Review of CCNU in clinical cancer. Cancer Treat. Rev. 1, 131 (1974).

135. WASSERMAN, T.H., SLAVIK, M., CARTER, S.K.: Methyl-CCNU in clinical cancer therapy. Cancer Treat. Rev. 1, 251 (1974).

136. LENHARD, R.E., POCOCK, S.: Combination chemotherapy in histiocytic lymphomas. A comparison of three multidrug regimens. Proc. Am. Soc. Clin. Oncol. 16, 236 (1975).

137. LUCE, J.K., GEHAN, E.A., GAMBLE, J.F., WILSON, H.E., MONTO, R.W., TALLEY, R.W.: High rate and long duration of complete remission in malignant lymphoma treated with combined oral cyclophosphamide and prednisone and IV vincristine. Proc. Am. Ass. Cancer Res. 16, 129 (1975).

138. SOLOMON, J., PUGH, R.P., GODFREY, T.E., SHEEHAN, W.W.: Comparison of two combination induction programs for non-Hodgkin's lymphomas. Proc. Am. Soc. Clin. Oncol. 16, 233 (1975).

139. PORTLOCK, C.S., ROSENBERG, S.A., GLATSTEIN, E., KAPLAN, H.S.: Stage IV non-Hodgkin's lymphoma: a prospective trial comparing CVP (cyclophosphamide, vincristine, prednisone) alone versus split course CVP with total lymphoid irradiation versus continuous single alkylating agent. Proc. Am. Soc. Clin. Oncol. 16, 266 (1975).

140. KENNEDY, B.J., HILL, J., BLOOMFIELD, C., KIANG, D., FORTUNY, I., THEOLOGIDES, A.: Combination (COP) versus successive single agent chemotherapy (C-O-P) in lymphocytic lymphoma. Proc. Am. Ass. Cancer Res. 16, 142 (1975).

141. BERD, D., CORNOG, J., DE CONTI, R.C., LEVITT, M., BERTINO, J.R.: Long-term remission in diffuse histiocytic lymphoma treated with combination sequential chemotherapy. Cancer 25, 1050 (1975).

142. McKELVEY, E.M., GOTTLIEB, J.A., HAUT, A., LANE, M.: Hydroxyldauno-mycin (adriamycin) combination chemotherapy in non-Hodgkin's lymphoma. Proc. Am. Soc. Clin. Oncol. 16, 233 (1975).

143. PECKHAM, M.J.: Radiation therapy of the non-Hodgkin's lymphomas. Seminars Hematol. 11, 41 (1974).

144. BOSTON, H.C., DAHLIN, D.C., IVINS, J.C., CUPPS, R.E.: Malignant lymphoma (so-called reticulum cell sarcoma) of bone. Cancer 34, 1131 (1974).

145. FAYOS, J.V., EDLUND, J.H., KNAPP, W.T., CAMPOS, J.L., LAMPE, I.: The lymphomas: response to irradiation. Cancer 34, 212 (1974).

146. LEVINE, P.H., CHO, B.R.: Burkitt lymphoma: Clinical features of North American cases. Cancer Res. 34, 1219 (1974).

147. MAGRATH, I.T., LWANGA, S., CARSWELL, W., HARRISON, N.: Surgical reduction of tumor bulk in the management of abdominal Burkitt's lymphoma. Brit. med. J. 2, 308 (1974).

148. ZIEGLER, J.L., YOUNG, R.C., POMEROY, T.C.: Combined modality treatment of American Burkitt's tumor. Proc. Am. Soc. Clin. Oncol. 16, 249 (1975).

149. LONG, J.C., MIHM, M.: Mycosis fungoides with extracutaneous dissemination: a distinct clinicopathologic entity. Cancer 34, 1745 (1974).

150. RAPPAPORT, H., THOMAS, L.B.: Mycosis fungoides: The pathology of extracutaneous involvement. Cancer 34, 1198 (1974).

151. VARIAKOJIS, D., ROSAS-URIBE, A., RAPPAPORT, H.: Mycosis fungoides: pathologic findings in staging laparotomies. Cancer 33, 1589 (1974).

152. KOMP, D.M., BRITTON, H.A., VIETTI, T.J., HUMPHREY, G.B.: Response of childhood histiocytosis X to procarbazine. Cancer Chemother. Rep. Part 1, 58, 719 (1974).

153. JONES, B.: Chemotherapy of reticuloendotheliosis. Cancer Chemother. Rep. 57, 110 (1973).

154. HELLMAN, S., ROSENTHAL, D.S., MOLONEY, W.C., CHAFFEY, J.T.: The treatment of non-Hodgkin's lymphoma. Cancer 36, 804 (1975).

155. MORGENFIELD, M.C., PAVLOVSKY, A., SUAREZ, A., SOMOZA, N., PAVLOVSKY, S., PALAU, M., BARROS, C.A.: Combined cyclophosphamide, vincristine, procarbazine, and prednisone (COPP) therapy of malignant lymphoma. Cancer 36, 1241 (1975).

156. MISSET, J.L., POUILLART, P., AMIEL, J.L., SCHWARZENBERG, L., HAYAT, M., DE VASSAL, F., MUSSET, M., BELPOMME, D., JASMIN, C., ALBAHARY, C., DEPIERRE, R., MATHE, G.: Combinaison d'adriamycine de VM 26, de cyclophosphamide et de prednisone (AVmCP) pour la chimiothérapie des lymphoréticulosarcomes disséminés. Nouv. Presse Méd. 4, 3117 (1975).

157. McKELVEY, E.M.: Cyclophosphamide versus arabinosyl cytosine combination maintenance chemotherapy in malignant lymphoma. Proc. Amer. Soc. Clin. Oncol. 17, 261 (1976).

158. RODRIGUEZ, V., BODEY, G.P., McKELVEY, E.M., FREIREICH, E.J.: Combination chemotherapy (CHOP-Bleo) of advanced diffuse histiocytic lymphoma. Proc. Amer. Soc. Clin. Oncol. 17, 249 (1976).

159. SWEET, D.L., GOLOMB, H.M., DRESSER, R.K., LESTER, E.P., BITRAN, J.D. et al.: Treatment of advanced histiocytic lymphoma with C.O.M.A. chemotherapy. Proc. Amer. Ass. Cancer Res. 17, 10 (1976).

Chapter 22
Skin Cancer and Malignant Melanoma

SKIN CANCER

The majority of malignant cutaneous lesions are derived from the epidermis. Basal-cell epithelioma, the most common skin cancer, is locally malignant and invasive but rarely metastasizes. Squamous-cell carcinoma, the second most frequent skin cancer, may spread to regional lymphatics. Most skin cancers are seen on exposed areas of the body in older people.

A. STRATEGY

1. Localized Skin Cancer

Treatment consists of thorough removal of the malignant lesion. Some local measures yield a cure rate of 95-98 percent when they are skilfully applied and the patients are carefully selected. Surgical excision, electrosurgery (electrosurgical excision, electrodesiccation, and electrocoagulation), chemosurgery (Mohs' technique), cryosurgery, and irradiation are all very effective. Correct selection of the most appropriate technique or combination of techniques depends on the skill of the treating physician, the location, extent and cell type of the lesion, and the nature of any previous therapy in the case of recurrent lesions.

Topical chemotherapy, especially with 5-fluorouracil (5-FU) has been very useful in multiple superficial lesions too extensive for treatment by local techniques (1-5). KLEIN has successfully (80 percent cure rate) treated premalignant keratoses (extensive multiple actinic keratoses, with or without squamous cell carcinoma in situ, or X-ray induced keratoses), multiple superficial basal-cell carcinomas and squamous-cell carcinomas and xeroderma pigmentosum (4, 5). 5-FU is less satisfactory in the treatment of nodular basal-cell carcinoma and infiltrating squamous-cell carcinoma. A 5 percent preparation in a cream base has been the most satisfactory. Application twice daily for approximately 4 weeks is usually required. The effect of topical 5-FU on epidermal neoplasms is selective. An inflammatory response is limited predominantly to sites of malignant or premalignant involvement, usually with minimal and readily reversible effects on the normal skin or other tissues, Large areas can thus be treated. Healing proceeds without scarring and normal skin color and texture are restored. There are virtually no serious systemic or local side-effects.

2. Advanced Skin Cancer

Bleomycin can be used for advanced cases that are no longer treatable by local therapy (6). In a recent review, 50 percent of such patients

were found to respond, but the response was incomplete and short-lived
in a large proportion of cases (7). Long-term therapy with this drug
is not recommended because of the cumulative risk of pulmonary toxicity.

MALIGNANT MELANOMA

Malignant melanoma is a relatively rare malignancy (1.3 percent of all
cancers), with a peak incidence in the 30-59 age group. There is a
slight preference for men. The variable biologic behavior of the
tumor makes it difficult to appraise the results of therapy. Spontaneous remissions are occasionally reported. Host factors seem to be important (8). The tumor spreads via the lymphatics, as shown by the appearance of satellite nodules around the main tumor and by early invasion of the regional lymph nodes. Following hematogenous dissemination,
all organs of the human body can be involved (9, 88).

A number of prognostic features have been recognized: sex, size, site,
clinical and pathologic characteristics of the primary lesion, duration
of symptoms, and the clinical stage (10, 11, 92). Females have a better
prognosis than males. In the case of occult lesions or primaries located on mucosal surfaces, the trunk or the anogenital area, prognosis
is less favorable than that for lesions of the head and neck area or of
the extremities (exposed sites). The prognosis is poor if the primary is
amelanotic, ulcerating, bulky, or diffuse, or if there are satellite
lesions in the skin. Immune responsiveness is important (12, 90). There
is a clear relationship between the depth of invasion (level) of the
primary and survival (13-16). Survival is most clearly related to the
clinical stage: in case with no metastases adequate treatment ensures
5-year survival in 60-80 percent of cases. With local skin metastases,
survival is 30-50 percent; with regional metastases (intradermal or
local node) 10-25 percent, and with distant metastases less than 5 percent (17). No staging system is universally accepted. The UICC-TNM
classification is based on the size and the local invasiveness of the
primary tumor, and presence of absence of nodal and distal metastases
(Table 22-1) (18). Others are based on 3- or 4-stage systems (Table 22-2)

Table 22-1. TNM staging for malignant melanoma

T	Primary tumor
TO	No primary tumor present
T1	Tumor 2 cm or less in its largest dimension, strictly superficial or exophytic. No satellite nodules
T2	Tumor more than 2 cm but not more than 5 cm in its largest dimension *or* with minimal infiltration of the dermis, irrespective of size. No satellite nodules
T3	Tumor more than 5 cm in its largest dimension *or* with deep infil-tration of the dermis, irrespective of size, *or* with satellite nodules within 5 cm of the borders of the primary tumor
NO	No palpable nodes
N1	Movable homolateral nodes N1a Nodes not considered to contain growth N1b Nodes considered to contain growth
N2	Movable contralateral or bilateral nodes N2a Nodes not considered to contain growth N2b Nodes considered to contain growth
MO	No evidence of distant metastases
M1	Distant metastases present including lymph nodes beyond the region in which the primary tumor is situated, *or* satellite nodules more than 5 cm from the border of the primary tumor

(17, 19, 92). Malignant melanoma occurs in three distinct clinicopathologic forms: lentigo maligna, superfacial spreading and nodular melanoma
(88).

Table 22-2. Staging of malignant melanoma (92)

A. Clinicopathologic staging

Stage
- I. Localized primary melanoma
- IA. Local recurrence
- II. Metastases to regional lymph nodes
- III. Disseminated melanoma (Visceral organs, distant lymph nodes, or distant cutaneous metastases)

B. Level of invasion

Level
- I. All tumor cells above basement membrane
- II. Invasion into loose connective tissue of papillary dermis
- III. Tumor cells at junction of papillary and reticular dermis
- IV. Invasion into reticular dermis
- V. Invasion into subcutaneous fat

A. CHEMOTHERAPY

1. Single-Agent Chemotherapy

Almost all cytotoxic agents have been tried at some time in the treatment of disseminated malignant melanoma (17, 20). This reflects the
fact that none has been consistently effective. Table 22-3 lists the
results compiled in 3 reviews (17, 20, 73). When strict criteria of
response are applied, none of the standard agents are retained. Cyclophosphamide (CPM) seems to be more active than other alkylating agents.
Melphalan is the most widely used agent for perfusion yet its activity
given by the systemic route is based on several old studies. Conventional antimetabolites are ineffective. The vinca alkaloids have marginal activity; vincristine (VCR) is thus often incorporated in combinations. Actinomycin D (ACD) is the only antibiotic with any effect. Activity, though inconsistent, has been claimed for hydroxyurea (HUR),
procarbazine (PCZ), and trimethylcolchicinic acid (TMCA). Initial reports are often not confirmed by subsequent studies (24-26). The nitrosoureas have some activity and are of particular interest in view of
the propensity of malignant melanoma to metastasise to the brain (74,
75). Hormones have occasionally been tried because of the more favorable
prognosis in women (17).

The only agent that has caused tumor regressions with any consistency is
imidazole carboxamide (DIC) (17, 27, 93) with an overall response rate
of 24 percent with 5-6 percent CR (73). Malignant melanoma is actually
the only tumor, with the exception of soft-tissue sarcomas, that responds to this drug (27-29). Female patients (26 percent) improve twice
as often as males (13 percent) (17). Regressions are noted more frequently in lymph node metastases (27 percent) than in liver (9 percent)
or brain metastases (17) and in previously untreated patients. Several
dose schedules have been evaluated, consisting either of high-dose
single injections 4 weeks apart (30), or of daily injections for 5 or
10 days every 3-4 weeks (17, 27-29, 31). The duration of response

Table 22-3. Effectiveness of single agents in malignant melanoma

Drug	Number treated	Total response (%)	Reference
Methotrexate	25	8	COMIS and CARTER (73)
6-Mercaptopurine	47	4	-
Imidazole carboxamide	853	24	-
TIC mustard	108	8	-
5-Fluorouracil	43	2	-
Cytosine arabinoside	52	2	
Hydroxyurea	127	23	-
BCNU	122	18	-
CCNU	133	13	-
MeCCNU	101	18	-
Procarbazine	50	16	-
Nitrogen mustard	45	7	-
Chlorambucil	22	9	-
Cylophosphamide	55	16	-
Melphalan	52	15	-
Hexamethylmelamine	42	5	-
Mitomycin C	65	14	-
Actinomycin D	55	35	-
Mithramycin	79	11	-
Adriamycin	19	0	-
Bleomycin	34	0	-
Vincristine	52	12	-
Vinblastine	71	15	-
TMCA			-
Camptothecin	15	0	GOTTLIEB and LUCE (23)
Pregnenetrione	155	7	LUCE (17)

recorded ranges from 1.3 months to over 28 months, with a median duration of 5.7 months (17). Responders live longer than non-responders.

TIC mustard, a derivative of imidazole carboxamide that contains an alkylating group, has not been promising in the treatment of malignant melanoma (73, 94). Studies in progress may answer the question of whether drug combinations including a nitrosourea plus vincristine in fact increase the proportion of visceral disease response or yield overall results superior to DIC (73).

2. Combinations

Combination chemotherapy has been disappointing in malignant melanoma. Trials with combinations of conventional agents with marginal activity have failed to demonstrate any synergistic or additive effect (Table 22-4). Promising initial results with VCR plus BCNU (9/20 or 45 percent) (34) were not confirmed by subsequent studies (17, 35, 40, 49). Fifty percent tumor regressions were reported in a small series treated with VCR + ACD; however, in this trial a 25 percent reduction in tumor volume was considered an objective response (32).

Combination of DIC with one or more conventional or experimental agents has not significantly improved the response rate over that obtained with DIC alone (Table 22-4). However, some of the combinations have given a higher proportion of responses in visceral disease than DIC alone (76, 77). Preliminary results with combinations of DIC, BCNU, HUR and VCR (46) and CCNU, VCR, and BLM (36) are encouraging, but experience has taught us to be cautious in interpreting preliminary data relating to malignant melanoma.

3. Intra-Arterial Chemotherapy

The rationale, techniques, indications and complications of intra-arterial chemotherapy (perfusion and infusion) are discussed in Chapter 11. Since malignant melanoma frequently involves the extremities (45 percent) and the head and neck area (35 percent) (50), it often lends itself to this form of treatment. It can be used as an adjuvant to surgical excision in the treatment of primary melanoma, or in the palliative treatment of inoperable regional disease, where it may be a satisfactory alternative to amputation (51-54). Thio-TEPA, methotrexate, and especially melphalan have been injected intra-arterially. None of these agents is very effective in the treatment of malignant melanoma when given systemically and it is hoped that intra-arterial therapy with DIC will prove to give better results. Preliminary reports of trials with DIC by infusion seem to indicate that it can control disease in the area of the infusion (56).

Most studies on intra-arterial chemotherapy are difficult to evaluate because they are uncontrolled. STEHLIN noted an incidence of 6.4 percent for recurrence of tumors in the extremities treated with perfusions, compared to 34 percent after conventional therapy (57). In another uncontrolled trial, KREMENTZ et al. found that chemotherapy by regional perfusion increases the 5-year survival rate for Stage-I melanoma by 15 percent and doubles the survival rate for Stage-II disease (58). Not all surgeons share their enthusiasm (59). Intra-arterial chemotherapy should be considered as an experimental tool that must still prove its effectiveness in prospective randomized trials.

B. STRATEGY

1. Localized Malignant Melanoma

(i) Surgery
Localized primary lesions are treated by wide excision of the tumor and the underlying fascia (60), to include the satellite microfoci of neoplastic cells common in the immediate neighborhood of the tumor. Whether or not prophylactic lymph node dissections should be carried out at the time of the primary excision is still the subject of debate (16, 19, 60-62, 89, 96). In favor of this procedure it is stated that at least 25 percent of patients with clinically negative lymph nodes already have microscopic involvement. Opponents argue that lymph nodes provide an

Table 22-4. Results with combination chemotherapy in malignant melanoma

Combination	Number of patients	Objective regressions (%)	Reference
DIC, BCNU	61	19	COSTANZA and NATHANSON (42)
DIC, MeCCNU	26	23	COSTANZA and NATHANSON (43)
DIC, PCZ	62	16	EINHORN et al. (76)
DIC, HMM	16	12.5	STOLINSKY et al. (41)
DIC, ACD	69	20	GERNER et al. (40)
DIC, VCR	56	16	AHMANN et al. (77)
	20	10	AHMANN et al. (80)
FUdR, IUdR	15	0	MORTON et al. (38)
BCNU, VCR	20	45	MOON (34)
	51	16	MOON et al. (81)
	55	11	GAILANI and MOON (35)
	22	23	BELLET (95)
CCNU, VCR	16	13	PRIMACK et al. (49)
MeCCNU, CPM	87	20	PUGH et al. (82)
CPM, VCR	20	5	AHMANN et al. (80)
CPM, VCR	9	0	JOHNSON and JACOBS (33)
ACD, VCR	12	50+	CHANES et al. (32)
DIC, BCNU, VCR	16	62	COHEN et al. (44)
	27	44	LUCE et al. (45)
	113	28	LUCE (17)
	65	23	CARTER et al. (83)
DIC, CCNU, VCR	67	16	CARTER et al. (83)
DIC, HUR, BCNU	63	13	CARTER et al. (83)
	89	27	CONSTANZI et al. (84)
DIC, CPM, VCR	20	25	GARDERE (48)
MPH, MTC, VCR	12	8	NATHANSON et al. (86)
PCZ, ACD, VLB	13	38	PERLIN et al. (85)
CCNU, BLM, VCR	17	58	KENIS et al. (36)

Table 22-4. (continued)

Combination	Number of patients	Objective regressions (%)	Reference
DIC, HUR, BCNU, VCR	12	25	WAGENKNECHT (47)
	89	30	COSTANZI et al. (84)
MTX, 5-FU, CPM, VCR	27	26	LUCE (17)
MTX, 5-FU, CPM, VCR, PDN	23	22	RAMIREZ (37)

+ 25% tumor regression evaluated as a response in this study

important immunological defense mechanism and that there is no statistical evidence that block dissection of regional nodes benefits patients with Stage-I melanoma. No stand can be taken until a prospective randomized study has taken place (16). Block dissection is generally recommended when regional lymph nodes contain metastases (Stage-II disease). In stage-I melanoma it should be considered only for level 4 or 5 lesions (96).

(ii) Radiotherapy
Radiotherapy plays very little part in the radical treatment of the disease in the early stages. Assertions of the insensitivity of melanoma to irradiation have resulted in a neglect of its use for palliation (60). Worthwhile palliation of local problems can sometimes be achieved in disseminated disease, for example brain metastases (9).

(iii) Adjuvant Therapy
Since recurrences are not uncommun after "curative" resections for localized disease, malignant melanoma lends itself to adjuvant therapy. To our knowledge, no studies on systemic chemotherapy have been published, which is not surprising since no agent or combination has sufficient antitumor activity to justify clinical trials. In malignant melanoma in particular, there is ample evidence that host immune defenses are important (8), and the risk of immunosuppression may well outweigh any potential antitumor effect. For this reason, more studies are in progress with adjuvant immunotherapy (BCG) (63). Preliminary trials in patients with limited disease are encouraging (49, 78, 87, 90, 97). These studies also indicate that the method of immune stimulation (type, dose of BCG, mode of administration) may influence the therapeutic outcome.

2. Advanced Malignant Melanoma

Chemotherapy is the mainstay of treatment for patients with disseminated disease.

Some investigators have been experimenting with immunotherapy in advanced stages. Not all share our belief, based on experimental data, that immunotherapy should be reserved for the treatment of minimal residual disease (64). Active (specific and nonspecific) (65, 66) adoptive (60, 67) and passive immunotherapy, and also direct intralesional injections with BCG (38, 68) have all been tried. It is beyond the scope of this text to review these techniques and their rationale (64, 69, 71). Tumor regressions have been recorded in a minority of patients (17, 18, 78).

Other workers propose to administer chemotherapy and immunotherapy alternately, in order to reap the benefits of both (17, 72, 79, 90, 91).

REFERENCES

1. KLEIN, E.: Tumors of skin. VIII. Local chemotherapy of metastatic neoplasma. N.Y. St. J. Med. 68, 877 (1968).
2. SERRI, F.(Ed.): International Conference on 5% Fluorouracil Ointment in Dermatology. Dermatologica 140, suppl. 1 (1970).
3. ZACKHEIM, H.S., FARBER, E.M.: Topical antimetabolites. Ann. Rev. Med. 21, 59 (1970).
4. KLEIN, E., MILGROM, H., STOLL, H.L., HELM, F., WALKER, M.J., HOLTERMANN, O.A.: Topical 5-fluorouracil chemotherapy for premalignant and malignant epidermal neoplasms. In: Cancer Chemotherapy, p. 147 (eds. I. Brodsky, S.B. Kahn, J.H. Moyer) New York: Grune and Stratton 1972.
5. KLEIN, E., CASE, R.W., BURGESS, G.H.: Chemotherapy of skin cancer. CA 23, 228 (1973).
6. E.O.R.T.C. CLINICAL SCREENING CO-OPERATIVE GROUP: Study of the clinical efficiency of bleomycin in human cancer. Brit. med. J. 2, 643 (1970).
7. BLUM, R.H., CARTER, S.K., AGRE, K.: A clinical review of bleomycin - a new antineoplastic agent. Cancer 31, 903 (1973).
8. KOPF, A.W.: Host defenses against malignant melanoma. Hosp. Practice. Oct. 116 (1971).
9. GUPTA, T.D., BRASFIELD, R.: Metastatic melanoma. A clinicopathological study. Cancer 17, 1323 (1964).
10. COCHRAN, A.J.: Method of assessing prognosis in patients with maglignant melanoma. Lancet 2, 1062 (1968).
11. MACKIE, R.M., CARFRAF, D.C., COCHRAN, A.J.: Assessment of prognosis in patients with malignant melanoma. Lancet 2, 455 (1972).
12. GUTTERMAN, J.U., MAVLIGIT, G.M.: Chemoimmunotherapy of disseminated malignant melanoma with imidazole carboxamide (DTIC) and BCG. Proc. Amer. Ass. clin. Oncol. 15, 182 (1974).
13. MEHNERT, J.H., HEARD, J.L.: Staging of malignant melanoma by depth of invasion. J. Surg. Amer. 110, 168 (1965).
14. CLARK, W.H., FROM, L., BERNARDINO, E.A., MIHM, M.C.: The histogenesis and biologic behavior of primary human malignant melanomas of the skin. Cancer 29, 705 (1969).
15. McGOVERN, V.J.: The classification of melanoma and its relationship with prognosis. Pathology 2, 85 (1970).
16. DELLON, A.L., KETCHAM, A.S.: Surgical treatment of stage I melanoma. Arch. Surg. (Chic.) 106, 738 (1973).
17. LUCE, J.K.: Chemotherapy of malignant melanoma. Cancer 30, 1604 (1972).
18. UNION INTERNATIONALE CONTRE LE CANCER: T.N.M. classification of malignant tumours. Geneva: G. de Buren 1968.
19. GOLDSMITH, H.S., SHAH, J.P., KIM, D.H.: Prognostic significance of lymph node dissection in the treatment of malignant melanoma. Cancer 26, 606 (1970).
20. LIVINGSTON, R.B., CARTER, S.K.: Single Agents in Cancer Chemotherapy. New York: IFI/Plenum 1970.
21. BLUM, R.H., LIVINGSTON, R.B., CARTER, S.K.: Hexamethylmelamine. A new drug with activity in solid tumors. Europ. J. Cancer 9, 195 (1973).
22. O'BRYAN, R.M., LUCE, J.K., TALLEY, R.W., GOTTLIEB, J.A., BAKER, L.H., BONADONNA, G.: Phase II evaluation of adriamycin in human neoplasia. Cancer 32, 1 (1973).

23. GOTTLIEB, J.A., LUCE, J.K.: Treatment of malignant melanoma with camptothecin (NSC-100880). Cancer Chemother. Rep. 56, 103 (1972).
24. GOTTLIEB, J.A., FREI, E., III, LUCE, J.K.: Dose-schedule studies with hydroxyurea (NSC 32065) in malignant melanoma. Cancer Chemother. Rep. 55, 277 (1971).
25. STOLINKSKY, D.C., JACOBS, E.M., BRAUNWALD, J., BATEMAN, J.R.: Further study of trimethylcolchicinic acid, methyl ether, d-tartrate (TMCA; NSC-36354) in patients with malignant melanoma. Cancer Chemother. Rep. 56, 263 (1972).
26. AHMANN, D.L., HAHN, R.G., BISEL, H.F.: Clinical evaluation of 5-(3,3-dimethyl-1-triazeno)imidazole-4-carboxamide (NSC-45388), melphalan (NSC-8806), and hydroxyurea (NSC-32065) in the treatment of disseminated malignant melanoma. Cancer Chemother. Rep. 56, 369 (1972).
27. CARTER, S.K., FRIEDMAN, M.A.: 5-(3,3-dimethyl-1-triazeno)-imidazole-4-carboxamide (DTIC, DIC, NSC-45388) - A new antitumor agent with activity against malignant melanoma. Europ. J. Cancer 8, 85 (1972).
28. WAGNER, D.E., RAMIREZ, G., WEISS, A.J., HILL, Jr., G.: Combination phase 1-II study of imidazole carboxamide (NCS 45388). Oncology 26, 310 (1971).
29. LUCE, J.K., THURMAN, W.G., ISAACS, B.L., TALLEY, R.W.: Clinical trials with the antitumor agent 5-(3,3-dimethyl-1-triazeno)imidazole-4-carboxamide (NSC-45388). Cancer Chemother. Rep. 54, 119 (1970).
30. COWAN, D.H., BERGSAGEL, D.E.: Intermittent treatment of metastatic malignant melanoma with high dose (5-(3,3-dimethyl-1-triazeno)imidazole-4-carboxamide (NSC 45388). Cancer Chemother. Rep., 55, 175 (1971).
31. GERNER, R.E., MOORE, G.E.: Study of 5-(3,3-dimethyl-1-triazeno) imidazole 4 carboxamide (NSC-45388) in patients with disseminated melanoma. Cancer Chemother. Rep. 57, 83 (1973).
32. CHANES, R.E., CONDIT, P.T., BOTTOMLEY, R.H., NISIMBLAT, W.: Combined actinomycin D and vincristine in the treatment of patients with cancer. Cancer 27, 613 (1971).
33. JOHNSON, F.D., JACOBS, E.M.: Chemotherapy of metastatic malignant melanoma. Experience with 73 patients. Cancer 27, 1306 (1971).
34. MOON, J.H.: Combination chemotherapy in malignant melanoma. Cancer 25, 468 (1970).
35. GAILANI, S., MOON, J.: Comparative study of imidazole carboxamide dimethyl triazeno (ICDT) and combination of 1,3,bis(2-chloroethyl)-1-nitrosourea (BCNU) and vincristine (VCR) in treatment of metastatic melanoma. Amer. Soc. Clin. Oncol. abstr. 23 (1971).
36. KENIS, Y., et al.: unpublished observations.
37. RAMIREZ, G. (Clinical Oncology Group): Five-drug combination therapy in the treatment of solid tumor. Proc. Amer. Ass. Cancer Res. 14, 17 (1973).
38. MORTON, D.J., EIBLER, F.R., MALMGREN, R.A., WOOD, W.C.: Immunological factors which influence response to immunotherapy in malignant melanoma. Surgery 68, 158 (1970).
39. AHMANN, D.L., HAHN, R.G., BISEL, H.F.: Clinical evaluation of CCNU (NSC 79037) and a combination of imidazole carboxamide (NSC 45388) and vincristine (NSC 67572) in the treatment of disseminated malignant melanoma. Presented at Amer. Soc. Clin. Oncol. May 1972 (abstr.)
40. GERNER, R.E., MOORE, G.E., DIDOLKAR, M.S.: Chemotherapy of disseminated malignant melanoma with dimethyl triazeno imidazole carboxamide and dactinomycin. Cancer 32, 756 (1973).
41. STOLINSKY, D.C., BOGDON, D.L., SOLOMON, J., BATEMAN, J.R.: Hexamethylmelamine (NSC-13875) alone and in combination with 5-(3,3-dimethyl-triazeno) imidazole-4-carboxamide (NSC-45388) in the treatment of advanced cancer. Cancer 30, 654 (1972).

42. COSTANZA, M., NATHANSON, I.: Therapy of melanoma with dimethyl-triazeno-imidazole carboxamide (DTIC) and bis-chloroethylnitro-sourea (BCNU): Response with cerebral metastases. Presented at Amer. Soc. Clin. Oncol. May 1972 (abstr.).

43. CONSTANZA, M.E., NATHANSON, L.: Combination DTIC and methyl CCNU vs. single agents in disseminated malignant melanoma: preliminary report. Proc. Amer. Ass. Clin. Oncol. 15, 173 (1974).

44. COHEN, S.M., GREENSPAN, E.M., WEINER, M.J., KARAKOW, B.: Triple combination chemotherapy of disseminated melanoma. Cancer 29, 1489 (1972).

45. LUCE, J.K., TORIN, L.B., PRICE, H.: Combination dimethyl triazeno imidazole carboxamide (NSC-45388; DIC), vincristine (NSC-67574 : VCR) and 1,3-bis(2-chloroethyl)-1-nitrosourea (NSC-409962; BCNU) chemotherapy of disseminated malignant melanoma. Proc. Amer. Ass. Cancer Res. 11, 50 (1970).

46. CARTER, S.K.: An overview of the status of the nitrosoureas in other tumors. Cancer Chemother. Rep. 3, 4, 35 (1973).

47. WAGENKNECHT, L.: Chimiothérapie systémique du mélanome malin. Méd. et Hyg. (Genève), 30, 1615 (1972).

48. GARDERE, S., HUSSAIN, S., COWAN, D.H.: Treatment of metastatic malignant melanoma with a combination of 5-(3,3-dimethyl-1-triazeno) imidazole-4-carboxamide (NSC-45388), cyclophosphamide (NSC-26271), and vincristine (NSC-67574). Cancer Chemother. Rep. 56, 357 (1972).

49. PRIMACK, A., DHRU, D., KIRYABWIRE, J.W.M., VOGEL, C.L.: Clinical trials of combination chemotherapy with BCNU and vincristine in the treatment of malignant melanoma in Uganda. Cancer 31, 337 (1973).

50. KNUTSON, C.O., HORI, J.M., SPRATT, Jr., J.S.: Melanoma. Curr. Probl. Surg. Dec. 1971.

51. STEHLIN, J.r, J.S., CLARK, R.L., SMITH, J.L., WHITE, E.C.: Malig-nant melanoma of the extremities: experiences with conventional therapy; a new surgical and chemotherapeutic approach with regional perfusion. Cancer 13, 55 (1960).

52. LEBRUN, J., SMETS, E.: Perfusion régionale par circulation extra-corporelle. Premiers résultats. Acta Un. int. Cancr. 20, 459 (1964).

53. CREECH, Jr., O., KREMENTZ, E.: Regional perfusion for melanoma and sarcoma of the limbs. In: New Trends in the Treatment of Cancer. (eds. L. Manuila, S. Moles, P. Rentchnick). Recent Results in Can-cer Research, Vol. 8, p. 154. Berlin: Springer-Verlag 1967.

54. OBERFIELD, R.A., SULLIVAN, R.D.: Prolonged and continuous regional arterial infusion chemotherapy in patients with melanoma. J. Amer. med. Ass. 209, 75 (1969).

55. GOLOMB, F.M.: Perfusion of melanoma. Oncology 26, 197 (1972).

56. EINHORN, L.H., McBRIDE, C.M., LUCE, J.K., CAOILI, E., GOTTLIEB, J.A.: Intra-arterial infusion therapy with 5-(3,3-dimethyl-1-tria-zeno)imidazole-4-carboxamide (NSC 45388) for malignant melanoma. Cancer 32, 749 (1973).

57. STEHLIN, Jr., J.S., CLARK, R.L.: Melanoma of the extremities. Amer. J. Surg. 110, 366 (1965).

58. KREMENTZ, E.T., RYAN, R.F.: Chemotherapy of melanoma of the extremi-ties by perfusion: fourteen years clinical experience. Ann. Surg. 175, 900 (1972).

59. PATTERSON, W.B.: Contributions of surgeons to clinical cancer chemotherapy. Oncology 26, 277 (1972).

60. MOORE, G.E., GERNER, R.E.: Malignant melanoma. Surg. Gynec. and Obstet. 132, 428 (1971).

61. CONRAD, F.G.: Treatment of malignant melanoma. Arch. Surg. 104, 587 (1972).

62. DAVIS, N.C. et al.: Elective lymph node dissection for melanoma. Brit. J. Surg. 58, 830 (1971).

63. BLUMING, A.Z., VOGEL, C.L., ZIEGLER, J.L., MODY, N., KAMYA, G.: Immunological effects of BCG in malignant melanoma: two modes of administration compared. Ann. intern. Med. 76, 405 (1972).
64. MATHE, G.: Active immunotherapy. Advanc. Cancer Res. 14, 1 (1971).
65. McCARTHY, W.H., COTTON, G., CARLON, A., MILTON, G.W., KOSSARD, S.: Immunotherapy of malignant melanoma. A clinical trial. Cancer 32, 97 (1973).
66. HUNTER-CRAIG, I., NEWTON, K.A., WESTBURY, G., LACEY, B.W.: Use of Vaccinia virus in the treatment of metastatic malignant melanoma. Brit. med. J. 2, 512 (1970).
67. NADLER, S.H., MOORE, G.E.: Immunotherapy of malignant disease. Arch. Surg. 99, 376 (1969).
68. NATHANSON, L.: Regression of intradermal malignant melanoma after intralesional injection of mycobacterium bovis strain BCG. Cancer Chemother. Rep. 56, 659 (1972).
69. MORTON, D.L.: Immunotherapy of cancer. Present status and future potential. Cancer 30, 1647 (1972).
70. THOMPSON, R.B., MATHE, G.: Adoptive immunotherapy in malignant disease. Transpl. Rev. 9, 54 (1972).
71. OETTGEN, H.F., OLD, L.J., BOYSE, E.A.: Human tumor immunology. Med. clin. N. Amer. 55, 761 (1971).
72. GUTTERMAN, J.U., MAVLIGIT, G., McBRIDE, C., FREI, E. III, FREIREICH, E.J., HERSH, E.M.: Active immunotherapy with BCG for recurrent malignant melanoma. Lancet 1, 1208 (1973).
73. COMIS, R.L., CARTER, S.K.: Integration of chemotherapy into combined modality therapy of solid tumors. IV. Malignant melanoma. Cancer Treat. Rev. 1, 285 (1974).
74. WASSERMAN, T.H., SLAVIK, M., CARTER, S.K.: Review of CCNU in clinical cancer therapy. Cancer Treat. Rev. 1, 131 (1974).
75. WASSERMAN, T.H., SLAVIK, M., CARTER, S.K.: Methyl-CCNU in clinical cancer therapy. Cancer Treat. Rev. 1, 251 (1974).
76. EINHORN, L.H., BURGESS, M.A., VALLEJOS, C., BODEY, G.P., GUTTERMAN, J. et al.: Prognostic correlation and response to treatment in advanced metastatic malignant melanoma. Cancer Res. 34, 1995 (1974).
77. AHMANN, D.L., HAHN, R.G., BISEL, H.F.: Evaluation of 1-(2-chloroethyl-3-4methylcyclohexyl)-1-nitrosourea (methyl-CCNU) versus combined modality therapy of solid tumors. IV. Malignant melanoma. seminated malignant melanoma. Cancer 33, 615 (1974).
78. MORTON, D.L., EILBER, F.R., HOLMES, E.C., HUNT, J.S., KETCHAM, A.S., et al.: BCG immuno-therapy of malignant melanoma: summary of a seven-year experience. Ann. Surg. 180, 635 (1974).
79. GUTTERMAN, J.U., MAVLIGIT, G., GOTTLIEB, J.A., BURGESS, M.A., McBRIDE, C.E., et al.: Chemoimmunotherapy of disseminated malignant melanoma with DTIC and BCG. New Engl. J. Med. 291, 592 (1974).
80. AHMANN, D.L., HAHN, R.G., BISEL, H.F., EAGAN, R.T., EDMONSON, J.H.: Comparative trial of methyl-CCNU with cyclophosphamide and 5-(3,3-dimethyl-1-triazeno)imidazole-4-carboxamide with vincristine in patients with disseminated malignant melanoma. Cancer Chemother. Rep. Part 1, Vol. 59, 451 (1975).
81. MOON, J.H., GAILANI, S., COOPER, M.R., HAYES, D.M., REGE, V.B. et al.: Comparison of the combination of 1,3-bis(2-chloroethyl)-1-nitrosourea (BCNU) and vincristine with two dose schedules of 5-(3,3-dimethyl-1-triazeno)imidazole-4-carboxamide (DTIC) in the treatment of disseminated malignant melanoma. Cancer 35, 368 (1975).
82. PUGH, R.P., JACOBS, E.M., BATEMAN, J.R., BULL, F.E., SOLOMON, J.: CCNU versus CCNU plus vincristine in disseminated melanoma. Proc. Am. Soc. Clin. Oncol. 16, 246 (1975).
83. CARTER, R.D., KREMENTZ, E.T., HILL, G.J., METTER, G.E., FLETCHER, W.S. et al.: DTIC (NSC-45388) and combination therapy for melanoma. I. Studies with DTIC, BCNU (NSC-409962), CCNU (NSC-79037), vincristine (NSC-67574), and hydroxyurea (NSC-32065). Cancer Treat. Rep. 60, 601 (1976).

84. COSTANZI, J.J., VAITKEVICIUS, V.K., QUAGLIANA, J.M., HOOGSTRATEN, B., COLTMAN, C.A., DELANEY, F.C.: Combination chemotherapy for disseminated malignant melanoma. Cancer 35, 342 (1975).

85. PERLIN, E., ENGELER, J., REID, J.W., LOKEY, J.L., KOSTINAS, J.: Treatment of malignant melanoma with vinblastine (NSC-49842), procarbazine (NSC-77213), and Actinomycin D (NSC-3053). Cancer Chemotherapy Rep. Part 1, 59, 767 (1975).

86. NATHANSON, L., HALL, T.C., SCHILLING, A., MILLER, S.: Concurrent combination chemotherapy of human solid tumors; Experience with a three-drug regimen and review of the literature. Cancer Res. 29, 419 (1969).

87. EILBER, F.R., MORTON, D.L., HOLMES, E.C., SPARKS, F.C., RAMMING, K.P.: Immunotherapy with BCG for lymph-node metastases from malignant lymphoma. New Engl. J. Med. 294, 237 (1976).

88. CLARK, W.H., AINSWORTH, A.M., BERNADINO, E.A., CHANG-HSU YANG, MIHM, M.C., REED, R.J.: The developmental biology or primary human malignant melanomas. Semin. Oncol. 2, 83 (1975).

89. GOLDMAN, L.I.: The surgical therapy of malignant melanomas. Semin. Oncol. 2, 175 (1975).

90. GUTTERMAN, J.U., MAVLIGIT, G., REED, R., RICHMAN, S., McBRIDE, C.E., Hersh, E.M.: Immunology and immunotherapy of human malignant melanoma: historic review and perspectives for the future. Sem. Oncol. 2, 155 (1975).

91. GUTTERMAN, J.U., MAVLIGIT, G.M., REED, R., BURGESS, M.A., GOTTLIEB, J., HERSH, E.M.: Bacillus Calmette-Guérin immunotherapy in combination with DTIC (NSC-45388) for the treatment of malignant melanoma. Cancer Treat. Rep. 60, 177 (1976).

92. DeVITA, V.T., FISHER, R.I.: Natural history of malignant melanoma as related to therapy. Cancer Treat. Rep. 60, 153 (1976).

93. COMIS, R.L.: DITC (NSC-45388) in malignant melanoma: a perspective. Cancer Treat. Rep. 60, 165 (1976).

94. COSTANZA, M.E., NATHANSON, L., COSTELLO, W.G., WOLTER, J., BRUNK, F. et al.: Results of a randomized study comparing DTIC with TIC mustard in malignant melanoma. Cancer 37, 1654 (1976).

95. BELLET, R.E., MASTRANGELO, M.J., LAUCIUS, J.F., BODURTHA, A.J.: Randomized prospective trial of DTIC (NSC-45388) alone versus BCNU (NSC-409962) plus vincristine (NSC-67574) in the treatment of metastatic malignant melanoma. Cancer Treat. Rep. 60, 595 (1976).

96. ROSENBERG, S.A.: Surgical treatment of malignant melanoma. Cancer Treat. Rep. 60, 159 (1976).

97. MORTON, D.L., EILBER, F.R., HOLMES, E.C., SPARKUS, F.C., RAMMING, K.P.: Present status of BCG immunotherapy of malignant melanoma. Cancer Immunol. Immunother. 1, 93 (1976).

Chapter 23
Head and Neck Cancer

"Cancer of the head and neck" (H and N) is a misnomer since tumors of
the brain, orbit, and thyroid are by tradition not discussed under this
heading. In fact it covers a heterogeneous group of squamous carcinomas
arising from the nasal fossa, paranasal sinuses, oral cavity (lip,
tongue, buccal mucosa, gums, floor of the mouth, palate) nasopharynx,
oropharynx, hypopharynx, and larynx. A more precise name for these tumors would be "cancer of the upper respiratory and alimentary passages."
They have in common a propensity to spread locally into the surrounding
tissues and into the regional lymph nodes. Local extension often causes
death before metastases in vital organs. Distant metastases, if they
occur, are a late manifestation.

Only squamous-cell carcinomas, which constitute the vast majority of
tumors in this area, are dealt with in this Chapter. Tumors can also
arise, however, from glandular epithelium, melanoblasts, the odonto-
genic apparatus, lymphoid tissue, soft tissue, and bone or cartilage
(1).

Head and neck cancer incidence is related to tobacco and alcohol consumption (2, 3), which clearly explains the male preponderance. The
incidence of second primary tumors is high among patients who continue
to smoke (4-6).

The prognosis and the response to therapy depend especially on the
anatomic site and the clinical stage (extent). A shift of a few centi-
meters in the upper respiratory passage can alter the prognosis sharply.
Mobility of tissues and proximity of lymphatics influence the pattern
and timing of tumor spread. In general, tumors of the oral cavity tend
to be less aggressive than tumors of the oropharynx, hypopharynx, and
nasopharynx, with respect to both the degree of anaplasia and spread
to regional lymph nodes. The anatomic site is not only a major factor
to be considered in selection of the primary modality for local therapy,
but may also affect the response to chemotherapy (7, 8). For example,
the response rate to bleomycin ranges from 72% for squamous-cell carcinoma of the mouth to 12% for the tongue, with 30% for the nasopharynx,
tonsils, sinuses, and other sites (8).

The degree of tumor differentiation is also important: well-differentiated squamous-cell carcinoma of the head and neck seems to regress
much more frequently with bleomycin therapy than do tumors in which
differentiation is not pronounced (9). It thus seems useful to evaluate
the results of chemotherapeutic trials in terms of anatomic sites and
histologic grade.

The extent of the disease is best described by the UICC-TNM classification, which is becoming increasingly widely accepted especially for
oral cavity cancer, because of the accessibility of both the primary
growth and the lymph nodes (10, 11).

The 5-year survival rate of patients presenting with lymph-node involvement is poor.

A. CHEMOTHERAPY

1. Single-Agent Chemotherapy

While a number of cytotoxic agents have been employed against head and neck cancer, only a few, that is MTX, bleomycin, (BLM), 5-FU, and hydroxyurea (HUR), have been evaluated in large series (35, 78, 81). The last two drugs are often used concomitantly with radiotherapy (see below). Methotrexate appears to be the most effective drug for single-agent therapy, with an overall response rate of 43.5% lasting 1 to 5 months (Table 23-1). The relative value of the data listed in tables of this nature must be stressed; they are compiled from a number of studies in which patient selection, dosage schedules, and criteria of response are not necessarily comparable. Methotrexate has been employed in a variety of schedules: low dose daily; single large doses, given at intervals of 4, 7, or 14 days (27), or 5-10 day courses repeated at intervals of one month (28-32). Finally, in an attempt to improve the therapeutic index of MTX, folinic acid (FA) has been administered following large doses of MTX given by infusion over 24-48 hours (33-35). This can be repeated after adequate bone-marrow recovery. Comparison of the results

Table 23-1. Effectiveness of single agents in head and neck cancers

Drug	Number of patients	Overall response (%)	Reference
Methotrexate	232	43.5	LIVINGSTON and CARTER (12)
6-Mercaptopurine	45	13	-
5-Fluorouracil	118	15	-
Cytosine arabinoside	20	20	PAPAC and FISCHER (13)
Hydroxyurea	18	39	LIVINGSTON and CARTER (12)
BCNU	25	16	CARTER (14)
CCNU	50	8	WASSERMAN et al. (70)
MeCCNU	53	11	WASSERMAN et al. (71)
Procarbazine	31	10	KENIS et al. (16)
Nitrogen mustard	66	7.5	LIVINGSTON and CARTER (12)
Chlorambucil	34	15	MOORE et al. (17)
Cyclophosphamide	77	36	LIVINGSTON and CARTER (12)
Hexamethylmelamine	75	12	BLUM et al. (18)
Mitomycin C	23	17	KENIS and STRYCKMANS (19)
Actinomycin D	11	0	LIVINGSTON and CARTER (12)
Adriamycin	34	23	BLUM and CARTER (72)
Bleomycin	576	58	BLUM et al. (8)
Vinblastine	35	29	SMART et al. (21)
Porfiromycin	26	15	IZBICHI et al. (22)

Table 23-2. Effectiveness of methotrexate in head and neck cancers

Dose schedule	Number of patients	Number of regressions	References
Monthly courses			
25 mg/d x 4-5, p.o.	8	3	HUSEBY and DOWNING (1962) (28)
15 mg/d x 5, p.o.	24	4	PAPAC et al. (1963) (29)
25 mg/d x 5, i.v.	23	4	PAPAC et al. (1963) (29)
0.2 mg/kg/d x 5, i.v.	10	2	HELLMAN et al. (1964) (30)
idem	11	5	KLIGERMAN et al. (1966) (38)
5 mg/d x 5-10	13	7	ANDREWS and WILSON (1967) (31)
0.2 mg/kg/d x 4			
0.1 mg/kg every 2 days	11	3	SULLIVAN et al. (1967) (32)
Total	100	28 (28%)	
Weekly or twice-weekly dosage			
0.8 mg/kg every 4 days, i.v.	15	9	PAPAC et al. (1967) (23)
20-50 mg every 4-5 days, i.v.	27	14	LANE et al. (1968) (24)
60 mg/m^2/week i.v.	35	20	LEONE et al. (1968) (25)
2 mg/kg, 24 h[a] infusion	19	9	MITCHELL et al. (1968) (33)
240 mg/m^2, 24 h[a] infusion	21	13	CAPIZZI et al. (1970) (34)
Different intermittent schedules	15	5	KENIS et al. (1970) (39)
Total	132	70 (53%)	

[a] followed by folinic acid.

of the monthly courses with those obtained with weekly or biweekly schedules suggest that the latter are superior (Table 23-2).

European and Japanese investigators have reported better response rates for bleomycin than have been found in American studies. BLUM et al. recorded a 58% overall response rate for 576 cases reported in the literature (8). Analysis of the tumors studied in American trials by site also reveals a wide variation in tumor regression (Table 23-3) (8). Although the response rate for BLM is comparable to that for intermittent MTX, the degree and duration of response appear somewhat better with MTX. Furthermore, BLM is not suitable for maintenance therapy because of the risk of pulmonary toxicity at total doses above 200-300 mg/m^2 body surface.

Table 23-3. Effect of bleomycin, classified by anatomic site of head and neck cancers. (From BLUM et al. (8))

	Number of patients entered	Number of patients evaluable	Response rate	Mean duration (months)
Mouth	21	18	72%	1.6
Tongue	34	26	12%	2
Nasopharynx	22	19	32%	4
Tonsils	25	20	30%	2
Sinuses	11	10	30%	2.7
Larynx	46	37	24%	1.8
Other sites	31	28	32%	-
	190	158	31%	2

Cyclophosphamide and hydroxyurea yield tumor regressions in approximately one-third of patients (Table 23-1). More data are required for the nitrosoureas (70, 71) and adriamycin (20, 72, 73). No significant remissions were recorded with either cytosine arabinoside or imidazole carboxamide (73).

2. Combinations

Combination chemotherapy has not been tried in large enough numbers of patients to permit any conclusions (Table 23-4). The availability of several effective single agents with different mechanisms of action and toxicity should make it possible to design effective combinations. One logical attempt at sequential MTX-BLM therapy was discontinued because of toxicity (35, 36). Severe mucosal and marrow effects resulted from the sequential use of doses of the two agents though the same doses of each agent alone are usually well tolerated. At the I.C.I.G., we are investigating a synchronization protocol with VCR, MTX-FA, and BLM (see Chap. 7, p. 148).

PRIESTMAN (26) was unimpressed with a 4-drug combination (CPM, MTX, VCR, 5-FU) (3/27 RR) which yielded eight regressions in ten patients in HANHAM's experience (37).

3. Intra-Arterial Chemotherapy

Most investigators interested in intra-arterial chemotherapy have applied this technique to head and neck cancers at some time (47-52) (see Chap. 11).

Table 23-5 lists results with intra-arterial therapy compiled by BER-TINO (35). LIVINGSTON et al., reviewing the value of MTX in head and neck cancers, concluded that intra-arterial MTX yields no better results than MTX by the systemic route (12). Overall response rates are higher for intra-arterial than for systemic 5-FU (cf. Table 23-1 and Table 23-5). Experience with intra-arterial bleomycin is unsufficient to permit comparison with systemic BLM (35, 51, 53).

Table 23-4. Response rates to combination chemotherapy in head and neck cancers

Combinations	Number evaluable	Number with ≥ 50% re- gression	Reference
MTX, BLM	4	2	MOSHER et al. (36)
	15	8	YAGODA et al. (74)
MTX, VCR	28	15 (53%)	NERVI et al. (40)
DBD, BLM	20	5 (25%)	OHNUMA et al. (9)
ADM, BLM	8	4	CORTES et al. (41)
ADM, CCNU	4	3	EINHORN et al. (75)
MeCCNU, CPM, BLM, VCR (COMB)	32	11 (35%)	LIVINGSTON et al. (44)
MTX, 5-FU, CPM, VCR (modified COMF)	10	8	HANHAM et al. (37)
	27	3 (11%)	PRIESTMAN (26)
MTX, 5-FU, CPM, VCR, PDN (Cooper's regimen)	18	4 (22%)	RAMIREZ (43)
CCNU, HN-2, ADM, BLM, VCR (BACON)	13	7	LIVINGSTON et al. (46)
MTX, 6-MP, PCZ, CLB, thioTEPA, STN, RFC, VLB	82	45 (55%)	JACQUILLAT et al. (45)

Table 23-5. Responses to intra-arterial chemotherapy in head and neck cancer (From BERTINO (35))

Drug	Number evaluated	Tumor regression > 50%	Overall response rate
Methotrexate	806	356	44%
5-Fluorouracil	28	21	75%
Nitrogen mustard	20	10	50%
Cyclophosphamide	100	28	28%
Bleomycin	24	6	25%
Vinblastine	24	6	25%

Most experts think that intra-arterial chemotherapy plays only a modest role in the treatment of head and neck cancers. Although tumor regressions are frequently noted, they are rarely sustained, and overall survival is not improved. Most importantly, the (theoretical) benefits of the method do not outweigh the concomitant risk of morbidity (up to 80%) (54) and mortality (51, 55). General results are not remarkably different from those obtained with systemic chemotherapy, which is safer (56). It remains for the time being an experimental tool that has still to be perfected.

B. STRATEGY

1. Localized Head and Neck Cancer

(i) Surgery and Radiotherapy
Surgery and radiotherapy are the primary modalities for treatment intended to cure H and N cancers. Therapy should be directed against the primary and its lymphatic drainage. In no area in oncology is there more need for individual decisions and a multidisciplinary approach (57). Many H and N tumors can be treated equally well by either surgery or radiotherapy. For others, a combination of the two is indicated (58, 59, 76, 79, 80). The selection of therapy depends mainly on the anatomic location and the extent of the disease. Cosmetic results and the preservation of essential functions (clear upper airway, swallowing, speech) must also be considered.

(ii) Chemotherapy - Radiotherapy with or without Surgery
A number of investigators have used chemotherapy immediately before or in conjunction with radiotherapy in H and N cancer in a attempt to improve the results over those achieved with radiotherapy alone. Such an initial approach can be followed in selected advanced cases by a definitive surgical procedure (60, 61). This approach is based on the following rationale: (1) the drug itself has a cytotoxic effect, (2) drug-induced reduction in tumor volume increases the effectiveness of radiotherapy (reduced cell number, improved oxygenation), (3) the drug may have a radiosensitizing effect (62). VERMUND et al. have reviewed the mechanisms of the last phenomenon (63). HN2 (64) MTX (65, 66) 5-FU (7), and HUR (60-62) are the drugs that have most often been used in combination with radiotherapy, administered either systematically (7, 60, 61, 63, 65, 66) or by intra-arterial injection (67, 68, 77). More references are given in BERTINO's (35, 78) and GOLDSMITH's (81) review articles.

Most investigators (but not all) have the impression that the combined approach improves the quality of response to radiotherapy (62), and some report improved survival while others have failed to observe such an effect (67). Unfortunately, the majority of these studies are uncontrolled, so that no definite conclusions can be drawn. ANSFIELD noted in a randomized controlled trial that the median survival was significantly increased by combined 5-FU and radiotherapy in patients with advanced tonsil and intra-oral cancer, but not in patients with more posterior lesions (7). Additional controlled studies, with evaluation of results according to stage an anatomic sites, may help to select patient categories likely to benefit from this approach. LIPSHUTZ's work indicates that a combined approach using chemotherapy, radiotherapy, and surgery is feasible in advanced H and N cancer, and may result in prolonged disease-free survival (60).

(iii) Adjuvant Chemotherapy and Immunotherapy
To our knowledge, there are no studies on chemotherapy or immunotherapy as an adjuvant to "curative" surgery and/or radiotherapy.

2. Advanced Head and Neck Cancer

Chemotherapy is the only course left when the disease is no longer
amenable to further local measures or after dissemination has occured.
Several authors are investigating combined chemo-immunotherapy (BCG +
INH) in advanced disease (18, 69).

REFERENCES

1. TOTTEN, R.S.: Tumors of the oral cavity, pharynx and larynx. J.
   Amer. med. Ass. 215, 454 (1971).
2. WYNDER, E.L.: Etiological aspects of squamous cancers of the head
   and neck. J. Amer. med. Ass. 215, 452 (1971).
3. KISSIN, B., KALEY, M.M., SU, W.H., LERNER, R.: Head and neck cancer
   in alcoholics. J. Amer. med. Ass. 224, 1174 (1973).
4. WYNDER, E.L., DODO, H., BLOCH, D.A., GANTT, R.C., MOORE, O.S.: Epidemiologic investigation of multiple primary cancer of the upper
   alimentary and respiratory tracts. Cancer 24, 730 (1969).
5. FARR, H.W., ARTHUR, K.: Epidermoid carcinoma of the mouth and pharynx, 1960-1964. Clin. Bull. 1, 130 (1971).
6. MOORE, C.: Cigarette smoking and cancer of the mouth, pharynx and
   larynx. A continuing study. J. Amer. med. Ass. 218, 553 (1971).
7. ANSFIELD, F.J., RAMIREZ, G., DAVIS, H.L., KORBITZ, B.C., VERMUND,
   H., GOLLIN, F.F.: Treatment of advanced cancer of the head and
   neck. Cancer 25, 78 (1970).
8. BLUM, R.H., CARTER, S.K., AGRE, K.: A clinical review of bleomycin -
   a new antineoplastic agent. Cancer 31, 903 (1973).
9. OHNUMA, T., HOLLAND, J.F., SAKO, K., SHEDD, D.P.: Effects of combination therapy with bleomycin (NSC-125066) and dibromodulcitol
   (NSC-104800) on squamous cell carcinoma in man. Cancer Chemother.
   Rep. 56, 625 (1972).
10. UICC: T.N.M. classification of malignant tumours. Geneva: G. de
    Buren 1968.
11. UICC Committee on Professional Education: Clinical Oncology. A
    manual for students and doctors. Berlin-Heidelberg-New York:
    Springer 1973.
12. LIVINGSTON, R.B., CARTER, S.K.: Single agents in cancer chemother-
    apy. New York: IFI/Plenum 1970.
13. PAPAC, R.J., FISCHER, J.J.: Cytosine arabinoside in the treatment
    of epidermoid carcinomas of the head and neck. Cancer Chemother. Rep.
    55, 193 (1971).
14. CARTER, S.K.: An overview of the status of the nitrosoureas in other
    tumors. Cancer Chemother. Rep. 3: 4, 35 (1973).
15. HOOGSTRATEN, B., GOTTLIEB, J.A., CAOILI, E., TUCKER, W.G., TALLEY,
    R.W., HAUT, A.: CCNU (1-(2-chloroethyl)-3-cyclohexyl-1-nitrosourea,
    NSC-79037) in the treatment of cancer. Phase II study. Cancer 32,
    38 (1973).
16. KENIS, Y., De SMEDT, J., TAGNON, H.: Action du Natulan dans 94
    cas de tumeurs solides. Europ. J. Cancer 2, 51 (1966).
17. MOORE, G.E., BROSS, I.D.J., AUSMAN, R., NADLER, S., JONES, Jr., R.,
    SLACK, N., RIMM, A.A.: Effects of chlorambucil (NSC-3088) in 374
    patients with advanced cancer. Eastern clinical drug evaluation
    program. Cancer Chemother. Rep. 52, 661 (1968).
18. RICHMAN, S.P., LIVINGSTON, R.B., GUTTERMAN, J.U., SUEN, J.Y., HERSH,
    E.M.: Chemotherapy versus chemoimmunotherapy of head and neck can-
    cer: report of a randomized study. Cancer Treat. Rep. 60, 535 (1976).
19. KENIS, Y., STRYCKMANS, P.: Action de la mitomycine C dans 65 cas
    de tumeurs malignes. Comparaison de l'effet de doses faibles,
    répétées et de doses "massives". Chemotherapia 8, 114 (1964).

20. O'BRYAN, R.M., LUCE, J.K., TALLEY, R.W., GOTTLIEB, J.A., BAKER, L. H., BONADONNA, G.: Phase II evaluation of adriamycin in human neoplasia. Cancer 32, 1 (1973).

21. SMART, C., ROCHLIN, D., NAHUM, A.: Clinical experience with vinblastine sulfate in squamous cell carcinoma and other malignancies. Cancer Chemother. Rep. 34, 31 (1964).

22. IZBICKI, R., AL-SARRAF, M., REED, M.L., VAUGHN, C.B., VAITKEVICIUS, V.K.: Further clinical trials with porfiromycin (NSC-56410) (large intermittent doses). Cancer Chemother. Rep. 56, 615 (1972).

23. PAPAC, R., LEFKOWITZ, E., BERTINO, J.R.: Methotrexate (NSC-740) in squamous cell carcinoma of the head and neck. II. Intermittent intravenous therapy. Cancer Chemother. Rep. 51, 69 (1967).

24. LANE, M., MOORE, J.E. III, LEVIN, H., SMITH, F.E.: Methotrexate therapy for squamous cell carcinoma of the head and neck. J. Amer. med. Ass. 204, 561 (1968).

25. LEONE, L.A., ALBALA, M.M., REGE, V.B.: Treatment of carcinomas of the head and neck with intravenous methotrexate. Cancer 21, 828 (1968).

26. PRIESTMAN, T.J.: Results in fifty cases of advanced squamous cell carcinoma of the head and neck treated by intravenous chemotherapy. Brit. J. Cancer 27, 400 (1973).

27. CONDIT, P.T.: Chemotherapy of squamous cell carcinoma of the upper air passages. In: Oncology 1970, Vol. 4, p. 32. (eds. R.L. Clark, R.W. Cumley, J.E. McKay) Chicago: Year Book Medical Publishers 1971.

28. HUSEBY, R.A., DOWNING, V.: The use of methotrexate orally in treatment of squamous cancers of the head and neck. Cancer Chemother. Rep. 16, 611 (1962).

29. PAPAC, R.J., JACOBS, E.M., FOYE, Jr., L.V., DONOHUE, D.M.: Systemic therapy with amethopterin in squamous carcinoma of the head and neck. Cancer Chemother. Rep. 32, 47 (1963).

30. HELLMAN, S., IANOTTI, A., BERTINO, J.: Determinations of the levels of serum folate in patients with carcinoma of the head and neck treated with methotrexate. Cancer Res. 24, 105 (1964).

31. ANDEWS, N., WILSON, W.: Phase II study of methotrexate in solid tumors. Cancer Chemother. Rep. 51, 471 (1967).

32. SULLIVAN, R., MILLER, E., ZUREK, W., OBERFIELD, R., OJIMA, Y.: Re-evaluation of methotrexate as an anticancer drug. Surg. Gynec. Obstet. 125, 819 (1967).

33. MITCHELL, M.S., WAWRO, N.W., DECONTI, R.C., KAPLAN, S.R., PAPAC, R., BERTINO, J.R.: Effectiveness of high-dose infusions of methotrexate followed by leucovorin in carcinoma of the head and neck. Cancer Res. 28, 1088 (1968).

34. CAPIZZI, R.L., DECONTI, R.C., MARSH, J.C., BERTINO, J.R.: Methotrexate therapy of head and neck cancer: improvement in therapeutic index by the use of leucovorin "rescue". Cancer Res. 30, 1782 (1970).

35. BERTINO, J.R., MOSHER, M.B., DECONTI, R.C.: Chemotherapy of cancer of the head and neck. Cancer 31, 1141 (1973).

36. MOSHER, M.B., DECONTI, R.C., BERTINO, J.R.: Bleomycin therapy in advanced Hodgkin's disease and epidermoid cancers. Cancer 30, 56 (1972).

37. HANHAM, I.W.F., NEWTON, K.A., WESTBURY, G.: Seventy-five cases of solid tumours treated by a modified quadruple chemotherapy regime. Brit. J. Cancer 25, 462 (1971).

38. KLIGERMAN, M., HELLMAN, M., VON ESSEN, C., BERTINO, J.: Sequential chemotherapy and radiotherapy. Preliminary results of clinical trial with methotrexate in head and neck cancer. Radiology 86, 247 (1966).

39. KENIS, Y., MICHEL, J., DEBUSSCHER, L., LACHAPELLE, F.: Action pharmacologique et thérapeutique de l'administration intermittente de méthotrexate dans les tumeurs solides. Corso Superiore sulla Chemoterapia dei Tumori, Milan., March 1970.

40. NERVI, C., PERRINO, A., VALENTE, V., CORTESE, M.: Chemioterapia intraateriosa prolungata con associazione di antimitotici e radioterapia nei tumori inoperabili del distretto orocervico facciale. Tumori 54, 199 (1968).
41. CORTES, E.P., SHEDD, D., ALBERT, D.J., OHNUMA, T., HRESHCHYSHYN, M.: Adriamycin and bleomycin in advanced cancer. Proc. Amer. Ass. Cancer Res. 13, 86 (1972).
42. OHNUMA, T., HOLLAND, J.F., SAKO, K., SHEDD, D.P.: Effects of combination therapy with bleomycin (NSC-125066) and dibromodulcitol (NSC-104800) on squamous cell carcinoma in man. Cancer Chemother. Rep. 56, 625 (1972).
43. RAMIREZ, G. (Clinical Oncology Group): Five-drug combination therapy in the treatment of solid tumors. Proc. Amer. Ass. Cancer Res. 14, 17 (1973).
44. LIVINGSTON, R.B., EINHORN, L.H., BODEY, G.P., BURGESS, M.A., FREIREICH, E.J., GOTTLIEB, J.A.: COMB (cyclophosphamide, oncovin, methyl-CCNU, and bleomycin): a four drug combination in solid tumors. Cancer 36, 327 (1975).
45. JACQUILLAT, C., SZIRGLAS, H., WEIL, M., et al.: Polychimiotherapie des cancers. Press Méd. 75, 321 (1967).
46. LIVINGSTON, R.B., BURGESS, M.A., GOTTLIEB, J.A., BODEY, Jr., G.P., RODRIGUEZ, V.: Bleomycin, adriamycin, CCNU, oncovin and nitrogen mustard (BACON) in squamous cancer. Proc. Amer. Ass. clin. Oncol. 15, 173 (1974).
47. SULLIVAN, R.D., MILLER, E., SYKES, M.P.: Antimetabolite-metabolite combination cancer chemotherapy. Effects of intra-arterial methotrexate - intramuscular citrovorum factor therapy in human cancer. Cancer 12, 1248 (1959).
48. LAWRENCE, Jr., W.: Current status of regional chemotherapy. N.Y. St. J. Med 63, 2359 (1963).
49. LACHAPELE, A.P., LAGARDE, C., HUGHES, A., CHAUVERGNE, J.: Notre expérience de la chimiothérapie par infusions continues de méthotrexate dans le système carotide externe (56 observations). Bull. Cancer 51, 329 (1964).
50. JEWELL, W.R.: Treatment of squamous cell carcinoma of the head and neck by chemotherapy. Oncology 26, 238 (1972).
51. DONEGAN, W.L., HARRIS, H.S.: Factors influencing the success of arterial infusion chemotherapy for cancer of the head and neck. Amer. J. Surg. 123, 549 (1972).
52. OBERFIELD, R.A., DADY, B., BOOTH, J.C.: Regional arterial chemotherapy for advanced carcinoma of the head and neck. Cancer 32, 82 (1973).
53. E.O.R.T.C., CLINICAL SCREENING CO-OPERATIVE GROUP: Study of the clinical efficiency of bleomycin in human cancer. Brit. med. J. 2, 643 (1970).
54. DUFF, J.K., SULLIVAN, R.D., MILLER, F., ULM, A.H., CLARKSON, B.D., CLIFFORD, P.: Antimetabolite metabolite cancer chemotherapy using continuous intra-arterial methotrexate with intermittent intramuscular citrovorum factor. Cancer 14, 744 (1961).
55. TINDEL, S.: Intra-arterial chemotherapy for recurrent neoplasms. J. Amer. med. Ass. 200, 105 (1967).
56. CREECH, Jr., O.: Intra-arterial chemotherapy for recurrent neoplasms. J. Amer. med. Ass. 200, 175 (1967).
57. RUBIN, P.: Cancer of the head and neck: general aspects. Comment: The undisciplinary vs- the multidisciplinary approach to oncology. J. Amer. med. Ass. 215, 461 (1971).
58. FLETCHER, G.H., JESSE, R.H.: Interaction of surgery and irradiation in head and neck cancers. Current Problems in Radiology 1, 1 (1971).
59. BEATTLE, Jr., E.J.: Therapeutic attitudes: cooperators and competitors. Cancer of the head and neck: general aspects. J. Amer. med. Ass. 215, 459 (1971).

60. LIPSHUTZ, H., LERNER, H.J.: Six-year survival in the combined treatment of far advanced head and neck cancer under a combined therapy program. Amer. J. Surg. 126, 519 (1973).

61. RICHARDS, Jr., G.J., CHAMBERS, R.G.: Hydroxyurea in the treatment of neoplasms of the head and neck. A resurvey. Amer. J. Surg. 126, 513 (1973).

62. RICHARDS, Jr., G.J., CHAMBERS, R.G.: Hydroxyurea: a radiosensitizer in the treatment of neoplasms of the head and neck. Amer. J. Roentgenol. 105, 555 (1969).

63. VERMUND, H., GOLLIN, F.F.: Mechanisms of action of radiotherapy and chemotherapy adjuvants. A review. Cancer 21, 58 (1965).

64. HENRY, J., LEBRUN, J., SOMIN, S., SMETS, W.: Perfusion intraartérielle régionale d'ypérite azotée de cancer étendus de la tête et du cou. Acta chir. belg. 59, 581 (1960).

65. FRIEDMAN, M., DENARVAES, F.N., DALY, J.F.: Treatment of squamous cell carcinoma of the head and neck with combined methotrexate and irradiation. Cancer 26, 711 (1970).

66. HARDINGHAM, M., HULBERT, M.H.E., WALSH-WARING, G.P.: Treatment of advanced carcinoma of the head and neck with a combination of high dose infusions of methotrexate (NSC-740) and radiotherapy: a preliminary report on eleven cases. Cancer Chemother. Rep. 56, 745 (1972).

67. GOLLIN, F.F., JOHNSON, R.O.: Pre-irradiation 5-fluorouracil infusion in advanced head and neck carcinomas. Cancer 27, 768 (1971).

68. LAWTON, R.L., GULESSERIAN, H.P., SHARZER, L.A.: Intra-arterial infusion. A seven-year study. Oncology 26, 259 (1972).

69. DONALDSON, R.C.: Chemoimmunotherapy for cancer of the head and neck. Amer. J. Surg. 126, 507 (1973).

70. WASSERMAN, T.H., SLAVIK, M., CARTER, S.K.: Review of CCNU in clinical cancer therapy. Cancer Treat. Rev. 1, 131 (1974).

71. WASSERMAN, T.H., SLAVIK, M., CARTER, S.K.: Methyl-CCNU in clinical cancer therapy. Cancer Treat. Rev. 1, 251 (1974).

72. BLUM, R.H., CARTER, S.K.: Adriamycin. Ann. intern. Med. 80, 249 (1974).

73. DOWELL, K.E., ARMSTRONG, D.M., AUST, J.B., CRUZ, A.B.: Systemic chemotherapy of advanced head and neck malignancies. Cancer 35, 1116 (1975).

74. YAGODA, A., LIPPMAN, A.J., WINN, R.J., SCHULMAN, P., COHEN, F.B.: Combination chemotherapy with bleomycin and methotrexate in patients with advanced epidermoid carcinomas. Proc. Am. Soc. Clin. Oncol. 16, 247 (1975).

75. EINHORN, L.H., LIVINGSTON, R.B., GOTTLIEB, J.A.: Combination chemotherapy with adriamycin and 1-(2-chloroethyl)-3-cyclohexyl-1-nitrosourea. Cancer Chemother. Rep. 57, 437 (1973).

76. JESSE, R.H., LINDBERG, R.D.: The efficacy of combining radiation therapy with a surgical procedure in patients with cervical metastasis from squamous cancer of the oropharynx and hypopharynx. Cancer 35, 1163 (1975).

77. RICHARD, J.M., SANCHO, H., LEPINTRE, Y., RODARY, J., PIERQUIN, B.: Intra-arterial methotrexate chemotherapy and telecobalt therapy in cancer of the oral cavity and oropharynx. Cancer 34, 491 (1974).

78. BERTINO, J.R., BOSTON, B., CAPIZZI, R.L.: The role of chemotherapy in the management of cancer of the head and neck: a review. Cancer 36, 752 (1975).

79. WANG, C.C.: Radiation therapy for head and neck cancers. Cancer 36, 748 (1975).

80. CACHIN, Y., ESCHWEGE, F.: Combination of radiotherapy and surgery in the treatment of head and neck cancers. Cancer Treat. Rev. 2, 177 (1975).

81. GOLDSMITH, M.A., CARTER, S.K.: The integration of chemotherapy into a combined modality approach to cancer therapy. Cancer Treat. Rev. 2, 137 (1975).

Chapter 24
Lung Cancer

Lung cancer remains the most pressing problem for oncologists and the most frequent cause of cancer deaths. The disease is fatal in 90-95% of diagnosed cases. Fewer than 10% of these survive 5 years. The results with surgery, radiotherapy, and chemotherapy alike are frustrating. Surgery is essentially the only method that can cure lung cancer, but 85% of cases are beyond the scope of surgical resection by the time of diagnosis. Of those undergoing an attempt at "curative" resection, only 25% are still alive after 5 years. These results are all the more regrettable because lung cancer is largely preventable.

Several features influence the prognosis and the selection of therapy. The histologic variant and the extent of the disease are the most important. The WHO histologic classification is generally used (Table 24-1) (1, 2, 100). It is important that results of any type of therapy be broken down according to histologic types. In placebo-treated patients, the median survival is longest for large-cell carcinoma, and progressively shorter for squamous-cell carcinoma, adenocarcinoma, and small-cell carcinoma, in that order, for both limited and extensive disease. Lung cancer must be considered a systemic disease at diagnosis in the majority of cases (3). Disappointed as they are with their results, even surgeons have come to accept this concept.

At present, no one classification is uniformly used to stage the extent of the disease (4-6). A practical clinical classification distinguishes localized operable cases and localized inoperable but radiotreatable ones (cases in which the primary lesion and the central lymphatics can be adequately covered by an irradiation field). The remaining cases, those confined to the chest but too extensive to be treated by either surgery or radiotherapy, and those of disseminated disease rely on chemotherapy. The American Joint Committee for Cancer Staging and End Results Reporting recently proposed a TNM classification for lung cancer (101). Current methods (6-8, 102, 103) for the determination of the extent of the disease are unsatisfactory, as has been demonstrated by autopsy studies of patients dying shortly after an operation expected to be curative. In 35% of these cases tumor was identified either as local spread or as distant metastases within one month of definitive surgery.

Other prognostic features that influence median survival include performance status, 5 kg weight loss, CNS involvement, hepatomegaly (9, 104), immunologic status of the host (10-13), size of tumor (14, 15), and previous therapy.

The survival rate is the most objective criterion available for measurement of response. The measurement of tumor regression on serial chest roentgenograms may be unreliable because of additional changes due to an inflammatory reaction or atelectasis. Different aspects of the lung

Table 24-1. WHO pathologic classification of lung tumors

I.   Epidermoid carcinoma

II.   Small-cell anaplastic carcinoma

    1. Fusiform cell type

    2. Polygonal cell type

    3. Lymphocyte-like ("oat-cell") type

    4. Others

III.   Adenocarcinoma

    1. Bronchogenic
      a. Acinar
      b. Papillary

    2. Bronchioloalveolar

IV.   Large-cell carcinoma

    1. Solid tumors with mucin-like content

    2. Solid tumors without mucin-like content

    3. Giant-cell carcinomas

    4. "Clear"-cell carcinomas

V.-VIII.   Others

---

cancer problem were discussed at the First International Workshop for Therapy of Lung Cancer held at Airline, Virginia, October 1972, and published in March 1973 (105).

A. CHEMOTHERAPY

1. Single-Agent Chemotherapy

A number of cytotoxic agents can induce tumor regressions in lung cancer. These are usually incomplete and of short duration, and occur in at best one-third of all patients (Table 24-2) (16-20, 106). Higher response rates are recorded for small-cell carcinoma, the histologic variant most sensitive to chemotherapy (Table 24-3). At least three agents have response rates over 20% in each of the major cell types. The alkylating agents are the most active drugs. Nitrogen mustard (HN2) is superior to cyclophosphamide (CPM) for epidermoid carcinoma, while CPM is superior in small-cell anaplastic carcinoma (21, 106). High-dose intermittent cyclophosphamide has been the most popular drug in recent years for the treatment of lung cancer (22), and has been proposed as the standard treatment for all types of lung cancer in controlled clinical trials (7). Other alkylating agents have no advantage over nitrogen mustard and cyclophosphamide. Methotrexate (MTX) is the only antimetabolite with any activity, at least when administered in high-dose "pulses" (23-26). 5-FU has not been adequately evaluated in adenocarcinoma, in spite of its activity in this cell type in cancer of the breast and gastrointestinal tract. Procarbazine (19, 27, 28) and hydroxyurea (19, 29) have definite activity. Vinca alkaloids have only

Table 24-2. Effectiveness of single agents in lung cancer (modified from SELAWRY, O.S. (106))

Drug	Number available	Percentage of objective responses	Range of responses
Methotrexate	416	22	3-43
6-Mercaptopurine	105	3	0- 4
Imidazole carboxamide (DIC)	132	11	10-25
5-Fluorouracil	157	7	0-36
5-FUdR	25	12	-
Cytosine arabinoside	19	0	0
Hydroxyurea	88	16	0-26
BCNU	91	11	0-21
CCNU	96	27	18-40
MeCCNU	51	21	17-19
1-Methyl-1-nitrosourea	89	36	22-63
Procarbazine	166	19	6-27
Nitrogen mustard	1266	36	0-68
Chlorambucil	21	5	-
Cyclophosphamide	1260	20	0-63
Melphalan	67	7	3-11
Busulfan	169	9	7-21
Thio-TEPA	141	15	7-32
Hexamethylmelamine	372	20	10-30
Mitomycin C	203	23	8-27
Actinomycin D	16	0	-
Mithramycin	23	0	-
Daunorubicin	14	7	-
Adriamycin	231	21	0-50
Bleomycin	315	13	0-20
Streptonigrin	53	11	0-29
Porfiromycin	42	7	-
Vincristine	43	14	5-33
Vinblastine	239	7	0-20

marginal activity (18, 19). Corticosteroids and hormones were initially studied by the Veterans Administration Lung Cancer Study Group (VALCSG) because the disease occurs mostly in males. Cortisone, in particular, was found to have an adverse effect (30).

Several experimental agents appear promising, especially the nitrosoureas because of their apparent lack of cross-resistance to the bifunctional agents and because of marked enhancement of effect when combined with CPM in certain experimental tumors. Preliminary data indicate

Table 24-3. Lung cancer: response rates to single-agent chemotherapy, analyzed with reference to histology. (From SELAWRY ([19]))

Objective response of epidermoid carcinoma

Drug	Responses (%)	No. of patients treated
CCNU	41	29
Nitrogen mustard	33	111
Methotrexate	25	140
Adriamycin	24	45
Procarbazine	20	30
Cyclophosphamide	19	183
Vinblastine	16	20
1-Methyl-1-nitrosourea	15	13
Hexamethylmelamine	11	99
Bleomycin	9	75
Busulfan	7	61
BCNU	3	33
Colchicine	0	11
6-Mercaptopurine	0	16
Mitomycin C	0	22
Streptonigrin	0	10

Objective response of small-cell carcinoma

Drug	Responses (%)	No. of patients treated
1-Methyl-1-nitrosourea	78	18[a]
Procarbazine	67	12
Cyclophosphamide	50	120
Methotrexate	50	20
Nitrogen mustard	39	51
Hexamethylmelamine	36	67
Adriamycin	29	17
BCNU	20	15
Busulfan	18	17
CCNU	13	15
Bleomycin	0	24

Objective response of adenocarcinoma

Drug	Responses (%)	No. of patients treated
Methotrexate	32	25
Nitrogen mustard	29	80
Mitomycin C	27	11
CCNU	24	21
Hexamethylmelamine	20	34
Procarbazine	19	16
Cyclophosphamide	17	12
Busulfan	4	28
BCNU	0	14

[a] Includes large cell anaplastic carcinoma.

Table 24-3. (continued)

Objective response of large-cell carcinoma

Drug	Responses (%)	Number of patients treated
Procarbazine	35	17
Mechlorethamine	27	129
Cyclophosphamide	23	22
Hexamethylmelamine	17	37
CCNU	15	19
Methotrexate	12	104
BCNU	7	15
6-Mercaptopurine	3	29
Colchicine	0	12

that CCNU is twice as active as BCNU (12, 18, 31-34, 107) but none of
the studies was controlled. MeCCNU is superior to the other nitrosoureas in Lewis lung tumor but seems to be only as active as CCNU in preliminary clinical reports (13, 108). One experimental agent, 1-methyl-
1-nitrosourea, has been reported in two Russian reports (19, 109) to
have shown response rates of 22 percent and 43 percent. Hexamethylmelamine (HMM) will be of interest if it can be established that it
lacks cross-resistance with alkylating agents (18, 35). Mitomycin C
(MTC) (36) and adriamycin (ADM) (37, 38, 110, 111, 126) head the list of
the antibiotics. Bleomycin (BLM), in spite of its reputation as an effective agent against epidermoid carcinomas and its selective concentration in lung tissue, has had disappointing results (19, 39). Imidazole carboxamide (40, 41) and ICRF 159 (42) appear to have some activity.

Some of the newest agents subjected to phase-I evaluation and awaiting
trial in lung cancer are discussed by CARTER (18, 20). Ifosfamide has
been promising in a small number of patients with small-cell carcinoma
quoted by SELAWRY (106). Emetine and dehydroemetine are of potential
interest for combination chemotherapy since they are non-myelosuppres-
sive.

2. Combinations

Single-agent therapy has undoubtedly been disappointing in lung cancer.
Now that a few agents that cause tumor regressions in one-third of patients have become available, it is hoped that effective combinations
will be possible, especially for small-cell carcinoma (44). Most of
the combinations so far tested have been empirical selections not adapted to the characteristics of specific types of lung cancer.

The results obtained with several combinations are listed in Table 23-4.
Unfortunately the patient populations and methods of reporting are not
always comparable. It appears that a response can be obtained in approximately one half of all patients treated. As in the case of single-
agent therapy, these responses are rarely complete; they are of short
duration and their effect on survival is disappointing. No particular
combination is clearly superior to the others. Some of them have the
theoretical advantage of having been rationally designed (46, 49, 54).
At the I.C.I.G., we have used a combination of VCR, 5-FU, and CCNU
(CISG II) (53). The published reports of simultaneous or sequential
use of cytotoxic drugs suggest superiority of combinations over single

Table 23-4. Reponse rates to combinations in lung cancer

Combinations	Number evaluated	Regressions (%)	Remarks	Reference
MTX, CPM	30	31	small-cell carcinoma	SELAWRY et al., 1974 (45), SELAWRY 1974 (106)
	28	6	adenocarcinoma	
5-FU, PCZ	31	6	2/19 squamous-cell carcinoma	ALBERTO, 1973 (46)
	24	62	0/6 small-cell carcinoma	BONADONNA et al., 1973 (47)
CCNU, ADM	33	9	1/1 large cell carcinoma	WOLF and ZELEN, 1975 (112)
			0/5 adenocarcinoma	
CCNU, CPM		35	small-cell carcinoma	EDMONSON and LAGAKOS, 1974 (51)
CCNU, CPM	38	5	0/17 squamous-cell carcinoma	WOLF and ZELEN, 1975 (112)
			1/4 small-cell carcinoma	
			1/8 large-cell carcinoma	
			0/6 adenocarcinoma	
MeCCNU, CPM	12	25		BODEY et al. 1973 (49)
CPM, ADM	36	8	1/15 squamous-cell carcinoma	WOLF and ZELEN 1975 (112)
			2/8 small-cell carcinoma	
			0/4 large-cell carcinoma	
			0/6 adenocarcinoma	
CPM, VCR (following XRT)	41	75	35% CR, oat-cell carcinoma	HOLOYE, et al. 1974 (50)
ACD, VCR	34	60		CHANES, et al. 1971 (48)
BLM, VCR	25	4		BITRAN, et al. (132)
	12	25		BODEY, et al. 1973 (49)

Table 23-4. (continued)

MTX(FA), CPM, VCR	47		median survival 7.5 months	MANNES et al., 1970 (56)
MTX, CCNU, CPM	31	57	small-cell carcinoma	SELAWRY, et al., 1974 (45)
	28	30	adenocarcinoma	
MeCCNU, CPM, VCR	15	27	3/3 adenocarcinoma	REDDY et al., 1974 (52)
			1/7 epidermoid carcinoma	
			0/5 large-cell anaplastic carcinoma	
CPM, ADM, VCR	32	70	small-cell carcinoma 13 CR, 9 PR (plus radiotherapy for limited disease)	HOLOYE et al., 1975 (113)
CPM, ADM, VCR	16	43		MUNDIA et al., 1975 (114)
5-FU, CCNU, VCR	16	56.5		POUILLART et al., 1974 (53)
MTX, HN2, ADM/	13	46	longer duration of remission	BONADONNA et al., 1973 (47)
+ 5-FU, HUR, PCZ	13	46		
MTX, CPM, VCR, PDN	235	15	10 cr, 29 PR	BEARDEN and COLTMAN 1975 (115)
MTX, PCZ, CPM, VCR combined	49	51		ALBERTO, 1973 (46)
sequentially	43	21		
BCNU, PCZ, CPM, VCR	31	58	small-cell carcinoma 3 CR, 15 PR	ABELOFF et al., 1975 (116)
MeCCNU, CPM, BLM, VCR	23	52		LIVINGSTON et al., 1973 (54)
MeCCNU, CPM, BLM, VCR	30	36	3/13 squamous-cell carcinoma	ARMENTROUT et al., 1975 (117)
			6/10 oat-cell carcinoma	
			2/4 large-cell carcinoma	
			0/3 adenocarcinoma	

411

Table 23-4. (continued)

Combinations	Number evaluated	Regres- sions (%)	Remarks	Reference[a]
CCNU, CPM, BLM, VCR	29	20	2/15 squamous-cell carcinoma 3/5 oat-cell carcinoma 0/4 large-cell carcinoma 1/5 adenocarcinoma	ARMENTROUT et al., 1975 (117)
MTX, 5-FU, CPM, VCR, PDN	23	47		RAMIREZ, 1973 (55)
MTX, 5-FU, CPM, BLM, VCR	38	39	non-oat cell carcinoma	LANZOTTI et al., 1975 (118)
5-FU, PCZ, CPM, MTC, VLB	78		median survival 6.5 months	MANNES et al., 1970 (56)
MTX, BCNU, PCZ, CPM, VCR	9	2/9	regional small-cell carci- noma 1 CR, 1 PR	HOLROYDE et al., 1975 (119)
	10	8/10	extensive small-cell carcinoma 8 PR	
MTX, DIC, HUR, CPM, ADM, VCR	23	56	12/13 undifferentiated carcinoma (5 CR, 7 PR) 1/8 squamous carcinoma	LOWENBRAUN, 1974 (57)

[a] For additional combinations: see ref. 127-130, 133-135.

agents. ELIAS, using a 5-drug combination in inoperable lung cancer, reported an effect of prior anticoagulation with heparin (58, 59). Two subsequent studies failed to confirm the effect of anticogulation (136, 137).

B. STRATEGY

1. Localized Lung Cancer

(i) Surgery
Surgery is the only treatment modality with a curative potential in lung cancer (120). Unfortunately, the great majority of cases are no longer resectable at the time of diagnosis. More than half the patients who have undergone resections for "cure" have already had unrecognized distal metastases at the time of surgery (3). Lung cancer should be treated as a systemic disease from diagnosis. Some type of regional and/or systemic therapy must be used as an adjunct to surgery if survival is to be improved in the future. Most surgeons agree that surgery is not justified in oat-cell carcinoma (except in the presence of a coin lesion).

(ii) Radiotherapy
Studies of operative and postmortem specimens after preoperative or radical radiotherapy have established that radiotherapy can accomplish local tumor ablation and nodal sterilization (60, 61, 121, 122). However, irradiation alone as the primary treatment for localized but unresectable tumor has proved only slightly better than placebo as far as length of survival is concerned (median survival 142 days compared to 112 days for controls) (62). Radiation therapy can be curative and quite effective in alleviating the distressing symptomatology in these patients (61, 121, 122) and remains the mainstay of palliation in patients with limited disease.

Routine use of preoperative irradiation in patients with lung cancer considered clinically to be resectable is not beneficial and may well be harmful (60, 63, 131). Nor is there any evidence that postoperative irradiation prolongs survival in patients treated surgically for bronchogenic carcinoma (61, 64, 65). Because of the high frequency of distant metastases, prophylactic irradiation of occult metastases in high-risk organs, especially the brain, is being considered in selected groups of patients such as those with oat-cell carcinoma (61, 66-68).

(iii) Adjuvant Chemotherapy and Immunotherapy
Neither surgery nor radiotherapy has been able to cure more than a minority of patients with limited lung cancer. Failure to control the local tumor or intrathoracic dissemination and the high incidence of distant metastases are the major reasons for these poor results. Surgeons and radiotherapists recognize the need for adjunctive therapy (chemotherapy and/or immunotherapy) for localized disease (Table 24-5).

The Veterans Administration (VALCSG) has been studying different drugs as adjuvants to surgery in lung cancer since 1957. Short-term adjuvant therapy with HN2 (69, 70) or CPM (69) has had no benificial effect after curative or palliative resections. One exception to these generally negative findings has been substantially longer survival in patients with oat-cell carcinoma after surgical resection followed by the administration of CPM (69). Long-term (18 months) intermittent adjuvant therapy with CPM or CPM alternating with MTX had neither a beneficial nor a

Table 24-5. Lung cancer; postoperative adjuvant chemotherapy (controlled trials)

Type of chemotherapy	Results	References
HN2 during and immediately after surgery	Survival not prolonged	HUGHES et al., 1966 (79)
HN2 during and immediately after surgery	Survival not prolonged	SLACK, 1970 (70)
CPM, 2 courses, postoperative	Survival not prolonged	HIGGINS et al., 1969 (80)
CPM for 2 years, postoperative	Survival not prolonged	M.R.C. Working Party 1971 (75)
CPM, 6 courses over 2 years	Shorter disease-free interval and probably shorter survival	BRUNNER et al., 1971 (72-74)
CPM, intermittent courses over 18 months	Survival not prolonged	SHIELDS et al., 1973 (71)
CPM alternating with MTX, intermittent courses over 18 months	Survival not prolonged	SHIELDS et al., 1973 (71)
BSF for 2 years, postoperative	Survival not prolonged	M.R.C. working Party 1971 (75)
VLB for 3 months, postoperative	Survival not prolonged	CROSBIE et al., 1966 (81)

detrimental effect in patients in whom all visible tumor had been resected but who had other poor prognostic features (69, 71). BRUNNER et al. actually observed a higher recurrence and death rate in patients treated with long-term (2 years) intermittent CPM after "curative" surgery (72-74). Immunosuppression may have favored tumor growth in CPM-treated patients. Survival was no longer in patients who received long-term daily therapy with CPM or busulfan after "curative" resections than in placebo-treated patients (75).

KARRER published encouraging preliminary results with high-dose intermittent CPM and a 5-drug combination (76, 77).

In summary, the data on adjuvant chemotherapy with the drugs and the schedules reported in the literature are contradictory, some reporting beneficial, others no or adverse effects (106). The need for controlled trials is obvious. CARTER suggests that it is time to test some of the newer agents rather than conventional alkylating agents for adjuvant therapy (78).

A number of investigators have combined radiotherapy with simultaneous single-agent chemotherapy in the hope of obtaining a more pronounced effect than is achieved with radiotherapy alone (Table 24-6). Most studies with a variety of drugs, such as 5 FU (82-86), MTX (83), HN2 (87, 88), CPM (89), HUR (123), ACD (85), and VLB (90), have failed to substantiate an additive effect. Among the exceptions are studies by COHEN (91) and GOLLIN (92) with 5-FU.

Chemotherapy has also been used as adjuvant following radiotherapy. HØST reports a possible benefit of daily oral CPM in undifferentiated

Table 24-6. Combined radiotherapy and chemotherapy for inoperable lung cancer (controlled trials)

Results	Agents used during and after radiotherapy	References
Negative	Methotrexate	HOSLEY et al., 1962 (83)
	5-Fluorouracil	HOSLEY et al., 1962 (83)
	5-Fluorouracil	HALL et al., 1967 (85)
	5-Fluorouracil 10 mg/kg/day	CARR et al., 1972 (86)
	Nitrogen mustard	KRANT et al., 1963 (87)
	Nitrogen mustard	DURRANT et al., 1971 (88)
	Nitromine	EWING et al., 1965 (95)
	Cyclophosphamide	EORTC, 1968 (89)
	Actinomycin D	HALL et al., 1967 (85)
	Vinblastine	COY, 1970 (90)
Positive	5-Fluorouracil 15 mg/kg/day	GOLLIN et al., 1964 (84) 1967 (92)
	Cyclophosphamide	BERGSAGEL et al., 1972 (94)

small-cell carcinoma but not in epidermoid-cell carcinoma (93). BERGS-AGEL et al. noted that intermittent courses of CPM following irradiation of the primary tumor and mediastinum delayed the progression of metas-tatic lesions outside the irradiation field in patients with nonresec-table lung cancer confined to the central area of the thorax (94). This resulted in a modest prolongation of survival (306 days versus 216 days with irradiation alone), which was calculated to be the result of a tumor-cell kill of only $10^{1.5}$. This indicates that CPM, though considered one of the better agents, is only minimally effective in the treatment of lung cancer.

Trials incorporating immunotherapy are still in the preliminary stages (68, 96, 124, 125). In line with our concept of the limited cell kill effected by immunologic stimulation, we anticipate that this treatment modality will be used mainly as an adjuvant to "curative" surgery or radical radiotherapy for limited disease.

(iv) Combined Chemotherapy-Radiotherapy
Protocols combining chemotherapy and radiotherapy as the primary thera-py for patients with unresectable but limited disease (68) or for small-cell carcinoma (97-99) or both localized and metastatic disease (68) are also under investigation.

2. Disseminated Disease

Patients who present with disseminated disease are usually treated with chemotherapy. Some investigators are evaluating protocols that combine chemotherapy with immunotherapy (10, 96). Radiotherapy may offer worth-while palliation of local symptoms. However, the indications for pal-liative resection are definitely limited (3, 6).

Table 24-7. Summary of strategy in lung cancer

Extent Histologic type	Operable	Inoperable	
		Limited (to chest)	Disseminated [a]
Epidermoid	Surgery + Adjuvant chemotherapy (theoretically but none effective thus far)	Radiotherapy or Radiotherapy + Chemotherapy	Cyclophosphamide Nitrogen mustard Methotrexate Adriamycin Nitrosoureas Hexamethylmelamine
Anaplastic	Radiotherapy + Adjuvant chemotherapy	Radiotherapy or Chemotherapy or Radiotherapy + Chemotherapy	Combinations

[a] See text.

416

3. Discussion

It is not possible to be dogmatic in making recommendations for the treatment of lung cancer (Table 24-7). No particular treatment modality, drug, or combination is significantly better than any of the others. At present, any type of therapy is unsatisfactory.

Surgery is the only method that can cure localized, resectable tumors. There is no evidence that postoperative adjuvant chemotherapy as practiced up to now is beneficial or not harmful. Radiotherapy remains the mainstay for palliative therapy of limited disease. At least one study indicates that adjuvant CPM following radiotherapy for limited but unresectable disease may delay progression and prolong survival (94). Single-agent chemotherapy is not very effective in metastatic disease. Intermittent high-dose cyclophosphamide (22) and MTX (24-26) appear to be the most active of the conventional agents. It is hoped that studies currently in progress with new agents, new combinations of drugs, or combinations of various treatment modalities will soon improve the dismal results of lung cancer therapy. The poor results obtained so far should not induce us to adopt a negative attitude towards the treatment of lung cancer (88), but must stimulate us all the more to take part in badly needed protocol studies.

REFERENCES

1. KREYBERG, K.: Histological Typing of Lung Tumours. International Histological Classification of Tumours. Geneva: WHO 1967.
2. MATTHEWS, M.J.: Morphologic classification of bronchogenic carcinoma. Cancer Chemother. Rep. Part 3, 4, 299 (1973).
3. MOUNTAIN, C.F.: Keynote address on surgery in the therapy for lung cancer: surgical prospects and priorities for clinical research. Cancer Chemother. Rep. Part 3, 4, 19 (1973).
4. UICC: T.N.M. Classification of Malignant Tumours. Geneva: G. de Buren 1968.
5. CARR, D.T.: Keynote address on diagnosis, staging, and criteria of response to therapy for lung cancer. Cancer Chemother. Rep. Part 3, 4, 17 (1973).
6. CARR, D.T.: Diagnosis, staging and criteria of response to therapy for lung cancer. Cancer Chemother. Rep. Part 3, 4, 303 (1973).
7. SELAWRY, O.S.: Initial therapeutic trial of new drugs in lung cancer. Cancer Chemother. Rep., Part 3, 4, 215 (1973).
8. HANSEN, H.H., MUGGIA, F.M.: Staging of inoperable patients with bronchogenic carcinoma with special reference to bone marrow examination and peritoneoscopy. Cancer 30, 1395 (1972).
9. ZELEN, M.: Keynote address on biostatistics and data retrieval. Cancer Chemother. Rep. Part 3, 4, 31 (1973).
10. ISRAEL, L.: Keynote address on immunology and immunotherapy. Cancer Chemother. Rep. Part 3, 4, 29 (1973).
11. ISRAEL, L.: Cell-mediated immunity in lung cancer patients: data, problems, and propositions. Cancer Chemother. Rep. Part 3, 4, 279 (1973).
12. TAKITA, H., BRUGAROLAS, A.: Effect of CCNU (NSC-79037) on bronchogenic carcinoma. J. nat. Cancer Inst. 50, 49 (1973).
13. TAKITA, H., BRUGAROLAS, A., MITTELMAN, A., VINCENT, R.: Phase II study of the effect of methyl-CCNU (NSC-95441) on bronchogenic carcinoma. Cancer Chemother. Rep. Part 3, 4, 257 (1973).
14. STEELE, J.D., KLEITSCH, W.P., DUNN, Jr., J.E., BUELL, P.: Survival in males with bronchogenic carcinomas resected as asymptomatic solitary pulmonary nodules. Ann. thor. Surg. 2, 368 (1966).

15. CARTER, S.K.: Some thoughts on surgical adjuvant studies in lung cancer. Cancer Chemother. Rep. Part 3, 4, 109 (1973).

16. CARBONE, P.P., FROST, J.K., FEINSTEIN, A.R., HIGGINS, Jr., G.A., SELAWRY, O.S.: Lung cancer: Perspectives and prospects. Ann. intern. Med. 73, 1003 (1970).

17. LIVINGSTON, R.B., CARTER, S.K.: Single Agents in Cancer Chemotherapy. New York-Washington-London: IFI-Plenum 1970.

18. CARTER, S.K.: New drugs on the horizon in bronchogenic carcinoma. Cancer 30, 1402 (1972).

19. SELAWRY, O.S.: Monochemotherapy of bronchogenic carcinoma with special reference to cell type. Cancer Chemother. Rep. Part 3, 4, 177 (1973).

20. SLAVIK, M., CARTER, S.K.: Bronchogenic carcinoma: New drugs available for study. Cancer Chemother. Rep. Part 3, 4, 265 (1973).

21. GREEN, R.A., HUMPHREY, E., CLOSE, H., PATNO, M.E.: Alkylating agents in bronchogenic carcinoma. Amer. J. Med. 46, 516 (1969).

22. BERGSAGEL, D.E., ROBERTSON, G.L., HASSELBACK, R.: Effect of cyclophosphamide on advanced lung cancer and the hematological toxicity of large, intermittent intravenous doses. Canad. med. Ass. J. 98, 532 (1968).

23. REED, L.J., MUGGIA, F.M., KLIPSTEIN, F.A., GELLHORN, A.: Intermittent parenteral methotrexate (NSC-740) therapy for carcinoma of the lung. Cancer Chemother. Rep. 51, 475 (1967).

24. BONADONNA, G., CUNSOLO, A., DE PALO, G.M., MONFARDINI, S., DE LENA, M., DI PIETRO, S., GUZZON, A.: Sperimentazione clinical con alte dose intermittenti di methotrexate nel carcinoma polmonare avanzato. Tumori 55, 387 (1969).

25. KENIS, Y., MICHEL, J., DEBUSSCHER, L., LACHAPELLE, F.: Action pharmacologique et thérapeutique de l'administration intermittente de méthotrexate dans les tumeurs solides. Corso Superiore sulla Chemiotherapia dei Tumori, p. 165. Milano 1970.

26. DJERASSI, I., ROMINGER, C.J., KIM, J.S., TURCHI, J., SUVANSRI, U., HUGHES, D.: Phase I study of high doses of methotrexate with citrovorum factor in patiens with lung cancer. Cancer 30, 22 (1972).

27. KENIS, Y., DESMEDT, J., TAGNON, H.J.: Action du Natulan dans 94 cas de tumeurs solides. Europ. J. Cancer 2, 51 (1966).

28. O.E.R.T.C., GROUPE COOPERATIVE D'ESSAIS THERAPEUTIQUES SUR LES CANCERS BRONCHO-PULMONAIRES: Résultats d'un essai d'une méthylhydrazine dans le traitement des cancers épidermoides et anaplasiques des bronches. Europ. J. Cancer 4, 129 (1968).

29. KAUNG, D.T., SBAR, S., PATNO, M.E.: Treatment of nonresectable cancer of the lung with hydroxyurea (NSC-32065) given intermittently. Cancer Chemother. Rep. Part 1, 55, 87 (1971).

30. WOLF, J., SPEAR, P., YESNER, R., PATNO, M.E.: Nitrogen mustard and the steroid hormones in the treatment of inoperable bronchogenic carcinoma. Amer. J. Med. 29, 100 (1960).

31. HANSEN, H.H., SELAWRY, O.S., MUGGIA, F.M., WALKER, M.D.: Clinical studies with 1-(2-chloroethyl)-3-cyclohexyl-1-nitrosourea (NSC-79037). Cancer Res. 31, 223 (1971).

32. OLSHIN, S., SIDDIQUI, S., FIRAT, D.: Phase II study of 1,3-bis(2-chloroethyl)-1-nitrosourea (BCNU; NSC-409962) in the treatment of bronchogenic carcinoma. Cancer Chemother. Rep. Part 1, 56, 259 (1972).

33. AHMANN, D.L., CARR, D.T., COLES, D.T., HAHN, R.G.: Evaluation of cyclophosphamide (NSC-26271) and 1,3-bis(2-chloroethyl)-1-nitrosourea (BCNU; NSC-409962) in the treatment of patients with inoperable or disseminated lung cancer. Cancer Chemother. Rep. Part 3, 56, 401 (1972).

34. CARTER, S.K.: An overview of the status of the nitrosoureas in other tumors. Cancer Chemother. Rep. Part 3, 4, 35 (1973).

35. BLUM, R.H., LIVINGSTON, R.B., CARTER, S.K.: Hexamethylmelamine. a new drug with activity in solid tumors. Europ. J. Cancer 9, 195 (1973).
36. KENIS, Y., STRYCKMANS, P.: Action de la mitomycin C dans 65 cas de tumeurs malignes. Comparaison de l'effet de doses faibles, répétées et de doses "massives". Chemotherapia 8, 114 (1974).
37. KENIS, Y., BRULE, G.: Preliminary clinical screening with daunorubicin in lung cancer. Europ. J. Cancer 6, 155 (1970).
38. KENIS, Y., MICHEL, J., RIMOLDI, R., ISRAEL, L., LEVY, P.: Results of a clinical trial with intermittent doses of adriamycin in lung cancer. Europ. J. Cancer 8, 485 (1972).
39. BLUM, R.H., CARTER, S.K., AGRE, K.: A clinical review of bleomycin - a new antineoplastic agent. Cancer 31, 903 (1973).
40. LUCE, J.K., THURMAN, W.G., ISAACS, B.L., TALLEY, R.W.: Clinical trials with the antitumor agent 5-(3,3-dimethyl-1-triazeno)imidazole-4-carboxamide (NSC-45388). Cancer Chemother. Rep. 54, 119 (1970).
41. MIZGERD, J.B., AMICK, R.M., HILAL, H.M., PATNO, M.E.: Clinical study of 5-(3,3-dimethyl-1-triazeno)imidazole-4-carboxamide (NSC-45388) in carcinoma of the lung. Cancer Chemother. Rep. Part 1, 55, 83 (1971).
42. HELLMANN, K.: Preliminary clinical assessment of ICRF 159 (NSC-129943) in bronchogenic carcinoma - abstract. Cancer Chemother. Rep. Part 3, 4, 243 (1973).
43. CLIFFTON, E.E.: Bronchial artery perfusion for treatment of advanced lung cancer. Cancer 23, 1151 (1969).
44. HANSEN, H.H.: Keynote address on chemotherapy for lung cancer. Cancer Chemother. Rep. Part 3, 4, 25 (1973).
45. SELAWRY, O., HANSEN, H., CARR, B., SEALY, R., SIMON, R.: Improved chemotherapy for advanced bronchogenic carcinoma. Proc. Amer. Ass. Cancer Res. 15, 118 (1974).
46. ALBERTO, P.: Remission rates, survival, and prognostic factors in combination chemotherapy for bronchogenic carcinoma. Cancer Chemother. Rep. Part 3, 4, 199 (1973).
47. BONADONNA, G., TANCINI, G., BAJETTA, E.: Chemotherapy of lung cancer: The experience of the National Cancer Institute of Milan. Cancer Chemother. Rep. Part 3, 4, 231 (1973).
48. CHANES, R.E., CONDIT, P.T., BOTTOMLEY, R.H., NISIMBLAT, W.: Combined actinomycin D and vincristine in the treatment of patients with cancer. Cancer 27, 614 (1971).
49. BODEY, G.P., GOTTLIEB, J.A., LIVINGSTON, R., FREI, E. III: New agents and combinations in the treatment of bronchogenic carcinoma. Cancer Chemother. Rep. Part 3, 4, 227 (1973).
50. HOLOYE, P.Y., HUSSEY, D., BARKELY, H., SAMUELS, M.L., WARD, D.: Combination intensive chemotherapy and radiotherapy in oat cell bronchogenic carcinoma. Proc. Amer. Ass. Cancer Res. 15, 43 (1974).
51. EDMONSON, J.H., LAGAKOS, S.W.: Combination chemotherapy for metastatic lung cancer. Proc. Amer. Ass. clin. Oncol. 15, 180 (1974).
52. REDDY, P., CORTES, E.P., CHITKARA, R., OLSHIN, S.: Combination of cyclophosphamide (CTX), vincristine (VCR), and methyl-CCNU (MeCCNU) in patients with advanced cancer. Proc. Amer. Ass. clin. Oncol. 15, 178 (1974).
53. POUILLART, P., SCHWARZENBERG, L., AMIEL, J.L., MATHE, G., et al.: Chimiothérapies séquentielles. II. Application au traitement des cancer bronchiques. Nouv. Press. méd., in press (1974).
54. LIVINGSTON, J.A., BODEY, G.P., GOTTLIEB, J.A., BURGESS, M.A.: Cytoxan, oncovin, methyl CCNU and bleomycin (COMB) in lung cancer and other solid tumors. Proc. Amer. Ass. clin. Oncol., Abstract 61 (1973).
55. RAMIREZ, G. (Clinical Oncology Group): Five-drug combination therapy in the treatment of solid tumors. Proc. Amer. Ass. Cancer Res. 14, 17 (1973).

56. MANNES, P., DERRIS, R., MOENS, R., HEYNEN, E.: La polychimiotherapie des cancers bronchiques inopérable. X. International Cancer Congress Abstracts, p. 450. Houston: Medicar Arts Publishing Co. 1970.

57. LOWENBRAUN, S.: Cycle-nonspecific preceding cycle-specific chemotherapy in metastatic lung carcinoma (CA). Proc. Amer. Ass. clin. Oncol. 15, 162 (1974).

58. ELIAS, E.G.: Heparin as an adjuvant to chemotherapy in lung carcinoma. Proc. Amer. Ass. Cancer Res. 14, 26 (1973).

59. ELIAS, E.G., SHUKLA, S.K., MINK, I.B.: Heparin and chemotherapy in the management of inoperable lung carcinoma. Cancer 36, 129 (1975).

60. SHIELDS, T.W.: Preoperative radiation therapy in the treatment of bronchial carcinoma. Cancer 30, 1388 (1972).

61. PEREZ, C.A.: Radiation therapy for cancer of the lung: previous experience and definition of current issues. Cancer Chemother. Rep. Part 3, 4, 145 (1973).

62. WOLF, J., PATNO, M.E., D'ESOPO, N.: Controlled study of survival of patients with clinically inoperable lung cancer treated with radiation therapy. Amer. J. Med. 40, 360 (1966).

63. WIDOW, W.: Preoperative irradiation of bronchial carcinoma. In: Oncology 1970 (Tenth International Cancer Congress, Houston), p. 513. Chicago: Year Book Medical Publishers 1970.

64. SHERRAH-DAVIES, E.: Does postoperative irradiation improve survival in lung cancer? J. Amer. med. Ass. 196, 133 (1966).

65. BANGMA, P.J.: Post-operative radiotherapy. In: Modern Radiotherapy - Carcinoma of the bronchus, p. 163 (ed. T.J. Deeley). New York: Appleton-Century-Crofts 1971.

66. HANSEN, H.H.: Should initial treatment of small cell carcinoma include systemic chemotherapy and brain irradiation? Cancer Chemother. Rep. Part 3, 4, 239 (1973).

67. RUBIN, P.: Radiotherapy for lung cancer. Cancer Chemother. Rep. Part 3, 4, 311 (1973).

68. DANA, M.: Radiotherapy for bronchogenic carcinoma: actual difficulties and plans for the future. Cancer Chemother. Rep. Part 3, 153 (1973).

69. HIGGINS, Jr., G.A.: Use of chemotherapy as an adjuvant to surgery for bronchogenic carcinoma. Cancer 30, 1383 (1972).

70. SLACK, N.H.: Bronchogenic carcinoma: nitrogen mustard as a surgical adjuvant and factors influencing survival. Cancer 25, 987 (1970).

71. SHIELDS, T.W.: Status report of adjuvant cancer chemotherapy trials in the treatment of bronchial carcinoma. Cancer Chemother. Rep. Part 3, 4, 119 (1973).

72. BRUNNER, K.W.: chemotherapy in the management of bronchogenic carcinoma. In: Cancer Chemotherapy, p. 138 (eds. F. Elkerbout, P. Thomas, A. Zwaveling). Leiden: University Press 1971.

73. BRUNNER, K.W., MARTHALER, T., MÜLLER, W.: Unfavorable effects of long-term adjuvant chemotherapy with endoxan in radically operated bronchogenic carcinoma. Europ. J. Cancer 7, 285 (1971).

74. BRUNNER, K.W., MARTHALER, T., MÜLLER, W.: Effects of long-term adjuvant chemotherapy with cyclophosphamide (NSC-26271) for radically resected bronchogenic carcinoma. Cancer Chemother. Rep. Part 3, 4, 125 (1973).

75. MEDICAL RESEARCH COUNCIL: Study of cytotoxic chemotherapy as an adjuvant to surgery in carcinoma of the bronchus. Brit. med. J. 2, 421 (1971).

76. KARRER, K.: Importance of dose schedules in adjuvant chemotherapy. Cancer Chemother. Rep. 56, 35 (1972).

77. KARRER, K., PRIDUN, N., ZWINTZ, E.: Chemotherapeutic studies in bronchogenic carcinoma by the Austrian Study Group. Cancer Chemother. Rep. Part 3, 4, 207 (1973).

78. CARTER, S.K.: Some thoughts on surgical adjuvant studies in lung cancer. Cancer Chemother. Rep. Part 3, 4, 109 (1973).
79. HUGHES, Jr., F.A., HIGGINS, G., BEEBE, G.W.: Present status of surgical adjuvant lung-cancer chemotherapy. J. Amer. med. Ass. 196, 131 (1966).
80. HIGGINS, G.A., HUMPHREY, E.W., HUGHES, F.A., KEEHN, R.J.: Cytoxan as an adjuvant to surgery for lung cancer. J. Surg. Oncol. 1, 221 (1969).
81. CROSBIE, W.A., KAMDAR, H.H., BELCHER, J.R.: A controlled·trial of vinblastine sulphate in the treatment of cancer of the lung. Brit. J. Dis. Chest 60, 28 (1966).
82. VON ESSEN, G.E., KLIGERMAN, M.M., CALABRESI, P.: Radiation and fluorouracil, a controlled clinical study. Radiology 81, 1018 (1963).
83. HOSLEY, H.F., MARANGOUDAKIS, S., ROSS, C.A., MURPHEY, W.T., HOLLAND, J.F.: Combined radiation-chemotherapy for bronchogenic carcinoma - pilot study. Cancer Chemother. Rep. 16, 467 (1962).
84. GOLLIN, F.F., ANSFIELD, F.J., VERMUND, H.: Continued studies of combined chemotherapy and irradiation in inoperable bronchogenic carcinoma. Cancer Chemother. Rep. 51, 189 (1967).
85. HALL, T.C., DEDERICK, M.M., CHALMERS, T.C., et al.: A clinical pharmacologic study of chemotherapy and X-ray therapy in lung cancer. Amer. J. Med. 43, 186 (1967).
86. CARR, D.T., CHILDS, Jr, D.S., LEE, R.E.: Radiotherapy plus 5-FU compared to radiotherapy alone for inoperable and unresectable bronchogenic carcinoma. Cancer 29, 375 (1972).
87. KRANT, M.J., CHALMERS, T.C., DEDERICK, M.M., et al.: Comparative trial of chemotherapy and radiotherapy in patients with non-resectable cancer of the lung. Amer. J. Med. 35, 363 (1963).
88. DURRANT, K.R., ELLIS, F., BLACK, J.M., BERRY, R.J., RIDEHALGH, F.R., HAMILTON, W.S.: Comparison of treatment policies in inoperable bronchial carcinoma. Lancet 1, 715 (1971).
89. O.E.R.T.C., GROUPE COOPERATEUR D'ESSAIS THERAPEUTIQUES SUR LES CANCERS BRONCHO-PULMONAIRES: Résultats d'un essai thérapeutique clinique sur une association radiothérapie et chimiothérapie dans les cancers broncho-pulmonaires. Europ. J. Cancer 4, 437 (1968).
90. COY, P.: A randomized study of irradiation and vinblastine in lung cancer. Cancer 26, 803 (1970).
91. COHEN, J.L., KRANT, M.J., SHNIDER, B.I., MARIAS, P.I., HORTON, J., BAXTER, D.: Radiation plus 5-fluoro-uracil (NSC-19893): clinical demonstration of an additive effect in bronchogenic carcinoma. Cancer Chemother. Rep. Part 1, 55, 253 (1971).
92. GOLLIN, F.F., ANSFIELD, F.J., VERMUND, H.: Clinical studies of combined chemotherapy and irradiation in inoperable bronchogenic carcinoma. Amer. J. Roentgen. 92, 22 (1964).
93. HØST, H.: Cyclophosphamide (NSC-26271) as adjuvant to radiotherapy in the treatment of unresectable bronchogenic carcinoma. Cancer Chemother. Rep. Part 3, 4, 161 (1973).
94. BERGSAGEL, D.E., JENKIN, R.D.T., PRINGLE, J.F., WHITE, D.M., FETTERLY, J.C.M., KLAASEN, D.J., McDERMOT, R.S.R.: Lung cancer: clinical trial of radiotherapy alone vs. radiotherapy plus cyclo-phosphamide. Cancer 30, 621 (1972).
95. EWING, D.P., McEWEN, B.W., ATKINSON, L.: Combined chemotherapy and radiotherapy in carcinoma of the lung. Med. J. Aust. 2, 397 (1965).
96. ISRAEL, L.: Preliminary results of nonspecific immunotherapy for lung cancer. Cancer Chemother. Rep. Part 3, 4, 283 (1973).
97. MAURES, L.H., TULLOH, M., EAGAN, R.T., FORCIER, R.J., HOUSE, R.: Combination chemotherapy and radiation for small cell carcinoma of the lung. Cancer Chemother. Rep. Part 3, 4, 171 (1973).

98. EAGON, R.T., MAURER, L.H., FORCIER, R.J., TULLOH, M.: Combination chemotherapy and radiation therapy in small cell carcinoma of the lung. Cancer 32, 371 (1973).

99. EAGON, R.T., MAURER, L.H., FORCIER, R.J., TULLOH, M.: Small cell carcinoma of the lung: Staging, paraneoplastic syndromes, treatment and survival. Cancer 33, 527 (1974).

100. MATTHEWS, M.L.: Morphology of lung cancer. Semin. Oncol. 1, 175 (1974).

101. CARR, D.T., MOUNTAIN, C.F.: The staging of lung cancer. Semin. Oncol. 1, 229 (1974).

102. MARGOLIS, R., HANSEN, H.H., MUGGIA, F.M., KANHOUWA, S.: Diagnosis of liver metastases in bronchogenic carcinoma. Cancer 34, 1825 (1974).

103. MUGGIA, F.M., CHERVU, L.R.: Lung cancer: diagnosis in metastatic sites. Semin. Oncol. 1, 217 (1974).

104. KAUNG, D.T., WOLF, J., HYDE, L., ZELEN, M.: Preliminary report on the treatment of nonresectable cancer of the lung. Cancer Chemother. Rep. Part 1, 58, 359 (1974).

105. SELAWRY, O.S., PRIMACK, A.: First International Workshop of Therapy of Lung Cancer, Airlie, Virginia, October 16-20, 1972. Cancer Chemother. Rep., Part 3, 4, 1 (1973).

106. SELAWRY, O.S.: The role of chemotherapy in the treatment of lung cancer. Semin. Oncol. 1, 259 (1974).

107. WASSERMAN, T.H., SLAVIK, M., CARTER, S.K.: Review of CCNU in clinical cancer therapy. Cancer Treat. Rev. 1, 131 (1974).

108. WASSERMAN, T.H., SLAVIK, M., CARTER, S.K.: Methyl-CCNU in clinical cancer therapy. Cancer Treat, Rev. 1, 251 (1974).

109. EMANUEL, N.M., VERMEL, E.M., OSTROVSKAYA, L.A., KORMAN, N.P.: Experimental and clinical studies of the antitumor activity of 1-methyl-1-nitrosourea. Cancer Chemother. Rep. Part 1, 58, 135 (1974).

110. CORTES, E.P., TAKITA, H., HOLLAND, J.F.: Adriamycin in advanced bronchogenic carcinoma. Cancer 34, 518 (1974).

111. KENIS, Y.: Adriamycin in lung cancer. In: Adriamycin Review, EORTC International Symposium, p. 268 (eds. M. Staquet, H. Tagnon, Y. Kenis et al.). Ghent: European Press Medikon 1975.

112. WOLF, J., ZELEN, M.: Comparative trial of two drug combinations in pulmonary cancer. Proc. Am. Soc. Clin. Oncol. 16, 272 (1975).

113. HOLOYE, P.Y., SAMUELS, M.L., BARKLEY, H.T., HOWE, C.D.: Cytoxan, adriamycin, and vincristine combination with radiation therapy in the treatment of small cell carcinoma of the lung. Proc. Am. Ass. Cancer Res. 16, 112 (1975).

114. MUNDIA, A., CORTES, E.P., CHITKARA, R., SERIFF, N., OLSHIN, S.: Combination of adriamycin, cyclophosphamide, and vincristine in inoperable lung cancer. Proc. Am. Soc. Clin. Oncol. 16, 241 (1975).

115. BEARDEN, J.D., COLTMAN, C.A.: Combination chemotherapy in disseminated lung cancer. Proc. Am. Soc. Clin. Oncol. 16, 250 (1975).

116. ABELOFF, M.D., ETTINGER, D.S., INALSINGH, D.S., HAZRA, T.A.: Combination chemotherapy of small cell carcinoma of the lung. Proc. Am. Ass. Cancer Res. 16, 80 (1975).

117. ARMENTROUT, S., BATEMAN, J., PAJAK, T., GUNNELL, J.: Oral nitrosoureas in multiple drug programs for bronchogenic carcinomas. Proc. Am. Soc. Clin. Oncol. 16, 242 (1975).

118. LANZOTTI, V.J., WARD, D.N., BOYLES, L.E., THOMAS, D.R., SMITH, T.L., SAMUELS, M.L.: Bleomycin followed by cyclophosphamide, vincristine, methotrexate, and 5-fluorouracil for non-oat cell bronchogenic carcinoma. Proc. Am. Ass. Cancer Res. 16, 112 (1975).

119. HOLROYDE, C.P., ENGSTROM, P.F., CREECH, R.H.: Combination chemotherapy in small cell carcinoma of the lung. Proc. Am. Soc. Clin. Oncol. 16, 223 (1975).

120. MOUNTAIN, C.F.: Surgical therapy in lung cancer: biologic, physiologic, and technical determinants. Semin. Oncol. 1, 253 (1974).

121. DEELEY, J.: Radiotherapy for carcinoma of the bronchus. Cancer Treat. Rev. 1, 39 (1974).

122. LEE, R.E.: Radiotherapy of bronchogenic carcinoma. Semin. Oncol. 1, 245 (1974).

123. LANDGREN, R.C., HUSSEY, D.H., BARKLEY, H.T., SAMUELS, M.L.: Split-course irradiation compared to split-course irradiation plus hydroxyurea in inoperable bronchogenic carcinoma - a randomized study of 53 patients. Cancer 34, 1598 (1974).

124. HERSH, E.M., GUTTERMAN, J.U., MAVLIGIT, G.M.: Perspectives in immunotherapy of lung cancer. Cancer Treatment Rev. 1, 65 (1974).

125. HERSH, E.M., MAVLIGIT, G.M., GUTTERMAN, J.U.: Immunotherapy as related to lung cancer: a review. Semin. Oncol. 1, 273 (1974).

126. SELAWRY, O.S.: Response of bronchogenic carcinoma to adriamycin (NSC-123127). Cancer Chemother. Rep. Part 3, 6, 349 (1975).

127. SELAWRY, O.S.: Polychemotherapy with adriamycin (NSC-123127) in bronchogenic carcinoma. Cancer Chemother. Rep. Part 3, 6, 353 (1975).

128. LIVINGSTON, R.B., EINHORN, L.H., BURGESS, M.A., FREIREICH, E.J., GOTTLIEB, J.A.: Combination chemotherapy with bleomycin (NSC-125066), adriamycin (NSC-123127), CCNU (NSC-79037), vincristine (NSC-67574), and mechlorethamine (NSC-762) (BACON) in squamous cell lung cancer: experience with 50 patients. Cancer Chemother. Rep. Part 3, 6, 361 (1975).

129. NIXON, D.W., CAREY, R.W., SUIT, H.D., AISENBERG, A.C.: Combination chemotherapy in oat cell carcinoma of the lung. Cancer 36, 867 (1975).

130. LIVINGSTON, R.B., EINHORN, L.H., BODEY, G.P., BURGESS, M.A., FREIREICH, E.J., GOTTLIEB, J.A.: COMB (cyclophosphamide, oncovin, methyl-CCNU, and bleomycin): a four-drug combination in solid tumors. Cancer 36, 327 (1975).

131. WARRAM, J.: Preoperative irradiation of cancer of the lung: final report of a therapeutic trial. A collaborative study. Cancer 36, 914 (1975).

132. BITRAN, J., BILLINGS, A., DRESSER, R.K., COHEN, L., COLMAN, M., SHAPIRO, C.: Survival of patients with lung cancer treated with vincristine and actinomycin D. Cancer 37, 1669 (1976).

133. COHEN, M.H., FOSSIECK, B.E., CREAVEN, P.J., MINNA, J.D.: Intensive chemotherapy of small cell bronchogenic carcinoma. Proc. Amer. Soc. Clin. Oncol. 17, 273 (1976).

134. STRAUS, M.J.: A design for combination chemotherapy in lung cancer with increased survival. Proc. Amer. Soc. Clin. Oncol. 17, 239 (1976).

135. HANSEN, H.H., HANSEN, M.: A comparison of 3 and 4 drug-combination chemotherapy for advanced small cell anaplastic carcinoma of the lung. Proc. Amer. Ass. Cancer Res. 17, 129 (1976).

136. CONROY, J., BRODSKY, I., KAHN, S.B., ELIAS, E.: Anticogulation in the treatment of inoperable lung cancer. Proc. Amer. Soc. Clin. Oncol. 17, 277 (1976).

137. EDLIS, H.E., GOUDSMIT, A., BRINDLEY, C., NIEMETZ, J.: Trial of heparin and cyclophosphamide in the treatment of lung cancer. Cancer Treat. Rep. 60, 575 (1976).

Chapter 25
Gastrointestinal Cancer

Most gastrointestinal cancers are diagnosed late in their course. The prognosis is worst for esophageal cancer and improves progressively with increasing proximity to the colon. Five-year survival rates are 2% for cancer of the pancreas, 4% for cancer of the esophagus, 10% for cancer of the stomach, and 35% when the colon and rectum are affected. The majority are adenocarcinomas, except in the esophagus and the anus, where the lesions are epidermoid. Gastrointestinal cancers are most prevalent in older patients. The incidence varies considerably in different parts of the world. No staging classification is presently uniformly accepted.

A. CANCER OF THE ESOPHAGUS

The incidence of carcinoma of the esophagus varies widely in different countries. It is most common in the sixth and seventh decades and more prevalent in men. Alcoholism, peptic and caustic esophagitis, and Plummer-Vinson's syndrome are thought to be predisposing factors. The majority of esophageal carcinomas are epidermoid, but adenocarcinomas are seen in the lower part of the esophagus. The tumor extends locally to the thoracic organs and lymph nodes, and less commonly spreads via the blood stream. Local spread is facilitated by the absence of a serosa. Prognosis is poor with 5-year survival of under 5%. A clinical staging system (TNM) has been proposed (81).

1. Chemotherapy

Few agents have significant therapeutic activity. No data on esophageal carcinoma are included in LIVINGSTON's and CARTER's review of single-agent therapy (1). A wide range of responses has been reported for bleomycin (10-100%), with an overall response rate of 33% (2). Methotrexate has also been used, because of the epithelial nature of esophageal carcinomas. A recent study reported 10 tumor regressions in 21 patients treated with methyl-GAG (3).

2. Strategy

The treatment to be used is selected with reference to histologic type and especially to the location (20% of esophageal tumors are in the upper third, 35% in the middle, and 45% in the lower third) and the extent of the tumor.

(i) Localized Esophageal Carcinoma

Radical surgery offers the best chance of a cure. It is most often feasible for lower-third tumors, and rarely for an upper-third lesion. Radiotherapy is reserved for cases that are not suitable for operation (the majority of upper- and middle-third carcinomas). It occasionally results in long survival. Some authors are investigating the value of preoperative radiotherapy.

(ii) Advanced Esophageal Carcinoma

Therapy of esophageal carcinoma is often limited to the palliation of dysphagia, which is achieved by means of radiotherapy in approximately 75% of cases. Several surgical techniques can be used to bypass the obstructing tumor.

B. CANCER OF THE STOMACH

Stomach cancer is most common among the Japanese. For reasons that remain obscure, the incidence has decreased in the United States, Australia, Canada, and England in recent decades. It is a disease of later life, particularly common in the 6th and 7th decade, and men are affected twice as often as women. The predisposing factors include achlorhydria. Over 95% of stomach cancers are adenocarcinomas. The five year survival rate is approximately 5-10%. The location and the size of the primary tumor, gross and microscopic pathologic findings, and lymph node involvement are important factors that influence prognosis. The American Joint Committee on Cancer Staging and End Results Reporting has developed a classification and staging system applying the TNM principle. (82).

1. Chemotherapy

(i) Single-Agent Chemotherapy

Few drugs have been adequately evaluated in gastric carcinoma (83). 5-FU is the agent that has most often been used. Reported response rates vary from 7.5 to 31% with an overall rate of 23% and an average duration of response lasting 4 to 5 months (1, 4-7, 83). Response rates for some other agents are listed in Table 25-1. Mitomycin C has been popular in Japan but its toxicity has precluded widespread use in the United States (10, 83). The overall response rate in 211 patients, most of whom had prior therapy, is 30%, lasting 1 to 3 months (83). An intermittent dose schedule is recommended. Porfiromycin seems to have some activity (11). Adriamycin is not particularly effective (83); BRUGAROLAS et al. (84) and FRYTAK et al. (103), however obtained 50% regressions in small series of patients. BCNU is the only compound of the nitrosoureas with a useful response rate (18%) (8, 31, 65, 83, 85, 86). In a randomized comparison, the response rate was 44% for 5-FU versus 19% for BCNU. The average duration of response was 5.3 months for 5-FU and 4.7 months for BCNU (31).

(ii) Combinations

Most reports on combination chemotherapy in gastric carcinoma involve too few patients to allow any conclusions (Table 25-2). Since there are few effective single agents, the potential for combination chemotherapy is limited. Two studies suggest that BCNU with 5-FU (5, 8, 13)

Table 25-1. Effectiveness of single agents in stomach cancer

Drug	Number evaluated	Responses	Reference
5-Fluorouracil	261	27%	LIVINGSTON and CARTER (1)
5-FUdR	10	6/10	DeCONTI et al. (7)
Cytosine arabinoside	11	3/11	COMIS and CARTER (83)
Hydroxyurea	31	19%	DeCONTI et al. (7)
BCNU	23	17.5%	KOVACH et al. (8)
CCNU	35	3%	WASSERMAN et al. (85)
MeCCNU	30	O	WASSERMAN et al. (86)
Nitrogen mustard	20	30%	LIVINGSTON and CARTER (1)
Chlorambucil	18	16.5%	LIVINGSTON and CARTER (1)
Hexamethylmelamine	12	2/12	BLUM et al. (9)
Mitomycin C	211	30%	COMIS and CARTER (83)
Porfiromycin	12	4/12	IZBICKI et al. (11)
Adriamycin	17	12%	COMIS and CARTER (83)

Table 25-2. Response rates to combinations in stomach cancer

Combination	Number evaluated	Number of responses	REFERENCE
5-FU, CAR	18	4	GAILANI et al. (12)
5-FU, BCNU	6	4	REITEMEIER et al. (13)
	34	14 (41%)	KOVACH et al. (8)
5-FU, MeCCNU	not given	(52%)	MOERTEL and HANLEY (87)
5-FU, MTC	5	2	REITEMEIER et al. (13)
5-FU, VLB	11	4 (36%)	AL-SARRAF et al. (14)
BCNU, MTC	4	2	REITEMEIER et al. (13)
MeCCNU, CPM	3	O	RIVA (65)
ACD, CPM	3	O	MOERTEL and REITEMEIER (15)
5-FU, CAR, MTC	27	15 (55%)	OTA et al. (16)
	4	1	YAGODA et al. (17)
	16	6 (37.5%)	DeJAGER et al. (18)
5-FU, BCNU, MTC	1	O	REITEMEIER and MOERTEL (13)
5-FU, MTC, ADM	18	9 (50%)	MAC DONALD et al. (19)
MTX, 5-FU, CPM, VCR (COMF)	2	2	HANHAM et al. (20)
DIC, 5-FU, BCNU, VCR	4	O	VAN EDEN et al. (21)

and MeCCNU combined with 5-FU (87) may be more effective than 5-FU alone. Japanese investigators obtained 15 regressions in 27 patients (55%) with a combination of MTC, 5-FU, and CAR (16), while DeJAGER et al. in the United States, reported a 37% response rate with this combination (18). KIM et al. obtained more regressions with 5-FU combined with MTC than with MTC alone (88). The combination of 5-FU, MTC plus ADM is also effective (19).

2. Strategy

(i) Localized Stomach Cancer
Surgery is the only curative therapy. The 5-year survival rate is up to 50% as long as only patients with no involvement of the adjacent lymph nodes are considered, as against under 15% with nodal involvement. Most gastric carcinomas are radio-resistant.

(ii) Adjuvant Chemotherapy
There is no evidence that adjuvant chemotherapy with thio-TEPA (22, 23), FUdR (24), or CPM (25) significantly prolongs survival (83). Most of the adjuvant studies used short-term chemotherapy of moderate intensity and were designed to eliminate circulating tumor cells released at surgery. Long-term, intensive, intermittent schedules designed to eliminate microscopic, disseminated metastases need to be studied.

(iii) Advanced Stomach Cancer
Satisfactory palliation can be achieved by means of various surgical procedures. Radiation therapy has been useful in chronically bleeding gastric cancers and in relieving localized areas of obstruction. Palliation with radiotherapy can be improved by simultaneous 5-FU therapy (4, 26).

C. CANCER OF THE COLON AND RECTUM

Cancers of the colon and rectum make up 14% and 15% of all cancers in men and women respectively. Familial polyposis of the colon, Gardners' syndrome and ulcerative colitis are predisposing diseases. Debate rages as to whether adenomatous polyps are premalignant. The likelihood of invasive cancer is considerably higher with villous adenomas. In 75% of cases the tumor is situated in the lower 25 cm of the colon and rectum.

Dukes' classification or modifications of this system are often used (Table 25-3). The 5-year survival rate for Type A lesions ranges from 61 to 81%, for Type B from 25 to 64%, and for Type C lesions 6 to 28%.

1. Chemotherapy

(i) Single-Agent Chemotherapy
The majority of cytotoxic agents have been adequately evaluated in colon cancer (5, 89, 90). Response rates for various single agents are listed in Table 25-4. 5-FU has been and remains the most popular agent for gastrointestinal carcinomas. Its popularity is not the result of outstanding effectiveness. Objective reponse rates reported have varied from 8% to 85%, which illustrates the difficulties in evaluating the

Table 25-3. Dukes' classification of colon cancers

Type A -	Lesions limited to the mucosa
Type B -	1. Lesions extending into the muscularis but not penetrating it, with negative nodes
	2. Lesions penetrating the muscularis, with negative nodes
Type C -	1. Tumor penetrating all layers lower nodes positive: but highest node negative
	2. As above but highest node positive (i.e., excision incomplete)

results of chemotherapy (4). MOERTEL has stressed the striking effect of the performance status on the objective reponse rate (91). The over-all response rate derived from several studies is approximately 20%, with a median duration of 3 months (1, 4, 5, 89, 92). The optimal do-sage schedule has not yet been determined (37, 38). Most authors agree that the toxicity of the original regimen proposed by CURRERI et al. (39) (15 mg/kg/d for 5 days, followed by 7.5 mg/kg every other day until toxicity effects are noted) is too high. Current brochure in-structions recommend, as suggested by ANSFIELD (40), 12 mg/kg, i.v. (maximum daily dose of 800 mg), daily for 4 successive days, followed by 4 doses of 6 mg/kg administered on alternate days unless toxic ef-fects appear. Several authors have recently proposed weekly injections (15-20 mg/kg or 500-600 mg/m²) with or without an initial loading dose, claiming similar effectiveness to that of earlier schedules with re-duced toxicity (41, 42). Comparative trials are in progress. Other wor-kers have proposed infusions of 5-FU rather than i.v. injections, to reduce toxicity. Earlier clinical reports were contradictory (43-45), and two recent randomized trials have not resolved the issue. BAKER et al. reported that continuous i.v. infusion of 5-FU (30 mg/kg/d) over 120 hours were superior in both rate of remission (44 percent versus 22 percent) and tolerance to bolus injections (12 mg/kg/d x 5) (46). MOERTEL et al., however, found no difference in effect between i.v. bolus injections and 2-hour infusions of equitoxic doses of 5-FU (47). JOHNSON et al. have been favorably impressed with the results of multiple daily injections for loading courses (in disseminated breast cancer) (48). Renewed interest in the oral administration of 5-FU has been aroused by LAHIRI et al. (49) and BATEMAN et al. (50). In a com-parative trial of 5-FU (15 mg/kg qw) by the i.v. route and the oral route, BATEMAN's group found no difference in effect. Serum levels of 5-FU are much more variable after oral administration than after i.v. injection (51, 52). More recently the Western Cancer Study Group re-ported that weekly 5-FU p.o. is inferior to 5-FU i.v. at equivalent doses (93). The Group at the Mayo Clinic reached the same conclusion for 5-FU administered in intensive courses (94). No conventional or experimental agents have been consistently superior to 5-FU in rate or duration of responses (Table 25-4) (5).

FUdR seems to be equally effective but is no longer used, except in perfusion therapy. Other antimetabolites are essentially inactive. Pre-liminary experience with Ftorafur is encouraging (95). Cyclophosphamide in intermittent high doses causes tumor regressions in 20% of cases with five out of thirteen previously untreated patients responding in one study, but in all these cases regression was of short duration (53). Antitumor antibiotics are without effect with the exception of mito-mycin C (16% RR). Actinomycin D (15% RR) deserves further study (83). The use of Vinca alkaloids is not indicated in colon cancer.

Table 25-4. Effectiveness of single agents in large bowel cancers

Drug	Number evaluated	Percentage of responses	Reference
Methotrexate	111	17	CARTER and FRIEDMAN (89)
6-Mercaptopurine	50	4	CARTER and FRIEDMAN (89)
6-Thioguanine	54	8	ECOG (27)
Imidazole carboxamide (DIC)	17	6	MOERTEL et al. (28)
	71	11	CARTER and FRIEDMAN (89)
TIC mustard	22	O	MOERTEL et al. (29)
5-Fluorouracil	2107	21	CARTER and FRIEDMAN (89)
FUdR	617	23	CARTER and FRIEDMAN (89)
Cytosine arabinoside	137	9.5	CARTER and FRIEDMAN (89)
5-Azacytidine	27	4	MOERTEL et al. (30)
Hydroxyurea	151	1o	CARTER and FRIEDMAN (89)
BCNU	64	12.5	MOERTEL (31)
CCNU	75	1o	MOERTEL (31)
	55	1o	ECOG (27)
	199	7	WASSERMAN et al. (85)
MeCCNU	40	17.5	MOERTEL (31)
	168	11	WASSERMAN et al. (86)
Streptozotocin	32	6	MOERTEL et al. (32)
	50	1o	ECOG (27)
Procarbazine	38	3	ECOG (27)
Nitrogen mustard	58	15.5	CARTER and FRIEDMAN (89)
Chlorambucil	37	13.5	CARTER and FRIEDMAN (89)
Cyclophosphamide	89	27	CARTER and FRIEDMAN (89)
Melphalan	110	17	CARTER and FRIEDMAN (89)
Thio-TEPA	27	22	CARTER and FRIEDMAN (89)
Hexamethylmelamine	86	11.5	CARTER and FRIEDMAN (89)
Dibromodulcitol	15	O	CARTER and FRIEDMAN (89)
Mitomycin C	57	14	REITEMEIER et al. (33)
Actinomycin D	48	15	CARTER and FRIEDMAN (89)
Mithramycin	28	14	CARTER and FRIEDMAN (89)
Daunorubicin	9	O	CARTER and FRIEDMAN (89)
Adriamycin	92	9	CARTER and FRIEDMAN (89)
Bleomycin	15	O	MOERTEL et al. (34)
Porfiromycin	38	17	IZBICKI et al. (11)
Vincristine	26	O	CARTER and FRIEDMAN (89)
Vinblastine	64	5	CARTER and FRIEDMAN (89)
Azotomycin	85	16	ANSFIELD (35)
Camptothecin	61	3	MOERTEL et al. (36)
T.M.C.A.	28	4	CARTER and FRIEDMAN (89)

The nitrosoureas are still under investigation. BCNU and CCNU are distinctly inferior to 5-FU in terms of both the response rate and duration of response (83, 85). In a prospective, randomized trial, MeCCNU seemed to be at least equal or perhaps slightly better than 5-FU (83). There appears to be a cross-resistance between the fluorinated pyrimidines and the nitrosoureas. MOERTEL, who has had the most experience with nitrosoureas in colon cancer concluded that MeCCNU appears to be the best nitrosourea; however, as single agents the nitrosoureas offer at best only a small therapeutic contribution but they may be beneficial in combination therapy (31). Further studies in progress, using MeCCNU, are discussed by WASSERMAN et al. (86). Most of the newer experimental agents, such as emetine (96), 5-aza-cytidine, imidazole carboxamide, TIC mustard, camptothecin, and porfiromycin have had no significant effect (5). Corticosteroid therapy has no antineoplastic activity but produces some symptomatic improvement in patients with preterminal gastrointestinal cancer (97). ICRF-159 deserves further evaluation (21).

(ii) Combinations
Since few agents other than 5-FU produce tumor regression in at least 20 percent of cases, a multitude of highly effective combinations for colon cancer cannot be expected, and it is not surprising that dual combinations of 5-FU with cytosine arabinoside (12), vinblastine (14), BCNU (13), and mitomycin C (13) have not been more effective than 5-FU; the same is true of the triple combinations of 5-FU, BCNU, MTC (13) and 5-FU, CPM, VCR (19), and also of Cooper's regimen (5-FU, MTX, CPM, VCR, PDN) (56) (Table 25-5). Encouraging reports on two combinations need confirmation by means of studies with larger numbers of patients: 5-FU, CAR, MTC (9/15 or 60 percent regression rate) (16) and 5-FU , DIC, VCR, BCNU (12/28) (98). A synchronization protocol with VCR, 5-FU, and MTC is under study at the I.C.I.G. (see p. 148). In contrast to an earlier report (13), VAUGHN et al. reports significant responses with the combination of 5-FU + MTC (68 percent) and of 5-FU + MeCCNU (99). MOERTEL recently reported 43.5% objective regressions in 39 patients treated with 5-FU + MeCCNU + VCR (5). Intra-arterial chemotherapy is discussed in Chapter 12.

2. Strategy

(i) Localized Cancer of Colon and Rectum
The only curative procedure is surgical removal of the bowel containing the cancer and the lymph nodes draining it. Special surgical techniques (e.g., the "no-touch" approach) have been recommended to prevent local recurrence at the anastomosis and any dissemination of tumor cells during surgery.

Preoperative radiation sometimes has a favorable effect on rectal lesions (57, 100). It has been used by several groups to improve resectability rate by reducing the bulk of tumor, minimizing regional node metastases, minimizing distant metastases and reducing the rate of local recurrences at the anastomosis. Some survival gain has been claimed by some investigators but definitive studies are still in progress (100).

(ii) Adjuvant Chemotherapy
ROUSSELOT was able to improve the five-year survival of Dukes'C carcinoma from 27% to 64% by short-term adjuvant chemotherapy (58, 59). He instilled 5-FU intraluminally during surgery and also gave 5-FU intravenously for two days. Systemic adjuvant FUdR (60, 61) or thio-TEPA (22) was of no benefit in prolonging survival of patients after curative resection of the large bowel. Several studies are still in progress but thus far it does not appear that the course of the disease has been signifi-

Table 25-5. Response rates to combinations in large bowel cancers

Combination	Number evaluated	Number of reponses	Reference
5-FU, CAR	43	10 (23%)	GAILANI et al. (12)
5-FU, BCNU	20	1 (5%)	REITEMEIER et al. (13)
5-FU, MeCCNU	not given	(55%)	VAUGHN et al. (99)
5-FU, MTC	17	3 (17%)	REITEMEIER et al. (13)
	not given	(68%)	VAUGHN et al. (99)
5-FU, VLB	17	1 (6%)	AL-SARRAF et al. (14)
BCNU, MTC	19	2 (10%)	REITEMEIER et al. (13)
MeCCNU, CPM	11	3 (27%)	RIVA (65)
CPM, ACD	8	O	MOERTEL and REITEMEIER (15)
5-FU, CAR, MTC	15	9 (60%)	OTA et al. (16)
	21	5 (23%)	YAGODA et al. (17)
	31	3 (10%)	DeJAGER et al. (18)
5-FU, BCNU, MTC	18	1 (5.5%)	REITEMEIER et al. (13)
5-FU, CCNU, CPM	8	5	STAAB et al. (54)
5-FU, MeCCNU, VCR	39	17 (43.5%)	MOERTEL (5)
DIC, 5-FU, BCNU, VCR	28	12 (43%)	FALKSON et al. (98)
MTX, 5-FU, CPM, VCR (COMF)	3	2	HANHAM et al. (20)
MTX, 5-FU, CPM, VCR	4	1	LOKICH and SKARIN (55)
PDN (Cooper's)	44	10 (23%)	RAMIREZ (56)

cantly altered (89). Some surgeons have advocated the use of adjuvant chemotherapy (5-FU) following potentially curative surgery in patients in whom the risk of recurrences is high. Some months after the operation a "second-look" reexploration is carried out, in the hope that any nests of neoplastic cells not recognized at the primary operation and refractory to chemotherapy can be recognized and totally excised (62). The value of this approach remains uncertain.

(iii) Advanced Cancer of Colon and Rectum
Both surgery and radiotherapy (63, 64) can offer palliation in selected patients with advanced (or recurrent) colorectal cancers. The topic of "second-look surgery" for suspected recurrences in cancer of the large bowel has been reviewed by ELLIS (101). As in the case of gastric cancers, MOERTEL improved on the survival rate by adding 5-FU to radiotherapy (4, 36). CARTER and FRIEDMAN recently reviewed nine studies evaluating the combination of chemotherapy with radiotherapy and concluded that statistically valid superiority of one treatment mode over another was not achieved in any of the studies (89).

D. CANCER OF THE PANCREAS

Pancreas cancers are usually not detected until they are far advanced. Even in advanced cases the diagnosis is difficult to establish. The incidence in increasing, but no predisposing or etiological factors have yet been recognized.

1. Chemotherapy

As this is an adenocarcinoma of gastrointestinal origin, it is not surprising that 5-FU is the agent that has been used most often (Table 25-6). The response rate (8-22%) is rather lower than that for colon and stomach cancers (4, 5). Mitomycin C has produced response rates comparable to 5-FU. Experience with other agents and combination chemotherapy is too limited to permit any valid conclusions (Table 25-7) (5, 104). Combinations of 5-FU with BCNU (6, 7, 67, 102), testolactone, or spirolactone (68) appear to deserve further investigation to confirm preliminary results. Additional studies in progress are discussed by COMIS and CARTER (104).

Table 25-6. Effectiveness of single agents in pancreas carcinoma

Drug	Number evaluated	Number of responses	Reference
TIC mustard	4	0	MOERTEL et al. (29)
5-Fluorouracil	212	60 (28%)	CARTER and COMIS (104)
	31	5 (16%)	KOVACH et al. (8)
BCNU	37	0	CARTER and COMIS (104)
CCNU	19	3 (16%)	-
MeCCNU	13	0	-
Streptozotocin	27	3 (11%)	-
Nitrogen mustard	7	1	-
Chlorambucil	6	4	-
Cyclophosphamide	5	1	-
Hexamethylmelamine	6	0	BLUM et al. (9)
Mitomycin C	44	12 (27%)	CARTER and COMIS (104)
Mithramycin	4	0	LIVINGSTON and CARTER (1)
Porfiromycin	6	0	IZBICKI et al. (11)

2. Strategy

Radical surgery, the only procedure offering any hope of a cure, is rarely possible by the time the diagnosis is made (69, 104). Five-year survival rates are depressinly low (2-3%). Surgery and radiotherapy can offer some palliation. Concomitant 5-FU sometimes seems to improve the results of radiotherapy (4).

E. PRIMARY LIVER CANCER

The incidence of primary liver cancer (70, 71) varies widely in different countries. It is a rare tumor among the peoples of Western Europe and North America but not infrequent among inhabitants of Africa and parts of Asia. Liver cirrhosis, hemochromatosis, intestinal parasi-

Table 25-7. Response rates to combinations in pancreas carcinoma

Combination	Number evaluated	Number of responses	Reference
5-FU, CAR	1	1	GAILANI et al. (12)
5-FU, BCNU	30	10 (33%)	KOVACH et al. (6)
	15	4 (26%)	LOKICH et al. (101)
5-FU, CAR, MTC	3	0	DeJAGER et al. (18)
MTX, 5-FU, CPM, VCR	3	2	COSTANZI and COLTMAN (66)

tism and possibly aflatoxins are etiological factors. The development of hepatic angiosarcoma has been linked to exposure to vinyl chloride gas in the manufacture of polyvinyl chloride.

1. Chemotherapy

Few cytotoxic agents have been evaluated in large numbers of patients (5, 105). The overall response rate noted for 5-FU in one study was 40% in 28 patients treated (1). However, the ALGB noted only 2 regressions in 58 patients treated with 5-FU with or without cytosine arabinoside (12). AL-SARRAF noted no objective regressions in 16 patients treated with systemic chemotherapy (mostly 5-FU) (71). Systemic dichloromethotrexate, a folic-acid antagonist which is concentrated in the liver and converted to an inactive metabolite by normal liver cells but not by certain liver tumors, has not been effective (72). Adriamycin appears promising (106).

The proponents of intra-arterial chemotherapy have been favorably impressed (uncontrolled studies) by their results; in experienced hands this form of treatment can offer palliation for primary hepatomas as well as metastatic deposits (70, 71, 73-78).

2. Strategy

Major hepatic resection offers the only chance of cure but is possible in only 25% of cases, and is associated with considerable mortality (71, 77, 79, 80). Radiotherapy is of limited value since most lesions are not very radiosensitive and liver tolerance is limited (105).

REFERENCES

1. LIVINGSTON, R.B., CARTER, S.K.: Single agents in cancer chemotherapy. New York-Washington-London: IFI/Plenum 1970.
2. BLUM, CARTER, S.K., AGRE, K.: A clinical review of bleomycin. A new antineoplastic agent. Cancer 31, 903 (1973).
3. FALKSON, G.: Methyl-GAG (NSC-32946) in the treatment of esophagus cancer. Cancer Chemother. Rep. 55, 209 (1971).
4. MOERTEL, C.G., REITEMEIER, R.J.: Chemotherapy of gastrointestinal cancer. Surg. Clin. N. Amer. 47, 929 (1967).
5. MOERTEL, C.G.: Clinical management of advanced gastrointestinal cancer. Cancer 36, 675 (1975).

6. KOVACH, J.S., SCHUTT, A.J., HAHN, R.G., REITEMEIER, R.J., MOERTEL, C.G.: A controlled evaluation of 5-fluorouracil and 1-3-bis-(2-chlorethyl)-1-nitrosourea used alone and in combination for thera- py of advanced gastrointestinal cancer. Proc. Amer. Soc. clin. Oncol. 1973 (abstract 46).

7. DeCONTI, R.C., KAPLAN, S.R., PAPAC, R.J., CALABRESI, P.: Continuous intravenous infusions of 5-Fluoro-2'-deoxyuridine in the treatment of solid tumors. Cancer 31, 894 (1973).

8. KOVACH, J.S., MOERTEL, C.G., SCHUTT, A.J., HAHN, R.G., REITEMEIER, R.J.: A controlled study of combined 1,3-bis-(2-chloroethyl)-1-nitrosourea and 5-fluorouracil therapy for advanced gastric and pancreatic cancer. Cancer 33, 563 (1974).

9. BLUM, R.H., LIVINGSTON, R.B., CARTER, S.K.: Hexamethylmelamine. A new drug with activity in solid tumors. Europ. J. Cancer 9, 195 (1973).

10. FRANK, W., OSTERBERG, A.E.: Mitomycin C (NSC-26980) - an evaluation of the Japanese reports. Cancer Chemother. Rep. 9, 114 (1960).

11. IZBICKI, R., AL-SARRAF, M., REED, M.L., VAUGHN, C.B., VAITKEVICIUS, V.K.: Further clinical trials with porfiromycin (NSC-56410) (large intermittent doses). Cancer Chemother. Rep. 56, 615 (1972).

12. GAILANI, S., HOLLAND, J.F., FALKSON, G., LEONE, L., BURNINGHAM, R., LARSEN, V.: Comparison of treatment of metastatic gastrointes- tinal cancer with 5-fluorouracil (5FU) to a combination of 5-FU with cytosine arabinoside. Cancer 29, 1308 (1972).

13. REITEMEIER, R.J., MOERTEL, C.G., HAHN, R.G.: Combination chemo- therapy in gastrointestinal cancer. Cancer Res. 30, 1425 (1970).

14. AL-SARRAF, M., VAUGHN, C.B., REED, M.L., VAITKEVICIUS, V.K.: Com- bined 5-fluorouracil and vinblastine therapy for gastrointestinal and other solid tumors. Oncology 26, 99 (1972).

15. MOERTEL, G., REITEMEIER, R.J.: An evaluation of combined cyclo- phosphamide and actinomycin D in advanced gastrointestinal carcino- ma. Cancer Chemother. Rep. 28, 35 (1963).

16. OTA, K., KURITA, S., NISHIMURA, M., OGAWA, M., KAMEI, Y., IMAI, K., ARIYOSHI, Y., KATAOKA, K., MURAKAMI, M., OYAMA, A., HOSHINO, A., AMO, H., KATO, T.: Combination therapy with mitomycin C (NSC- 26980), 5-fluorouracil (NSC-19893), and cytosine arabinoside (NSC- 63878) for advanced cancer in man. Cancer Chemother. Rep. 56, 373 (1972).

17. YAGODA, A., LIPPMAN, A., WINN, R., ROSENBERG, A., SCHULMAN, P.: Mitomycin-C, 5-FU and cytosine (MiFuca) in adenocarcinomas. Proc. Amer. Ass. Cancer Res. 15, 190 (1974).

18. DEJAGER, R., MAGILL, G.B., GOLBEY, R.B., KRAKOFF, I.H.: Mitomycin C, 5-fluorouracil and cytosine arabinoside (MFC) in gastrointes- tinal cancer. Proc. Amer. Ass. Cancer Res. 15, 178 (1974).

19. MACDONALD, J., SCHEIN, P., UENO, W., WOOLLEY, P.: 5-fluorouracil, mitomycin-C and adriamycin (FAM): a new combination chemotherapy program for advanced gastric carcinoma. Proc. Amer. Soc. Clin. Oncol. 17, 264 (1976).

20. HANHAM, I.W.F., NEWTON, K.A., WESTBURY, G.: Seventy-five cases of solid tumours treated by a modified quadruple chemotherapy regime. Brit. J. Cancer 25, 462 (1971).

21. MARCINIAK, T.A., MOERTEL, C.G., SCHUTT, A.J., HAHN, R.G., REITE- MEIER, R.J.: Phase II study of ICRF-159 (NSC-129943) in advanced colorectal carcinoma. Cancer Chemother. Rep. Part 1, 59, 761 (1975).

22. DIXON, W.J., LONGMIRE, Jr., W.P., HOLDEN, W.D.: Use of triethylene- thiophosphoramide as an adjuvant to the surgical treatment of gastric and colorectal carcinoma: ten-year follow-up. Ann. Surg. 173, 26 (1971).

23. V.A. COOPERATIVE SURGICAL ADJUVANT GROUP: Use of thioTEPA as an adjuvant to the surgical management of carcinoma of the stomach. Cancer 18, 291 (1965).

24. SERLIN, O., WOLKOFF, J.S., AMADEO, J.M., KEEHN, R.J.: Use of 5-fluorodeoxyuridine (FUDR) as an adjuvant to the surgical management of carcinoma of the stomach. Cancer 24, 223 (1969).

25. BLIXENKRONE-MØLLER, N.: Long-term results of chemotherapy of operable cancer of the gastro-intestinal tract. Acta chir. scand. 133, 157 (1967).

26. MOERTEL, C.G., REITEMEIER, F.R.: Advanced gastrointestinal cancer. Clinical management and chemotherapy. New York-Evanston-London: Harper & Row 1969.

27. HORTON, J., MITTELMAN, A., TAYLOR III, S.G., et al.: Phase II trials with procarbazine (NSC-77213), streptozotocin (NSC-85998), 6-thioguanine (NSC-752), and CCNU (NSC-79037) in patients with metastatic cancer of the large bowel. Cancer Chemother. Rep. Part 1, 59, 333 (1975).

28. MOERTEL, C.G., REITEIMEIER, R.J., HAHN, R.G., SCHUTT, A.: Study of 5-(3,3-dimethyl-1-triazeno)imidazole-4-carboxamide (NSC-45388) in patients with gastrointestinal carcinoma. Cancer Chemother. Rep. 54, 471 (1970).

29. MOERTEL, C.G., SCHUTT, A.J., REITEMEIER, R.J., HAHN, R.G.: Phase II study of 5-(3,3-bis(2-chloroethyl)-1-triazeno)imidazole-4-carboxamide (NSC-82196) in advanced gastrointestinal cancer. Cancer Chemother. Rep. 56, 267 (1972).

30. MOERTEL, C.G., SCHUTT, A.J., REITEMEIER, R.J., HAHN, R.G.: Phase II study of 5-azacytidine (NSC-102816) in the treatment of advanced gastrointestinal cancer. Cancer Chemother. Rep. 56, 649 (1972).

31. MOERTEL, C.G.: Therapy of advanced gastrointestinal cancer with the nitrosoureas. Cancer Chemother. Rep. Part 3, 4, 27 (1973).

32. MOERTEL, C.G., REITEMEIER, R.J., SCHUTT, A.J., HAHN, R.G.: Phase II study of streptozotocin (NSC-85998) in the treatment of advanced gastrointestinal cancer. Cancer Chemother. Rep. 55, 303 (1971).

33. REITEMEIER, R.J., MOERTEL, C.G., HAHN, R.G.: Mitomycin C therapy of advanced gastrointestinal adenocarcinoma. Comparison of short and long treatment schedules. Proc. Amer. Ass. Cancer Res. 8, 56 (1967).

34. MOERTEL, C.G., ARENA, P.J., SCHUTT, A.J., REITEMEIER, R.J., HAHN, R.G.: Phase II study of bleomycin (NSC-125066) therapy for large bowel cancer. Cancer Chemother. Rep. 56, 207 (1972).

35. ANSFIELD, F.J.: Carcinoma of the digestive tract. In: Cancer Chemotherapy, p. 132 (eds. F. Elkerbout, P. Thomas, A. Zwaveling). Leiden: Leiden University Press 1971.

36. MOERTEL, C.G., SCHUTT, A.J., REITEMEIER, R.J., HAHN, R.G.: Phase II study of camptothecin (NSC-100880) in the treatment of advanced gastrointestinal cancer. Cancer Chemother. Rep. Part 1, 56, 95 (1972).

37. KAUFMAN, S.: 5-Fluorouracil in the treatment of gastrointestinal meoplasia. New Engl. J. Med. 288, 199 (1973).

38. Correspondence: 5-Fluorouracil in the treatment of gastrointestinal neoplasia. New Engl. J. Med. 288, 910 (1973).

39. CURRERI, A.R., ANSFIELD, F.J., McIVER, F.A., WAISMAN, H.A., HEIDELBERGER, C.: Clinical studies with 5-fluorouracil. Cancer Res. 18, 478 (1958).

40. ANSFIELD, F.J.: A less toxic fluorouracil dosage schedule. J. Amer. med. Ass. 190, 686 (1964).

41. HORTON, J., OLSON, K.B., SULLIVAN, J., REILLY, C., SHNIDER, B.: 5-Fluorouracil in cancer: an improved regimen. Ann. intern. Med. 73, 897 (1970).

42. JACOBS, E., LUCE, J., WOOD, D.: Treatment of cancer with weekly intravenous 5-fluorouracil. Cancer 22, 1233 (1968).

43. KRANT, M.J.: Alterations in the administration of 5-fluorouracil experiences with two-hour infusions. Cancer Chemother. Rep. 15, 35 (1961).

44. REITEMEIER, R.J., MOERTEL, C.G.: Comparison of rapid and slow intravenous administration of 5-fluorouracil in treating patients with advanced carcinoma of the large intestin. Cancer Chemother. Rep. 25, 87 (1962).
45. CRESSY, N.L., SCHELL, H.W.: Effectiveness and toxicity of prolonged infusions of 5-fluorouracil in the treatment of cancer. Amer. J. med. Sci. 249, 52 (1965).
46. SEIFERT, P., BAKER, L.H., REED, M.L., VAITKEVICIUS, V.K.: Comparison of continuously infused 5-fluorouracil with bolus injection in treatment of patients with colorectal adenocarcinoma. Cancer 36, 123 (1975).
47. MOERTEL, C.G., SCHUTT, A.J., REITEMEIER, R.J., HAHN, R.G.: A comparison of 5-fluorouracil administration by slow infusion and rapid injection. Cancer Res. 32, 2717 (1972).
48. JOHNSON, E.C., ANSFIELD, F.J., RAMIREZ, G., DAVIS, Jr., H.L.: Further clinical studies of 5-fluorouracil (5-FU; NSC-19893) given by the multiple daily dose method in disseminated breast cancer. Cancer Chemother. Rep. 57, 59 (1973).
49. LAHIRI, S.R., BOILEAU, G., HALL, T.C.: Treatment of metastatic colorectal carcinoma with 5-fluorouracil by mouth. Cancer 28, 902 (1971).
50. BATEMAN, J.R., PUGH, R.P., CASSIDY, F.R., MARSHALL, G.J., IRWIN, L.E.: 5-Fluorouracil given once weekly: comparison of intravenous and oral administration. Cancer 28, 907 (1971).
51. BRUCKNER, H.W., CREASEY, W.A.: The administration of 5-fluorouracil by mouth. Cancer 33, 14 (1974).
52. HAHN, R.G., MOERTEL, C.G., SCHUTT, A.J., BRUCKNER, H.W.: A controlled comparison of intensive 5-FU by oral vs. IV route in colorectal carcinoma. Proc. amer. Ass. Cancer Res. 15, 191 (1974).
53. SCHUTT, A.J., HAHN, R.G., REITEMEIER, R.J., MOERTEL, C.G.: A phase 2 study of intermittent high-dose cyclophosphamide therapy of advanced gastrointestinal cancer. Cancer Res. 33, 2218 (1973).
54. STAAB, R.C., RODRIGUEZ, V., HART, J.S.: FCC (5-fluorouracil, cyclophosphamide and CCNU) for metastatic adenocarcinoma. Proc. amer. Ass. Cancer Res. 15, 174 (1974).
55. LOKICH, J.J., SKARIN, A.T.: Five-drug combination chemotherapy for disseminated adenocarcinoma. Cancer Chemother. Rep. 56, 761 (1972).
56. RAMIREZ, G. (Clinical Oncology Group): Five-drug combination therapy in the treatment of solid tumors. Proc. Amer. Ass. Cancer Res. 14, 17 (1973).
57. ROSWIT, B., HIGGINS, G.A., KEEHN, R.J.: Preoperative irradiation for carcinoma of the rectum and rectosigmoid colon: report of a National Veterans Administration randomized study. Cancer 35, 1597 (1975).
58. ROUSSELOT, L.M., COLE, D.R., GROSSI, C.E., CONTE, A.J., GONZALEZ, E.M., PASTERNACK, B.S.: A five-year progress report on the effectiveness of intraluminal chemotherapy (5-fluorouracil) adjuvant to surgery for colon rectal cancer. Amer. J. Surg. 115, 140 (1968).
59. ROUSSELOT, L.M., COLE, D.R., GROSSI, C.E., CONTE, A.J., GONZALEZ, E.M., PASTERNACK, B.S.: Adjuvant chemotherapy with 5-fluorouracil in surgery for colorectal cancer. Dis. Colon Rect. 15, 169 (1972).
60. HIGGINS, G.A., WHITE, G.E.: Adjuvant chemotherapy and cancer surgery. Surgery Annual, p. 305 (ed. P. Cooper) 1969.
61. DWIGHT, R.W., HUMPHREY, E.W., HIGGINS, G.A., KEEHN, R.J.: FUDR as an adjuvant to surgery in cancer of the large bowel. J. Surg. Oncol. 5, 243 (1973).
62. MACKMANN, S., CURRERI, A.R., ANSFIELD, F.J.: Second-look operation for colon carcinoma after fluorouracil therapy. Arch. Surg. 100, 527 (1970).
63. WHITELEY, Jr., H.W., STEAR, Jr., M.W., LEAMING, R.H., DEDDISH, M.R.: Radiation therapy in the palliative management of patients with recurrent cancer of the rectum and colon. Surg. Clin. N. Amer. 49, 381 (1969).

64. URDANETA-LAFEE, N., KLIGERMAN, M.M., KNOWITON, A.H.: Evaluation of palliative irradiation in rectal carcinoma. Radiology 104, 673 (1972).
65. RIVA, A.: Me-CCNU versus Me-CCNU and cyclophosphamide (CTX) in gastrointestinal carcinoma. Proc. Amer. Ass. Cancer Res. 15, 91 (1974).
66. COSTANZI, J.J., COLTMAN, Jr., C.A.: Combination chemotherapy using cyclophosphamide, vincristine, methotrexate and 5-fluorouracil in solid tumors. Cancer 23, 590 (1969).
67. LOKICH, J.L., SKARIN, A.T.: Combination therapy with 5-fluorouracil and 1,3-bis(2-chloroethyl)-1-nitrosoureas (BCNU) for disseminated gastrointestinal carcinoma. Cancer Chemother. Rep. 56, 653 (1972).
68. WADDELL, W.R.: Chemotherapy for carcinoma of the pancreas. Surgery 74, 420 (1973).
69. BOWDEN, L.: Cancer of the pancreas. CA, 22, 274 (1972).
70. EL-DOMEIRI, A.A., HUVOS, A.G., GOLDSMITH, H.S., FOOTE, Jr., F.W.: Primary malignant tumors of the liver. Cancer 27, 7 (1971).
71. Al-SARRAF, M., KIHIER, K., VAITKEVICIUS, V.K.: Primary liver cancer. A review of the clinical features, blood groups, serum enzymes, therapy, and survival of 65 cases. Cancer 33, 574 (1974).
72. VOGEL, C.L., ADAMSON, R.H., DeVITA, V.T., JOHNS, D.G., KYALWAZI, S.K.: Preliminary clinical trials of dichloromethotrexate (NSC-29630) in hepatocellular carcinoma. Cancer Chemother. Rep. 56, 249 (1972).
73. CLARKSON, B., YOUNG, C., DIERICK, W., KUEHN, P., KIM, W., BERRETT, A., CLAPP, P., LAWRENCE, Jr., W.: Effects of continuous hepatic artery infusion of antimetabolites on primary and metastatic cancer of the liver. Cancer 15, 472 (1962).
74. ARIEL, I.M., PACK, G.T.: Intra-arterial chemotherapy for cancer metastatic liver. Arch. Surg. 91, 851 (1965).
75. ROCHLIN, D.B., SMART, C.R.: An evaluation of 51 patients with hepatic artery infusion. Surg. Gynec. Obstet. 123, 535 (1966).
76. ARIEL, I.M., PACK, G.T.: Treatment of inoperable cancer of the liver by intra-arterial radioactive isotopes and chemotherapy. Cancer 20, 793 (1967).
77. FORTNER, J.G., MULCARE, R.J., SOLIS, A., WATSON, R.C., GOLBEY, R.B.: Treatment of primary and secondary liver cancer by hepatic artery ligation and infusion chemotherapy. Ann. Surg. 178, 162 (1973).
78. FORTNER, J.G., EL-CASTRO, B., GOLBEY, R., KRAKOFF, I.H., CAIRD WATSON, R., YEH, S.D.J., SHIU, M.H., KINNE, D.W., LISE, M., MABOGUNJE, O.: Quadruple drug therapy combined with surgery for hepatoma and metastatic colon cancer. Proc. Amer. Ass. Cancer Res. 15, 193 (1974).
79. CHAN, K.T.: The management of primary liver carcinoma. Ann. roy. Coll. Surg. Engl. 41, 253 (1967).
80. BRASFIELD, R.D., BOWDEN, L., McPEAK, C.J.: Major hepatic resection for malignant neoplasms of the liver. Ann. Surg. 176, 171 (1972).
81. AMERICAN JOINT COMMITTEE FOR CANCER STAGING AND END RESULTS REPORTING: Clinical staging system for carcinoma of the esophagus. CA 25, 50 (1975).
82. KENNEDY, B.J.: TNM classification for stomach cancer. Cancer 26, 317 (1970).
83. COMIS, R.L., CARTER, S.K.: A review of chemotherapy in gastric cancer. Cancer 34, 1576 (1974).
84. BRUGAROLAS, A., GARCIA, M., LACAVE, A.J.: Chemotherapy in advanced gastric cancer. A controlled clinical study. Proc. Am. Ass. Cancer Res. 16, 169 (1975).
85. WASSERMAN, T.H., SLAVIK, M., CARTER, S.K.: Review of CCNU in clinical cancer therapy. Cancer Treat. Rev. 1, 131 (1974).
86. WASSERMAN, T.H., SLAVIK, M., CARTER, S.K.: Methyl-CCNU in clinical cancer therapy. Cancer Treat. Rev. 1, 251 (1974).

87. MOERTEL, C.G., HANLEY, J.A.: Phase II-III studies in chemotherapy of advanced gastric cancer. Proc. Am. Soc. Clin. Oncol. 16, 260 (1975).

88. KIM, P.M., DE MATTIA, M., BUROKER, T., VAITKEVICIUS, V.K.: Mitomycin C alone and in combination with infused 5-fluorouracil in treatment of disseminated gastrointestinal carcinomas. Proc. Am. Soc. Clin. Oncol. 16, 230 (1975).

89. CARTER, S.K., FRIEDMAN, M.: Integration of chemotherapy into combined modality treatment of solid tumors. II. Large bowel cancer. Cancer Treat. Rev. 1, 111 (1974).

90. LEONE, L.A.: The chemotherapy of colorectal cancer. Cancer 34, 972 (1974).

91. MOERTEL, C.H., SCHUTT, A.J., REITEMEIER, R.J.: Effects of patient selection on results of phase II chemotherapy trials in gastrointestinal cancer. Cancer Chemother. Rep. Part 1, 58, 257 (1974).

92. MOERTEL, G.C.: Sequential 1-(2-chloroethyl)-3-cyclohexyl-1-nitrosourea and 5-fluoro-uracil therapy of gastrointestinal cancer. Cancer Res. 32, 1280 (1972).

93. BATEMAN, J., IRWIN, L., PUGH, R., CASSIDY, F., WEINER, J.: Comparison of intravenous and oral administration of 5-fluorouracil for colorectal carcinoma. Proc. Am. Soc. Clin. Oncol. 16, 242 (1975).

94. HAHN, R.G., MOERTEL, C.G., SCHUTT, A.J., BRUCKNER, H.W.: A double-blind comparison of intensive course 5-fluorouracil by oral versus intravenous route in the treatment of colorectal carcinoma. Cancer 35, 1031 (1975).

95. VALDIVIESO, M., BODEY, G.P., McKELVEY, E.M., GOTTLIEB, J.A.: Initial clinical studies with Ftorafur. Proc. Am. Ass. Cancer Res. 16, 86 (1975).

96. MOERTEL, C.G., SCHUTT, A.J., HAHN, R.G., REITEMEIER, R.J.: Treatment of advanced gastrointestinal cancer with emetine. Cancer Chemother. Rep. Part 1, 58, 229 (1974).

97. MOERTEL, C.G., SCHUTT, A.J., REITEMEIER, R.J., HAHN, R.G.: Corticosteroid therapy of preterminal gastrointestinal cancer. Cancer 33, 1607 (1974).

98. FALKSON, G., van EDEN, E.B., FALKSON, H.C.: Fluorouracil, imidazole carboxamide, dimethyl triazeno, vincristine, and bis-chloroethyl nitrosourea in colon cancer. Cancer 33, 1207 (1974).

99. VAUGHN, C.B., CHINN, B.J., DAVERSA, G., PARZUCHOWSKI, J.: Comparison of combination chemotherapy in advanced gastrointestinal malignancy. Proc. Amer. Soc. Clin. Oncol. 16, 252 (1975).

100. BRADY, L.W., ANTONIADES, J., PRASASVINICHAI, S., TORPIE, R.J., ASBELL, S.O., GLASSBURN, J.R.: Preoperative radiation therapy. Cancer 34, 960 (1974).

101. ELLIS, H.: "Second look surgery" for suspected recurrences in cancer of the large bowel. Cancer Treat. Rev. 1, 205 (1974).

102. LOKICH, J., CHAWLA, P.L., BROOKS, J., FREI, E.: Chemotherapy in pancreatic carcinoma: 5-fluorouracil and 1,3 bis-(2-chloroethyl)-1-nitrosourea. Ann. Surg. 179, 450 (1974).

103. FRYTAK, S., MOERTEL, C.G. SCHUTT, A.J., et al.: Adriamycin (NSC-123127) therapy for advanced gastrointestinal cancer. Cancer Chemother. Rep. Part 1, 59, 405 (1975).

104. CARTER, S.K., COMIS, R.L.: The integration of chemotherapy into a combined modality approach for cancer treatment. VI. Pancreatic adenocarcinoma. Cancer Treat. Rev. 2, 193 (1975).

105. FALKSON, G.: Therapeutic approaches to hepatoma. Cancer Treat. Rev. 2, 73 (1975).

106. OLWENY, C.L.M., TOYA, T., KATONGOLE-MBIDDE, E., et al.: Treatment of hepatocellular carcinoma with adriamycin. Cancer 36, 1250 (1975).

Chapter 26

Breast Cancer

Breast cancer is the most common cancer in women, accounting for almost 25% of all malignancies recorded in female patients. It is the major cause of death among middle-aged women in America. Two thirds of patients develop disseminated disease and require systemic therapy. Two major phases can be distinguished in the management of breast cancer. The primary tumor is first treated locally by surgery with or without radiotherapy. Only 40% of those presenting with localized disease are cured. After a clinically disease-free interval, disseminated disease requiring hormonal or cytotoxic therapy, is noted in the other 60%. Approximately one sixth of patients present with disseminated disease. A number of features influence the prognosis of the disease (1-6). Most important is the clinical stage.

Different systems are in use to classify the disease into various stages. The most popular ones are the TNM classification (7, 8, 150), and the Columbia classification (Tables 26-1, 26-2). They take into account several features that influence survival: the size of the primary tumor (9), its fixation to the skin and underlying tissues, presence, size and fixation of axillary lymph nodes, the histology of the regional lymph nodes (151), and distant metastases. The cell type and grade of malignancy (10, 11) and the disease-free interval between the diagnosis of the primary and subsequent dissemination (5) are also important, as is the location of metastasis (soft tissues, visceral, osseous) (10). The age and the menstrual status (premenopause, menopause, postmenopause) influence prognosis (5), and the menstrual status constitutes a dividing line in the management of patients with recurrent breast cancer in view of the hormone dependency of breast tumors.

A. HORMONE THERAPY

Figure 26-1, borrowed from STOLL (12, 13) illustrates the relationship between various hormones and the growth of mammary carcinoma. The growth can be influenced by estrogens and progesterone of either ovarian or adrenal origin. It is probably influenced by androgens secreted by the ovary and the adrenal gland, and possibly by adrenal corticosteroids and the thyroid hormones. These hormones in turn alter the pituitary secretion of gonadotrophin and ACTH, which affect the growth of the tumor indirectly. The pituitary has a direct influence through its secretion of prolactin. Prolactin stimulates the induction and growth of experimental tumors but there is no clear evidence that this hormone plays a significant role in human breast cancer (152, 153).

Table 26-1. TNM staging for breast cancer

T1S Pre-invasive carcinoma, so-called carcinoma in situ, non-infiltra-
     ting intraductal carcinoma or Paget's disease of the nipple with
     no demonstrable tumor
     Note: Paget's disease associated with a demonstrable tumor is
           classified according to the size of the tumor

T0   No demonstrable tumor in the breast

T1   Tumor of 2 cm or less in its greatest dimension
     T1a With no fixation to underlying pectoral fascia and/or muscle
     T1b With fixation to underlying pectoral fascia and/or muscle

T2   Tumor more than 2 cm but not more than 5 cm in its greatest
     dimension
     T2a With no fixation to underlying pectoral fascia and/or muscle
     T2b With fixation to underlying pectoral and/or muscle

T3   Tumor more than 5 cm in its greatest dimension
     T3a With no fixation to underlying pectoral fascia and/or muscle
     T3b With fixation to underlying pectoral fascia and/or muscle
      Note: Dimpling of the skin, nipple retraction or any other skin
            changes except those in T4b may occur in T1, T2, or T3
            without affecting the classification.

T4   Tumor of any size with direct extension to chest wall or skin
      Note: Chest wall includes ribs, intercostal muscles, and serratus
            anterior muscle but not pectoral muscle.
     T4a With fixation to chest wall
     T4b With edema, infiltration or ulceration of skin of breast
          (including peau d'orange), or satellite skin nodules con-
          fined to the same breast
     T4c Both of above

N0   No palpable homolateral axillary nodes
N1   Movable homolateral axillary nodes
     N1a Nodes not considered to contain growth
     N1b Nodes considered to contain growth

N2   Homolateral axillary nodes fixed to one another or to other
     structures

N3   Homolateral supraclavicular or infraclavicular nodes or edema
     of the arm
      Note: Edema of the arm may be caused by lymphatic obstruction;
            lymph nodes may not then be palpable.

M0   No evidence of distant metastases
M1   Distant metastases present including skin involvement beyond the
     breast area

Stage Grouping

TIS   Carcinoma in situ
With M0 Stage grouping is as follows:

Stage I	T1a	N0 or N1a		Stage III	Any T3 with any N	
	T1b	N0 or N1a			Any T4 with any N	
Stage II	T0	N1b			Any T with	N2
	T1a	N1b			Any T with	N3
	T1b	N1b				
	T2a or T2b	NO or N1a				
	T2a	N1b				
	T2b	N1b				

With M1 Stage must be IV

Table 26-2. Columbia staging for breast cancer (From HAAGENSEN)

Clinical Stage	Clinical Features
A	1. No clinically involved axillary nodes 2. No grave signs as in clinical stage C
B	1. Clinically involved axillary nodes less than 2,5 cm transverse diameter 2. No grave signs as in clinical stage C

C	Any one of five signs
	  1. Edema of skin limited extent (less than one third of skin involved)
	  2. Ulceration of skin
	  3. Solid fixation primary tumor to chest wall
	  4. Axillary nodes 2.5 cm or more transverse diameter
	  5. Fixation axillary nodes to overlying or surrounding tissues

D	All more advanced cases

Hypothalamic centers control the release of pituitary trophic hormones. They secrete an inhibiting factor for prolactin but a releasing factor for growth hormone, adenocorticotrophin, and gonadotrophin. Catecholamines have been shown to play a major role in the function of the hypothalamo-hypophyseal axis (14, 15); dopamine and its precurcors, L-dopa, increase catecholamine levels in the hypothalamus and depress the blood level of prolactin, which may explain the tumor regressions noted in some patients treated with L-dopa. A beneficial effect seems to depend on adequate levels of either endogenous or administered estrogen.

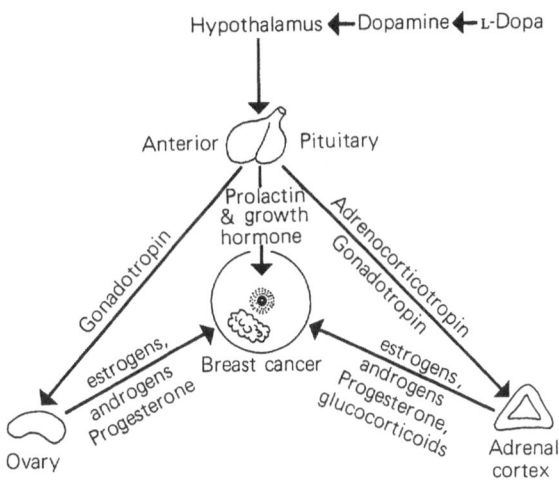

Fig. 26-1. Diagrammatic representation of the hormonal factors which influence the growth of breast cancer in the female. ⟶ Denotes a controlling effect. (Modified from STOLL (23))

Two types of hormone therapy are commonly used in breast cancer (12, 13, 154). Additive therapy consists of the administration of estrogens, progesterone, or androgens. Ablative therapy removes the organs that produce the hormones thought to influence the growth of the tumor. In many cases of disseminated breast cancer, oophorectomy, adrenalectomy, or hypophysectomy is thus carried out at some stage in the management (6, 16, 17). Estrogens suppress pituitary secretion of gonadotrophin, and, at certain dose levels, of prolactin. Thus the effect of steroid hormones may be a direct one on the tumor and an indirect one via the pituitary. Glucocorticosteroids effect a medical adrenalectomy. The effect of hormone manipulation (additive or ablative) cannot always be easily explained. For instance, ablation of the ovaries or adrenals and the administration of their hormonal secretion, two diametrically opposite methods, have both been used successfully in many patients. Other mechanisms may be involved, such as the transformation of androgens into estrogens, possibly by the tumor itself (18).

Androgens may achieve an anti-estrogen effect by blockade of the receptors in the tumor. Specific estrogen receptors are in fact present in the cytoplasm of certain mammary carcinoma cells (19-21), and the responsiveness of human breast cancer to estrogen has been correlated with the presence of estrogen receptors.

It would be logical to suppose that tumors showing estrogen binding would be the ones likely to respond to ablative therapy. Some investigators (19, 21, 155, 156), but not all (22), have confirmed this hypothesis.

1. Estrogens

Treatment with estrogens results in 20-40% objective responses. No comparative study has demonstrated the superiority of one estrogen over another. Diethylstilbestrol and ethinyl estradiol are the most popular preparations (see Chapt. 5) (Table 26-3).

Table 26-3. Effectiveness of estrogens in advanced breast cancer

Drug	Number treated	Objective responses (%)	References
Various estrogen preparations	364	36	Council on Drugs (AMA) (23)
	407	31	STOLL (12)
Diethylstilbestrol	261	18	Co-operative Breast Cancer Group (24)
	55	29	KENNEDY (25)

Estrogen administration is a simple initial method of endocrine therapy recommended in postmenopausal women with advanced disease and in whom vaginal smear reveals no evidence of estrogen secretion. The reponse rate rises with increasing interval since menopause and with increasing duration of the disease-free interval (13). Cutaneous and bone metastases respond better than visceral lesions (liver, lung, brain). The average duration of response is 16.5 months and the survival of responding patients is prolonged (13). Estrogen therapy should be tried for 2 to 3 months unless there is definite exacerbation of the disease. The first evidence of tumor regression usually appears within 6 weeks but can be delayed even longer. Patients must be watched carefully in the early weeks of estrogen administration for hypercalcemia, estrogen intolerance (especially gastrointestinal), fluid retention or, rarely, tumor stimulation. Estrogens are generally continued as long as the disease is under control. STOLL prefers intermittent administration with discontinuation of estrogens as soon as complete regression of visible tumor has occurred (13). When tumor activity recurs after prolonged control by means of estrogen maintenance, withdrawal of therapy may lead to another regression in 10-30% of cases by inducing another

Table 26-4. Effectiveness of androgens in advanced breast cancer

Drug	Number treated	Objective response (%)	References
Testosterone propionate, i.m.	521	21.5[a]	Co-operative Breast Cancer Group (33)
	518	13.5[b]	Co-operative Breast Cancer Group (24)
	269	11	STOLL (12)
	59	10	KENNEDY (25)
	49	16	EORTC (34)
	65	14	EORTC (35)
	40	18	Japanese co-operative Group (30)
Drostanolone propionate	96	26[a]	Co-operative Breast Cancer Group (36)
	193	20[b]	Co-operative Breast Cancer Group (24)
	165	19	TALLEY et al. (32)
Fluoxymesterone, p.o.	106	15[a]	Co-operative Breast Cancer Group (36)
	160	15[b]	Co-operative Breast Cancer Group (24)
	116	20	STOLL (14)
Delta-1-testololactone i.m.	70	13	Co-operative Breast Cancer Group (24)
	59	15	EORTC (34)
	24	8	TALLEY et al. (32)
p.o.	65	20	Co-operative Breast Cancer Group (24)
	32	12.5	CANTINO and GORDAN (37)
	115	18	Co-operative Breast Cancer Group (29)
Calusterone	99	43	GORDAN et al. (31)
	109	28	Co-operative Breast Cancer Group (29)

[a] Studies carried out in 1956-1960.
[b] Studies carried out in 1961-1963.

abrupt change in the internal milieu (26, 27). Thus an observation period of 6-8 weeks without therapy can be useful, except in the presence
of rapidly advancing disease.

2. Androgens

Androgens are generally used after other endocrine manipulations. They
can be prescribed in postmenopausal women who no longer respond to
estrogen (or withdrawal of estrogens) or in premenopausal women in whom
exacerbation is observed after regression induced by castration (28).
Androgens (RR 10-25%) are generally less effective than estrogens in
postmenopausal women (20-40%) (Tables 26-4, 26-5). As with estrogens,
the response rate improves with increasing length of time since menopause and increasing duration of disease-free intervals (13). Bone
metastases and local lesions respond more frequently than visceral metastases (13, 29, 30). Stimulation of erythropoiesis and an anabolic
effect (weight gain, improved appetite, and energy) are useful additional effects that occur in some cases. Six weeks of therapy are usually required before signs of a tumor regression become evident. An androgen trial should not be abandoned after less than 2-3 months unless
disease is rapidly advancing. A withdrawal reponse is seen in approximately 10% of patients who have responded to androgens.

The greatest problem with androgen therapy is virilization. Many ste-
roidal compounds have been examined in the hope that a compound more
effective and less masculinizing than the standard testosterone propionate might be found (Table 26-4). While some are less virilizing
their response rates are not much better than that of testosterone propionate. Calusterone deserves further trials (29, 31).

Androgen therapy is best started with a parenteral preparation, preferably a quick-acting one, so that its effect can be promptly terminated
if deterioration or hypercalcemia is observed shortly after the initiation of androgen therapy. If the hormone is tolerated, a switch can be
made to the longer-acting parenteral esters. The oral preparations
(methyltestosterone, fluoxymesterone) may not be sufficiently potent
to induce a remission, but can be used to maintain a remission. Studies
are in progress to determine whether calusterone will be more effective

Table 26-5. Comparison of estrogens and androgens in advanced breast
cancer

Drugs	Objective response		References
	Estrogens	Androgens	
Estrogens vs. androgens	37%	21%	Council on Drugs (23)
Estrogens vs. androgens	31%	15%	STOLL (12)
DES[a] vs. testosterone propionate[b]	16%	10%	Co-operative Breast Cancer Group (24)
DES[a] vs. testosterone propionate[b]	29%	10%	KENNEDY (25)
Stilbestrol vs. methyl-testosterone	23%	24%	JONES et al. (38)

[a] DES = diethylstilbestrol.
[b] Controlled comparative trials.

444

in the induction of remission (29, 31). Androgen therapy can be either continuous or intermittent (see p. 443) (13). The response rate may be dose-related (32).

3. Progestational Agents

The place of progestational agents in the treatment of advanced breast cancer is less well defined than that of other hormones (154). The most effective preparation and the most suitable phase for progestational agents in the sequence of hormone manipulations are not known. A wide range of response rates has been published (Table 26-6). Progestational agents are not as active as estrogens, and in one controlled trial the response rate was lower than that for androgens (38). From this study, the authors concluded that progestins (17α-hydroxyprogesterone caproate, Primolut, 250 mg i.m., three times weekly) have no place in the treatment of patients with generalized disease since only 1/24 patients (4%) responded. A 19% (3/16) response rate was obtained in patients with localized disease. STOLL has observed that women whose vaginal smears are characterized by a predominance of intermediate cells probably show the best response (12, 13, 39). This suggests that some estrogen priming effect is necessary for their function. Combinations of progestins and estrogens can be more effective than progestins alone. Some patients who fail to improve with estrogens alone (5, 47, 49) or after adrenalectomy and hypophysectomy (28, 48, 50) still respond to the combination. Soft-tissue metastases improve more often than bone or visceral lesions (13, 46). The regression rate is higher when progestins are used as the first method of hormone manipulation and with long disease-free intervals; age, however, has no significant influence on the response rate (13). AHMANN et al. failed to demonstrate the superiority of a stilbestrol-medrogestone (an oral progesterone) combination over stilbestrol alone (157).

Table 26-6. Effectiveness of progestins in advanced breast cancer

Drug	Number treated	Objective reponse (%)	References
Various progestins	115	16	Co-operative Breast Cancer Group (36)
	80	20	STOLL (39)
17α-Hydroxy-progesterone caproate	20	0	
	40	10	JONES et al. (38)
Medroxyprogesterone	24	25	Co-operative Breast Cancer Group (24)
	23	0	SEGALOFF et al. (40)
	34	20	MUGGIA et al. (41)
	30	37	BUCALOSSI et al. (42)
Norethisterone	121	43	CURWEN (43)
	45	38	DARGENT et al. (44)
	28	28	GORINS and NETTER (45)
	154	41	EDELSTYN (46)

4. Corticosteroid and Other Agents

It is thought that corticosteroid exert their action in disseminated breast cancer by effecting a "medical" adrenalectomy; however, they are less effective than surgical adrenalectomy (51, 52). STOLL reports significant tumor regression in only 15% of cases, and this is usually incomplete and of short duration (about six months) (13, 53). Corticosteroids sometimes have a striking effect in seriously ill patients. Dyspnea associated with lymphangitic pulmonary involvement, intracranial hypertension due to cerebral metastases, jaundice due to hepatic metastases and hypercalcemia often respond to steroid therapy. They are useful in patients who have documented hormone-dependent tumors and could not tolerate ablative therapy or chemotherapy. Corticosteroid therapy has been suspected of facilitating tumor dissemination, especially in the form of gastroduodenal metastases (54).

Thyroid hormones have been used in the past but recent studies fail to confirm their efficacy (55).

Several estrogen antagonists have been the subject of preliminary trials. The EORTC Breast Cancer Group obtained 8 objective regressions in 23 evaluable patients (35%) with nafoxidine (56). COLE noted 10 regressions in 46 patients treated with tamoxifen (57). The effectiveness of these drugs was confirmed by WARD (148) and BLOOM (149).

Inhibitors of prolactin secretion, which are effective in rat mammary carcinoma (58), have been ineffective in women with breast cancer (59, 60). Some tumor regressions have already been reported with L-dopa, another agent that inhibits prolactin secretion (selective "medical hyophysectomy") (14, 15). When combined with estrogens, it seems to produce objective tumor regressions in 50% of patients treated (15). PAPAIOANNOU does not believe that the benifit derived from L-dopa is caused by inhibition of prolactin release (61); he suggests that its action may be achieved through a stimulation of the immune response.

B. CHEMOTHERAPY

1. Single-Agent Chemotherapy

Breast cancer is one of the more responsive solid tumors. Several classes of cytotoxic agents have significant activity. This subject has been reviewed by CARTER (62, 158) and BRODER and TORMEY (159).

Alkylating agents were the first drugs shown to be effective, causing tumor regressions in one-third of patients (Table 26-7). Cyclophosphamide (CPM) is the drug of choice among the alkylating agents. The overall response for CPM administered daily, with or without an initial loading dose, is 35%. The activity ·of high-dose intermittent CPM, the more effective schedule in the experimental situation, has not yet been adequately evaluated but is under study (63). Soft-tissue lesions respond more often (43%) than visceral (28%) or osseous metastases (24%) (62). In contrast to hormones, CPM achieves higher response rates when menopause has occurred less than 1 year before (38% versus 18% when menopause has occurred 5-10 years earlier) and in patients with short disease-free intervals. The response rate for other alkylating agents is approximately the same.

5-Fluorouracil (5-FU) has been used more often than any other agent in mammary carcinoma (62, 64, 65). The standard schedule devised by ANSFIELD (15 mg/kg, qd x 5 followed by 7.5 mg/kg every other day until toxicity, repeated with 30-day intervals) (27% RR) does not appear to be more effective than weekly administration (20 mg/kg) with (45%) (66) or without (36%) (67) a loading dose (62). Methotrexate yields the best response rates of all single agents (Table 26-7). The vinca alkaloids result in a 20% response rate.

The data are more sparse for antibiotics (Table 26-7.) A low therapeutic index has precluded more extensive trials with mitomycin C (62, 70).

Table 26-7. Effectiveness of single agents in breast cancer

Drug	Number evaluable	Response rate (%)	References
Methotrexate, daily	106	41.5	CARTER (62)
twice weekly	38	40	-
6-Mercaptopurine	45	13	-
Imidazole carboxamide (DIC)	29	7	-
5-Fluorouracil, "standard"	983	27	-
weekly	58	30	-
Cytosine arabinoside	64	9	-
Hydroxyurea	21	19	-
BCNU	97	20	-
CCNU	170	12	WASSERMAN et al. (162)
MeCCNU	100	4	WASSERMAN et al. (163)
Streptozotocin	19	10.5	BAND et al. (78)
Procarbazine	21	5	CARTER (62)
Nitrogen mustard	92	35	-
Chlorambucil	54	20.5	-
Cyclophosphamide, daily	106	35	-
Melphalan	86	23	-
thio-TEPA	162	30	-
Hexamethylmelamine	54	20	BLUM et al. (82)
Dibromodulcitol	22	27	CARTER (62)
Mitomycin C	60	38	-
Actinomycin D	44	11	-
Mithramycin	32	16	-
Daunorubicin	40	38	-
Adriamycin	121	36	BLUM (160)
Bleomycin	18	16	BAND et al. (78)
Streptonigrin	13	23	-
Vincristine	226	20	CARTER (62)
Vinblastine	95	20	-

Adriamycin appears to be perhaps the most effective single agent (71, 75, 160, 161, 179), with an overall response rate of 36% (160) among 121 patients, most of whom had failed to respond on combination chemotherapy with many of the standard agents. The response rate attains 50% in previously untreated patients (161). Bleomycin (76-78), actinomycin D and mithramycin seem to be ineffective (158).

BCNU is active (RR 21%) (62, 71, 79), but not in end-stage disease; the other nitrosoureas (CCNU and MeCCNU) are under study (63, 71, 72, 78, 80, 81, 162, 163) but reports so far indicate that nitrosoureas are less valuable than ADM in breast cancer (158).

Hexamethylmelamine (HMM) (30% RR) (62, 70, 82)·, dibromodulcitol (DBD) (27% RR) (62, 70) and Ftorafur (8/17) (83) appear to be effective. Imidazole carboxamide (DIC) (5/37) (70), 5-azacytidine (2/21) (80), VM 26 (84), and carbestrol (a synthetic estrogen which has antitumor activity) (85) do not appear to be promising. Phenestrin (an alkylating group bound to cholesterol) (86) and estracyt, a compound resulting from chemical binding of non-nitrogen mustard to estradiol phosphate (87), have also been disappointing. It was hoped that with the last compound a selective concentration of alkylating agent would be obtained in the breast tissue that contains specific receptors for estrogens. Dose scheduling and various pre-therapeutic factors seem to influence the response rate and the survival duration of single-agent chemotherapy and deserves further study (159).

2. Combinations

With a large variety of active single agents, it is not surprising that combination chemotherapy has been relatively successful in breast cancer (Table 26-8) (159). GREENSPAN obtained a tumor regression rate of 60 percent with thio-TEPA and MTX and of 81 percent with a combination of thio-TEPA or CPM with MTX, 5-FU, PDN, and testosterone (88). However, interest in combination chemotherapy was not very great until COOPER reported an 88 percent regression rate in 60 hormone-resistant patients with advanced breast cancer when he used a 5-drug combination (89). COOPER combined five of the most active agents, 5-FU, MTX, VRC, CPM, and PDN. Other investigators, though less successful, have obtained tumor regression in more than half the patients treated with the same regimen (overall response rate 160/210 = 72.7 percent) (62, 93-95, 158, 159). The response rate is not influenced by the menopausal status, prior response to hormone manipulation or disease-free interval (95) Liver metastases, rarely benefited by hormone therapy, regress quite frequently. It is by no means certain that COOPER's schedule is the most effective way of combining these five agents in breast cancer, or that five agents are better than three or four (Table 26-8). The contribution of each individual component to the combination is not known. The rationale for use of two agents (5-FU and MTX) acting on the same phase of the cell cycle is questionable. COOPER's regimen was not designed to exploit the phenomena of cell synchronization, recruitment, or potentiation, and the effect of drugs on cell-cycle traverse (Chapters 5, 6, and 7). Our own results at the I.C.I.G. (96) with a three-drug combination (VCR, CPM, and 5-FU) based on such concepts are encouraging (33 percent CR, 41 percent PR, 22<50 percent regression and 4 percent F in 27 patients). Several co-operative groups are in the process of comparing COOPER's regimen with the same regimen minus one or two drugs, with intermittent cycles of the same five drugs or their sequential use (62). Preliminary reports are conflicting. The Southeastern Cancer Study Group has confirmed the superiority of the 5-drug combination over the same agents used sequentially (97), while LEMKIN et al. ob-

Table 26-8. Response rates to combinations in breast cancer

Combinations	Number evaluated	Proportion of regressions		References
MTX, CPM	39	49%	5% CR	BRUNNER et al.
MTX, CLB	23	52%	4% CR	(1975) (91)
MTX, CPM or thio-TEPA	31	70%	CR 13	DEEMARSKY (1970) (112)
MTX, thio-TEPA	40	60%		GREENSPAN (1966) (88)
MTX, ADM	24	38%		AHMANN (1975) (181)
CLB, PDN	87	20.5%		GOLDENBERG et al. (1973) (102)
ADM, MeCCNU	22	18%		LOKICH et al. (1974) (165)
ADM, CPM	51	78%	22% CR	JONES et al. (1975) (178)
ADM, VCR	40	48%	8% CR	DE LENA et al. (1975) (166)
5-FU, VCR, PDN	92	36%		GOLDENBERG et al. (1973) (102)
5-FU, VCR, PDN	64	42%	Median duration: 4,5 mo.	LEONE (1973) (99)
5-FU, CPM, PDN	49	59%		AHMANN et al. (1975) (180)
5-FU, CPM, VCR	27	74%	33% CR, 41% PR 22%<50%, 4% F	POUILLART et al. (1974) (96)
5-FU, CPM, VCR	46	43.5%	mean survival 8.6 mo.	VAUGHN et al. (1973) (100)
Same drugs sequentially	30	53.5%	mean survival 10.2 mo.	VAUGHN et al. (1973) (100)
5-FU, CPM, VCR	19	58%	8>50% regression; 3: 25-50%	TUCKER et al. (1968) (108)
5-FU, CPM, ADM (C.A.F.)	17	50%		SMALLEY (1975) (168)
5-FU, CPM, ADM	31	61%	no prior ther.	DE JAGER et al. (1975) (167)
5-FU, CPM, ADM	13	23%	prior ther.	
5-FU, CPM, ADM	39	70%		GOTTLIEB et al. (1974) (161)

Table 26-8. (continued)

Combinations	Number evaluated	Proportion of regressions		References
5-FU, CPM, ADM	30	66%	median duration 40 weeks	BULL et al. (1975) (109)
MTX, 5-FU, CPM (C.M.F.)	32	64%	median duration 24 weeks	–
MTX, 5-FU, CPM	88	52%		TAYLOR et al. (1974) (110)
MTX, 5-FU, CPM	40	48%	10% CR	DE LENA et al. (1975) (166)
MTX, 5-FU, CPM (C.M.F. low dose)	46	46%	13% CR, 33% PR 26% stable	CREECH et al. (1975) (111)
MTX, CPM, PDN	18	64%	4% CR	BRUNNER et al. (1975) (91)
	49	61%	6% CR	—
MTX, CPM, VCR	46	48%	7% CR	—
MTX, ADM, VCR	23	48%		EAGAN et al. (1975) (182)
ADM, VCR, PDN	21	57%	9% CR	BRAMBILLA et al. (1974) (164)
MTX, 5-FU, CPM, VCR (COMF)	14	14/14	6 CR, 8PR	HANHAM et al. (1971) (104)
MTX, 5-FU, CPM, PDN	28	64%	7/18 CR	CANELLOS et al. (1974) (105)
5-FU, CPM, VCR, PDN	41	46%		AHMANN et al. (1975) (180)
DIC, 5-FU, BCNU, VCR	12	6/12	6 PR	VAN EDEN et al. (1972) (107)
MTX, 5-FU, CPM, VCR, PDN	60	90%		COOPER (1969) (89)
	9	7/9	2 CR, 5 PR	LOKICH (1972) (90)
	91	75%	7% CR	BRUNNER et al. (1975) (91)
Continuously	85	66%		GOTTLIEB et al. (1974) (161)
intermittently	75	60%		GOTTLIEB et al. (1974) (161)

Table 26-8. (continued)

Combinations	Number evaluated	Proportion of regressions		References
	74	41%		DAVIS et al. (1974) (92)
	16	69%	no prior ther.	-
	64	63%	median duration: 8 months	LEONE (1973) (99)
COMF + PDN	16	62%	4 CR, 6 PR	SPIGEL et al. (1973) (93)
	18	61%		ANSFIELD et al. (1971) (94)
	42	53%		KAUFMAN (1973) (95)
	88	50%		GOLDENBERG et al. (1973) (102)
	31	35%		SMALLEY et al. (1973) (97)
	11	O		KISTER (1971) (103)
Same drugs sequentially	21	O		SMALLEY et al. (1973) (97)
MTX, 5-FU, CLB, VCR, PDN	20	30%		LEMKIN (1973) (98)

tained the same results with a 5-drug combination as with 5-FU alone
(98). The ALGB noted a longer duration of response and a better survival
with five drugs than with three drugs (VCR, 5-FU, PDN) though the
response rate was of the same order (99). VAUGHN reported no significant difference in tumor response or patient survival with 5-FU, CPM,
and VCR used in sequence or in combination (100, 101).

Adriamycin is being incorporated in combination therapy (161, 164, 165,
166). Several two- and three-drug combinations are undergoing intensive
trials: C.M.F.(CPM, MTX, 5-FU) (109, 111, 166), C.A.F.(CPM, ADM, 5-FU)
(109, 161, 167, 168), VCR, ADM (164, 166), and 5-FU, CPM, PDN (73, 81,
106, 180). It seems reasonable to use two of these combinations in sequence in an attempt to delay resistance and to permit the use of ADM
during a longer period of time without reaching cardiotoxic doses (166,
169, 170).

No definite conclusions can be drawn from the data listed in Table 26-8,
except that most investigators obtain higher response rates with combination chemotherapy than with single agents (cf. Table 26-7). Furthermore, concomitant use of drugs seems to be superior to their sequential
use (155). Skin and soft tissue metastases seem to be more responsive
to combination therapy than visceral disease while osseous metastases
respond the least. It is not clear, however, which combination is
best. With effective agents in all major classes of antitumor agents,
a large number of combinations and schedules is possible. High response

rates have been reported with COOPER's regimen, but it is quite likely
that this is not the best conceivable combination. Its toxicity is
high, and it should be used only by specialists experienced in combination therapy . We prefer a three-drug combination which is less toxic
and apparently equally effective (96). Table 26-8 does not take into
consideration toxicity, duration of remission, or the effect on survival, which are very important factors when the practicing oncologist
has to select a particular protocol from a large number with similar
initial response rates.

C. STRATEGY

1. Localized Breast Cancer

Each of the four treatment modalities for cancer has a place in the
management of the different stages of mammary carcinoma (Table 26-9).

(i) Surgery and Radiotherapy
Surgery (171) and radiotherapy constitute the primary therapy for localized disease (Stages I, II, and III). A detailed discussion of the
many controversies surrounding their relative merits is beyond the
scope of this text. Many more prospective trials are needed if decisions are to be based on facts rather than on impressions and emotions
(113, 172, 185).

Few people will deny that Stage-I breast cancer is predominantly a surgical disease. The debate centers around the extent of surgery and the
need for postoperative radiotherapy. Radical mastectomy is still considered the procedure of choice by the majority of surgeons. However,
many breast cancers are now diagnosed while smaller in size than a
century ago, when HALSTED introduced a radical procedure intended to
remove the tumor and its lymph drainage. Some surgeons advocate less
radical procedures for Stage-I lesions: for example simple mastectomy,
modified radical mastectomy, wide excision with postoperative radiotherapy. The proponents of these less radical operative procedures hope
to attain better cosmetic results without compromising the patient's
chance of cure. Others propose a "supraradical" or extended" radical
mastectomy (this includes excision of the internal mammary lymph node
chain), especially for medial and central lesions, which tend to metastasize to the internal mammary nodes (186). A few defend preoperative
radiotherapy or radiotherapy as the sole treatment for Stage-I.

It is more generally (but not universally) accepted that nothing less
than a radical mastectomy is required for Stage-II disease. However
the role of postoperative radiotherapy is also a matter of controversy.
Several controlled studies failed to show any benefit and an increased
mortality rate has been reported (187).

Stage-III disease is primarily referred to the radiotherapist (188). A
simple mastectomy may, however, be advisable to facilitate radiotherapy
in women with large pendulous breasts. This procedure may also be indicated if the tumor persists of reactivates after radiotherapy.

A discussion of the treatment of primary (localized) breast cancer is
nowadays incomplete without mentioning the role of adjuvant chemotherapy (183, 184, 188).

(ii) Adjuvant Chemotherapy

Surgeons and radiotherapists have not been able to improve significantly the overall cure rate of breast cancer in the past decades in spite of various approaches. A large proportion of their failures are caused by patients harboring distant microscopic metastases that are not affected by their local therapeutic modalities. By 10 years, 65% and 86% of patients found to have 1 to 3 and 4 or more involved lymph nodes respectively will demonstrate a treatment failure and only 25% are still alive (37.5% with 1 to 3 and 13.4% of these with 4 and more positive nodes). Some 50% of patients operated upon have positive nodes. Thus primary breast cancer cannot be considered as a local disease in the majority of patients. Some form of systemic therapy is often indicated in addition to local measures.

The rationale for adjuvant chemotherapy has been discussed in chapter 13. Results of early studies were contradictory. Most of these were short-term cytotoxic treatments aimed at malignant cells circulating in the blood following operative manipulation. This approach resulted in either an adverse (121), no (113, 115, 117) or a benificial effect (120) (at least in some subgroups). A long-term treatment study with postoperative thio-TEPA (118) was without effect, while another with nitrogen mustard (119) showed no recurrences or death related to cancer in the treated patients, while the recurrence rate was 36% in the controls and survival only 57%.

More recently two random, well controlled studies have demontrated the value of adjuvant chemotherapy. The National Surgical Adjuvant Breast Project (NSABP) undertook a long-term adjuvant study with melphalan (MPH) as an adjuvant to radical mastectomy (conventional or modofied) in patients with positive axillary lymph nodes. MPH-treated patients received 0.15 mg/kg per day for five consecutive days every six weeks, until evidence of recurrence or for two years, whichever occurred first. Treatment failures occurred in 22% of 108 control patients and in 9.7% of 103 MPH-treated patients, indicating a statistically significant difference (173). The beneficial effect was more striking in premenopausal women (30% relapse in controls versus 3% in MPH-treated patients) than in postmenopausal women (21% versus 11%).

BONADONNA et al. at the NCI-Milan evaluated the CMF (12 monthly cycles) (see p. 451) combination as an adjuvant to radical or supraradical mastectomy (without postoperative radiotherapy) in patients with positive lymph nodes (175). This combination was shown to be more effective in far-advanced breast cancer than melphalan. Indeed the ECOG randomly compared in previously untreated patients the CMF program (52% response rate) to melphalan (24%) (110). Since CMF has a higher order of anti-tumor activity in advanced disease, it would also be expected to be superior to melphalan. After 27 months of study, treatment failure occurred in 24% of 179 control patients and in 5.3% of CMF-treated patients (Fig. 26-2). Toxicity has been acceptable. The failure rate was most prominently affected by the number of positive axillary lymph nodes but not by the menopausal status as was the case in the melphalan study. The observation that more than three fourths of recurrences occurred at distant sites confirms that a large number of patients with involved axillary lymph nodes have microscopic disseminated metastases at the time of radical mastectomy.

A longer follow-up is required before it will be known whether current adjuvant therapy improves survival rate in addition to the disease-free interval. BONADONNA's study already seems to indicate that CMF is destroying micrometastases not merely suppressing them.

Table 26-9. Treatment strategy for breast cancer

Stage	Standard therapy	Comments, controversies
Stage I (A)	a. Outer quadrant lesion: surgery b. Inner quadrant lesion: surgery + radiotherapy	1. Extent of surgery radical mastectomy (HALSTED) simple mastectomy -/+ radiotherapy wide excision ("lumpectomy") + radio-therapy partial mastectomy modified radical mastectomy supraradical or extended radical mastectomy 2. Extent of treated fields (+/- chest wall) optimum dose radiation as primary treatment modality preoperative irradiation	3. Adjuvant therapy chemotherapy hormonal-additive -ablative immunotherapy 4. Prophylactic therapy of opposite breast
Stage II (B)	Surgery (radical mastec-tomy) + Radiotherapy	1. Extent of surgery radical mastectomy for outer quadrants radical or supraradical for inner quadrants	idem
Stage III (C)	Radiotherapy +/- surgery (simple mastectomy) +/- systemic therapy hormonal - additive - ablative chemotherapy	1. Radiotherapy is primary treatment modality 2. Indication for surgery: large, pendulous breasts, to facilitate radiotherapy simple mastectomy post-radiotherapy for: residual tumor for recurrent local tumor mastectomy "de toilette"	idem

Table 26-9. (continued)

Stage	Standard therapy	Comments, controversies
Stage IV	Systemic therapy Hormonal – additive – ablative Chemotherapy	1. Sequential or simulataneous use of hormonal and cytotoxic therapy 2. If sequential: order of sequence 3. Chemotherapy: sequential single agent or combination therapy 4. Ablative procedures: adrenalectomy or hypophysectomy

Obviously we are only witnessing the beginning of succesful adjuvant chemotherapy. Better and more effective schedules will undoubtedly be developed, while new questions will be raised; for example concerning the optimal schedule and duration of therapy, the long-term side-effects, risks of carcinogenesis, and the selection of patients as candidates for adjuvant therapy. Whether immunotherapy will play a significant part is not yet known. GOTTLIEB et al. have initiated an adjuvant program combining chemotherapy with immunotherapy (161).

The introduction of effective adjuvant therapy will also require a re-evaluation of the extent of surgery and the role of radiotherapy. If chemotherapy is equally effective against microscopic residual local and regional disease, lesser surgical procedures (plus adjuvant therapy) may be as effective, and yield better cosmetic results than more radical ones and costly postoperative radiotherapy may become unnecessary.

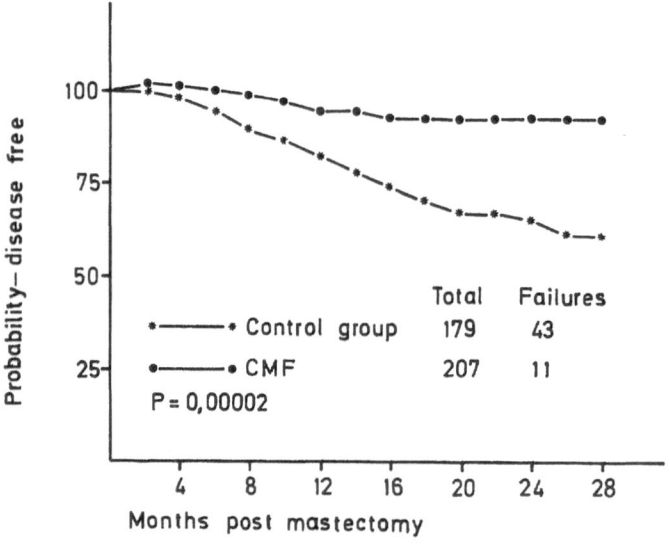

Fig. 26-2. *Adjuvant chemotherapy with CMF following radical mastectomy; treatment-failure time distribution in all evaluable patients (from BONADONNA et al. (175))*

(iii) Prophylactic Versus Therapeutic Castration
The relative merits of prophylactic (at the time of primary treatment) versus therapeutic (at the time of recurrence and dissemination) oophorectomy also remain controversial. FISHER has reviewed this subject, and concludes that there is no justification for prophylactic castration in the treatment of operable breast cancer (113, 116). A controlled study by the NSABP failed to demonstrate that prophylactic oophorectomy confers any advantage by lengthening the time from operation to recurrence, nor did it delay death (123). KENNEDY et al. arrived at the same conclusions (124). Prophylactic oophorectomy retards the appearance of metastases but survival after dissemination is shorter than in patients castrated at the time of dissemination. Total length of survival is the same for both groups. He does not recommend prophylactic castration in premenopausal women because it deprives the therapist of valuable information regarding the hormone responsiveness of a particular tumor, information that normally guides the selection of subsequent therapies.

The postponement of castration until evidence of dissemination avoids unnecessary operations on patients who are actually cured. In spite of two studies that suggest some advantage of prophylactic castration (125, 126), this is no longer recommended (113, 123, 154). Furthermore the introduction of effective adjuvant chemotherapy makes prophylactic castration obsolete. However a combination of prophylactic castration plus adjuvant chemotherapy may be worth investigating in estrogen receptor positive patients (184).

2. Disseminated Breast Cancer

(i) Hormone Therapy Versus Chemotherapy

The treatment of metastatic breast cancer is more complicated than that of other disseminated malignancies, since there are three therapeutic approaches to be considered at different phases of the disease: chemotherapy, and additive or ablative hormonotherapy (Fig. 26-3). The selection is determined mainly by the patient's age and menopausal status, the rapidity of progression, the anatomic location and extent of metastatic disease, and the response to prior therapy. It used to be customary to begin with hormone manipulations, reserving chemotherapy for later in the course of the disease or for hormone-resistant patients. Endocrine therapy was preferred to chemotherapy because it tended to produce longer remissions and was better tolerated by the patient. This was true as long as chemotherapy consisted of single agent therapy. The 20 to 30% regression rates using anyone of the single agents were not higher than those achieved with classical hormonal therapy.

Some 30 to 40% of patients respond to initial hormone manipulation, but improvement is slow. Local or regional recurrences and skeletal metastases regress more often than visceral involvement (regression rate under 20%). Furthermore the effectiveness of hormone therapy depends upon the patient's age, being less effective in younger patients, menopause (the poorest results are in the five years after menopause) and the disease-free interval, more regressions occurring the longer this interval, i.e., slow growing tumors. In contrast, the effect of chemotherapy does not appear to be dependant on the patient's age, location of the metastases or disease-free interval. Chemotherapy is often successful where hormone therapy fails most frequently. Since the introduction of combination chemotherapy, the regression rates are distinctly higher than those obtained with hormone therapy and tumor reponses occur more rapidly. Several authors have warned that chemotherapy may be associated with sudden death after hypophysectomy or adrenalectomy and should be used with extreme caution (140, 141). These considerations provide the basis for a fundamental change in the place of chemotherapy in the management of breast cancer. Patients with rapidly progressing disease, inflammatory carcinomatosis or essential organ involvement (brain, liver, lymphangitic pulmonary involvement) should be treated promptly with chemotherapy.

Hormone therapy should only be considered for slowly progressing cases, with a long estimated survival, preferably older patients, with a long disease-free interval and predominantly local or regional recurrences or skeletal metastases. Most importantly, the presence or absence of estrogen receptor should be taken into consideration. Estrogen receptor assays can be helpful to predict the results of endocrine therapy for metastatic breast cancer. In patients without detectable estrogen receptor, the chances of tumor regression in response to endocrine therapy

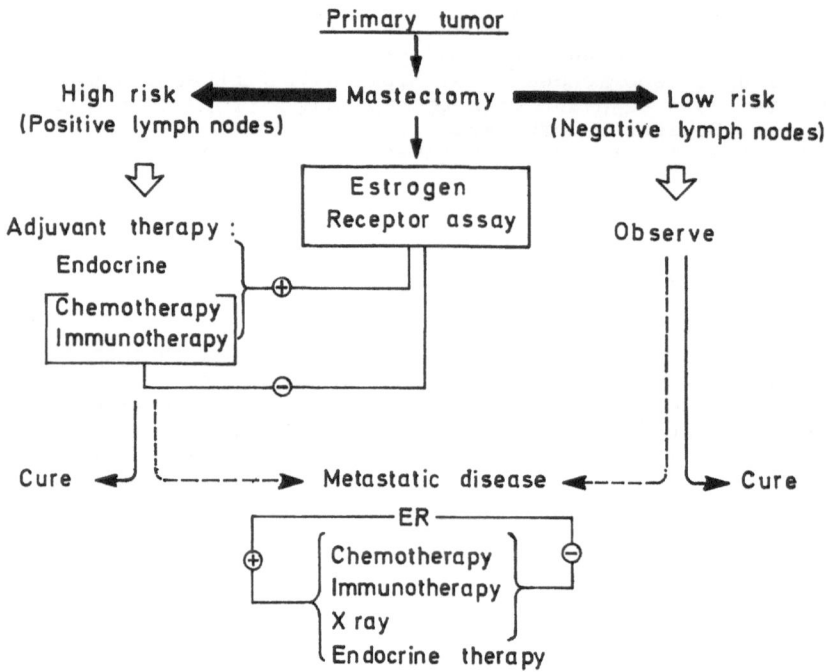

Fig. 26-3. Treatment scheme for breast cancer (from McGUIRE) (19)

are minimal, while the response rate to hormone therapy is 55 to 60% in patients with detectable estrogen receptor. This together with the factors mentioned above should permit the oncologist to select patients most likely to benefit from hormone therapy. Occasionally the disease will exacerbate rather than regress after initiation of hormone therapy. We have already referred to the risk of hypercalcemia occurring shortly after hormone therapy is instituted (130).

Recently, antagonists of hormones have been introduced in the oncology clinic. They block the binding of estrogen to hormone receptors and may accomplish the same therapeutic result as ablative hormonal procedures (oophorectomy, adrenalectomy and hypophysectomy). The latter also reduce estrogen production but they require major surgery with its attendant morbidity and mortality. Some studies in progress combine chemotherapy with hormone therapy (176).

(ii) Hormone Therapy in Premenopausal Women
The initial endocrine therapy is determined by the patient's menopausal status. The important factor is whether physiologic amounts of estro-gens are still being secreted. This can be determined by vaginal cyto-logy. Since there is some residual ovarian function after the cessation of menses, women in whom menopause has occurred less than one year be-fore are treated as premenopausal for the purpose of hormone treatment.

It is generally agreed that castration is the first step in the endo-crine treatment in premenopausal women. Good palliation can be expected in 30 - 47.5% (131), lasting 6-12 months and sometimes several years. More than a third of patients aged 46-50 obtain a remission, whereas only one-fifth of those who are 35 years of age or younger respond (6).

Patients with irregular menses respond less frequently than those with regular menses (6). Surgical castration is preferable to castration by radiation, being quicker and more reliable (16). Variations in the position of the ovaries and the size of the patient frequently make accurate radiotherapy difficult, and total suppression of ovarian hormonal activity can take up to two or three months.

Nowadays many oncologists prefer to switch to chemotherapy rather than resorting to further ablative surgery in premenopausal women no-longer responding to castration.

It is unlikely that primary castration failures will benefit from hormonal manipulation. The response rate to subsequent hypophysectomy or adrenalectomy is only 10 to 17% (6, 132, 137). Here too, chemotherapy is the next preferred step.

(iii) Hormone Therapy in Postmenopausal Women
Most oncologists precribe estrogens as the primary endocrine therapy in postmenopausal women in the absence of any significant estrogen secretion (Fig. 26-3). This can be determined by the vaginal smear pattern of the urinary estrogen excretion. Cornification of over 15% of the cells in the vaginal smear is due to the presence of ovarian estrogens. Cyclic fluctuation in estrogen secretion is not uncommon in women within five years following menopause. This is a difficult group of patients to treat with any type of endocrine therapy.

The risk of tumor aggravation is low when more than five years have elapsed since the menopause.

Approximately one third of patients respond to this type of treatment, the remission rate increasing with increasing number of years since menopause (12, 13, 28). The average duration of tumor control is 12 to 15 months.

Preliminary results with antiestrogens are also encouraging. They may even be more effective than estrogens (189).

After relapse following an initial response to the primary endocrine therapy (estrogens or antiestrogens) in postmenopausal women several options are open for further management. Further along the line of endocrine manipulations there remain androgens and ablative surgery (bilateral adrenalectomy or hypophysectomy). Approximately 50% of patients can be expexted to show an additional response to ablative surgery. However most oncologists will rather switch to chemotherapy instead.

Patients in whom the menopause has occurred 1 to 5 years earlier constitute a difficult group for any type of endocrine therapy and are best treated with cytotoxic therapy.

Both radiotherapy and surgery can still be useful in disseminated disease for the palliation of local symptoms. Radiotherapy is used for bone metastases, cerebral metastases, cord comression (with or without prior laminectomy), and orthopedic procedures for pathologic or impending fractures (143).

Cancer of the male breast is a rare disease, which is not surprising
in view of the small amount of mammary gland tissue. The lobular variety does not seem to occur in males (144). The only predisposing factor recognized is Klinefelter's syndrome. It is often said that the
prognosis is more ominous in men than in women. HOLLEB made a careful
comparison and did not confirm this impression (145). Many cases are
dependent on androgens for continued growth. Androgens are thus contraindicated. Endocrine manipulation is aimed at the removal of androgens
or at an anti-androgenic action (as in cancer of the prostate).

A. STRATEGY

1. Localized Breast Cancer

The management of early cases is the same as that of localized breast
cancer in women. Radical mastectomy with axillary nodal dissection
yields a 5-year survival rate of 43-57% (145). Postoperative radiotherapy is given to patients with histologically positive nodes.

2. Recurrent and Disseminated Disease

Local soft-tissue and nodal recurrence are best treated by radiotherapy,
while disseminated disease is usually treated by endocrine manipulations
or chemotherapy (Fig. 26-4) (177, 190).

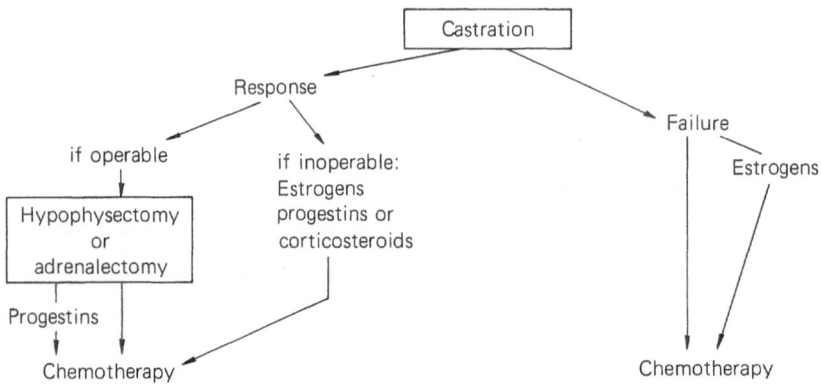

Fig. 26-4. Treatment scheme for metastatic breast cancer in males

STOLL (13), KENNEDY (28), and HOLLEB (145) recommend castration (surgical rather than radiotherapeutic) as the primary endocrine therapy.
Objective tumor regressions occur in 45 to 68% (13, 145, 146) and are
of relatively long duration (6-40 months). Patients with long disease-
free survival between mastectomy and recurrence are the most likely to
benefit. Palliation is most frequent for bone involvement but is not
uncommon for soft tissue and visceral metastases. STOLL (12, 13) and

HOLLEB (145) have not been impressed with the effect of estrogens in breast cancer of the male. KENNEDY, in contrast, suggests that they can be used either as primary therapy or as secondary hormone therapy (147).

Secondary therapy for patients who respond to initial castration consists of: (1) bilateral adrenalectomy, (2) hypophysectomy, (3) estrogens, or (4) corticosteroids. It should be remembered that few authors have much experience with this type of tumor, so that recommendations cannot be backed up with actual clinical data. Major ablative surgery should be reserved for patients who are neither too old or not too ill. Significant regressions lasting several years have been reported in small series. The exact role of prolactin in male breast carcinoma is not known, and it cannot be stated which of the two major ablative procedures (adrenalectomy and hypophysectomy), if either, is more effective. As already mentioned, several authors have not been satisfied with estrogens, while others consider them part of the therapeutic armamentarium for this malignancy. Corticosteroids are useful for palliation in patients who are not candidates for major ablative surgery. The value of progestins is not known.

Chemotherapy is reserved for patients who have failed to or no longer respond to endocrine therapy. It may also be the treatment of choice in rapidly progressing disease, and for patients with extensive liver involvement, cerebral metastases or pulmonary lymphangitic carcinomatosis. We assume that the same drugs are effective as are recommended for female breast cancer.

REFERENCES

1. FORREST, A.P.M., KUNKLER, P.B.: Prognostic Factors in Breast Cancer. (eds. A.P.M. Forrest, P.B. Kunkler). Edinburgh-London: Livingstone 1968.
2. HAAGENSEN, C.D.: Diseases of the Breast. Philadelphia-London-Toronto: Saunders 1971.
3. CUTLER, S.J.: The prognosis of treated breast cancer. In: Prognostic Factors in Breast Cancer, p. 20 (eds. A.P.M. Forrest, P.B. Kinkler). Edinburgh-London: Livingstone 1968.
4. CUTLER, S.J., BLACK, M.M., MORK, T., HARVEI, S., FREEMAN, C.: Further observations on prognostic factors in cancer of the female breast. Cancer 24, 653 (1969).
5. CUTLER, S.J., ASIRE, A.J., TAYLOR, S.G.III: An evaluation of ovarian status as a prognostic factor in disseminated cancer of the breast. Cancer 26, 938 (1970).
6. FRACCHIA, A.A.: Indications for castration and adrenalectomy for advanced breast cancer. Cancer 28, 1699 (1971).
7. UICC: T.N.M. classification of malignant tumours. Geneva: G. de Buren 1968.
8. UICC Commitee on Professional Education: Clinical Oncology. A manual for students and doctors. Berlin-Heidelberg-New York: Springer-Verlag 1973.
9. FISHER, B., SLACK, N.H., BROSS, I.D.J., and cooperating investigators: Cancer of the breast: size of neoplasm and prognosis. Cancer 24, 1071 (1969).
10. BLOOM, H.J.G.: Survival of women with untreated breast cancer - past and present. In: Prognostic Factors in Breast Cancer, p. 3 (eds. A.P.M. Forrest, P.B. Kinkler). Edinburgh-London: Livingstone 1968.
11. BUTCHER, Jr., H.R.: Mammary carcinoma. A discussion of therapeutic methods. Cancer 24, 1273 (1969).

12. STOLL, B.A.: Hormonal Management in Breast Cancer. London: Pitman Medical 1969.
13. STOLL, B.A.: Endocrine therapy in malignant disease. London-Philadelphia-Toronto: Saunders 1972.
14. STOLL, B.A.: Brain catecholamines and breast cancer: a hypothesis. Lancet 1, 431 (1972).
15. FRIESEN, H.G.: Prolactin: its physiologic role and therapeutic potential. Hosp. Prac. Sept. 123 (1972).
16. DAO, T.L.: Ablation therapy for hormone-dependent tumors. Ann. Rev. Med. 23, 1 (1972).
17. STOLL, B.A.: Hypothesis: breast cancer regression under oestrogen therapy. Brit. Med. J. 3, 446 (1973).
18. ADAMS, J.B., WONG, M.S.F.: Paraendocrine behavior of human breast cancer. In vitro transformation of steroids to physiologically active hormones. J. Endoc. 41, 41 (1968).
19. MC GUIRE, W.L.: Current status of estrogen receptors in human breast cancer. Cancer 36, 638 (1975).
20. DESHPANDE, N., JENSEN, V., BULBROOK, R.D., BERNE, T., ELLIS, F.: Accumulation of tritiated oestradiol by human breast tissue. Steroids 10, 219 (1967).
21. JENSEN, E.V., BLOCK, G.E., SMITH, S., KYSER, K., DESOMBRE, E.R.: Estrogen receptors and breast cancer response to adrenalectomy. In: Prediction of Response in Cancer Therapy. (ed. T.C. Hall) Nat. Cancer Inst. Monogr. 34, 55 (1971).
22. BRAUNSBERG, H., JAMES, V.H.T., IRVINE, W.T., JAMES, F., JAMIESON, C.W., SELLWOOD, R.A., CARTER, A.E., HULBERT, M.: Prognostic significance of oestrogen uptake by human breast-cancer tissue. Lancet 1, 163 1973.
23. COUNCIL ON DRUGS: Androgens and estrogens in the treatment of disseminated mammary carcinoma. Retrospective study of nine hundred forty-four patients. J. Amer. med. Ass. 172, 1271 (1960).
24. COOPERATIVE BREAST CANCER GROUP: Results of studies of the cooperative breast cancer group - 1961-63. Cancer Chemother. Rep. Suppl. 1, 41, 1 (1964).
25. KENNEDY, B.J.: Diethylstilbestrol versus testosterone therapy in advanced breast cancer. Surg. Gynec. Obstet. 120, 1246 (1965).
26. KAUFMAN, R.J., ESCHER, G.C.: Rebound regression in advanced mammary carcinoma. Surg. Gynec. Obstet. 113, 635 (1961).
27. BAKER, L.H., VAITKEVICIUS, V.K.: Reevaluation of rebound regression in disseminated carcinoma of the breast. Cancer 29, 1268 (1972).
28. KENNEDY, B.J.: Endocrine therapy of breast cancer. J. Amer. med. Ass. 200, 971 (1967).
29. GOLDENBERG, I.S., WATERS, M.N., RAVDIN, R.S., ANSFIELD, F.J., SEGALOFF, A.: Androgenic therapy for advanced breast cancer in women. J. Amer. med. Ass. 223, 1267 (1973).
30. JAPANESE COOPERATIVE GROUP OF HORMONAL TREATMENT FOR BREAST CANCER: 2α, 3α epithio-5α-androstan-17β-OL in the treatment of advanced breast cancer. Cancer 31, 789 (1973).
31. GORDAN, G.S., WESSLER, S., AVIOLI, L.V.: Calusterone in the therapy for advanced breast cancer. J. Amer. med. Ass. 219, 483 (1972).
32. TALLEY, R.W., HAINES, C.R., WATERS, M.N., GOLDENBERG, I.S., OLSON, K.B., BISEL, H.F.: A dose-response evaluation of androgens in the treatment of metastatic breast cancer. Cancer 32, 315 (1973).
33. COOPERATIVE BREAST CANCER GROUP: Testosterone propionate therapy in breast cancer. J. Amer. Med. Ass. 188, 1069 (1964).
34. GROUPE EUROPEEN DU CANCER DU SEIN: Le traitement hormonal du cancer du sein en phase avancée. Comparaison des résultat obtenus au moyen de la Δ-testololactone et du propionate de testostérone. Rev. franc. Etud. clin. biol. 7, 1067 (1962).

35. GROUPE EUROPEEN DU CANCER DU SEIN: Le traitement hormonal du cancer du sein en phase avancée. Comparaison entre le propionate de testostérone et la combinaison propionate de testostérone-delta-1-testololactone. Rev. franc. Etud. Clin. biol. 9, 88 (1964).
36. COOPERATIVE BREAST CANCER GROUP: Progress Report: results of studies by the cooperative breast cancer group - 1956-60. Cancer Chemother. Rep. 11, 109 (1961).
37. CANTINO, T.J., GORDAN, G.S.: High-dosage Δ1-testololactone therapy of disseminated carcinoma of the breast. Cancer 20, 458 (1967).
38. JONES, V., JOSLIN, C.A.F., JONES, R.E., DAVIES, D.K.L., ROBERTS, M.M., GLEAVE, E.N., CAMPBELL, H., FORREST, A.P.M.: Progestagens and advanced breast cancer. Lancet 1, 1049 (1971).
39. STOLL, B.A.: Vaginal cytology as an aid to hormone therapy in postpausal cancer of the breast. Cancer 20, 1807 (1967).
40. SEGALOFF, A., CUNINGHAM, M., RICE, B.F., WEETH, J.B.: Hormonal therapy in cancer of the breast. XXIV. Effect of corticosteroids or medroxyprogesterone acetate on clinical course and hormonal excretion. Cancer 20, 1673 (1967).
41. MUGGIA, F.M., CASSILETH, P.A., OCHOA, Jr., M., FLATOW, F.A., GELLHORN, A., HYMAN, G.A.: Treatment of breast cancer with medroxyprogesterone acetate. Ann. intern. Med. 68, 328 (1968).
42. BUCALOSSI, P., DIPIETRO, S., GENNARI, L.: Hormone treatment of diffuse breast carcinoma with a synthetic progestional agent: 6α-methyl-17α-acetoxyprogesterone. Minerva chir. 18, 358 (1963).
43. CURWEN, S.: The treatment of advanced carcinoma of the breast with SH 420. Clin. Radiol. 21, 218 (1970).
44. DARGENT, M., POMMATAU, E., SERVONNAT, F.: Résultats du traitement par le noréthindrone (norluten) des cancers du sein en phase de diffusion. Bull. Acad. nat. Méd. (Paris) 152, 163 (1968).
45. GORINS, A., NETTER, A.: L'apport des norstéroides dans le traitement des cancers du sein en phase avancée. Presse méd. 77, 817 (1969).
46. EDELSTYN, G.A.: Norethisterone acetate (SH420) in advanced breast cancer. Cancer 32, 1317 (1973).
47. CROWLEY, L.G., MacDONALD, L.: Delalutin and estrogens for the treatment of advanced mammary carcinoma in the postmenopausal women. Cancer 18, 436 (1965).
48. KENNEDY, B.J.: Hormone therapy for advanced breast cancer. Cancer 18, 1551 (1965).
49. STOLL, B.A.: Effect of lyndiol, an oral contraceptive, on breast cancer. Brit. med. J. 1, 150 (1967).
50. LANDAU, R.L.: Can endorine therapy be expected to replace the surgical treatment of advanced breast cancer? In: Major Endorine Surgery for the Treatment of Cancer of the Breast in Advanced Stages, p. 263 (eds. M. Dargent, C.I. Romieu). Lyons: Simep 1967.
51. DAO, T.L., TAN, E., BROOKS, V.: A comparative evaluation of adrenalectomy and cortisone in the treatment of advanced mammary carcinoma. Cancer 14, 1259 (1961).
52. FORREST, A.P.M., STEWART, H.J., BENSON, E.A., KER, H., JONES, V., KUNKLER, P.B., CAMPELL, H.: Controlled studies in advanced breast cancer. In: Prognostic Factors in Breast Cancer, p. 186 (eds. A.P.M. Forrest, P.B. Kunkler). Edinburgh-London: Livingstone 1968.
53. MOORE, F.D., WOODROW, S.I., ALIAPOULIOS, M.A., WILSON, R.E.: Carcinoma of the breast. A decade of new results with old concepts. New Engl. J. Med. 277, 293 (1967).
54. HARTMAN, W.H., SHERLOCK, P.: Gastroduodenal metastases from carcinoma of the breast. An adrenal steroid-induced phenomenon. Cancer (Philad.) 14, 426 (1961).
55. LYONS, A.R.: Thyroid hormones and breast cancer. In: Prognostic Factors in Breast Cancer, p. 164 (eds. A.P.M. Forrest, P.B. Kunkler). Edinburgh-London: Livingstone 1968.

56. E.O.R.T.C. Breast Cancer Group: Clinical trial of nafoxidine, an oestrogen antagonist in advanced breast cancer. Europ. J. Cancer **8**, 387 (1972).

57. COLE, M.P., JONES, C.T.A., TODD, I.D.H.: A new anti-oestrogenic agent in late breast cancer. An early clinical appraisal of ICI 46474. Brit. J. Cancer **25**, 270 (1971).

58. HEUSON, J.C., WAELBROECK-VAN GAVER, C., LEGROS, N.: Growth inhibition of rat mammary carcinoma and endocrine changes produced by 2-Br-α-Ergocryptine, a suppressor of lactation and nidation. Europ. J. Cancer **6**, 353 (1970).

59. European Breast Cancer Group: Clinical trial of 2-Br-α-ergocryptine (CB 154) in advanced breast cancer. Europ. J. Cancer **8**, 155 (1972).

60. European Breast Cancer Group: Clinical trial of the cyclic imide 1-(morpholinomethyl)-4-phtalimido-piperidindione-2,6 (CG 603) in advanced breast cancer. Europ. J. Cancer **8**, 157 (1972).

61. PAPAIOANNOU, A.N.: Prolactin, levodopa, and immune response in breast cancer. Lancet **2**, 226 (1972).

62. CARTER, S.K.: Single and combination nonhormonal chemotherapy in breast cancer. Cancer **30**, 1543 (1972).

63. CARTER, S.K.: An overview of the status of the nitrosoureas in other tumors. Cancer Chemother. Rep. Part 3, **4**, 35 (1973).

64. AHMANN, D.L., BISEL, H.F., HANH, R.G.: An evaluation of 5-fluorouracil in the treatment of advanced cancer. Mayo Clin. Proc. **42**, 193 (1967).

65. ANSFIELD, F.J.: Current status of 5-fluorouracil in the therapy of breast cancer. In: Proceedings of the Chemotherapy Conference on the Chemotherapy of Solid Tumors. An appraisal of 5-Fluorouracil and BCNU. (ed. S.K. Carter). Bethesda: National Cancer Institute 1970.

66. JACOBS, E.M., LUCE, J.K., WOOD, D.A: Treatment of cancer with weekly intravenous 5-fluorouracil. Cancer **22**, 1233 (1968).

67. HORTON, J., OLSON, K.B., SULLIVAN, J., REILLY, C., SHNIDER, B.: 5-Fluorouracil in cancer: an improved regimen. Ann. intern. Med. **73**, 897 (1970).

68. BRENNAN, M.J., TALLEY, R.W.: Implications of treatment sequence effects on responsiveness to 5-fluorouracil and Cytoxan. In: Current Concepts in Breast Cancer, p. 225 (eds. A. Segaloff, K.K. Meyer, S. Debakey). Baltimore: Wilkins 1967.

69. SEARS, M.: Effectiveness of various schedules of methotrexate in advanced breast carcinoma. Cancer Chemother. Rep. **53**, 93 (1969).

70. SHINGLETON, W.W., SEDRANSK, N., JOHNSON, R.O.: Chemotherapy of breast carcinoma. Oncology **26**, 287 (1972).

71. GOTTLIEB, J.A., BONNET, J.D., HOOGSTRATEN, B., O'BRYAN, R.M.: Superiority of adriamycin over oral nitrosoureas in patients with breast cancer. Proc. Amer. Soc. clin. Oncol. abstr. **37** (1973).

72. GOTTLIEB, J.A., RIVKIN, S.E., SPIGEL, S.C., HOOGSTRATEN, B., O'BRYAN, R.M., DELANEY, F.C., SINGHAKOWINTA, A.: Superiority of adriamycin over oral nitrosoureas in patients with advanced breast carcinoma. A Southwest Cancer Chemotherapy Study Group Study. Cancer **33**, 519 (1974).

73. AHMANN, D.L., BISEL, H.F., HAHN, R.G.: A phase II evaluation of adriamycin (NSC-123127) as treatment for disseminated breast cancer. Proc. Amer. Ass. Cancer Res. **15**, 100 (1974).

74. ROSNER, D., DAO, T.L., HORTON, J., CUNNINGHAM, T., DIAZ, R., TAYLOR, S., ROSENBAUM, C., VATANASAPT, V.: Randomized study of adriamycin vs. combined therapy (FCP) vs. adrenalectomy in breast cancer. Proc. Amer. Ass. Cancer Res. **15**, 63 (1974).

75. O'BRYAN, R.M., LUCE, J.K., TALLEY, R.W., GOTTLIEB, J.A., BAKER, L.H., BONADONNA, G.: Phase II evaluation of adriamycin in human neoplasia. Cancer **32**, 1 (1973).

76. E.O.R.T.C. Clinical Screening Co-operative Group: Study of the clinical efficiency of bleomycin in human cancer. Brit. med. J. 2, 643 (1970).
77. BLUM, R.H., CARTER, S.K., AGRE, K.: A clinical review of bleomycin - a new antineoplastic agent. Cancer 31, 903 (1973).
78. BAND, P.R., SEARS, M., CANELLOS, G.P., SCHEIN, P.: Bleomycin, streptozotocin and CCNU in the treatment of breast cancer. Proc. Amer. Ass. Cancer Res. 15, 22 (1974).
79. AHMANN, D.L., HAHN, R.G., BISEL, H.F.: Evaluation of 1,3-bis(2-chloroethyl)-1-nitrosourea (BCNU; NSC-409962) in the management of patients with advanced breast cancer. Cancer Chemother. Rep. 56, 93 (1972).
80. CUNNINGHAM, T.J., NEMOTO, T., ROSNER, D., KNIGHT, E., TAYLOR, S., ROSENBAUM, C., HORTON, J., DAO, T.: Comparison of 5-azacytidine with CCNU in the treatment of patients with breast cancer and evaluation of the subsequent use of cyclophosphamide. Cancer Chemother. Rep. Part 1, 58, 677 (1974).
81. AHMANN, D.L., BISEL, H.F., HAHN, R.G.: A phase 2 evaluation of 1-(2-chloroethyl)-3-(4-methylcyclohexyl)-1-nitrosourea (NSC 95441) in patients with advanced breast cancer. Cancer Res. 34, 27 (1974).
82. BLUM, R.H., LIVINGSTONE, R.B., CARTER, S.K.: Hexamethylmelamine. A new drug with activity in solid tumors. Europ. J. Cancer 9, 195 (1973).
83. BLOKHINA, N.G., VOZNY, E.K., GARIN, A.M.: Results of treatment of malignant tumors with ftorafur. Cancer 30, 390 (1972).
84. E.O.R.T.C. Co-operative Group for Leukemia and Hematosarcoma: Clinical screening of epipodophyllotoxin VM 26 in malignant lymphomas and solid tumors. Brit. med. J. 2, 744 (1972).
85. KOGLER, J., HILL, G., SEDRANSK, N., COLE, D.R., WEISS, A.J., WILSON, W.: Phase II study of carbestrol (NSC-19962) in patients with solid tumors. Cancer Chemother. Rep. 56, 641 (1972).
86. ANSFIELD, F.J., CARTER, A.C., GOLDENBERG, I.S., SEGALOFF, A.: Phase I study of phenesterin (NSC-104469). Cancer Chemother. Rep. 55, 259 (1971).
87. GROUPE EUROPEEN DU CANCER DU SEIN: Essai clinique du phénol bis (2-chloroéthyl) carbamate d'oestradiol dans le cancer mammaire en phase avancée. Europ. J. Cancer 5, 1 (1969).
88. GREENSPAN, E.M.: Combination of cytotoxic chemotherapy in advanced disseminated breast carcinoma. J. Mt. Sinai Hosp. 33, 1 (1966).
89. COOPER, B.G.: Combination chemotherapy in hormone resistant breast cancer. Proc. Amer. Ass. Cancer Res. 10, 15 (1969).
90. LOKICH, J.J., SKARIN, A.T.: Five-drug combination chemotherapy for disseminated adenocarcinoma. Cancer Chemother. Rep. 56, 761 (1972).
91. BRUNNER, K.W., SONNTAG, R.W., MARTZ, G., et al.: A controlled study in the use of combined drug therapy for metastatic breast cancer. Cancer 36, 1208 (1975).
92. DAVIS, H.L., RAMIREZ, G., ELLERBY, R.A., ANSFIELD, F.J.: Five drug therapy in advanced breast cancer. Cancer 34, 239 (1974).
93. SPIGEL, M.S.C., COLTMAN, Jr., C.C.A., COSTANZI, J.J.: Disseminated breast carcinoma. Arch. intern. Med. 132, 575 (1973).
94. ANSFIELD, F.J., RAMIREZ, G., KORBITZ, B.C., DAVIS, Jr., H.L.: Five-drug therapy for advanced breast cancer. Cancer Chemother. Rep. Part 1, 55, 183 (1971).
95. KAUFMAN, S., GOLDSTEIN, M.: Combination chemotherapy in disseminated carcinoma of the breast. Surg. Gynec. Obstet. 137, 83 (1973).
96. POUILLART, P., SCHWARZENBERG, L., AMIEL, J.L., MATHE, G. et al.: Chimiothérapies sequentielles. I. Application au traitement des cancers du sein. Nouv. Presse Méd. 4, 713 (1975).
97. SMALLEY, R.V., MURPHEY, S., CHAN, Y.-K., HUGULEY, Jr., C.M.: Comparison of two five drug regimens versus sequential chemotherapy in metastatic breast carcinoma. Proc. Amer. Soc. clin. Oncol. Abstr. 82 (1973).

98. LEMKIN, S.R., DOLLINGER, M.R.: Combination vs. single-drug therapy in advanced breast cancer. Proc. Amer. Ass. Cancer Res. 14, 37 (1973).
99. LEONE, L.A., REGE, V.: Treatment of metastatic, recurrent or inoperable carcinoma of breast with VCR/Pred/5-FU/MTX/Cyclo (reg.1) vs. VCR/Pred/5-FU (reg. II). Proc. Amer. Ass. Cancer Res. 14, 125 (1973).
100. VAUGHN, C.B., BAKER, L.H., AL-SARRAF, M., VAITKEVICIUS, V.K.: Combination versus sequential cytotoxic chemotherapy in the treatment of advanced breast cancer. Proc. Amer. Soc. clin. Oncol. Abstr. 87 (1973).
101. BAKER, L.H., VAUGHN, C.B., AL-SARRAF, M., REED, M.L., VAITKEVICIUS, V.K.: Evaluation of combination vs. sequential cytotoxic chemotherapy in the treatment of advanced breast cancer. Cancer 33, 513 (1974).
102. GOLDENBERG, I.S., McMAHAN, C.A., ESCHER, G.C., VOLK, H., ANSFIELD, F.J., OLSON, K.B.: Secondary chemotherapy of advanced breast cancer. Cancer 31, 660 (1973).
103. KISTER, S.J.: The chemotherapy of breast cancer. In: Disease of the Breast, p. 769 (ed. C.H. Haagensen). Philadelphia-London-Toronto: Saunders 1971.
104. HANHAM, I.W.F., NEWTON, K.A., WESTBURY, G.: Seventy-five cases of solid tumours treated by a modified quadruple chemotherapy regime. Brit. J. Cancer 25, 462 (1971).
105. CANELLOS, G.P., DeVITA, V.T., GOLD, G.L., CHABNER, B.A., SCHEIN, P.S., YOUNG, R.C.: Cyclical combination chemotherapy in the treatment of advanced breast carcinoma. Proc. Amer. Ass. Cancer Res. 15, 37 (1974).
106. AHMANN, D.L., HAHN, R.G., BISEL, H.F.: A phase II evaluation of ifosfamide (NSC-109724) treatment of disseminated breast cancer. Proc. Amer. Ass. clin. Oncol. 15, 182 (1974).
107. VAN EDEN, FLAKSON, G., VAN DYK, J.J., VAN DER MERWE, A.M., FALKSON, H.C.: 5-Fluorouracil (5-FU; NSC-19893), 5-(3,3-Dimethyl-1-triazeno)-imidazole-4-carboxamide (NSC-45388), vincristine (NSC-67574) and 1,3-bis(2-chloroethyl)-1-nitrosourea (BCNU; NSC-409962) given concomitantly in the treatment of solid tumors in man. Cancer Chemother. Rep. 56, 107 (1972).
108. TUCKER, W.G., TALLEY, R.W., BROWNLEE, R.W., BURROWS, J.H., STOTT, P.B., MOORHEAD, E.L., II, SAN DIEGO, E.L.: Preliminary trials with combination therapy of cyclophosphamide (NSC-26271), vincristine (NSC-67574), and 5-fluorouracil (NSC-19893). Cancer Chemother. Rep. 52, 593 (1968).
109. BULL, J., TORMEY, D., FALKSON, G., BLOM, J., PERLIN, E., CARBONE, P.: A comparison of cyclophosphamide, adriamycin, and 5-fluorouracil versus cyclophosphamide, methotrexate, and 5-fluorouracil in metastatic breast cancer. Proc. Am. Soc. clin. Oncol. 16, 246 (1975).
110. TAYLOR, S.G., CANELLOS, G.P., BAND, P., POCOCK, S.: Combination chemotherapy for advanced breast cancer: randomized comparison with single drug therapy. Proc. Amer. Ass. clin. oncol. 15, 175 (1974).
111. CREECH, R.H., CATALANO, R.B., MASTRANGELO, M.J., ENGSTROM, P.F.: An effective low-dose intermittent cyclophosphamide, methotrexate, and 5-fluorouracil treatment regimen for metastatic breast cancer. Cancer 35, 1101 (1975).
112. DEEMARSKY, L.Y., CHERNOMORDIKOVA, M.F.: Combination chemotherapy in the management of breast cancer metastases. Cancer 26, 771 (1970).
113. FISHER, B.: Cooperative clinical trials in primary breast cancer: a critical appraisal. Cancer 31, 1271 (1973).

114. DAO, T.L., NEMOTO, T.: Clinical significance of skin recurrence after radical mastectomy in women with cancer of breast. Surg. Gynec. Obstet. 117, 447 (1963).

115. FISHER, B.: Systemic chemotherapy as an adjuvant to surgery in the treatment of breast cancer. Cancer 24, 1286 (1969).

116. FISHER, B.: Status of adjuvant therapy: results of the national surgical adjuvant breast studies on oophorectomy, postoperative radiation therapy, and chemotherapy. Cancer 28, 1654 (1971).

117. FISHER, B.: Surgical adjuvant therapy for breast cancer. Cancer 30, 1556 (1972).

118. DONEGAN, W.L.: Extended surgical adjuvant thiotepa for mammary carcinoma. Arch. Surg. 109, 187 (1974).

119. MRAZEK, R.G., McDONALD, G.O.: Surgery and adjuvant chemotherapy in the treatment for breast carcinoma. Xth International Cancer Congress, Houston 1970.

120. NISSEN-MEYER, R., KJELLGREN, K., MANSSON, B.: Preliminary report from the Scandinavian Adjuvant Chemotherapy Study Group. Cancer Chemother. Rep. Part 1, 55, 561 (1971).

121. FINNEY, R.: Adjuvant chemotherapy in the radical treatment of carcinoma of the breast - a clinical trial. Amer. J. Roentgenol. 111, 137 (1971).

122. MEAKIN, J.W. et al.: A preliminary report of two studies of adjuvant treatment of primary breast cancer. In: Prognostic Factors in Breast Cancer. p. 157 (eds. A.P.M. Forrest, P.B. Kunkler). (from Proceedings of First Tenovus Symposium, Cardiff 1967). Edinburgh: Livingstone 1968.

123. RAVDIN, R.G., LEWISON, E.F., SLACK, N.H., DAO, T.L., GARDNER, B., STATE, D., FISHER, B.: Results of a clinical trial concerning the worth of prophylactic oophorectomy for breast carcinoma. Surg. Gynec. Obstet. 131, 1055 (1970).

124. KENNEDY, B.J., MIELKE, Jr., P.W., FORTUNY, I.E.: Therapeutic castration versus prophylactic castration in breast cancer. Surg. Gynec. Obstet. 118, 524 (1964).

125. NISSEN-MEYER, R.: Suppression of ovarian function in primary breast cancer. In: Prognostic Factors in Breast Cancer, p. 139. (eds. A.P.M. Forrest, P.B. Kunkler). Edinburgh-London: Livingstone 1968.

126. COLE, M.P.: Suppression of ovarian function in primary breast cancer. In: Prognostic Factors in Breast Cancer, p. 146 (eds. A.P.M. Forrest, P.B. Kunkler). Edinburgh-London: Livingstone 1968.

127. HAYWARD, J.L., BULBROOK, R.D.: Urinary steroids and prognosis in breast cancer. In: Prognostic Factors in Breast Cancer, p. 383 (eds. A.P.M. Forrest, P.B. Kunkler). Edinburgh-London: Livingstone 1968.

128. ATKINS, H., BULBROOK, R.D., FALCONER, M.A., HAYWARD, J.L., Mac LENA, K.S., SCHURR, P.H.: Ten years' experience of steroid assays in the management of breast cancer. Lancet 2, 7581 (1968).

129. AHLQUIST, K.A., JACKSON, A.W., STEWART, J.G.: Urinary steroid values as a guide to prognosis in breast cancer. Brit. med. J. 1, 217 (1968).

130. KENNEDY, B.J., TIBBETTS, D.M., NATHANSON, I.T., AUB, J.C.: Hypercalcemia, a complication of hormone therapy of advanced breast cancer. Cancer Res. 13, 445 (1953).

131. STEIN, J.J.: Management of disseminated breast cancer. Cancer 28, 1679 (1971).

132. MacDONALD, I.: Endocrine ablation in disseminated mammary carcinoma. Surg. Gynec. Obstet. 115, 215 (1972).

133. HAYWARD, J.: Ablative endocrine therapy. In: Oncology 1970, Vol. 4, p. 55 (eds. R.L. Clark, R.W. Cumley, J.E. McCay). Chicago: Year Book Medical Publishers 1971.

134. EDITORIAL: Prolactin and breast cancer. Lancet 1129 (1972).
135. HAYWARD, J.: Hormones and human breast cancer. An account of 15 years study. In: Recent Results in Cancer Research, Vol. 24. Berlin: Springer-Verlag 1970.
136. ATKINS, H., FALCONER, M.A., HAYWARD, J.L., MacLEAN, K.S., SCHURR, P.H.: The timing of adrenalectomy and of hypophysectomy in the treatment of advanced breast cancer. Lancet 1, 827 (1966).
137. PEARSON, O.H., RAY, B.S.: Hypophysectomy in the treatment of metastatic breast cancer. Amer. J. Surg. 99, 544 (1960).
138. SEGALOFF, A.: Hormonal therapy of breast cancer. Cancer 30, 1541 (1972).
139. DAO, T.L., NEMOTO, T.: An evaluation of adrenalectomy and androgen in disseminated mammary carcinoma. Surg. Gynec. Obstet. 121, 1257 (1965).
140. HALL, T.C., WILSON, R.E.: Safe and effective method of administering 5-fluorouracil to adrenalectomized patients. Surg. Gynec. Obstet. 123, 978 (1966).
141. NEMOTO, T., DAO, T.: 5-Fluorouracil and cyclophosphamide in disseminated breast cancer. New York J. Med. 71, 554 (1971).
142. SALIH, H., FLAX, H., BRANDNER, W., HOBBS, J.R.: Prolactin dependence in human breast cancers. Lancet 2, 1103 (1972).
143. PARRISH, F.F., MURRAY, J.A.: Orthopedic aspects of breast carcinoma. In: Breast Cancer: Early and Late, p. 355. Chicago: Year Book Medical Publishers 1970.
144. VISFELDT, J., SCHEIKE, O.: Male breast cancer. I. Histologic typing and grading of 187 cases. Cancer 32, 985 (1973).
145. HOLLEB, A.I.: Cancer of the male breast. In: Breast Cancer: Early and Late, p. 245. Chicago: Year Book Medical Publishers 1970.
146. TREVES, N., HOLLEB, A.I.: Cancer of the male breast. A report of 146 cases. Cancer 8, 1249 (1955).
147. KENNEDY, B.J.: Hormone therapy in cancer. Geriatrics 25, 106 (1970).
148. WARD, H.W.C.: Anti-oestrogen therapy for breast cancer: A trial of tamoxifen at two dose levels. Brit. med. J. 1, 13 (1973).
149. BLOOM, H.J.G., BOESEN, E.: Antioestrogens in the treatment of breast cancer: value of nafoxidine in 52 advanced cases. Brit. med. J. 2, 7 (1974).
150. CUTLER, S.J.: Classification of extent of disease in breast cancer. Sem. Oncol. 1, 91 (1974).
151. TSAKRAKLIDES, V., OLSON, P., KERSEY, J.H., GOOD, R.A.: Prognostic significance of the regional lymph node histology of the breast. Cancer 34, 1259 (1974).
152. WILSON, R.G., BUCHAN, R., ROBERTS, M.M., FORREST, A.P.M., BOYNS, A.R., COLE, E.N., GRIFFITHS, K.: Plasma prolactin and breast cancer. Cancer 33, 1325 (1974).
153. SMITHLINE, F., SHERMAN, L., KOLODNY, H.D.: Prolactin and breast carcinoma. New Engl. J. Med. 292, 784 (1975).
154. KENNEDY, B.J.: Hormonal therapies in breast cancer. Semin. Oncol. 1, 119 (1974).
155. MOSELEY, H.S., FLETCHER, W.S., LEUNG, B.S., KRIPPAEHNE, W.W.: Predictive criteria for the selection of breast cancer patients for adrenalectomy. Amer. J. Surg. 128, 143 (1974).
156. DeSOMBRE, E.R., SMITH, S., BLOCK, G.E., FERGUSON, D.J., VENSEN. E.V.: Prediction of breast cancer response to endocrine therapy. Cancer Chemother. Rep. Part 1, 58, 513 (1974).
157. AHMANN, D.L., HAHN, R., BISEL, H.F.: Disseminated breast cancer: evaluation of hormonal therapy utilizing stilbestrol and medrogestone singly and in combination. Cancer 30, 651 (1972).
158. CARTER, S.K.: The chemical therapy of breast cancer. Semin. Oncol. 1, 131 (1974).
159. BRODER, L.E., TORMEY, D.C.: Combination chemotherapy of carcinoma of the breast. Cancer Treat. Rev. 1, 183 (1974).

160. BLUM, R.H., CARTER, S.K.: Adriamycin Ann. intern. Med. <u>80</u>, 249 (1974).
161. GOTTLIEB, J.A., BLUMENSCHEIN, G.B., GUTTERMAN, J.U., FREIREICH, E.J., CARDENAS, J.: Adriamycin in the treatment of breast cancer. In: Adriamycin review. EORTC International Symposium, p. 249 (eds. M. Staquet, H. Tagnon, Y. Kenis et al.) Ghent: European Press Medikon 1975.
162. WASSERMAN, T.H., SLAVIK, M., CARTER, S.K.: Review of CCNU in clinical cancer. Cancer Treat. Rev. <u>1</u>, 131 (1974).
163. WASSERMAN, T.H., SLAVIK, M., CARTER, S.K.: Methyl-CCNU in clinical cancer therapy. Cancer Treat. Rev. <u>1</u>, 251 (1974).
164. BRAMBILLA, C., DE LENA, M., BONADONNA, G.: Combination chemotherapy with adriamycin in metastatic mammary carcinoma. Cancer Chemother. Rep. Part 1, <u>58</u>, 251 (1974).
165. LOKICH, J.J., SKARIN, A.T., FREI, E.: 1,-(2-chloroethyl)-3-cyclo-hexyl-1-nitrosourea (methyl CCNU) and adriamycin combination therapy. Cancer <u>34</u>, 1593 (1974).
166. De LENA, M., BRAMBILLA, C., MORABITO, A., BONADONNA, G.: Adriamycin plus vincristine compared to and combined with cyclophosphamide, methotrexate, and 5-fluorouracil for advanced breast carcinoma. Cancer <u>35</u>, 1108 (1975).
167. DeJAGER, R., KAUFMAN, R., OCHOA, M., KRAKOFF, T.H.: Chemotherapy of advanced breast cancer with a combination of cytoxan, adria-mycin, and 5-fluorouracil. Proc. Am. Soc. Clin. Oncol. <u>16</u>, 273 (1975).
168. SMALLEY, R., BORNSTEIN, R.: C-A-F treatment of metastatic breast cancer. Proc. Am. Soc. Clin. Oncol. <u>16</u>, 265 (1975).
169. CANELLOS, G.P., DE VITA, V.T., GOLD, G.L., CHABNER, B.A., SCHEIN, P.S., YOUNG, R.C.: Cyclical combination chemotherapy for advanced breast cancer. Brit. Med. J. <u>1</u>, 218 (1974).
170. E.O.R.T.C. Protocol 10743.
171. ROSEMUND, G.P., MAIER, W.P.: Role of mastectomy in breast cancer. Sem. Oncol. <u>1</u>, 97 (1974).
172. BAUM, M.: Surgery and radiotherapy in breast cancer. Sem. Oncol. <u>1</u>, 101 (1974).
173. FISHER, B., CARBONE, P., ECONOMOU, S.G., FRELICK, R., GLASS, A., LERNER, H., REDMOND, C., ZELEN, M., BAND, P., KATRYCH, D.L., WOLMARK, N., FISHER, E.R.: L-Phenylalanine mustard in the management of primary breast cancer. New Engl. J. Med. <u>292</u>, 117 (1975).
174. RAMIREZ, G.: Combined chemotherapy-radiotherapy as an adjuvant to mastectomy in patients with positive nodes. Proc. Am. Soc. clin. Oncol. <u>16</u>, 224 (1975).
175. BONADONNA, G., BRUSAMOLINO, E., VALAGUSSA, P., et al.: Combination chemotherapy as an adjuvant treatment in operable breast cancer. New Engl. J. Med. <u>294</u>, 404 (1976).
176. E.O.R.T.C. Protocol 10741
177. BRICHLOW, R.W.: Breast cancer in men. Semin. Oncol. <u>1</u>, 145 (1974).
178 JONES, S.E., DURIE, B.G.M., SALMON, S.E.: Combination chemotherapy with adriamycin and cyclophosphamide for advanced breast cancer. Cancer <u>36</u>, 90 (1975).
179. TORMEY, D.C.: Adriamycin (NSC-123127) in breast cancer: an overview of studies. Cancer Chemother. Rep. Part 3, <u>6</u>, 319 (1975).
180. AHMANN, D.L., BISEL, H.F., HAHN, R.G., EAGAN, R.T., EDMONSON, J. H., et al.: An analysis of a multiple-drug program in the treatment of patients with advanced breast cancer utilizing 5-fluorouracil, cyclophosphamide, and prednisone with or without vincristine. Cancer <u>36</u>, 1925 (1975).
181. AHMANN, D.L., EAGAN, R.T., BISEL, H.F., HAHN, R.G., O'CONNELL, M.J., EDMONSON, J.H.: Evaluation of combination therapy with adriamycin (NSC-123127) and methotrexate (NSC-740) in patients with disseminated breast cancer. Cancer Chemother. Rep. Part 3, <u>6</u>, 335 (1975).

182. EAGAN, R.T., AHMANN, D.L., EDMONSON, J.H., HAHN, R.G., BISEL, H. F.: Controlled evaluation of the combination of adriamycin (NSC-123127), vincristine (NSC-67574), and methotrexate (NSC-740Z) in patients with disseminated breast cancer. Cancer Chemother. Rep. Part 3, _6_, 339 (1975).
183. FISHER, B., WOLMARK, N.: New concepts in the management of primary breast cancer. Cancer _36_, 627 (1975).
184. CARBONE, P.P.: Chemotherapy in the treatment strategy of breast cancer. Cancer _36_, 633 (1975).
185. URBAN, J.A.: Changing pattern of breast cancer. Lucy Wortham James Lecture (Clinical). Cancer _37_, 111 (1976).
186. LACOUR, J., BUCALOSSI, P., CACERS, E., JACOBELLI, G., KOSZAROWSKI, T., LE, M., et al.: Radical mastectomy versus radical mastectomy plus internal mammary dissection. Cancer _37_, 206 (1976).
187. STJERNSWARD, J.: Decreased survival related to irradiation post-operatively in early operable breast cancer. Lancet _2_, 1285 (1974).
188. ZUCALI, R., USLENGHI, C., KENDA, R., BONADONNA, G.: Natural history and survival of inoperable breast cancer treated with radiotherapy and radiotherapy followed by radical mastectomy. Cancer _37_, 1422 (1976).
189. HEUSON, J.C., ENGELSMAN, E, BLONK-VAN DER WIJST, J., MAASS, H., DROCHMANS, A., MICHEL, J., NOWAKOWSKI, H., GORINS, A.: Comparative trial of nafoxidine and ethinyloestradiol in advanced breast cancer: an EORTC study. Brit. J. Med. _2_, 711 (1975).
190. MEYSKENS, F.L., Jr., TORMEY, D.C., NEIFELD, J.P.: Male breast cancer: a review. Cancer Treat. Rev. _3_, 83 (1976).

Chapter 27
Gynecologic Cancer and Trophoblastic Disease

A. CANCER OF THE OVARY

Ovarian carcinoma now causes more deaths than any other gynecologic malignancy in the United States. The age at diagnosis is very variable but most patients are between the ages of 40 and 60 years. No etiologic factors have been recognized. The disease is usually diagnosed late in its course. Less than 30% of all ovarian malignancies can be cured by surgery alone by the time of the initial exploration.

The many histologic types of ovarian tumors are best classified according to their embryonic origin: (1) coelomic epithelial, (2) germinal cell, and (3) gonadal mesenchyme (or sex cord) origin (Table 27-1). The majority (+ 85%) of ovarian tumors are of epithelial origin. These are further subdivided into serous (52%) and mucinous (13%) cystadenocarcinomas and endometroid (17%), undifferentiated (18%) and mesonephroid (8%) adenocarcinomas. Among the tumors of germinal origin we distinguish dysgerminomas (a homologue of testicular seminoma) and the teratocarcinomas (developed from embryonal pluripotential tissue capable of forming elements from all three embryonal layers). Tumors of mesenchymal origin can differentiate into male (arrhenoblastoma, Sertoli-cell tumors) or female (granulosa-cell tumor, theca-cell tumor) gonadal structures.

In addition to the usual local lymphatic (relatively rare) and hematogenous spread, ovarian cancers are characterized by a tendency to implant in the peritoneal cavity, resulting in ascites formation. These implants can cause recurrences after apparent total excision. This mode of spread makes it imperative that the entire abdomen and pelvis be treated by either radiation or chemotherapy. Involvement of both ovaries is not uncommon.

Most authorities have adopted the staging system of the International Federation of Gynecologists and Obstetricians (FIGO) (Table 27-2). The TNM staging is listed in Table 27-3 (1).

The prognosis is largely dependent on the clinical stage, and to a lesser extent on the cell type and the grade of malignancy (3, 4). The FIGO system does not attribute any prognostic significance to penetration of the ovarian capsule by the tumor (5), nor is the influence of ascites or tumor spill at the time of surgery on prognosis well defined. The overall 5-year survival rate is 25-30%.

Table 27-1. Histologic classification of ovarian carcinomas (according to their embryonic origin)

I. Coelomic epithelial origin		($\pm$ 85%)
	Serous cystadenocarcinoma	52%
	Mucinous cystadenocarcinoma	13%
	Endometroid adenocarcinoma	17%
	Undifferentiated adenocarcinoma	18%
	Mesonephroid adenocarcinoma	8%

II. Germinal cell origin

    Dysgerminomas
    Teratocarcinomas

III. Gonadal mesenchyme or sex cord origin, capable of differentiating into:

    (a) Male gonadal structures - masculinizing
        Arrhenoblastomas
        Sertoli cell tumors

    (b) Female gonadal structures - feminizing
        Granulosa-cell tumors
        Theca-cell tumors

Table 27-2. F.I.G.O. Staging of carcinoma of the ovary

Stage Ia - Growth limited to one ovary; no ascites
     Ib - Growth limited to both ovaries; no ascites
     Ic - Growth limited to one or both ovaries; ascites present, with malignant cells in the fluid

Stage IIa - Growth involving one or both ovaries with extension and/or metastasis to uterus and/or tubes only
      IIb - Growth involving one or both ovaries with extension to other pelvic tissues

Stage III - Growth involving one or both ovaries with widespread intraperitoneal metastasis to the abdomen[a]

Stage IV - Growth involving one or both ovaries, with distant metastasis outside the peritoneal cavity

[a] Including omentum, intestine, mesentery, liver, retroperitoneal glands, and other viscera.

1. Chemotherapy

(i) Single-Agent Chemotherapy

Alkylating agents are definitely the most active group of cytotoxic compounds in ovarian carcinomas, yielding a response rate of 45-65 with 5-15 percent of all treated patients continuing to respond two years after initiation of therapy (Table 27-4) (4, 6-15, 95, 96). Most authorities are of the opinion that there is little to distinguish one alkylating agent from another, and no particular dose schedule appears to be superior. The final selection is determined by personal experience, differences in toxicity, ease of administration, and the urgency of the

Table 27-3. TNM staging of carcinoma of the ovary

T1S Pre-invasive carcinoma, so-called carcinoma in situ
T1 Tumor limited to one ovary
T2 Tumor limited to both ovaries
T3 Tumor extending into the uterus and/or fallopian tubes
T4 Tumor extending directly to other surrounding anatomical structures
TX Tumor cannot be assessed (laparotomy not done)
    N.B. - No regard is paid to the presence of ascites
NX When it is not possible to assess the regional lymph nodes, the
    symbol NX will be used permitting eventual addition of histological
    information, thus: NX - or NX+
NO No abnormal regional lymph nodes demonstrated
N1 Abnormal regional lymph nodes demonstrated
MO No evidence of distant metastases
M1 Implantation or other metastases present
    M1a In the true pelvis only
    M1b Within the abdomen
    M1c Beyond the abdomen and pelvis
The TNM Classification must be supplemented by histological grading

---

Stage Grouping

Stage Ia   T1NOMO
Stage Ib   T2NOMO
Stage IIa   T3NOMO
Stage IIb   T4 NOMO   Any M1a
Stage III   Any N1
             Any M1b
Stage IV   Any M1c
Special category: Any TX

Table 27-4. Effectiveness of single agents in ovarian carcinoma

Drug	Number evaluated	Response (%)	Reference
Methotrexate	16	25	SULLIVAN et al. (16)
5-Fluorouracil	141	26.5	BAGLEY et al. (4)
Cytosine arabinoside	6	0	BAGLEY et al. (4)
BCNU	34	6	YOUNG et al. (95)
CCNU	22	32	WASSERMAN et al. (97)
MeCCNU	25	0	WASSERMAN et al. (98)
Chlorambucil	422	52.5	LIVINGSTON and CARTER (6)
Cyclophosphamide	262	44	LIVINGSTON and CARTER (6)
Melphalan	367	47	LIVINGSTON and CARTER (6)
Uracil mustard	17	29	BAGLEY et al. (4)
Thio-TEPA	574	31	BAGLEY et al. (4)
Hexamethylmelamine	32	38	BLUM et al. (17)
Actinomycin D	6	0	BAGLEY et al. (4)
Adriamycin	18	28	YOUNG et al. (95)
Bleomycin	12	0	BLUM et al. (20)
Porfiromycin	14	14	ISBICKI et al. (21)
Vincristine	17	0	YOUNG et al. (95)
Vinblastine	20	15	LIVINGSTONE and CARTER (6)

situation. Some authors thus recommend an i.v. injection of thio-TEPA
in rapidly progressing or extensive disease where prompt control of
symptoms and tumor masses is desirable, while chlorambucil (CLB) is reserved for less urgent cases. SMITH and RUTLEDGE, at the M.D. Anderson

Hospital, have had extensive experience with melphalan (10, 15) given i.v. (1 mg/kg infused over 8 hours) every three weeks or orally (0.2 mg/kg qd for 5 days) every 4 weeks. They obtained objective tumor regressions in 47% (20% CR, 27% PR) in 494 patients. The response rates for the different histologic types of epithelial origin were similar but complete remissions are significantly less common with undifferentiated tumors and appear to be of shorter duration. Forty-two percent of responders were alive 2 years after the initiation of chemotherapy, as against 10 percent nonresponders.

There seems to be little evidence that switching from one alkylating agent to another is of any value in patients who fail to respond or who have become resistant to the initial alkylating agent. The second-choice drugs for ovarian carcinoma include 5-FU (10-30% RR) (4, 6, 9, 12, 95), MTX (4/16) (16), adriamycin (28%) (19, 95), vinblastine (15%) (6), and hexamethylmelamine (38%) (17) (Table 27-3). Few data are available on the nitrosoureas (18, 95, 97, 98). Most patient receiving these agents had already failed or become resistant to alkylating agents and often to radiotherapy as well. Therefore no direct comparison can be made with alkylating agents to judge their value. Prospective randomized trials of chemotherapy with 5-FU, hexamethylmelamine, and melphalan and of methotrexate and thio-TEPA in previously untreated patients with advanced ovarian cancer (FIGO Stages III and IV) are now in progress and should provide needed information on the relative activity of these agents in advanced ovarian cancer (95).

Hormonal agents have been evaluated infrequently in ovarian carcinomas. A few regressions have been reported with progestational agents or estrogen (3, 4, 8, 11, 12). A recent report suggests that high-dose progestins warrant further evaluation (22).

(ii) Combinations
Since only one class of agents has any significant activity in ovarian cancers it is not surprising that combinations have not been much more effective than single alkylating agents (Table 27-5). The combination of actinomycin D (ACD), 5-FU, and cyclophosphamide, although more toxic, was not more effective in ovarian carcinoma than melphalan alone (15). The value of ACD alone in this cancer is not known. A 39% response rate is obtained with this combination in patients who have become resistant to melphalan (10). GREENSPAN reported good responses in 63% of patients treated with thio-TEPA combined with MTX (23). BRANDL obtained 80% regressions in 26 previously untreated patients with a combination of cyclophosphamide, vinblastine, and triaziquone (Trenimon) given in intermittent cycles (24). LLOYD et al. obtained 61% objective regressions with a combination of ADM plus CPM (99) and YOUNG et al. (29) in 79% with MTX, 5-FU, CPM, HMM. Few other combinations have been evaluated in large enough numbers to allow any conclusions to be drawn (95).

LI recommends a combination of chlorambucil and 5-FU for tumors of epithelial origin and of vincristine, actinomycin D, chlorambucil, and methotrexate for germinal mesenchymal tumors (9). If mesenchymal tumors fail to respond to the quadruple therapy, mithramycin can be tried. WIDER et al. obtained sustained remissions in 3 out of 4 patients with ovarian carcinoma containing choriocarcinoma who were treated with a combination of MTX, CLB, and ACD (31). Adriamycin appears promising in some of the unusual ovarian cancers, including ovarian teratoma (32).

474

Table 27-5. Response rates to combinations in ovarian carcinoma

Combination	Number evaluated	Response		Reference
MTX, thio-TEPA	96	63%	43: 80-99% 17: 58-80% regression	GREENSPAN (23) (1968)
MTX, VCR	5	2/5		LOUIS (25) (1974)
MTX-FA, CPM	18	43%		BARLOW and PIVER (18) (1976)
CPM, ADM	23	61%		LLOYD et al. (99) (1976)
CPM, triaziquone, VLB	26	80%	2 CR	BRANDL (24) (1970)
5-FU, CPM, ACD	47	45%	30% CR 15% PR	SMITH et al. (15) (1972)
MTX, 5-FU, CPM	25	32%	No CR	BRODOVSKY (26) (1974)
MTX, 5-FU, CPM, VCR	19	42%	1 CR, 7 PR	SWCCG (27) (1972)
MTX, 5-FU, CPM, VCR (COMF)	4	0/ 4		HANHAM et al. (28) (1971)
MTX, 5-FU, CPM, HMM	24	79%	8 CR 11 PR	YOUNG et al. (29) (1976)

2. Strategy

There is a great deal of controversy over the management of the different stages of ovarian carcinoma. Lack of uniformity in staging and histologic classification in therapeutic schemes, and especially the lack of controlled trials are responsible for this confusion. The following discussion is applicable to ovarian epithelial tumors.

(i) Stage-I Ovarian Carcinoma

The initial step is an exploratory laparotomy. It is generally accepted that a total abdominal hysterectomy with bilateral salpingo-oophorectomy (TAH + BSO) is the surgical procedure of choice (2, 4, 5, 12-14). Less radical procedures are occasionally used for well-differentiated tumors localized to the ovary (3). The value of prophylactic omentectomy in decreasing the chance of subsequent troublesome tumor masses and ascites formation has not been documented in comparative trials.

Since approximately one-third of patients develop recurrent disease after surgery alone (5-year survival 32-78%, mean 67% (4)), various forms of adjuvant therapy have been proposed. The value of short-term or long-term systemic adjuvant chemotherapy has not been documented (7) but several studies are in progress (95). The high response rate to alkylating agents in advanced stages suggests that their use in early stages may be indicated. The justification for i.p. chemotherapy following surgery, to kill small numbers of floating cells and microscopic implants is questionable and the results are inconclusive (7).

Postoperative radiotherapy has been of two types: (1) external radiotherapy to the pelvis or the whole abdomen, and (2) radioactive isotopes (14, 33). These two methods have been advocated because of the tendency of ovarian carcinoma to spread by implantation over the entire abdominal cavity. Most studies suggest that external radiation (7, 34, 35) has no beneficial effect, while i.p. isotopes might have some effect on survival (36-38). PEREZ, reviewing trends in treatment methods, noted that radioactive isotopes are rarely used at present because of a significant complication rate (33). He recommends postoperative pelvic irradiation in the less well-differentiated adenocarcinomas. Adjuvant immunotherapy has not yet been evaluated. In Stage I disease (Ia and Ib) the question remains whether adjuvant therapy after primary resection is beneficial and what type (chemotherapy, radiotherapy, or immunotherapy) is to be recommended.

(ii) Stage-II Ovarian Carcinoma

Most authorities agree that adjuvant radiotherapy following surgery (preferably TAH + BSO) improves 5-year survival rates (39% (27-69%) versus 27% (0-33%) for surgery alone (2, 4)). However, there is some controversy as to what type of radiotherapy is best: irradiation of the pelvis only, external irradiation of the whole abdomen (14), or i.p. isotopes. PEREZ recommends treatment of the entire abdomen with ^{60}Co by the strip technique in Stage-II patients with ascites, those in whom gross spillage of tumor contents occurred at the time of removal of a completely resectable tumor, and those with unfavorable histology (33). Since the relapse rate remains relatively high even after combined surgery and radiotherapy it seems logical to evaluate long-term adjuvant chemotherapy with or without optimal radiotherapy.

The management of the locally advanced case that cannot be completely resected because the tumor is fixed to adjacent structures is the subject of debate. Some authors advocate resection of as much tumor as possible, followed by radiotherapy and/or chemotherapy (2). Other propose biopsy only, followed by radiotherapy (33) or chemotherapy (15) or a combination (13, 39) to reduce the tumor mass. If tumor regression occurs, a "second-look" operation is carried out, in the hope that complete resection will be possible (14, 15, 33, 39).

(iii) Stage-III Ovarian Carcinoma

The tumor is completely removed if possible. There are at least three options for further, postoperative treatment: radiotherapy (pelvis + external total abdomen), chemotherapy alone, and a combination of radiotherapy and chemotherapy (13). No prospective trials comparing these different treatment modalities have been published. Several authors recommend that total-abdomen radiotherapy be used only if there is no residual tumor or if remaining tumor masses are less than 3 cm in diameter (14, 15, 33).

In patients with extensive tumors that are not completely resectable, the remarks made on the management of nonresectable Stage-II tumors (see above) are applicable.

(iv) Stage-IV Ovarian Carcinoma

Most patients with Stage-IV disease are women who have not responded as hoped to treatment in earlier stages, and they are likely to have been treated previously with surgery, radiotherapy, and/or chemotherapy. In these cases management must be individually decided to suit each patient.

It is obvious that no clear-cut guidelines can be given for the treatment of the various stages of ovarian carcinoma until appropriate prospective comparative trials have been carried out (95). Gynecologic co-operative groups have a great deal of work before them. Surgical resection alone is clearly inadequate in the majority of cases. The most effective adjuvant therapy following complete resection of tumor, and the optimal management of tumors unsuited to complete resection at the time of initial exploration have still to be determined.

B. CANCER OF THE ENDOMETRIUM

Endometrial carcinoma is the second most common female genital malignancy. It occurs predominantly in older women (75% of patients are postmenopausal). A frequent association has been noted with obesity, diabetes, hypertension, and a late onset of menopause. Prolonged episodes of anovulation and unopposed estrogen stimulation are thought to be predisposing factors for its development. GUSBERG reported that 12% of patients with adenomatous hyperplasia develop endometrial cancer (40). Endometrial carcinoma is not uncommonly associated with estrogen-secreting tumors and Stein-Leventhal syndrome. A gradual progression from endometrial cystic hyperplasia through various stages of adenomatous hyperplasia, anaplasia, carcinoma in situ to invasive carcinoma has been described (41). Any one of these pathologic processes can regress when the constant stimulation by estrogen is removed or if progestins are prescribed. The majority of tumors of the corpus uteri arise in the endometrium, and they are generally well-differentiated, slowly growing adenocarcinomas which retain histological similarity to the parent tissue. More rarely malignant tumors arise in the myometrium (sarcomas).

The staging approved by the FIGO is the system most often used in the Anglo-American literature (Table 27-6). The TNM classification is shown in Table 27-7 (1). The prognosis is greatly influenced by the extent of the disease, and to a lesser extent by the degree of cellular differentiation. In at least 75% of cases the tumor is still limited to the corpus at the time of diagnosis. Without pronounced involvement of the myometrium 5-year survivals as high as 80% have been reported. The prognosis is poor once extrauterine spread has occurred.

1. Hormone Therapy

Progestins have been tried in endometrial carcinoma because of the maturing effect of progesterone on the normal endometrium and the sensitivity of the well-differentiated neoplastic counterpart to hormonal stimuli. Response rates ranging from 19% to over 50% have been reported, with an average of one-third of patients showing objective tumor regression (42-51). Subjective responses are more common. Slow-growing, well-differentiated tumors, with a long disease-free interval between the primary and recurrence, tend to respond more often than others. Some investigators report that recurrences in previously irradiated areas are less likely to respond, while pulmonary metastases are the ones that regress most often. Remissions last 12-18 months, and occasionally much longer. Survival is considerably longer in responders (21.6 months) than in nonresponders (7.8 months) (45). The fact that the survival rate of the responders has remained constant at 31.4% for over 4 years (50) is most encouraging. These may be the patients in whom the malignant disease has been "cured." Evidence of objective regression is usually detectable within 1 to 3 months of the initiation of therapy. Progestins should be prescribed for a minimum of 3 months and should then be maintained in responding patients. There appear to be no contraindications, and side-effects are rare (50, 100). Regressions have been reported with 17α-hydroxyprogesterone caproate (Delalutin) (42, 43, 50), medroxyprogesterone acetate (44-46), and megestrol acetate (49). These

Table 27-6. Staging for endometrial carcinoma (recommended by the American Joint Committee for Cancer Staging and End-Results Reporting)

Stage O	Pre-invasive, carcinoma in situ
Stage I	Confined to corpus uteri
Stage II	Confined to corpus and cervix uteri
Stage III	Outside the uterus but not outside the true pelvis
Stage IV A	Outside true pelvis and/or involving mucosa of bladder or bowel
Stage IV B	Distant metastasis

Table 27-7. TNM Staging of endometrial carcinoma

T1S	Pre-invasive carcinoma, so-called in situ
T1	Carcinoma confined to the corpus
	T1a The uterine cavity is not enlarged
	T1b The uterine cavity is enlarged (enlargement is judged on whether the sound passes more than 8 cm beyond the cervical os: the distance to be recorded)
T2	Carcinoma involving the cervix
T3	Carcinoma extending outside the uterus, including spread to vagina, but remaining within the true pelvis
T4	Carcinoma involving the mucosa of the bladder or the rectum or extending beyond the true pelvis (the presence of bullous edema is not sufficient evidence to classify the tumor as T4)
	T4a Carcinoma involving the bladder or the rectum only and histologically proved
	T4b Carcinoma extending beyond the true pelvis
	N.B.-Enlargement of the uterus alone does not constitute grounds for assignment to T4
NX	When it is impossible to assess the regional lymph nodes the symbol NX will be used, permitting eventual addition of histological information, thus NX - or NX+
NO	No deformity of regional nodes as shown by available diagnostic methods
N1	Pelvic nodes distal to the bifurcation of the common iliac arteries deformed as shown by available diagnostic methods
N2	Intra-abdominal para-aortic nodes proximal to the bifurcation of the common iliac arteries deformed as shown by available diagnostic methods
MO	No evidence of distant metastases
M1	Distant metastases present, including involved inguinal lymph nodes

Stage Grouping

The categories NO and N1 are not taken into account in stage grouping:

Stage "O"	T1S
Stage Ia	T1aNXMO
Stage Ib	T1bNXMO
Stage II	T2NXMO
Stage III	T3NXMO, T1, T2 or T3N2MO
Stage IVa	Any T4MO
Stage IVb	Any M1

different preparations seem to yield similar results, but no comparative trials have been carried out.

KISTNER emphasizes the importance of a loading dose in producing remission (51). The optimum dosage seems to be in the range of 3 to 5 g
17α-hydroxyprogesterone caproate, or 3.5 g medroxyprogesterone acetate
weekly by i.m. injection. If a remission occurs the therapy is continued
with lower maintenance doses.

2. Chemotherapy

Endometrial carcinoma has not responded consistently to cytotoxic therapy (8, 11, 46, 101), Some responses have been reported in small series
with alkylating agents (46), 5-FU (6), hexamethylmelamine (2/6) (17),
adriamycin (3/8) (19), and hydroxyurea (2/6) (43). Adriamycin has been
combined with CPM (4/6) (99) or with 5-FU (5/5) (30).

3. Strategy

Surgical excision is the most important feature of the management of
endometrial carcinoma (46, 51-53). However, this is often preceded by
preoperative irradiation to facilitate total excision and to reduce
the risk of local recurrences. Intracavitary radium is used to deliver
intensive irradiation to the tumor. This is supplemented by external
irradiation of the whole of the pelvis to treat the sites and pathways
of regional spread in cases where the uterus is greatly enlarged by
cancer or for anaplastic tumors, which are more likely to reach the
serosal surface of the uterus and to metastasize to surrounding organs.
BONTE et al. (54) have suggested that progestins may have a radiosensitizing effect. However the Endometrial Adjuvant Study Group did not
observe a significant improvement in the survival or local control rate
in patients receiving progestational therapy in addition to surgery
and radiation (102).

The extent of the operation ranges from simple hysterectomy for most
patients to radical hysterectomy when the cervix is involved or when
spread is more advanced and to pelvic exenteration when the bladder
or rectum is involved. Because of the increasing risk of positive nodes
in the pelvic wall in Stages II and III it is recommended that they be
treated by either external irradiation or pelvic lymphadenectomy. Surgery is best performed 6 to 8 weeks after completion of the course of
radium therapy.

Postoperative external irradiation is indicated for anaplastic tumors
and when extrauterine spread is found at surgery.

Inoperable tumors and operable tumors occurring in patients unfit for
surgery are treated by a combination of radium insertion and external
irradiation of the lateral pelvic areas.

C. CANCER OF THE CERVIX

Carcinoma of the cervix accounts for approximately 14% of all malignancies in females, making it the second most common cancer in women and
the most common gynecologic malignancy. Earlier diagnosis and advances
in therapy have led to a reduction in the death rate in recent years.
The average age of women with invasive cervical cancer is 50 years.

Several predisposing factors are recognized, the most striking being that of coitus. An association has been discovered between Herpes simplex virus type 2 and cervical cancer (55).

There is evidence that progression from minor dysplasia through major dysplasia, intraepithelial carcinoma, and microinvasive carcinoma to frank invasive carcinoma is the usual histogenetic sequence.

Over 90% of cervical cancers are epidermoid. Different degrees of differentiation are noted. The so-called small-cell type is the least differentiated and presumably the most malignant form (56). A minority are adenocarcinomas, arising from glandular elements of the cervix. The clinical behavior of adenocarcinomas is similar to that of the epidermoid cancers but the response to radiotherapy is less predictable.

Cervical carcinoma spreads mainly by local infiltration and by lymphatic routes. The vagina, corpus uteri, parametrium, pelvic walls, bladder, and rectum can thus become involved as the tumor progresses. Hematogenous dissemination is rare. The League of Nations classification is almost universally used (Table 27-8).

Table 27-8. Clinical staging and lymph node metastases of cancer of the cervix[a]

Stage	Direct extension	Lymph node metastases
O	Pre-invasive carcinoma (carcinoma in situ)	None
I	Carcinoma strictly confined to the cervix (extension to the corpus disregarded)	11%
Ia	Minimal stromal invasion (preclinical invasive carcinoma, i.e., cases which cannot be diagnosed by routine clinical examination)	
Ib	All other cases of Stage I	
II	Carcinoma extends beyond the cervix but has not extended to pelvic wall; vagina (but not the lower third) is involved	22%
IIa	Carcinoma has not infiltrated parametrium	
III	Carcinoma has extended to pelvic wall. Rectal examination shows no cancer-free space between tumor and pelvic wall. Lower third of vagina is involved	33%
IV	Carcinoma has extended beyond true pelvis or has involved the mucosa of the bladder or rectum. However, the presence of bullous edema is not sufficient evidence to classify a case as Stage IV	77%

[a] Approved by the International Federation of Obstetricians and Gynecologists.

The prognosis varies with the clinical stage at diagnosis and the cell type. Five-year survival rates are 100% for Stage O; 80% for Stage I, 50-60% for Stage II, 25% for Stage III, and 5-10% for Stage IV.

1. Chemotherapy

Cervical carcinoma is not very sensitive to cytotoxic agents ([8], [11], [57], [58]). Published response rates often vary significantly, probably due to difficulties in evaluating tumor regressions. Most conventional agents achieve tumor regressions in no more than 20%, and these are usually only of brief duration (Table 27-9). No one agent appears to be especially useful. Bleomycin is not more promising than conventional agents ([20]).

Table 27-9. Effect of single agents on cervix cancer

Drug	Number evaluated	Resonse	Reference
Methotrexate: systemic:	25	20%	LIVINGSTON and CARTER ([6])
	27	29%	LIVINGSTON and CARTER ([6])
intra-arterial:	71	46.5%	LIVINGSTON and CARTER ([6])
5-Fluorouracil	136	21%	LIVINGSTON and CARTER ([6])
Hydroxyurea	10	O	HOWE and SAMUELS ([62])
CCNU	5	1/ 5	WASSERMAN et al. ([97])
MeCCNU	32	13%	WASSERMAN et al. ([98])
Nitrogen mustard	12	O	LIVINGSTON and CARTER ([6])
Chlorambucil	44	25%	LIVINGSTON and CARTER ([6])
Cyclophosphamide	91	20%	SMITH ([60])
Hexamethylmelamine	17	29%	BLUM et al. ([17])
Mitomycin C	18	22%	MOORE et al. ([61])
Adriamycin	11	4/11	O'BRYAN et al. ([19]) and BARLOV et al. ([32])
Bleomycin	78	21%	BLUM et al. ([20])
Profiromycin	15	5/15	IZBICKI et al. ([21])

Few authors report their experience with combination chemotherapy (Table 27-10). Several two-drug combinations appear to be superior to single-agent therapy.

Although intra-arterial chemotherapy has resulted in both objective and subjective responses, it has been of limited practical use ([58]).

There is no evidence to implicate hormonal factors in the histogenesis of cervical carcinoma. Not surprisingly, objective remissions have not been obtained in advanced cervical cancer with the administration of hormonal agents.

2. Strategy

The management of cervix carcinoma is fairly well standardized. Radiotherapy is the primary treatment modality for invasive cancers. Intracavitary radium is applied to the vagina and uterine cavity to achieve high-dose local tumor irradiation, while supplementary external radiotherapy is necessary for treatment of the lateral pelvic structures

Table 27-10. Response rates to combinations in cancer of the cervix

Combination	Number evaluated	Number of regressions		Reference
CPM, VCR	9	7	7 Karnof. category I	EAGAN et al. (63) (1973)
	11	4		MONFARDINI et al. (64) (1974)
MTX, CPM	23	10	3 CR, 7 PR	PAPAVASILIOU et al. (65) (1969)
MTX, BLM	8	5	3 CR, 2 PR	PIEL et al. (66) (1973)
MTX, BLM	6	3		YAGODA et al. (105) (1975)
ADM, MTX	9	8		GUTHRIE and WAY (106) (1974)
ADM, BLM	8	5		MONFARDINI et al. (64) (1974)
	10	1		BARLOW et al. (32) (1973)
DIC, HMM	10	5	4: > 50% 1: 25-50%	STOLINSKY et al. (67) (1972)
MTC, BLM, VCR	26	13 (50%)		BAKER et al. (107) (1975)
MTX, 5-FU, CPM, VCR (COMF)	3	3	3 PR	HANHAM et al. (28) (1971)

and regional lymph nodes. This is the treatment of choice for the majority of cases in Stages I to III.

Surgery is used in carcinoma in situ (Stage O). Total hysterectomy with removal of a wide vaginal cuff (with preservation of ovaries in premenopausal women) is generally recommended, but deep conization with careful follow-up may be acceptable in young patients wishing to have children in the future. Some surgeons treat even Stage-I carcinoma with radical total hysterectomy and lymph-node dissection, with survival rates comparable to those of radiotherapy. Radical surgery in Stages II and III is reserved for selected cases, normally cases that prove to be resistant to or recur after radiotherapy.

Surgical and radiotherapeutic possibilities should be exhausted before chemotherapy is initiated in advanced carcinoma of the cervix.

The role of adjuvant chemotherapy or immunotherapy has not yet been evaluated.

D. GYNECOLOGIC SARCOMAS

1. Chemotherapy

Since these tumors are rare, few authors have accumulated extensive experience (11). MALKASIAN noted objective regressions in five out of ten patients treated with 5-FU (68). Preliminary results with adriamycin in uterine sarcomas (5/7 responses) are encouraging (32).

E. TROPHOBLASTIC DISEASE

The term trophoblastic disease refers to a spectrum of chorionic tumors that originate either from the placenta (gestational trophoblastic tumors) or from the germinal cells of the gonads of both sexes (nongestational (69-73). A trophoblastic tumor can arise from misplaced primordial cells in the pineal body, mediastinum, or retroperitoneal area, but this is rare. Gestational trophoblastic tumors include hydatidiform mole, chorioadenoma destruens, or invasive mole, and choriocarcinoma. All these neoplasms arise from and relate to the abnormal behavior of the epithelial elements of the chorionic villus and to vascular abnormalities in the chorionic villus. Hydatidiform mole is a benign lesion. It has large hydropic villi with variable trophoblastic proliferation which is noninvasive. An invasive mole can retain the chorionic villus structure but show microscopic signs of invasiveness by trophoblast into the surrounding uterine structure. There may also be metastases to the lungs or brain or other parts of the body. Such trophoblastic emboli, in which chorionic villi persist, produce a variety of symptoms, and can even result in death, depending on the particular site of impaction, the extent of further proliferation at the new site, and the extent of any resultant local hemorrhage. Both hydatidiform mole and invasive mole can be transformed into choriocarcinoma. This is an anaplastic tumor composed of syncytiotrophoblasts and cytotrophoblasts. No residual villous structure remains at any given focus; only trophoblast is present. It is highly invasive and highly malignant. It has spread almost always beyond the uterus to various vital structures, and it almost inevitably fatal (if untreated). It is often difficult to distinguish between invasive mole and choriocarcinoma. According to BAGSHAWE, trophoblastic proliferation occurring a few weeks or more after a delivery at term or a nonmole abortion has always proved to be choriocarcinoma (72). Approximately 50% of choriocarcinomas are preceded by a hydatiform mole, 25% by abortion, about 22% normal delivery and the rest by ectopic pregnancy. Approximately 85% of patients with molar pregnancy enter complete remission after uterine evacuation. Disease persits in the remaining 15%, either as inaccessible residual mole or as choriocarcinoma with or without metastatic spread.

The incidence of gestational trophoblastic disease is about 10 times as high in Asians and Mexicans than in Caucasians.

Gestational trophoblastic tumors are unique in that they are the products of the conceptus, and are therefore genetically made up of paternal as well as maternal transplantation antigens. The tumor-host relationship is similar to that with a homologous transplant, and is theoretically subject to an immunological rejection reaction, which could explain some of the unexpected tumor regressions. It is also possible, however, that antibodies produced in response to tumor antigens favor tumor growth (74, 75), a phenomenon that may correspond to the facilitaion or enhancement observed in animal experiments.

Another unique feature of trophoblastic disease is its consistent production of human chorionic gonadotropin (HCG). There is experimental and clinical evidence that the amount of HCG produced correlates closely with the amount of viable tumor. Thus the measurement of HCG can be used to monitor tumor response and to determine the optimal duration of therapy (70).

Nongestational or gonadal choriocarcinoma can exist singly or, more commonly, associated with embryonal choriocarcinoma, teratocarcinoma, seminoma, dysgerminoma, or any combination of these (71). These tumors are discussed in the chapter on ovarian and testicular tumors (see p. 474 and 495).

1. Chemotherapy

The initial report in 1956, by LI et al. (76) of the induction of complete and sustained remission in three patients with metastatic choriocarcinoma treated with methotrexate (MTX) was a major breakthrough for chemotherapy. For the first time it was shown that the hope of curing disseminated disease with cytotoxic agents had become a reality. Of the first three patients treated at the N.I.H., two are still alive and have received no chemotherapy for 15 years. The effectiveness of MTX was confirmed in subsequent studies with a response rate of 48% (77, 78) (Table 27-11). A similar response was reported for an alkylating agent (Mitomen) (79) and for 6-mercaptopurine (80).

Table 27-11. Effectiveness of single agents and combinations in trophoblastic disease

Drugs	Number evaluated	Response	Reference
Methotrexate	63	48%	HERTZ et al. (77) (1961)
	144	65%	UICC Trophoblast Neoplasia Study Group (86) (1970)
6-Mercaptopurine	93	56%	SUNG et al. (80) (1963)
Alkylating agents	19	48%	ISHIZUKA (79) (1950)
Actinomycin D	8	8/8	SHER et al. (94) (1974)
	32	90%	GOLDSTEIN et al. (93) (1972)
MTX, 6MP	100	78%	BAGSHAWE (70) (1969)
MTX, ACD sequentially	75	74%	HERTZ (78) (1967)
MTX, ACD sequentially	29	72%	HAMMOND and PARKER (90) (1969)
MTX, ACD	85	88%	BREWER et al. (91) (1970)

It was soon realized that following an initial favorable response, a number of patients (about 50%) (81) become refractory to MTX. BAGSHAWE attempted to delay or prevent the occurence of resistance by adding 6-MP to MTX (82), a combination that induces 78% remissions (70). A major advance in the treatment of MTX-resistant tumors was the demonstration that actinomycin D (ACD) is capable of inducing response rates as high as those achieved with MTX as the initial agent (81). Some authors recommend actinomycin as the initial agent, especially in the presence of impaired liver function (94, 95). Furthermore there is no evidence of cross-resistance between these two agents. Complete remissions were obtained in 74% of cases when MTX and ACD were used in sequence (i.e., beginning with one and changing to the other when the tumor no longer responded to the first) (78, 83) or 88% when they were used simultaneously (84). Occasional regressions have been reported with vinblastine (85) or 6-diozo-5-oxo-L-norleucine (69).

Most authors have prescribed cytotoxic drugs intermittently in large doses: MTX (15-25 mg p.o. or i.m. qd for 5 days) or ACD (0.5 mg i.v. qd. for 4 or 5 days) or MTX (25 mg p.o., qd) plus 6-MP (300 mg qd p.o.) for a total of 3 to 5 days, with cycles to be repeated after recovery from toxicity (2 to 3 weeks). Most patients attain normal HCG levels after 3 to 5 courses. One or two additional courses are added after the urinary HCG titer returns to normal. MTX is the preferred initial single agent unless there is impaired hepatic or renal function. HOLLAND et al. have shown that intermittent MTX (0.6 mg/kg twice weekly) is as effective as intermittent 5-days courses (86). It has the additional advantage that it allows out-patient treatment and higher drug dosages can be administered at equal cost in toxicity.

Intra-arterial chemotherapy has been used in patients who have no evidence of extrapelvic disease (69) and for liver metastases (87).

High response rates (100%) are obtained with MTX and ACD in patients with a short duration of disease (treated within 4 months of apparent onset), a urine HCG titer of less than 100,000 IU per 24 hours and metastases limited to the lung and pelvis (87, 88). A longer duration of disease, a urine titer above 100,000 IU and metastases to the liver or brain are unfavorable prognostic signs. The combination of MTX and ACD (65%-80% CR) is best in these high-risk patients (88, 103).

The state of complete remission should be defined on the basis of a sensitive assay for HCG, that is when a woman has three consecutive weekly gonadotrophin levels in a range consistent with pituitary origin (88). Of those achieving a remission according to this definition, 90% remained free of disease without further therapy; 8% relapsed within 8 weeks, 2% after 8 weeks, the longest temporary remission lasting 3 years 6 months. A patient with a gonadotropin excretion in the pituitary range for 3 months thus had a 98% chance of having no further trouble with her disease without further chemotherapy (88). After a waiting period of at least one year further childbearing is allowed. A large number of successful pregnancies have been possible and there has been no evidence of an increased incidence of abortions, congenital anomalies, or reactivation of trophoblastic disease.

2. Strategy

This section deals with the management of several clinical situations that may require chemotherapy. It is obvious that close co-operation between oncologist and gynecologist is essential to ensure optimal therapy.

(i) Molar Pregnancy and Nonmetastatic Trophoblastic Disease
Evacuation of the mole and curettage are indicated to end the disease process and prevent extension into malignant phases. The tissue removed should be examined to determine whether malignant tissue is present. Several studies have shown that evacuation under the protection of a course of chemotherapy effectively reduces the incidence of invasive and metastatic neoplastic disease (86, 87, 104). Both normal and neoplastic trophoblast have an inherent tendency to invade blood vessels and to be transported in the bloodstream. The danger of dissemination at the time of surgery is always present. LEWIS et al. proposed that evacuation be carried out halfway through a 5-day course of intensive chemotherapy with either MTX or ACD (93).

HOLLAND et al. effectively used MTX 0.6 mg/kg, given twice weekly for 3 weeks. Prophylactic chemotherapy is indicated especially in situations where no adequate follow-up with the proper HCG titers is guaranteed, in selected patients at high risk, particularly in those parts of the world where the proliferative complication rate of molar pregnancy is high (104). With adequate follow-up prophylactic cytotoxic therapy is not necessary. Only a few carefully observed patients require subsequent chemotherapy. The results of such a deferred regimen, reported by HERTZ et al., indicate that nothing is lost by delay and much unnecessary chemotherapy is obviated (73).

In patients who have had a mole evacuated elsewhere prior to consultation HCG titers should be monitored carefully each week, with a method to assay sufficiently sensitive to allow measurement of gonadotropins down to normal pituitary levels, and two-weekly chest roentgenograms should be taken. If the titer remains normal for 3-6 consecutive weeks, it should then be followed monthly for 6-12 months, while the patient continues to use contraception. Further therapy is indicated if clinical, roentogenographic, and hormonal evidence of persistent mole or trophoblastic disease develops. Treatment should be based on persistent activity of the disease, as demonstrated by an elevated HCG, and not on histologic diagnosis alone. A persistent mole or nonmetastatic trophoblastic disease should be suspected when uterine subinvolution, vaginal bleeding, or an elevated gonadotropin level (either at a plateau or rising) is noted. Pelvic arteriography is indicated to determine whether there is myometrial invasion (nonmetastatic trophoblastic disease) or not (retained mole). In addition, a dilatation and curettage is carried out under chemoprophylaxis. Hysterectomy can be performed instead of dilatation and curettage in women who have no wish for further pregnancies.

If there is evidence (obtained by arteriography or curettage) of nonmetastatic trophoblastic disease (which differs from retained mole in the degree of myometrial invasion), chemotherapy with MTX and ACD is recommended (87). This therapy should be continued longer if there is histologic evidence of choriocarcinoma. If preservation of fertility is of no importance to the patient a hysterectomy under chemotherapy can also be considered. The cure rate of 100% in patients with nonmetastatic choriocarcinoma with either chemotherapy alone or chemotherapy plus surgery (87) compares extremely well with the reported cure rate of 40% with hysterectomy alone (92). Hypogastric artery infusion has been used in some cases, for example choriocarcinoma in intramural nodule that does not respond to systemic chemotherapy.

(ii) Metastatic Trophoblastic Disease
Trophoblastic disease is considered metastatic once it is beyond the confines of the uterus. The definitive diagnosis and classification are based on histology, but biopsy does not always prove to be clinically practicable. Early therapy with combination chemotherapy is important as the prognosis worsens considerably with delay and more extensive disease (see high-risk groups, above). MTX-ACD therapy offers a 90% chance of cure in low-risk patients. Whole-brain irradiation (70, 87) and intrathecal MTX (70) have been used to treat brain metastases. More radical approaches are under study, with thoracotomy for a large solitary nodule or hepatic artery infusion, local resection and irradiation for hepatic metastases that fail to respond to systemic chemotherapy (87).

(iii) Immunotherapy
Immune mechanisms seem to influence the natural course of this disease and the response to therapy. It is thus logical to hypothesize that these responses might be rendered more effective by immunization procedures. Preliminary trials are in progress.

REFERENCES

1. UICC: T.N.M. classification of malignant tumours. Geneva: G. de
   Buren 1968.
2. TOBIAS, J.S., GRIFFITHS, C.T.: Management of ovarian carcinoma.
   New Engl. J. Med. 294, 818 and 877 (1976).
3. WEBB, M.J., DECKER, D.G., MUSSEY, E., WILLIAMS, T.J.: Factors influencing survival in Stage I ovarian cancer. Amer. J. Obstet.
   Gynecol. 116, 222 (1973).
   (1973).
4. BAGLEY, Jr., C.M., YOUNG, R.C., CANELLOS, G.P., DeVITA, V.T.:
   Treatment of ovarian carcinoma: possibilities for progress. New
   Engl. J. Med. 287, 856 (1972).
5. DRUKKER, B.H., HODGINSON, C.P.: Ovarian carcinoma - perspective
   for the 70's. Amer. J. Obstet. Gynec. 109, 825 (1971).
6. LIVINGSTON, R.B., CARTER, S.K.: Single agents in cancer chemotherapy.
   New York-Washington-London: IFI/Plenum 1970.
7. JULIAN, C.G., WOODRUFF, J.D.: The role of chemotherapy in the treatment of primary ovarian malignancy. A review. Obstet. gynec. Surv.
   24, 1307 (1969).
8. HALL, T.C.: The chemotherapy of gynecologic malignancy. Progr.
   Gynec. p. 370 (1970).
9. LI, M.C., HSU, K.P.: Combined drug therapy for ovarian carcinoma.
   Clin. Obstet. Gynec. 13, 928 (1970).
10. SMITH, J.P., RUTLEDGE, F.: Chemotherapy in the treatment of cancer
    of the ovary. Amer. J. Obstet. Gynec. 107, 691 (1970).
11. BLOOMFIELD, R.D.: Current cancer chemotherapy in obstetrics and
    gynecology. Amer. J. Obstet. Gynec. 109, 487 (1971).
12. KAUFMAN, R.J.: Ovarian carcinoma. In: Cancer Chemotherapy, p. 226
    (eds. F. Elkerbout, P. Thomas, A. Zwaveling). Leiden: Leiden Uni-
    versity Press 1971.
13. SPECKHARD, M.E., HURLEY, J.D., FETHERSON, W.C., GUENINGER, A.J.:
    Integrated therapy in the treatment of ovarian cancer with surgery,
    radiation and chemotherapy. Oncology 26, 297 (1972).
14. PIVER, M.S.: Guidelines for the management of patients with ovarian
    adenocarcinoma. Obstet. and Gynecol. 40, 411 (1972).
15. SMITH, J.P., RUTLEGE, F., WHARTON, J.T.: Chemotherapy of ovarian
    cancer. New approaches to treatment. Cancer 30, 1565 (1972).
16. SULLIVAN, R.D., MILLER, E., ZUREK, W.Z., et al.: Re-evaluation
    of methotrexate as an anticancer drug. Surg. Gynecol. Obstet.
    125, 819 (1967).
17. BLUM, R.H., LIVINGSTON, R.B., CARTER, S.K.: Hexamethylmelamine. A
    new drug with activity in solid tumors. Europ. J. Cancer 9, 195
    (1973).
18. BARLOW, J.J., PIVER, M.S.: Methotrexate (NSC-740) with citrovorum
    factor (NSC-3590) rescue, alone and in combination with cyclo-
    phosphamide (NSC-26271), in ovarian cancer. Cancer Treat. Rep.
    60, 527 (1976).
19. O'BRYAN, R.M., LUCE, J.K., TALLEY, R.W., GOTTLIEB, J.A., BAKER,
    L.H., BONADONNA, G.: Phase II evaluation of adriamycin in human
    neoplasia. Cancer 32, 1 (1973).
20. BLUM, R.H., CARTER, S.K., AGRE, K.: A clinical review of bleomycin -
    a new antineoplastic agent. Cancer 31, 903 (1973).
21. IZBICKI, R., AL-SARRAF, M., REED, M.L., VAUGHN, C.B., VAITKEVICIUS,
    V.K.: Further clinical trials with porfiromycin (NSC-56410) (large
    intermittent dose). Cancer Chemother. Rep. 56, 615 (1972).
22. MALKASIAN, Jr., G.D., DECKER, D.G., JORGENSEN, E.O., WEBB, M.J.:
    6-Dehydro-6,17α-dimethylprogesterone (NSC-123018) for the treatment
    of metastatic and recurrent ovarian carcinoma. Cancer Chemother.
    Rep. Part 1, 57, 241 (1973).

23. GREENSPAN, E.M.: Thio-TEPA and methotrexate chemotherapy of advanced ovarian carcinoma. J. Mt. Sinai Hosp. 35, 52 (1968).
24. BRANDL, K.: Über die versuchsweise Anwendung einer Kombination von Zytostatika bei fortgeschrittenen Fällen von Ovarialkarzinomen. Zentralbl. Gynaekol. 92, 233 (1970).
25. LOUIS, J.: Combination of methotrexate (MTX) and vincristine (VCR) in solid tumors. Proc. Amer. Ass. Cancer Res. 15, 119 (1974).
26. BRODOVSKY, H.S.: A comparison of melphalan with 5-fluorouracil, cytoxan and methotrexate in patiens with ovarian cancer. Proc. Amer, Ass. clin. Oncol. 15, 165 (1974).
27. SWCCG, New Orleans Meeting, October 1972.
28. HANHAM, I.W.F., NEWTON, K.A., WESTBURY, G.: Seventy-five cases of solid tumours treated by a modified quadruple chemotherapy regime. Brit. J. Cancer 25, 462 (1971).
29. YOUNG, R.C., DeVITA, V.T., CHABNER, B.A.: A prospective trial of melphalan (PAM) and combination chemotherapy in advanced ovarian cancer. Proc. Amer. Soc. Clin. Oncol. 17, 279 (1976).
30. RAMIREZ, G., WEISS, A.: A phase II study of adriamycin - 5-FU given weekly in the treatment of solid tumors. Proc. Amer. Soc. Clin. Oncol. 17, 248 (1976).
31. WIDER, J.A., MARSHALL, J.R., BARDIN, C.W., LIPSETT, M.B., ROSS, G.T.: Sustained remissions after chemotherapy for primary ovarian cancers containing choriocarcinoma. New Engl. J. Med. 280, 1439 (1969).
32. BARLOW, J.J., PIVER, M.S., CHUANG, J.T., CORTES, E.P., OHNUMA, T., HOLLAND, J.F.: Adriamycin and bleomycin, alone and in combination in gynecologic cancers. Cancer 32, 735 (1973).
33. PEREZ, C.A., BRADFIELD, J.S.: Radiation therapy in the treatment of carcinoma of the ovary. Cancer 29, 1027 (1972).
34. MUNNELL, E.W.: The changing prognosis and treatment in cancer of the ovary. Amer. J Obstet. Gynecol. 100, 790 (1968).
35. MAUS, J.J., MACKAY, E.N., SELLERS, C.D.: Cancer of the ovary. Amer. J. Roentgenol. 102, 603 (1968).
36. MULLER, J.H.: Curative aim and results of routine intraperitoneal radiocolloid administration in the treatment of ovarian cancer. Amer. J. Roentgenol. Radium Ther. Nucl. Med. 89, 533 (1963).
37. KEETTEL, W.C., FOX, M.R., LONGNECKER, D.S. et al.: Prophylactic use of radioactive gold in the treatment of primary ovarian cancer. Amer. J. Obstet. Gynecol. 94, 766 (1966).
38. HILARIS, B.S., CLARK, D.G.C.: The value of postoperative intraperitoneal injection of radiocolloids in early cancer of the ovary. Amer. J. Roentgenol. Radium Ther. Nucl. Med. 112, 749 (1971).
39. TEPPER, E., SANFILIPPO, L.J., GRAY, J., ROMNEY, S.L.: Second look surgery after radiation therapy for advanced stages of cancer of the ovary. Amer. J. Roentgenol. Radium Ther. nucl. Med. 112, 755 (1971).
40. GUSBERG, S.B., KAPLAN, A.L.: Precursors of corpus cancer. IV. Adenomatous hyperplasia as stage O carcinoma of the endometrium. Amer. J. Obstet. Gynec. 87, 662 (1963).
41. HERTIG, A.T., SOMMERS, S.C.: Genesis of endometrial carcinoma. I. Study of prior biopsies. Cancer 2, 946 (1949).
42. KELLEY, R.M., BAKER, W.H.: Progestational agents in the treatment of carcinoma of the endometrium. New Engl. J. Med. 264, 216 (1961).
43. KENNEDY, B.J.: A progestogen for treatment of advanced endometrial cancer. J. Amer. med. Ass. 184, 758 (1963).
44. ANDERSON, D.G.: Management of advanced endometrial adenocarcinoma with medroxyprogesterone acetate. Amer. J. Obstet. Gynec. 92, 87 (1965).
45. KISTNER, R.W., GRIFFITHS, C.T., CRAIG, J.M.: Use of progestional agents in the management of endometrial cancer. Cancer 18, 1563 (1965).

46. SYKES, M.P.: Management of endometrial cancer. Med. Clin. N. Amer. 50, 833 (1966).
47. BONTE, J., DROCHMANS, A., LASSANCE, M.: Traitement des adénocarcinomes du corps utérin par la médroxyprogestérone. Gynéc. et Obstét. 65, 179 (1966).
48. KENNEDY, B.J: Progestogens in the treatment of carcinoma of the endometrium. Surg. Pbstet. 127, 103˙ (1968).
49. KUIPERS, T.: Megestrol acetate in the treatment of recurrent endometrial carcinoma. Proceedings of the 2nd International Symposium "New developments in gynaecological endocrinology". R.C. Hospital, Sittard, The Netherlands, 3 October 1970.
50. REIFENSTEIN, Jr., E.C.: Hydroxyprogesterone caproate therapy in advanced endometrial cancer. Cancer 27, 485 (1971).
51. KISTNER, R.W.: Endometrial and cervical cancer. In: Endocrine therapy in malignant disease, p. 323 (ed. B.A. Stoll). London-Philadelphia-Toronto: Saunders 1972.
52. RUTLEDGE, F.: Treatment for cancer of the endometrium. In: Oncology 1970, Vol. 4, p. 263 (Eds. R.L. Clark, R.W. cumley, J.E. McCay, M.M. Copeland). Chicago: Year Book Medical Publishers 1970.
53. EASSON, E.C.: Cancer of the corpus uteri. In: Oncology 1970, Vol. 4, p. 267 (eds. R.L. Clark, R.W. Culmley, J.E. McCay, M.M. Copeland). Chicago: Year Book Medical Publisher 1970.
54. BONTE, J., DECOSTER, J.M., IDE, P.: Radiosensitization of endometrial adenocarcinoma by means of medroxyprogesterone. Cancer 25, 907 (1970).
55. Symposium'Herpesvirus and cervical cancer. Cancer Res. 33, 1345 (1973).
56. WENTZ, W.B., LEWIS, Jr., G.C.: Correlation of histologic morphology and survival in cervical cancer following radiation therapy. Obstet. Gynec. 26, 228 (1965).
57. HRESHCHYSHYN, M.M.: Experience with chemotherapy in gynecologic cancer. N.Y. St. J. Med. 64, 2431 (1964).
58. MALKASIAN, Jr., G.D., DECKER, D.G., MUSSEY, E., JOHNSON, C.R.: Chemotherapy of squamous cell carcinoma of the cervix, vagina, and vulva. Clin. Obstet. Gynec. 11, 367 (1968).
59. HAFFNER, W.H., FRICK, H.C.II.: Intermittent intravenous methotrexate in the treatment of advanced epidermoid carcinoma of the cervix and vulvovagina. Cancer 26, 812 (1970).
60. SMITH, J.P.: In: Cancer of the Uterus and Ovary, p. 345 (ed. R.L. Clark). Chicago: Year Book Medical Publishers 1969.
61. MOORE, G.E., BROSS, I.D., AUSMAN, R., NADLER, S., JONES, R., SLACK, N., RIMM, A.A.: Effects of mitomycin C (NSC-26980) in 346 patients with advanced cancer. Cancer Chemother. Rep. 52, 675 (1968).
62. HOWE, C.D., SAMUELS, M.L.: Phase II studies of hydroxyurea (NSC-32065) in adults: urologic and gynecologic neoplasms. Cancer Chemother. Rep. 40, 47 (1964).
63. EAGAN, R.T., MAURER, L.H., FORCIER, R.J.: Chemotherapy of recurrent carcinoma of the cervix: a preliminary report. Proc. Amer. Ass. clin. Oncol. Abstr. 6 (1973).
64. MONFARDINI, S., DE PALO, G.M., BAJETTA, E., VERONESI, U.: Adriamycin (ADM) plus bleomycin (BLM) versus CTX plus VCR in advanced carcinoma of the cervix. Proc. Amer. Ass. Cancer Res. 15, 91 (1974).
65. PAPAVASILIOU. C., ANGELAKIS, P., GOUVALIS, P., PAPAKYRIAKIDES, L.: Treatment of cervical carcinoma by methotrexate (NSC-740) combined with cyclophosphamide (NSC-26271). Cancer Chemother. Rep. Part 1, 53, 255 (1969).
66. PIEL, I.J., SLAYTON, R.E., PERLIA, C.P., WILBANKS, G.D.: Combination chemotherapy with bleomycin and methotrexate in recurrent and disseminated cervical carcinoma: A preliminary study. Gynecol. Oncol. 1, 184 (1973).

67. STOLINSKY, D.C., BOGDON, D.L., SOLOMON, J., BATEMAN, J.R.: Hexa-methylmelamine (NSC-13875) alone and in combination with 5-(3,3-dimethyl-1-triazeno)imidazole-4-carboxamide (NSC-45388) in the treatment of advanced cancer. Cancer 30, 654 (1972).

68. MALKASIAN, Jr., G.D., MUSSEY, E., DECKER, D.G., JOHNSON, C.R.: Chemotherapy of gynecologic sarcomas. Cancer Chemother. Rep. 51, 507 (1967).

69. HOLLAND, J.F., HRESHCHYSHYN, M.M.: Choriocarcinoma. Berlin: Springer-Verlag 1967 (UICC Monograph 3).

70. BAGSHAWE, K.D.: Choriocarcinoma. Baltimore: Williams and Wilkins 1969.

71. LI, M.C.: Trophoblastic disease: natural history, diagnosis, and treatment. Ann. inter. Med. 74, 102 (1971).

72. BAGSHAWE, K.D.: Choriocarcinoma. In: Cancer Chemotherapy, (eds. F. Elkerbout, P. Thomas, A. Zwaveling). p. 205. Leiden: Leiden University Press 1971.

73. HERTZ, R.: Gestational trophoblastic neoplasia. Hosp. Pract. Jan. 157 (1972).

74. MATHE, G., DAUSSET, J., HERVET, E., AMIEL, J.L., COLOMBANI, J., BRULE, G.: Immunological studies in patients with placental chorio-carcinoma. J. nat. Cancer Inst. 33, 193 (1964).

75. AMIEL, J.L., MERY, A.M., MATHE, G.: Les rêsponses immunitaires chez les patients atteintes de choriocarcinome placentaire. Corrêlation entre ces rêsponses et l'évolution de la maladie. In: Cell-bound Immunity with Special Reference to Anti-Lymphocyte Serum and Im-munotherapy of Cancer, p. 197. Liège: Univ. Ed. 1967.

76. LI, M.C., HERTZ, R., SPENCER, D.B.: Effect of methotrexate therapy upon choriocarcinoma and chorioadenoma. Proc. Soc. exp. biol. Med. 93, 361 (1956).

77. HERTZ, R., LEWIS, Jr., J., LIPSETT, M.B.: Five years' experience with the chemotherapy of metastatic choriocarcinoma and related trophoblastic tumors in women. Amer. J. Obstet. Gynec. 82, 631 (1961).

78. HERTZ, R.: Eight years' experience with the chemotherapy of chorio-carcinoma and related trophoblastic tumors in women. In: Chorio-carcinoma, p. 66 (eds. J.F. Holland, M. Hreshchyshyn). Berlin: Springer-Verlag 1967 (UICC Monograph 3).

79. ISHIZUKA, N.: Chemotherapy for chorioepithelioma. Gann 47, 460 (1956).

80. SUNG, H.C., WU, P.C., HO, T.H.: Treatment of choriocarcinoma and chorioadenoma destruens with 6-mercaptopurine and surgery: a clin-ical report of 93 cases. China Med. J. 82, 24 (1963).

81. ROSS, G.T., STOLBACH, L.L., HERTZ, R.: Actinomycin D in the treat-ment of methotrexate-resistant trophoblastic disease in women. Cancer Res. 22, 1015 (1962).

82. BAGSHAWE, K.D.: Trophoblastic tumors: chemotherapy developments. Brit. med. J. 2, 1303 (1963).

83. ROSS, G.T., GOLDSTEIN, D.P., HERTZ, R. et al.: Sequential use of methotrexate and actinomycin D in the treatment of metastatic choriocarcinomas and related trophoblastic diseases in women. Amer. J. Obstet. Gynec. 93, 223 (1965).

84. BREWER, J.I., DOLKART, R.E., TOROK, E.E., et al.: Gestational trophoblastic disease. In: Sixth National Cancer Conference Pro-ceedings, p. 387. Philadelphia: Lippincott 1970.

85. HERTZ, R., LIPSETT, M.B., MOY, R.H.: Effect of vincaleukoblastine on metastatic choriocarcinoma and related trophoblastic tumors in women. Cancer Res. 20, 1050 (1960).

86. HOLLAND, J.F., HRESHCHYSHYN, M.M., GLIDEWELL, O.: Controlled clinical trials of methotrexate in treatment and prophylaxis of trophoblastic neoplasia. In: Oncology 1970. Vol. 5, p. 220. Chicago: Year Book Medical Publishers 1970.

87. GOLDSTEIN, D.P.: The chemotherapy of gestational trophoblastic disease. Principles of clinical management. J. Amer. med. Ass. 220, 209 (1972).
88. LEWIS, Jr., J.L.: Chemotherapy of gestational choriocarcinoma. Cancer 30, 1517 (1972).
89. HOLLAND, J.E., HRESHCHYSHYN, M.M., GLIDEWELL, O.: Controlled clinical trials of methotrexate in the treatment and prophylaxis of trophoblastic neoplasia (abstract). In: Abstracts of the Tenth International Cancer Congress. Houston, May 1970. pp. 461-462.
90. HAMMOND, C.B., PARKER, R.I.: Diagnosis and treatment of trophoblastic disease. Obstet. Gynec. 35, 132 (1970).
91. BREWER, J.L., SMITH, R.T., PRATT, G.B.: Choriocarcinoma. Absolute 5 year survival rates of 122 patients treated by hysterectomy. Amer. J. Obstet. Gynec. 85, 841 (1964).
92. LEWIS, Jr., J., GORE, H., HERTIG, A.T. et al.: Treatment of trophoblastic disease, with rationale for the use of adjunctive chemotherapy at the time of indicated operation. Amer. J. Obstet. Gynec. 96, 710 (1966).
93. GOLDSTEIN, D.P., WINIG, F.P., SHIRLEY, R.L.: Actinomycin D as initial therapy of gestational trophoblastic disease. A reevaluation. Obstet. Gynec. 39, 341 (1972).
94. SHER, M.M., D'ERRICO, A., CARTNICK, E.: Dactinomycin as primary therapy for gestational trophoblastic disease. Proc. Amer. Ass. clin. Oncol. 191 (1974).
95. YOUNG, R.C., HUBBARD, S.P., DeVITA, V.T.: The chemotherapy of ovarian carcinoma. Cancer Treat. Rev. 1, 99 (1974).
96. BUCKNER, C.D., BRIGGS, R., CLIFT, R.A., FEFER, A., FUNK, D.D., GLUCKSBERG, H., NEIMAN, P.E., STORB, R., THOMAS, E.D.: Intermittent high-dose cyclophosphamide treatment of stage III ovarian carcinoma. Cancer Chemother. Rep. Part 1, 58, 697 (1974).
97. WASSERMAN, T.H., SLAVIK, M., CARTER, S.K.: Review of CCNU in clinical cancer therapy. Cancer Treat. Rev. 1, 131 (1974).
98. WASSERMAN, T.H., SLAVIK, M., CARTER, S.K.: Methyl-CCNU in clinical cancer therapy. Cancer Treat. Rev. 1, 251 (1974).
99. LLOYD, R.E., JONES, S.E., SALMON, S.E., DURIE, B.G.M., McMAHON, L.J.: Combination chemotherapy with adriamycin (NSC-123127) and cyclophosphamide (NSC-26271) for solid tumors: A phase II trial. Cancer Treat. Rep. 60, 77 (1976).
100. ROZIER, J.C., UNDERWOOD, P.B.: Use of progestational agents in endometrial adenocarcinoma. Obstet. Gynecol. 44, 60 (1974).
101. DONOVAN, J.F.: Nonhormonal chemotherapy of endometrial adenocarcinoma: a review. Cancer 34, 1587 (1974).
102. BRADY, L.W.: Combined modality therapy of gynecologic cancer. Cancer 35, 76 (1975).
103. JONES, W.B., LEWIS, J.L.: Treatment of gestational trophoblastic disease. Am. J. Obstet. Gynecol. 120, 14 (1974).
104. GOLDSTEIN, D.P.: Prevention of gestational trophoblastic disease by use of actinomycin D in molar pregnancies. Obstet. Gynecol. 43, 475 (1974).
105. YAGODA, A., LIPPMAN, A.J., WINN, R.J., SCHULMAN, P., COHEN, F.B.: Combination chemotherapy with bleomycin and methotrexate in patients with advanced epidermoid carcinomas. Proc. Am. Soc. Clin. Oncol. 16, 247 (1975).
106. GUTHRIE, D., WAY, S.: Treatment of advanced carcinoma of the cervix with adriamycin and methotrexate combined. Obstet. Gynecol. 44, 586 (1974)
107. BAKER, L.H., OPIPARI, M.: IZBICKI, R.: Mitomycin-C, vincristine and bleomycin combination treatment of disseminated cervical carcinoma. Proc. Am. Ass. Cancer. Res. 16, 35 (1975).

Chapter 28
Testicular Cancers

Testicular tumors are relatively rare. They constitute approximately 1% of all malignant tumors in males. Most of the men affected are young (aged 20-40 years). Undescended testes are prone to malignant degeneration.

The histology of the tumor has an important bearing on both prognosis and choice of initial therapy. Several classifications, most of a complex character, are used. The most popular in the United States is that of the Armed Forces Institute of Pathology (Table 28-1) (1, 2). The majority of testicular tumors arise from cells in the germ series (germinal tumors: 96.5%). Pure seminomas are malignant tumors of seminal epithelial origin, but possess little or no capacity for further differentiation. They have the best prognosis because they are very radiosensitive, are often detected in an early clinical stage and progress slowly, and the early spread is confined to lymphatic routes. Embryonal carcinoma is a primitive and undifferentiated neoplasm composed of pluripotential germ cells which have the potentiality for differentiation along either somatic (teratomas) or trophoblastic lines (choriocarcinoma) or both. Thus embryonal carcinomas, teratomas, and choriocarcinomas are closely related tumors with different degrees of cellular differentiation. It must be recognized that the term teratoma, as applied to testicular neoplasia, always denotes a malignant tumor. It is not uncommon to find different histologic types in the various metastases of a particular patient. Seminomatous elements can coexist with embryonal carcinoma, teratoma, and choriocarcinoma. In such cases treatment must be directed predominantly at the most malignant elements. The AFIP classification differs from the British classification, which requires that the presence of true choriocarcinomatous tissue, even if only in a small part of the tumor, be delineated as a separate entity (3). Most of these tumors are radioresistant. Testicular tumors containing trophoblastic elements secrete urinary gonadotrophins, and these should always be looked for. Endocrine signs (gynecomastia, feminization) are sometimes present.

Testicular tumors spread fairly early via the lymphatics. Hematogenous dissemination is also relatively common early in the course of choriocarcinomas, less so in seminomas.

No staging classification is uniformly accepted. The UICC TNM classification (4, 5) and the Walter Reed General Hospital system (often used in the United States) (6) are reproduced in Tables 28-2 and 28-3.

As with most tumors, the prognosis of testicular germinal tumors depends chiefly on the histology and clinical stage. Five- and 10-year survival rates decrease progressively for seminoma, teratocarcinoma, embryonal carcinoma to choriocarcinoma in that order. For all histologic types the presence of urinary chorionic gonadotrophins appears to worsen the prognosis (7).

Table 28-1. Armed Forces Institute of Pathology (AFIP) classification of testes neoplasms (partial). (From DIXON and MOORE (1))

	Frequency	Approximate 5-year survival (%)
I. Germinal origin	96.5	
1. Seminoma	40	70-90
2. Embryonal carcinoma ± seminoma	15-20	34
3. Teratoma ± seminoma	1- 5	100
4. Teratoma ± embryonal carcinoma or choriocarcinoma or both	20-25	45
5. Choriocarcinoma	1	0-14
6. Compound tumor	15-20	
II. Nongerminal origin		
1. Interstitial cell tumor		
2. Gonadal stromal tumors		
III. Miscellaneous		

Table 28-2. Walter Reed General Hospital Staging for testicular neoplasms (From MAIER et al. (34))

Stage IA.	Tumor confined to one testis; no clinical or roentgenographic evidence of spread beyond; may include excretory or retrograde urography, lymphangiography, inferior venacavography, and chest roentgenography
Stage IB.	Same as in stage IA. but found to have histologic evidence of metastases to iliac or paraaortic lymph nodes at time of retroperitoneal lymph node dissection
Stage II.	Clinical or roentgenographic evidence of metastases to femoral, inguinal, iliac, or paraaortic lymph nodes; no demonstrable metastases above the diaphragm or to visceral organs
Stage III.	Clinical or roentgenographic evidence of metastases above the diaphragm or other distant metastases to body organs

A. CHEMOTHERAPY

1. Single-Agent Chemotherapy

Most cytotoxic drugs have been evaluated at some time in testicular carcinoma, but few single agents have been consistently effective. There are few reports of the use of alkylating agents alone (8, 38).

Table 28-3. TNM Staging of testicular neoplasms

T1	Tumor occupying less than one half of the testis
T2	Tumor occupying one half or more of the testis
T3	Tumor confined to the testis and producing enlargement
T4	Tumor extending to the epididymis or beyond the testis
NX	When it is impossible to assess the regional nodes the symbol NX will be used, permitting eventual addition of histological information, thus: NX - or NX+
NO	No deformity of regional nodes on lymphangiography
N1	Regional nodes deformed on lymphangiography
N2	Fixed palpable abdominal nodes
MO	No evidence of distant metastases
M1	Distant metastases present

MACKENZIE observed regressions in four of eight patients treated with chlorambucil (CLB); all the responders had seminomas (9). Alkylating agents have therefore been recommended as the drugs of choice for seminoma (9, 10). Chlorambucil, nitrogen mustard (HN2), cyclophosphamide (CPM), and melphalan (MPH) have been used in combinations (see below). LI tried methotrexate (MTX) in testicular choriocarcinoma because of the effect of this drug in gestational trophoblastic disease but he found this tumor to be generally resistant to MTX and to 6-MP when these agents were given singly (11). The response rates for MTX and 5-FU in CARTER's review of the literature are listed in Table 28-4 (8). Vinblastine, especially at high dose levels (0.4-0.8 mg/kg, usually 0.5 to 0.6 mg/kg, given in 2 or 3 equal fractions daily for 2 or 3 days; repeat courses at 3-4 week intervals) as used by SAMUELS resulted in 50% tumor regressions (10 PR + 5 CR in 29 patients) (12-14). Though responses were seen in all histologic groups, embryonal carcinoma (8/19) and especially teratoma (9/11, of which 5 CR) proved most responsive.

Some of the antibiotics seem to be among the more promising agents. MACKENZIE believes that actinomycin D (ACD) is probably the most effective drug in metastatic testicular tumors other than seminoma (9). Germinal tumors of the testis are the only ones that have responded with any degree of consistency to mithramycin (MTM) (15, 16). The responses have been most evident in patients with embryonal-cell carcinoma (15). An alternate-day dosage regimen greatly improves the therapeutic index over that of the original daily schedule (15). Preliminary reports on bleomycin (BLM) are encouraging (32% PR in 37 patients) (17), with regressions in embryonal (8/21), choriocarcinoma (2/6), and teratocarcinoma (2/8). Unfortunately the duration of response has so far been short (1.5-2 months). Adriamycin shows an overall response of 18%, however most of the patients treated had already received conventional agents, indicating that ADM may have significant activity (8). We have no information on the effectiveness of CCNU. No regressions were recorded in 6 patients with MeCCNU (39). HIGBY et al. reported encouraging results with diamminodichloroplatinum (DDP) (40).

2. Combinations

Testicular tumors were among the first to respond to combination chemotherapy. A significant rate of remission has been obtained for a variety of combinations (Table 28-5) but in only a small percentage have complete remissions of long duration been achieved. However, in contrast to results with disseminated solid tumors, some of these long-term remissions are apparently cures. This alone justifies an attempt at chemotherapy.

Table 28-4. Effectiveness of single agents in testicular cancers

Drug	Number evaluated	Responses	Reference
Methotrexate	10	4	CARTER and WASSERMAN (8)
5-Fluorouracil	15	4	-
MeCCNU	6	O	WASSERMAN et al. (39)
Procarbazine	3	1	CARTER and WASSERMAN (8)
Chlorambucil	8	4	MACKENZIE (9)
Melphalan	86	57%	CARTER and WASSERMAN (8)
Diamminodichloroplatinum	15	10	HIGBY et al. (40)
Actinomycin D	31	52%	CARTER and WASSERMAN (8)
Mithramycin	431	36%	-
Adriamycin	60	20%	-
Bleomycin	57	42%	-
Porfiromycin	6	O	IZBICKI et al. (20)
Vinblastine			
conventional dose	9	2	WARWICK et al. (12)
large dose	29	51%	SAMUELS and HOWE (14)

Combination chemotherapy began with LI's report in 1960 (22). MACKENZIE reviewed the experience of the Memorial Hospital at New York, including the cases treated by LI et al. (9). This extended experience confirmed the earlier results: 50% regressions, with 12% complete remissions, for the triple combination of ACD, MTX, and CLB. The same results were obtained with the dual combination of ACD and CLB. MACKENZIE felt that ACD was the most effective drug of the triple combination. He obtained results similar to the triple combination by intermittent administration of high doses of ACD alone. LI, however, is of the opinion that combination therapy offers a better chance for a sustained remission. He has recently proposed a 4-drug combination (ACD, MTX, CLB, and VCR) (32). Attempts have been made to improve on the combination, for example by substituting CPM or MPH for CLB, and/or VCR for ACD, without any improvement in the results.

Reports have begun to appear on new combinations that include bleomycin (21, 30, 31). SAMUELS et al. reported 32% CR (16/50) and a 76% total response rate for a combination of VLB and BLM (31). Complete remissions were much more frequent in patients with minimal disease and all complete responders were alive at 2 years, 15 being free of disease. These results were confirmed by SPIGEL and COLTMAN (21, 41). SAMUELS improved on his results using continuous i.v. bleomycin therapy with vinblastine (31). CVITKOVIC et al. obtained 7 CR and 12 PR in 24 patients treated with a four-drug combination (VLB, BLM-infusion, ACD, and DDP) (43). Similar response rates have been obtained with a three-drug combination (ADM, VCR, BLM) (28% CR, 52% PR) (44). BLOM et al. confirmed the superiority of combination therapy (YCD, BLM, VCR) (29% CR, 50% PR) over single agent (ACD) therapy (12% CR, 10% PR) (45).

Table 28-5. Response rates to combinations in testicular cancers

Combination	Number evaluated	Response		Reference
CLB, ACD	31	45%	5 CR	MACKENZIE (9) (1966)
MPH, VLB	11	45%	2 CR, 3 PR	SAMUELS and HOWE (13) (1970)
BLM, VLB	50	76%	16 CR (32%) 22 PR	SAMUELS et al. (31) (1975)
	10	8	5 CR, 3 PR	SPIGEL and COLTMAN (21) (1974)
	40	72%	19 CR (47%) 10 PR	SAMUELS (42) (1975)
MTX, CLB, ACD	23	52%	7 CR	LI et al. (22) (1960)
	90	50%	11 CR	MACKENZIE (9) (1966)
	21	66%	4/5 chorio-carcinomas 7/10 embryo-nal ca. 3/6 terato-carcinomas	ANSFIELD et al. (23) (1969)
	11	72%	1 CR, 7 PR	MOORE (24) (1966)
MTX, CPM, VCR	11	54%	6 PR	SOLOMON et al. (25) (1967)
MTX, MPH, VCR	29	63%	4/4 semino-mas 1/2 terato-carcinomas 3/3 chorio-carcinomas 4/10 embryo-nal ca.	SOLOMON et al. (25) (1967)
CPM, ACD, VCR	10	5	1 CR, 5 PR	JACOBS (26) (1970)
ACD, BLM, VLB	16	50%	6>75% re-gressions	SILVAY et al. (27) (1973)
DDP, BLM, VLB	20	100%	15 CR, 5 PR	EINHORN et al. (33) (1976)
ACD, BLM, VCR	3	2	2 CR	SPIGEL and COLTMAN (21) (1974)
	42	69%	8 CR, 21 PR	BLOM and BRODOVSKY (45) (1976)
ADM, BLM, VCR	25	80%	7 CR, 13 PR	BURGESS et al. (44) (1975)
MTX, 5-FU, CPM, VCR (COMF)	4	0		HANHAM et al. (28) (1971)
	17	41%	5 CR (em-bryonal ca) 2 PR (em-bryonal ca)	MENDELSON and SERPICK (29) (1970)
ACD, BLM, VLB, DDP	24	79%	7 CR, 12 PR	CVITKOVIC et al. (43) (1975)
ACD, BLM, VLB, DDP, CPM	26	92%	18 CR, 6 PR	CVITKOVIC et al. (42) (1976)

Table 28-5. (continued)

Combination	Number evaluated	Response	Reference
CPM, ACD, alternate MTM, VCR	6	4	3/4 CR (emb- JACOBS (26) (1970) ryonal ca. 1/2 PR (tera- tocarcinoma
MeCCNU, CPM, BLM, VCR (COMB)	2	2	LIVINGSTON et al. (30) (1973)
MTX, 5-FU, CPM, BLM, VCR (COMF-B)	11	7	4 CR, 3 PR SAMUELS et al. (31) (1975)

B. STRATEGY

1. Seminoma

(i) Early Stages (I and II)
Biopsy should not be performed when clinical findings suggest a testicular tumor. A high inguinal orchiectomy is performed for both diagnosis
and treatment of the local disease. Comparative studies have shown that
there is no need for lymphadenectomy (34). Rather than this, since approximately one-third of patients with seminoma have lymphatic metastases (which are very radiosensitive) postoperative radiotherapy is recommended. Not all radiotherapists are agreed upon the total dose required to sterilize seminoma or upon the extent of the lymphatic areas
to be treated. The major controversy centers around the advisability
of prophylactic irradiation of the mediastinum and the supraclavicular
area(s). MAIER et al. who do advocate this, obtained 10-year survival
rates of 98% for Stage IA and approximately 78% for Stages IB and II
(35).

The results of surgery with postoperative radiotherapy are so good
(especially for Stage IA) that it would be difficult to prove the usefulness of adjuvant chemotherapy.

(ii) Advanced Stage (Stage III)
Radiotherapy, with fields individually selected according to the location of the metastases, is combined with chemotherapy. Alkylating
agents, for example CLB, are the drugs of choice for pure seminoma.
Actinomycin D is best added if the seminoma contains other pathologic
variants.

2. Nonseminomatous Germinal-Cell Tumors

(i) Early Stages (I, II)
There is no agreement as to what constitutes the best treatment after the
initial orchiectomy with high ligation of the spermatic cord (8). Many
patients have been subjected to lymphadenectomy of the retroperitoneal
lymph nodes as a second surgical procedure. It remains debatable whether

bilateral lymphadenectomy is more effective than a unilateral procedure (7, 36, 37, 46). Postoperative radiotherapy (to the inguinal and
para-aortic nodes, with or without prophylactic irradiation of the mediastinum and supraclavicular areas) is often given to patients found to
have positive nodes at surgery. MAIER, reviewing the experience of the
Walter Reed Hospital, concluded that it would be helpful to know what
results could be obtained with orchiectomy followed by retroperitoneal
lymphadenectomy alone versus orchiectomy followed by postoperative irradiation alone versus a combination of the two modalities in patients
with similar histologic types and in whom extent of the disease is also
similar (7). Retrospective studies indicate that there might be no difference. He is currently conducting a prospective study whereby patients
are allocated by random selection to receive a full course of irradiation to the lymphatic drainage areas alone, or preoperative irradiation
(3000 rads) to the iliac and abdominal para-aortic lymph nodes followed
by bilateral retroperitoneal lymphadenectomy. This is followed by an
additional 1500 rads to the abdominal lymphatics with subsequent prophylactic irradiation to the mediastinum and supraclavicular lymph node
areas.

Other workers do not favor the use of irradiation in these types of
testicular tumors, because they consider them to be radioresistant, and
there is as yet no proof that it improves prognosis (10, 36, 37). Furthermore, these tumors are less likely to disseminate solely by lymphatic routes. The more significant metastases are probably hematogenous.
Radiotherapy decreases the bone-marrow reserve, which limits subsequent
chemotherapy. Finally, they question the justification for supplementary radiotherapy if the positive nodes have been removed. GOLBEY does
not generally recommend retroperitoneal lymph node dissection for choriocarcinomas since they are usually in Stage III by the time of diagnosis.

Since the 5- and 10 year-survival rates (10) for these tumors are below 50% (except for Stages IA) adjuvant chemotherapy deserves consideration.

(ii) Advanced Stage (III)
Chemotherapy is the primary treatment modality, but surgical or radiotherapeutic reduction of large tumor masses can be included in the overall strategy (37, 47). In recent years promising regimens have been
introduced combining several of the more active agents: VLB, BLM, DDP,
ACD and an alkylating agent (Table 28-5). Some particular drugs or
combinations have been recommended for specific histologic variants.
Mithramycin has thus been suggested for the treatment of embryonal
carcinoma (15, 16), high-dose VLB for teratocarcinoma (14), and LI's
triple or quadruple combination of choriocarcinoma (32).

Patients who respond to chemotherapy should be treated for a total of
three years. Some 10-15% of patients with advanced disease are potentially curable when treated with aggressive chemotherapy.

REFERENCES

1. DIXON, F.J., MOORE, R.A. (eds.): Tumors of the male sex organs.
   In: Atlas of Tumor Pathology, Vol. 32, p. 48 Washington, D.C.: Armed
   Forces Institute of Pathology 1952.

2. MOSTOFI, F.K.: Testicular tumors: epidemiologic, etiologic, and pathologic features. Cancer 32, 1186 (1973).
3. COLLINS, D.H., PUGH, R.C.B.: The pathology of testicular tumors. Brit. J. Urol. 36, (Suppl. 2), 1 (1964).
4. UICC: T.N.M. classification of malignant tumours. Geneva: G. de Buren 1968.
5. UICC Committee on Professional Education: Clinical Oncology. A manual for students and doctors. Berlin-Heidelberg-New York: Springer-Verlag 1973.
6. RUBIN, P.: Cancer of the urogenital tract: testicular tumors. J. Amer. med. Ass. 213, 89 (1970).
7. MAIER, J.G., SULAK, M.H.: Radiation therapy in malignant testis tumors: Part II: carcinoma. Cancer 32, 1217 (1973).
8. CARTER, S.K., WASSERMAN, T.H.: The chemotherapy of urologic cancer. Cancer 36, 728 (1975).
9. MACKENZIE, A.R.: Chemotherapy of metastatic testis cancer. Cancer 19, 1369 (1966).
10. KAUFMAN, R.J.: Testicular carcinoma. In: Cancer Chemotherapy, p. 21 (eds. F. Elkerbout, P. Thomas, A. Zwaveling). Leiden: Leiden University Press 1971.
11. LI, M.C., HERTZ, R., BERGENSTAL, D.M.: Therapy of choriocarcinoma and related trophoblastic tumors with folic acid and purine antagonists. New Engl. J. Med. 259, 66 (1958).
12. WARWICK, O.H., DARTE, J.M.M., BROWN, T.C.: Some biological effects of vincaleukoblastine, an alkaloid in Vinca rosea Linn., in patients with malignant disease. Cancer Res. 30, 1032 (1960).
13. SAMUELS, M.L., HOWE, C.D.: Vinblastine in the management of testicular cancer. Cancer 25, 1009 (1970).
14. SAMUELS, M.L., HOWE, C.D.: Vinblastine sulfate in the treatment of germinal tumors of the testis. In: Oncology 1970, Vol. 4, p. 335 (eds. R.L. Clark, R.W. Cumley, J.E. McCay, M. Copeland). Chicago: Year Book Medical Publishers 1971.
15. KENNEDY, R.J.: Mithramycin therapy in advanced testicular neoplasms. Cancer 26, 755 (1970).
16. HILL, G.J., II, SEDRANSK, N., ROCHLIN, D., BISEL, H., ANDREWS, N.C., FLETCHER, X., SCHROEDER, J.M., WILSON, W.L.: Mithramycin (NSC-24559) therapy of testicular tumors. Cancer 30, 900 (1972).
17. BLUM, R.H., CARTER, S.K., AGRE, K.: A clinical review of bleomycin - a new antineoplastic agent. Cancer 31, 903 (1973).
18. BLUM, R.H., CARTER, S.K.: Adriamycin. Ann. intern. Med. 80, 249 (1974).
19. BLOKHIN, N., LARIONOV, L., PERENODCHIKOVA, L., CHEBOTAREVA, L., MERKULOVA, N.: Clinical experience with sarcolysin in neoplastic diseases. Ann. N.Y. Acad. Sci. 68, 1128 (1958).
20. IZBICKI, R., AL-SARRAF, M., REED, M.L., VAUGHN, C.B., VAITKEVICIUS, V.K.: Further clinical trials with porfiromycin (NSC-56410) (large intermittent doses). Cancer Chemother. Rep. 56, 615 (1972).
21. SPIGEL, S.C., COLTMAN, C.A.: Combination chemotherapy of testicular carcinoma. Proc. Amer. Soc. clin. Oncol. 15, 186 (1974).
22. LI, M.C., WHITMORE, Jr., W.F., GOLBEY, R., GRABSTALD, H.: Effects of combined drug therapy on metastatic cancer of the testis. J. Amer. med. Ass. 174, 1291 (1960).
23. ANSFIELD, F.J., KORBITZ, B.C., DAVIS, Jr., H.L., RAMIREZ, G.: Triple drug therapy in testicular tumors. Cancer 24, 442 (1969).
24. MOORE, C.A.: Triple chemotherapy in the treatment of metastatic testicular neoplasms. J. Urol. (Baltimore) 100, 527 (1968).
25. SOLOMON, J., STEINFELD, J.I., BATEMAN, J.R.: Chemotherapy of germinal tumors. Cancer 20, 747 (1967).
26. JACOBS, E.M.: Combination chemotherapy of metastatic testicular germinal cell tumors and soft part sarcomas. Cancer 25, 324 (1970).

27. SILVAY, O., YAGODA, A., WITTES, R., WHITMORE, W., GOLBEY, R.: Treatment of germ cell carcinomas with a combination of actinomycin D, vinblastine and bleomycin. Proc. Amer. Ass. Cancer Res. 14, 68 (1973).
28. HANHAM, I.W.F., NEWTON, K.A., WESTBURY, G.: Seventy-five cases of solid tumours treated by a modified quadruple chemotherapy regime. Brit. J. Cancer 25, 462 (1971).
29. MENDELSON, D., SERPICK, A.A.: Combination chemotherapy of testicular tumors. J. Urol. 103, 619 (1970).
30. LIVINGSTON, R.B., BODEY, G.P., GOTTLIEB, J.A., BURGESS, M.A.: Cytoxan, oncovin, methyl-CCNU and bleomycin (COMB) in lung cancer and other solid tumors. Proc. Amer. Soc. Clin. Oncol. 1973. (Abstr. 61).
31. SAMUELS, M.L., HOLOYE, P.Y., JOHNSON, D.E.: Bleomycin combination chemotherapy in the management of testicular neoplasia. Cancer 36, 318 (1975).
32. LI, M.C.: Trophoblastic disease: natural history, dyagnosis, and treatment. Ann. intern. Med. 74, 102 (1971).
33. EINHORN, L.H., FURNAS, B.E., POWELL, N.: Combination chemotherapy of disseminated testicular carcinoma with cis-platinum diammine dichloride, vinblastine and bleomycin. Proc. Amer. Soc. Clin. Oncol. 17, 240 (1976).
34. MAIER, J.G., MITTEMEYER, B.T., SULAK, M.H.: Treatment and prognosis in seminoma of the testis. J. Urol. 99, 72 (1968).
35. MAIER, J.G., SULAK, M.H.: Radiation therapy in malignant testis tumors: Part I: seminoma. Cancer 32, 1212 (1973).
36. WALSH, P.C., KAUFMAN, J.J., COULSON, W.F., GOODWIN, W.E.: Retroperitoneal lymphadenectomy for testicular tumors. J. Amer. med. Ass. 217, 309 (1971).
37. STAUBIZ, W.J., EARLY, K.S., MAGOSS, I.V., MURPHY, G.P.: Surgical treatment of non-seminomatous germinal testes tumors. Cancer 32, 1206 (1973).
38. BUCKNER, C.D., CLIFT, R.A., FEFER, A., FUNK, D.D., GLUCKSBERG, H., NEIMAN, P.E., PAULSON, A., STORB, R., THOMAS, E.D.: High-dose cyclophosphamide for the treatment of metastatic testicular neoplasms. Cancer Chemother. Rep. Part 1, 58, 709 (1974).
39. WASSERMAN, T.H., SLAVIK, M., CARTER, S.K.: Methyl-CCNU in clinical cancer therapy. Cancer Treat. Rev. 1, 251 (1974).
40. HIGBY, D.J., WALLACE, H.J., ALBERT, D., HOLLAND, J.F.: Diamminodichloroplatinum in the chemotherapy of testicular tumors. J. Urol. 112, 100 (1974).
41. SPIGEL, S.C., COLTMAN, C.A.: Vinblastine and bleomycin therapy for disseminated testicular tumors. Cancer Chemother. Rep. Part 1, 58, 213 (1974).
42. CVITKOVIC, E., HAYES, D., GOLBEY, R.: Primary combination chemotherapy (VAB III) for metastatic of unresectable germ cell tumors. Proc. Amer. Soc. Clin. Oncol. 17, 269 (1976).
43. CVITKOVIC, E., WITTES, R., GOLBEY, R., KRAKOFF, I.H.: Primary combination chemotherapy (VAB II) for metastatic or unresectable germ cell tumors. Proc. Am. Ass. Cancer Res. 16, 174 (1975).
44. BURGESS, M.A., EINHORN, L.H., GOTTLIEB, J.A.: Treatment of metastatic germ cell tumors with adriamycin, vincristine and bleomycin. Proc. Am. Soc. Clin. Oncol. 16, 244 (1975).
45. BLOM, J., BRODOVSKY, H.S.: Comparison of the treatment of metastatic testicular tumors with actinomycin-D or actinomycin-D, bleomycin, and vincristine. Proc. Amer. Soc. Clin. Oncol. 17, 290 (1976).
46. DURAND, J.C., BARRAT, F.: L'envahissement ganglionnaire lombo-aortique dans les dysenbryomes testiculaires. Nouv. Presse méd. 3, 1929 (1974).
47. MERRIN, C., TAKITA, H., WEBER, R., WAJSMAN, Z., BAUMGARTNER, G., MURPHY, G.P.: Combination radical surgery and multiple sequential chemotherapy for the treatment of advanced carcinoma of the testis (Stage III). Cancer 37, 20 (1976).

Chapter 29
Prostate, Renal and Bladder Cancer

Prostate cancer accounts for approximately one-tenth of male cancers. The true incidence is difficult to ascertain, since clinical cancers are less frequent than latent prostate cancers (found incidentally). No predisposing factors are recognized, but the incidence is age-associated and there are impressive racial and geographical differences in incidence. Prostate cancer is rare in mongoloid races (1).

Of the prostate cancers diagnosed, 95% are recognizable adenocarcinomas with varying degrees of differentiation, while 5% are undifferentiated. The majority arise in the peripheral portions of the prostate (in the outer prostatic glands), while the benign prostatic hypertrophy arises from the inner, central or peri-urethral portions of the gland. As a result, it is difficult to diagnose in an early stage because it does not cause symptoms (urinary) until later in its course. In addition, invasion of the capsule is common and early, and tumor cells soon invade perineural lymphatics and blood vessels in the periprostatic tissues. Distant metastases are common. Less than 10% are sufficiently localized at the time of diagnosis for radical prostatectomy to be considered.

Several staging systems are used. The UICC TNM classification is not very popular. The two systems in common use recognize 4 stages indicated either by roman numerals or by letters (Table 29-1). The first stage (A or I) is not clinically apparent and is found incidentally by the pathologic examination of prostatic tissue removed for the benign hyperplasia or at autopsy. Stage B or II represents clinically apparent prostatic cancer as a discrete firm nodule, confined within the prostatic capsule and with no evidence of metastases. Stage C or III has extended locally beyond the prostatic capsule but there is no evidence of metastases. Once metastases become clinically apparent the disease is staged as D or IV. Most clinicians realize that clinically manifest prostatic carcinoma is frequently understaged.

A. HORMONE THERAPY

The hormone dependency of prostate carcinoma was established experimentally and clinically more than 30 years ago by HUGGINS and HODGES (1941) (4) and by HERBST (1941) (5). These studies showed that the suppression of estrogen production by castration (and eventually by adrenalectomy or hypophysectomy) or by the administration of estrogens can result in objective tumor regressions. Alternatively, androgens can stimulate tumor growth, as demonstrated by studies of acid phosphatase and fi-

Table 29-1. Staging for prostate cancer

Stage	I:	Tumor confined to the prostate, not detectable by rectal examination
Stage	II.	Tumor confined to the prostate, but detectable by rectal examination
Stage	III.	Locally extended tumors
Stage	IV.	Tumors with evidence of distant metastasis obtained by biopsy, X-ray, or detection of acid phosphatase elevations in excess of 1.0 K.A.U.
Stage	A:	Occult tumor with microscopic foci found incidental to re-section for a benign condition or at autopsy
Stage	B:	Disease confined within the capsule, with no acid phospha-tase elevation
Stage	C:	Extracapsular cancer, regardless of acid phosphatase level, or intracapsular disease with enzyme elevation
Stage	D:	Demonstrable involvement beyond the pevis or demonstrable metastasis

brinolysis (4, 6). Thus, in cancer of the prostate at least some of the tumor cells retain their susceptibility to hormonal influence, and to this extent the disease remains hormone-sensitive (7-17).

On this basis, thousands of patients have been treated with additive or ablative hormone therapy. However, it was not until the Veterans Administration Cooperative Urological Research Group (VACURG) was organized in 1960 that the effectiveness of hormone manipulation was evaluated in controlled studies. Three consecutive clinical trials have been carried out (13). In the first study over 2000 patients were treated (13, 14). Stage-I and Stage-II patients undergoing radical prostatectomy were randomly allocated to a group to receive in addition either placebo or 5.0 mg daily of diethylstilbestrol (DES). In Stage-I patients survival was significantly better after prostatectomy plus placebo than after prostatectomy plus DES. No significant differences were noted in Stage II. Stage-III and Stage-IV patients were randomly allocated to placebo, 5.0 mg DES daily, orchiectomy plus placebo, or orchiectomy plus DES (5.0 mg/d.) In the two treatment groups involving DES there were fewer deaths from prostatic cancer but more cardiovascular deaths, while the reverse was true in the two groups receiving placebo. It was concluded that estrogen has some effect in retarding the course of prostatic cancer but that this is more than offset by a substantial increase in mortality from cardiovascular disease. The greatest difference in the risk of cardiovascular death appears to occur within the first year (13-15). If Stage-III and -IV patients submitted to castration (+ placebo) are compared with those treated with placebo alone, it is noticeable that the survival curves constructed for deaths from cancer alone are identical. In other words, castration has no influence on death from cancer in Stages III and IV, and the combination of orchiectomy plus estrogen has not much to offer beyond the benefits of estrogen alone (which is more effective than castration alone). As a result of this study it was recommended that estrogen therapy should be withheld until symptoms were severe enough to require relief (13, 14). By withholding hormonal treatment until symptoms develop, survival rates are not adversely affected. The second study was set up to compare radical prostatectomy plus placebo versus placebo alone in Stages I and II. Up

502

Table 29-2. Effectiveness of single agents in prostate cancer

Drug	Number evaluated	Number of responses	Reference
Methotrexate	3	1	YAGODA (23)
5-Fluorouracil	66	19 (29%)	CARTER and WASSERMAN (90)
FUdR	8	3	YAGODA (23)
Hydroxyurea	20	8 (40%)	LERNER and MALLOY (77)
BCNU	15	2 (14%)	CARTER and WASSERMAN (90)
MeCCNU	19	2 (11%)	-
Nitrogen mustard	31	12 (39%)	-
Cyclophosphamide	57	8 (14%)	-
Uracil mustard	1	O	SLAVIK and CARTER (24)
Busulfan	16	1 (6%)	SLAVIK and CARTER (24)
Alinine mustard	29	4 (14%)	YAGODA (23)
Degranol	16	2 (12.5%)	YAGODA (23)
Mitomycin C	8	1	CARTER and WASSERMAN (90)
Adriamycin	9	2	BLUM and CARTER (69)
Mithramycin	25	1 (4%)	YAGODA (23)
Chromomycin A3	1	1	SLAVIK and CARTER (24)
Vincristine	22	2 (9%)	CARTER and WASSERMAN (90)
Vinblastine	2	1	CARTER and WASSERMAN (90)

to the last report (November 1973) there was no difference in survival or development of progressive cancer between the 2 groups, but it was too early to analyze the data in detail (13). In Stages III and IV placebo was compared with 3 graded doses (0.2 mg, 1.0 mg, or 5.0 mg daily) of DES. In terms of survival, placebo seems to be as good as 1 mg of DES in Stage III, but significantly worse than 1 mg of DES in Stage IV disease. Thus far, the 1 mg dose of DES has been as effective as the 5 mg dose of DES in controlling prostatic cancer in both stages but has been associated with a lower incidence of cardiovascular deaths (70). Again it was concluded that estrogen therapy (which is only palliative) should be withheld until it is required for relief of symptoms. If DES is prescribed, the recommended daily dose is 1.0 mg.

In the third study the treatment for Stages I and II is the same as in study 2, while in Stages III and IV patients are randomized between 1 mg/day of Premarin for 1 month followed by 2.5 mg/day, 10 mg of medroxyprogesterone acetate three times daily, and 1 mg/day of DES plus 10 mg of medroxyprogesterone acetate three times daily (70). Up to now, Premarin, medroxyprogesterone acetate or the combination of DES and medroxyprogesterone acetate do not appear to be any better than DES alone in terms of survival or effects on the cancer (70).

A response rate of 40-80% has been reported in various publications for primary hormone therapy. The duration of benefit remains unpredictable. Remissions lasting 1-2 years are not uncommon. The response is most often subjective, with relief of pain, especially that related to bone metastases, and improved performance status. There may also be objective evidence of regression, such as a reduction in the size of primary tumors or metastases, recalcification of osteolytic lesions, and decrease in previously elevated acid phosphatase or calcium levels.

Endocrine manipulations eventually select out clones of malignant cells that are no longer hormone-dependent and exacerbations result. Secondary hormone manipulations have a beneficial effect in only 17-37% of patients, and this is generally of short duration. The following treatments have been tried: orchiectomy in patients who had estrogen as primary therapy (little benefit can be expected if the testes have already become small), estrogens in patients who initially underwent orchiectomy, an increase in the dose of estrogen, switching to other estrogens, androgens (8), progestins (16), and large doses of corticosteroids (9). Adrenalectomy or hypophysectomy have benefited 40% of carefully selected patients (18-21). Relief of bone pain is far more common than objective tumor regression. At present the role of chemotherapy is being studied more critically (see below). Some newer developments in hormone therapy deserve to be mentioned. Progestins, especially cyproterone acetate have been shown to inhibit endogenous and exogenous androgenic action in animal experiments (17, 22, 71, 72). It reduces the excretion of gonadotrophins and is thought to act as a competitor at the level of androgen receptors of the prostatic cell. Preliminary clinical trials were encouraging (17), but no comparative studies have been carried out with DES. Several other antiandrogens appear promising (17). SCOTT suggests that the combination of estrogens (acting largely through the pituitary) and progestins (acting at the local level) may provide maximum inhibition of androgenic action and may therefore deserve a clinical trial (17). Estracyt, an estradiol phosphate linked by a carbamate to nor-nitrogen mustard may be effective (17, 73, 74). The EORTC studied 2-bromo-α-ergocryptine, an inhibitor of prolactin since it appeared from in vitro and in vivo studies in animals that prolactin might play a role in controlling the activity of the prostate. The compound failed to induce remissions in 24 patients with Stage III and IV disease (75).

B. CHEMOTHERAPY

A review of nonhormonal cytotoxic therapy in prostatic cancer is necessarily brief, because it has never been adequately studied in this tumor and its value is thus not known. The lack of adequate trials is the result of the introduction of an effective palliative hormonal therapy shortly before cytotoxic agents became available. Since then estrogen administration or orchiectomy have remained the major form of initial therapy for disseminated prostatic cancer. When patients progress after an initial response, further endocrine manipulations (ablative or additive) are usually tried rather than chemotherapy, although their efficacy remains doubtful. Thus the few attempts at chemotherapy have often been carried out in terminal patients, resulting in the impression that they are of little value (23). The realization that hormone therapy fails to increase survival has led to a renewed interest in chemotherapy (23, 24). Preliminary results of a series of ongoing trials were reported at the National Prostate Cancer Project workshop (76). A review of the available results is listed in Table 29-2. Regressions have been reported with alkylating agents, 5-FU (23), and HUR (77). The National Prostate Project has activated a randomized comparative trial of 5-FU and cyclophosphamide (24, 78) with cross-over at progression. MTX, vincristine, actinomycin D, and procarbazine are also considered for evaluation. Other groups are trying 5-FU (79, 80), ADM (80, 81, 96), CCNU (79) and the combinations of 5-FU plus CPM (81, 96), and 5-FU plus DES (79).

The evaluation of chemotherapy has been hampered by the fact that many patients with prostate carcinoma do not have easily measurable lesions. The recent availability of methods to screen cytotoxic agents in animal models or in-vitro systems will hopefully be of great help in the selection of effective agents (17, 23, 82, 83). Vincristine, cyclophosphamide, hexamethylmelamine, and 5-FU, in that order, were the most effective agents in a test system devised by SANDBERG and SAROFF, quoted by SCOTT (17). Mithramycin and radioactive phosphorus have been shown to reduce bone pain due to metastatic involvement (25, 26).

C. STRATEGY

The management of localized prostate cancer is not standardized (2, 26, 91, 92). It is not known whether additional therapy is required for Stage-I (or-A) lesions after the initial surgery leading to the diagnosis. A Veterans Administration Cooperative Urological Research Group study suggested that radical prostatectomy may not be indicated for most patients with Stage I carcinoma (70). The majority of these lesions never become clinically manifest (3, 27). Adjuvant hormonal therapy has adverse effects (13). Some recommend that large lesions or poorly differentiated ones be treated by radical prostatectomy or radiotherapy (2).

Stage II or B has been treated by both radical prostatectomy (especially small and low-grade lesions), and external or interstitial irradiation. Each of these methods has its enthusiasts. Since 10-25% of patients subjected to surgery develop local recurrences or metastases, some workers recommend additional therapy, such as infiltration of the prostatic bed with chemotherapy (e.g., thio-TEPA), adjuvant interstitial or external irradiation, or massive doses of intravenous estrogens.

The majority of patients with locally extended disease (Stage C or III) have positive pelvic and paraaortic lymph nodes. Some specialists recommend radical or superradical surgery (28, 29), extended-field irradiation (84) or combinations of these methods with or without adjuvant hormonal therapy. Others, who no longer have the ambition, or do not see the need, to attempt a cure of prostatic cancer at this stage, direct their therapeutic efforts at palliation.

Metastatic disease (Stage IV or D) has generally been treated with hormone manipulations, as discussed earlier in this chapter. It is anticipated that chemotherapy will play a greater role in the future. Unfortunately extensive marrow involvement may frequently make it impossible to give effective dosages.

RENAL CARCINOMA

This discussion deals with malignant tumors of the renal tubular epithelium, which are referred to as renal-cell carcinomas, adenocarcinomas, hypernephromas, or Grawitz's tumor. Hypernephroma is a misnomer introduced at a time when it was thought that renal tumors arose from

adrenal remnants in the kidneys. Electron-microscope studies have demonstrated that cells of renal adenocarcinoma are almost identical to
normal epithelial cells of the proximal convoluted tubule (30).

The majority of renal tumors are adenocarcinomas (89%). Two cell types,
clear and granular, are identified. Clear cells are the more common
(75%), and are thought to be associated with a more indolent course
and a better prognosis.

The tumor spreads locally and via lymphatic and hematogenous routes.
Venous invasion and growth of the tumor into intrarenal veins are noted
in one-third of surgically obtained specimens, positive regional lymph
nodes in approximately one-fourth. Systemic effects (e.g., malaise,
anorexia, weight loss, fever, anemia, hepatopathy, amyloidosis, and
neuromyopathy) and endocrine effects (erythrocytosis, hypertension,
hypercalcemia, gonadotrophin production) are often present before local
symptoms (31). A variety of clinical syndromes can thus be mimicked
before the true nature of the disease is recognized. The diagnosis is
not often made early in the course of the disease. One-third of patients
already have metastases at the time of diagnosis.

Various staging systems are in use. The UICC TNM classification is supplemented by a P category, which is a histopathological staging deter-

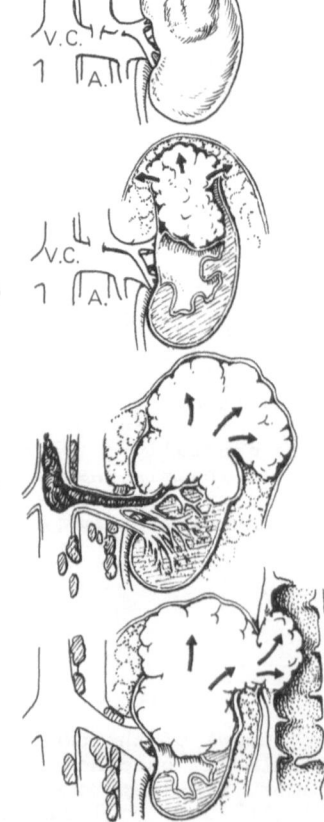

STAGE I
Tumor within capsule

STAGE II
Tumor invasion of
perinephric fat (con-
fined to Gerota's fascia)

STAGE III
Tumor involvement of
regional lymph nodes
and/or renal
vein and cava

STAGE IV
Adjacent organs or
distant metastases

*Fig. 29-1. Staging of renal
carcinoma (From HOLLAND (31))*

mined after surgery (32, 33). Most American authors use a four-stage system (Fig. 29-1) (31). Some renal carcinomas have a notoriously un-predictable clinical course. A number of spontaneous regressions of metastatic renal carcinoma (+ 40 acceptable cases) have been reported. BLOOM has reviewed the literature on this subject, and concluded that the incidence of marked spontaneous tumor regressions in this disease seems to be exceedingly rare (34). Generally, only pulmonary lesions seem to regress spontaneously. Such features as spontaneous regressions, delayed appearances of metastases (20-50 years after therapy for the primary tumors), prolonged survival or cure following removal of soli-tary metastases, suggest that host defense mechanisms are operative (immunologic, or possibly hormonal (see below), or both).

The prognosis of inoperable and metastatic cases is rather poor, with only 28% alive at 1 year and 7% at 2 years. The clinical stage is the main determinant of prognosis.

A. CHEMOTHERAPY

Cytotoxic agents have not achieved many tumor regressions in renal adeno-carcinomas. Two reviewers on this subject have failed to find either a single agent or a combination of agents which produces consistent response rates (Table 29-3) (35, 36). TALLEY concluded from his review that the only drugs for which any significant results had been reported were cyclophosphamide (CPM), 6-MP, vinblastine (VLB), and hydroxyurea (HUR) (36). Among the newer experimental agents CCNU deserves a mention. MITTELMAN et al. observed regressions in 4/20 patients treated with CCNU (37). Unfortunately the activity of CCNU or MeCCNU in renal cancer could not be confirmed by subsequent studies (85, 86). Adriamycin, though useful in bladder cancers, has no significant activity against renal carcinomas (94). Bleomycin is inactive (93); dibromodulcitol holds some promise (39, 90). There are no reports of very effective combination chemotherapy (43, 44, 97, 98).

B. HORMONE THERAPY

BLOOM has been the major proponent of hormone therapy for renal adeno-carcinomas (34, 42, 45). He cites as arguments for a possible hormonal influence the male predominance, the influence of gonadal hormones on the normal kidney in experimental animals, the successful induction of renal tumors in hamsters by estrogen and the inhibition of such tu-mors by estrogen antagonists or endocrine ablation procedures. He ini-tiates therapy with progestins (Provera 100 mg t.i.d., p.o.). If there is no response to this preparation within 8 weeks, or a shorter time if the patient is deteriorating rapidly a change is made to testosterone propionate, 100 mg i.m. on 5 days per week, later reduced to 3 days per week. Reviewing his own experience and that of 10 different centers with a total of 272 cases, BLOOM records an overall objective reponse rate of 15% (range 6-33%) for various progestins and androgen preparations prescribed in different schedules (34, 36, 45-49). About 50% of patients derive subjective benefit from hormone therapy. A favorable response is more frequent in men (21%) than in women (8%) and survival is pro-longed in responders (19.6 versus 5.2 months). Tumor regressions are more frequent with progestins than with androgens. TALLEY remarks that all regressions were noted in pulmonary metastases (none in brain or soft-tissue lesions) and occurred in patients who had previously under-gone nephrectomy (36). The development of suitable assays might help in the screening for hormone dependency prior to initiation of therapy.

507

Table 29-3. Effectiveness of single agents in renal carcinoma

Drug	Number evaluated	Number of responses	Reference
Methotrexate	16	1 (6%)	TALLEY (36)
6-Mercaptopurine	16	3 (19%)	TALLEY (36)
Imidazole carboxamide (DIC)	29	1	CARTER and WASSERMAN (90)
5-Fluorouracil	40	3 (8%)	CARTER and WASSERMAN (90)
5-FUdR	22	1 (4.5%)	TALLEY (36)
Cytosine arabinoside	2	0	TALLEY (36)
Hydroxyurea	25	6 (24%)	TALLEY (36)
CCNU	59	4 (7%)	CARTER and WASSERMAN (90)
MeCCNU	21	0	CARTER and WASSERMAN (90)
Chlorambucil	14	2 (14%)	TALLEY (36)
Cyclophosphamide	34	7 (20%)	TALLEY (36)
Hexamethylmelamine	17	1 (6%)	BLUM et al. (38)
Dibromodulcitol	19	4 (21%)	CARTER and WASSERMAN (90)
Mitomycin C	36	4 (11%)	CARTER and WASSERMAN (90)
Actinomycin D	5	1	TALLEY (36)
Mithramycin	3	0	TALLEY (36)
Adriamycin	94	5 (5%)	SLAVIK (94)
Bleomycin	7	3	BLUM et al. (60)
	20	2	JOHNSON et al. (93)
Porfiromycin	2	0	IZBICKI et al. (40)
Vincristine	3	0	TALLEY (36)
Vinblastine	12	1	CARTER and WASSERMAN (90)
VM-26	5	0	EORTC (41)

The Swiss Group for Clinical Cancer Research failed to confirm the beneficial effects of hormone therapy in renal carcinoma (87).

C. STRATEGY

1. Localized Renal Adenocarcinoma

Radical nephrectomy is considered to be the treatment of choice; however, there is no information available to suggest that it is superior to simple nephrectomy. The value of preoperative or postoperative radiotherapy is uncertain, few controlled studies having been carried out. One randomized trial of preoperative radiotherapy (3,000 rads in 3 weeks) failed to reveal any improvement of the 5-year prognosis (50). However, it was noted that more complete resections were possible (especially in locally advanced stages) in the irradiated group. This suggests that preoperative irradiation may have rendered some borderline cases completely operable. Since the incidence of metastases is significantly higher in patients with residual tumor, the authors thought that preoperative irradiation was valuable, especially in locally advanced cases.

Postoperative radiotherapy has been recommended for anaplastic tumors
and cases in which extrarenal spread is found at surgery; however, a
controlled trial showed that patients treated by surgery had better
survival figures than patients with hypernephroma treated by surgery
and postoperative radiotherapy (51).

Radiotherapy is not recommended as the primary therapy for operable
cases, since this tumor does not appear to be radiocurable.

Adjuvant hormone therapy studies are in progress (34).

2. Locally Advanced and Disseminated Renal Carcinoma

Nephrectomy may still be indicated in selected cases for palliation of
local or systemic symptoms that do not respond to conventional measures
(52). However, regression of metastatic disease following nephrectomy
is so rare that surgery is not indicated for this purpose alone (34,
53).

Approximately 2% of patients with renal adenocarcinoma have solitary
metastases. Some 60 cases are recorded in the literature of patients
undergoing surgery for the primary tumor and the metastasis, with 3-
and 5-year survival rates of 45% and 34% respectively after resection
of the metastasis (survival figures not unlike those recorded after
nephrectomy for nonmetastatic renal carcinoma).

Radiotherapy can provide worthwhile local palliation in inoperable
tumors.

Hormone therapy is currently the treatment of choice for disseminated
disease; cytotoxic agents are used in cases that fail to respond or no
longer respond to hormones. Several treatment modalities have also been
combined (99).

BLADDER CANCER

Malignant tumors of the bladder account for approximately 3% of all
malignant tumors and are three times more common in men than in women
(54-57). Peak incidence is in the seventh decade. Chemical carcinogens
in the aniline dye, synthetic rubber, and other industries, tobacco,
excessive consumption of analgesics (e.g., phenacetin), and chronic
irritation associated with bilharziasis have been considered as etiological factors. It has been suggested that spontaneous bladder cancer
may be due to carcinogenic substances produced by metabolic processes,
for example metabolites of tryptophan.

The majority (97%) are derived from epithelium, and are made up of
transitional cells (90%), or, less frequently, squamous cells (6-7%)
or adenocarcinomas (2%). The Jewitt-Marshall staging system is the most
popular (Table 29-4). The UICC system can also be used (Table 29-5).
Both systems are based on the depth of penetration into the bladder
wall. All staging is crude at best and no information about lymph node
involvement is available except in patient who are staged surgically.

Prognosis depends mainly on stage and grade. Recurrences are not uncommon. It has been suggested that they are the result of a multifocal
origin of bladder tumors or of seeding of cells from the primary tumor.

Table 29-4. Staging for bladder cancer (Jewett-Marshall classification)

Description of tumor	Jewett-Marshall classification
Superficial, confined to mucosa	O
Confined to submucosa	A
Infiltrated halfway through bladder muscle	B_1
Infiltrated more than halfway through bladder muscle	B_2
Extended to perivesical fat	C
Spread to regional lymph nodes	D_1
Spread to distant sites	D_2

Table 29-5. TNM Staging for bladder cancer

T1S	Pre-invasive carcinoma, so-called carcinoma in situ, either papillary or sessile
T1	Tumor with infiltration of subepithelial connective tissue
T2	Tumor with infiltration of superficial muscle
T3	Tumor with infiltration of deep muscle
T4	Tumor fixed or invading adjoining organs
NX	When it is impossible to assess the regional lymph nodes the symbol NX will be used
NO	No deformity of regional nodes on lymphangiography
N1	Regional nodes deformed on lymphangiography
MO	No evidence of distant metastases
M1	Distant metastases present

A. CHEMOTHERAPY

1. Systemic Chemotherapy

Most cytotoxic agents have not been very effective in bladder cancer. Except for 5-FU, few agents have been evaluated in large numbers (Table 29-6). 5-FU and hydroxyurea (HUR) appear to be the most effective of the conventional agents. However, it must be noted that in a comparative trial, 5-FU-treated patients did no better than placebo-treated controls (62). Several of the newer agents deserve to be mentioned: VP-213 (61), VM26 (41), mitomycin C (59), hexamethylmelamine (38), bleomycin (2 CR, 3 PR < 50 percent in 30 patients (88)), PDD (37% RR) (100), and especially adriamycin (69, 94).

2. Topical Chemotherapy

Intravesical instillation of thio-TEPA (63) has been useful for topical treatment of papillary lesions that have not invaded beyond the subepithelium (1/3 CR, 1/3 PR). SADOUGHI et al. report good results in one patient treated with intravesical bleomycin (64). ADM has also been used topically (101).

Table 29-6. Effectiveness of single agents in bladder cancers

Drug	Number evaluated	Number of responses	Reference
5-Fluorouracil	74	26 (35%)	LIVINGSTON and CARTER (58)
Hydroxyurea	8	5	-
Procarbazine	3	1	-
Chlorambucil	10	O	-
Cyclophosphamide	10	2	CARTER and WASSERMAN (90)
Hexamethylmelamine	10	3	BLUM et al. (38)
Mitomycin C	51	13 (25%)	CARTER and WASSERMAN (90)
Diamminodichloro-platinum	19	7 (37%)	YAGODA et al. (100)
Adriamycin	136	37 (27%)	SLAVIK (94)
Bleomycin	14	O	BLUM et al. (60)
VM-26	24	5 (20%)	EORTC (41)
VP-16216	5	1	EORTC (61)

B. STRATEGY

1. Early, Superficial Tumors (Stage O, A)

The need for a multidisciplinary approach and organized trials is clear-ly recognized (54-57, 65, 66, 90). Various local therapeutic measures have been employed, including transurethral resection, segmental resec-tion, excision and electrocoagulation through the opened bladder, local instillation of cytotoxic agents or isotopes, and interstitial radio-therapy. Selection of the most suitable of these methods depends on the size, location, degree of spread and nature of the tumor, and the expertise and personal convictions of the treating physician (55, 57). It must be realized that clinical staging, which is the principal de-terminant in the selection of a treatment modality, is often inaccurate, many cases being understaged (65).

2. Lesions Invading the Muscle Wall

These are likely to be of a higher grade and to have regional lymphatic involvement (in about 50%). Some advocate total cystectomy with or with-out pelvic lymphadenectomy (67). This procedure requires either bladder reconstruction or a supravesical type of urinary diversion. Others pre-fer radiation as the primary therapy. Finally, combinations of modali-ties, such as radiotherapy preceding surgery, are also possible (89, 95). One prospective trial has showed the superiority of this combined ap-proach in the intermediate group of tumors (B2 and C) (66). Another similar controlled trial is still in progress. It is hoped that pre-operative irradiation might seal off lymphatics, alter cell viabili-ty so that implants will not occur or grow, and sterilize microscopic and macroscopic foci in lymph nodes. Postoperative radiotherapy has been recommended when there is evidence of residual tumor either at the primary site or in the regional lymph nodes, and for high-grade tumors, that is situations in which it seems that recurrence would otherwise be likely .

The combination of radiotherapy with 5-FU did not result in a better regression rate or survival rate for advanced invasive carcinoma of the bladder than radiotherapy alone (68).

3. Locally Advanced and Disseminated Bladder Carcinoma

Chemotherapy is reserved for cases that can no longer be managed by surgery and/or radiotherapy.

REFERENCES

1. FRANKS, L.M.: Etiology, epidemiology and pathology of prostatic cancer. Cancer 32, 1092 (1973).
2. PROUT, Jr., G.R.: Diagnosis and staging of prostatic carcinoma. Cancer 32, 1096 (1973).
3. WHITMORE Jr., W.F.: The natural history of prostatic cancer. Cancer 32, 1104 (1973).
4. HUGGINS, C., HODGES, C.V.: Studies on prostatic cancer: In: The effect of castration, of estrogen and of androgen injection on serum phosphatases in metastatic carcinoma of the prostate. Cancer Res. 1, 292 (1941).
5. HERBST, W.P.: The effects of estradiol dipropionate and diethyl-stilbestrol on malignant prostatic tissue. Trans. Amer. Ass. genitourin. Surg. 34, 195 (1941).
6. TAGNON, H.J., SCHULMAN, P., WHITMORE, Jr., W.F., LEONE, L.A.: Prostatic fibrinolysin. Study of a case illustrating role in hemorrhagic diathesis of cancer of the prostate. Amer. J. Med. 15, 875 (1953).
7. FERGUSSON, J.D.: Cancer of the prostate (2 parts). Brit. med. J. 4, 475 and 539 (1970).
8. BRENDLER, H., CHASE, W.E., SCOTT, W.W.: Prostatic cancer. Further investigation of hormonal relationships. Arch. Surg. 61, 433 (1950).
9. HODGES, C.V., KIRCHHEIM, D.: Hormone treatment of cancer of the prostate. In: New Trends in the Treatment of Cancer, Vol. 8, p. 133 (eds. L. Manuila, S. Moles, P. Rentchick). Recent Results in Cancer Research. Berlin: Springer 1967.
10. RUBIN, P.: Cancer of the urogenital tract: prostatic cancer. Introduction. J. Amer. med. Ass. 209, 1695 (1969).
11. PROUT, G.R.: Hormone therapy in advanced prostatic carcinoma. In: Oncology 1970, Vol. 4, p. 301. Chicago: Year Book Medical Publishers 1970.
12. BAILAR, III, J.C., BYAR, D.P., and THE VETERANS ADMINISTRATION CO-OPERATIVE UROLOGICAL RESEARCH GROUP: Estrogen treatment for cancer of the prostate. Early results with 3 doses of diethylstilbestrol and placebo. Cancer 26, 257 (1970).
13. BYAR, D.P.: The Veterans Administration Cooperative Urological Research Group's studies of cancer of the prostate. Cancer 32, 1126 (1973).
14. VETERANS ADMINISTRATION COOPERATIVE UROLOGICAL RESEARCH GROUP. Treatment and survival of patients with cancer of the prostate. Surg. Obstet. Gynec. 124, 1011 (1967).
15. BLACKARD, C.E., DOE, R.P., MELLINGER, G.T., BYAR, D.P.: Incidence of cardiovascular disease and death in patients receiving diethyl-stilbestrol for carcinoma of the prostate. Cancer 26, 249 (1970)
16. GELLER, J., FRUCHTMAN, B., NEWMAN, H., ROBERTS, T., SILVA, R.: Effect of progestational agents on carcinoma of the prostate. Cancer Chemother. Rep. 51, 41 (1967).

17. SCOTT, W.W.: Rationale and results of primary endocrine therapy in patients with prostatic cancer. Cancer 32, 1119 (1973).
18. MURPHY, G.P., REYNOSO, G., SCHOONEES, R., GAILANI, S., BOURKE, R., KENNY, G.M., MIRAND, E.A., SCHALCH, D.S.: Hypophysectomy and adrenalectomy for disseminated prostatic carcinoma. J. Urol. 105, 817 (1971).
19. MADDY, J.A., WINTERNITZ, W.W., NORRELL, H.: Cryohypophysectomy in the management of advanced prostatic cancer. Cancer 28, 322 (9171).
20. MAHONEY, E.M., HARRISON, J.H.: Bilateral adrenalectomy for palliative treatment of prostatic cancer. J. Urol. 108, 936 (1972).
21. WEST, C.R., MURPHY, G.P.: Pituitary ablation and disseminated prostatic carcinoma. J. Amer. med. Ass. 225, 253 (1973).
22. GELLER, J., VAZAKAS, G., FRUCHTMAN, B., NEWMAN, H., NAKAO, K., LOH, A.: The effect of cyproterone acetate for advanced carcinoma of the prostate. Surg. Gynec. Obstet. 127, 748 (1968).
23. YAGODA, A.: Non-hormonal cytotoxic agents in the treatment of prostatic adenocarcinoma. Cancer 32, 1131 (1973).
24. MURPHY, G.P.: Cancer of the prostate. Cancer 32, 1089 (1973).
25. PERSKY, L., GUERRIER, K., RABIN, R., ALBERT, D.J.: Mithramycin and metastatic carcinoma of the prostate. J. Urol. 104, 884 (1970).
26. FLOCKS, R.H.: Carcinoma of the prostate. J. Urol. 101, 741 (1969).
27. BYAR, D.P., and the VETERANS ADMINISTRATION COOPERATIVE UROLOGICAL RESEARCH GROUP: Survival of patients with incidentally found microscopic cancer of the prostate: results of a clinical trial of conservative treatment. J. Urol. 108, 908 (1972).
28. CULP, O.S., MEYER, J.J.: Radical prostatectomy in the treatment of prostatic cancer. Cancer 32, 1113 (1973).
29. McCULLOUGH, D.L., LEADBETTER, W.: Radical pelvic surgery for locally extensive carcinoma of the prostate. J. Urol. 108, 939 (1972).
30. BENNINGTON, J.L.: Cancer of the kidney: etiology, epidemiology and pathology. Cancer 32, 1017 (1973).
31. HOLLAND, J.F.: Cancer of the kidney: natural history and staging. Cancer 32, 1030 1973.
32. UICC: T.N.M. classification of malignant tumors. Geneva: G. de Buten 1968.
33. UICC Committee on Professional Education: Clinical Oncology. A manual for students and doctors. Berlin-Heidelberg-New York: Springer-Verlag 1973.
34. BLOOM, H.J.G.: Hormone-induced and spontaneous regression of metastatic renal cancer. Cancer 32, 1066 (1973).
35. WOODRUFF, M.W., WAGLE, D., GAILANI, S.D., JONES, Jr., R.: The current status of chemotherapy for advanced renal carcinoma. J. Urol. 97, 611 (1967).
36. TALLEY, R.W.: Chemotherapy of adenocarcinoma of the kidney. Cancer 32, 1062 (1973).
37. MITTELMAN, A., ALBERT, D.J., MURPHY, G.P.: Lomustine treatment of metastatic renal cell carcinoma. J. Amer. med. Ass. 225, 32 (1973).
38. BLUM, R.H., LIVINGSTON, R.B., CARTER, S.K.: Hexamethylmelamine. A new drug with activity in solid tumors. Europ. J. Cancer 9, 195 (1973).
39. ANDREWS, N.C., WEISS, A.J., ANSFIELD, F.J., ROCHLIN, D.B., MASON, J.H.: Phase I study of dibromodulcitol (NSC-104800) Cancer Chemother. Rep. 55, 61 (1971).
40. IZBICKI, R., AL-SARRAF, M., REED, M.L., VAUGHN, C.B., VAITKEVICIUS, V.K.: Further clinical trials with porfiromycin (NSC-56410) (large intermittent doses). Cancer Chemother. Rep. 56, 615 (1972).
41. E.O.R.T.C. CLINICAL SCREENING COOPERATIVE GROUP: Clinical screening of epipodophyllotoxin VM26 in malignant lymphomas and solid tumors. Brit. med. J. 2, 774 (1972).

42. BLOOM, H.J.G.: Medroxyprogesterone acetate (Provera) in the treatment of metastatic renal cancer. Brit. J. Cancer 25, 250 (1971).
43. HANHAM, I.W.F., NEWTON, K.A., WESTBURY, G.: Seventy-five cases of solid tumours treated by a modified quadruple chemotherapy regime. Brit. J. Cancer 25, 462 (1971).
44. LOKICH, J.J., SKARIN, A.T.: Five-drug combination chemotherapy for disseminated adenocarcinoma. Cancer Chemother. Rep. 56, 761 (1972).
45. BLOOM, H.J.G.: Renal Cancer. In: Endocrine therapy in malignant disease, p. 339 (ed. B.A. Stoll). London-Philadelphia-Toronto: Saunders 1972.
46. SAMUELS, M.L., SULLIVAN, P., HOWE, C.D.: Medroxyprogesterone acetate in the treatment of renal cell carcinoma (hypernephroma). Cancer 22, 525 (1968).
47. PAPAC, R.C.: Hormonal therapy of renal carcinoma. Proc. Amer. Ass. Cancer. Res. 10, 67 (1969).
48. PAINE, C.H., WRIGHT, F.W., ELLIS, F.: The use of progestogen in the treatment of metastatic carcinoma of the kidney and uterin body. Brit. J. Cancer 24, 277 (1970).
49. VAN DER WERF-MESSING, B., VAN GILSE, H.A.: Hormonal treatment of metastases of renal carcinoma. Brit. J. Cancer 25, 423 (1971).
50. VAN DER WERF-MESSING, B.: Carcinoma of the kidney. Cancer 32, 1056 (1973).
51. FINNEY, R.: An evaluation of postoperative radiotherapy in hypernephroma treatment - a clinical trial. Cancer 32, 1332 (1973).
52. MIDDLETON, R.G.: Surgery for metastatic renal cell carcinoma. J. Urol. 97, 973 (1967).
53. MARKEWITZ, M., TAYLOR, D.A., VEENEMA, R.J.: Spontaneous regression of pulmonary metastases following palliative nephrectomy. Cancer 20, 1147 (1967).
54. AD-HOC BLADDER CANCER COMMITTEE OF THE CCIR: Tumors of the bladder. J. Urol. 108, 414 (1972).
55. JEWETT, H.J.: Cancer of the bladder: diagnosis and staging. Cancer 32, 1072 (1973).
56. SOUTHCOTT, R.D.C.: Bladder tumors. Brit. J. clin. Pract. 26, 543 (1972).
57. KAUFMAN, J.J.: Current therapy for carcinoma of the bladder. Postgrad. Med. 96 (1969).
58. LIVINGSTON, R.B., CARTER, S.K.: Single agents in cancer chemotherapy. New York-Washington-London: IFI/Plenum 1970.
59. EARLY, K., ELIAS, E.G., MITTELMAN, A., ALBERT, D., MURPHY, G.P.: Mitomycin C in the treatment of metastatic transitional cell carcinoma of urinary bladder. Cancer 31, 1150 (1973).
60. BLUM, R.H., CARTER, S.K., AGRE, K.: A clinical review of bleomycin - a new antineoplastic agent. Cancer 31, 903 (1973).
61. E.O.R.T.C. Clinical Screening Group: Epipodophyllotoxin VP 16213 in the treatment of acute leukaemias, haematosarcomas and solid tumors. Brit. med. J. 3, 199 (1973).
62. PROUT, Jr., G.R., BROSS, I.D.J., SLACK, N.H., AUSMAN, R.K.: Carcinoma of the bladder, 5-fluorouracil and the critical role of a placebo. A cooperative group report. I. Cancer 22, 926 (1968).
63. ABBASSIAN, A., WALLACE, D.M.: Intracavitary chemotherapy of diffuse non-infiltrating papillary carcinoma of the bladder. J. Urol. (Baltimore) 96, 461 (1966).
64. SADOUGHI, N., JOHNSON, R.A., EZDINLI, E.Z., BUSH, I.M., GIUNAN, P.: Intravesical bleomycin in treatment of carcinoma of the bladder. J. Amer. med. Ass. 226, 465 (1973).
65. BAGSHAW, M., CALDWELL, W.L., GRABSTALD, H., WIZENBERG, M.: Rx of bladder cancer: Complex and Controversial. CA 23, 81 (1973).
66. MILLER, L.S.:Bladder cancer. Cancer Bull. 25, 57 (1973).
67. WALLACE, D.M.: Total cystectomy: an editorial overview. Cancer 32, 1078 (1973).

68. EDLAND, R.W., WEAR, Jr., J.B., ANSFIELD, F.J.: Advanced cancer of the urinary bladder. An analysis of the results of radiotherapy alone vs. radiotherapy and concomitant 5-Fluorouracil; a prospective randomized study of 36 cases. Amer. J. Roentgenol. 108, 124 (1970).
69. BLUM, R.H., CARTER, S.K.: Adriamycin Ann. intern. Med. 80, 249 (1974).
70. BLACKARD, C.E.: The Veterans Administration Cooperative Urological Research Group studies of carcinoma of the prostate; a review. Cancer Chemother. Rep. Part 1, 59, 225 (1975).
71. WEIN, A.J., MURPHY, J.J.: Experience in the treatment of prostatic carcinoma with cyproterone acetate- J. Urol. 109, 68 (1973).
72. SMITH, R.B., WALSH, P.C., GOODWIN, W.E.: Cyproterone acetate in the treatment of advanced carcinoma of the prostate. J. Urol. 110, 106 (1973).
73. MITTELMAN, A., SHUKLA, S.K., WELVAART, K., MURPHY, G.P.: Oral estramustine phosphate in the treatment of advanced (stage D) carcinoma of the prostate. Cancer Chemother. Rep. Part, 59, 219 (1975).
74. NILSSON, T., JONSSON, G.: Clinical results with estramustine phosphate: a comparison of the intravenous and oral preparations. Cancer Chemother. Rep. Part 1, 59, 229 (1975).
75. COUNE, A., SMITH, P.: Clinical trial of 2-bromo-α-ergocryptine in human prostatic cancer. Cancer Chemother. Rep. Part 1, 59, 209 (1975).
76. NATIONAL PROSTATIC CANCER PROJECT WORKSHOP, Proceedings. Cancer Chemother. Rep. Part 1, 59, 1-254 (1975).
77. LERNER, H.J., MALLOY, T.: Hydroxyurea for stage D carcinoma of the prostate: a preliminary report. Proc. Am. Soc. Clin. Oncol. 16, 221 (1975).
78. SCOTT, W.W., GIBBONS, R.P., JOHNSON, D.E., PROUT, G.R., SCHMITDT, J.D., CHU, T.M., GAETA, J.F., JOINER, J., SAROFF, J., MURPHY, G.P.: Comparison of 5-fluorouracil and cyclophosphamide in patients with advanced carcinoma of the prostate. Cancer Chemother. Rep. Part 1, 59, 195 (1975).
79. TEJADA, F., COHEN, M.H.: Initial chemotherapeutic trials in patients with inoperable or recurrent cancer of the prostate. Cancer Chemother. Rep. Part 1, 59, 243 (1975).
80. DeWYS, W.D.: Comparison of adriamycin and 5-fluorouracil in advanced prostatic cancer. Cancer Chemother. Rep. Part 1, 59, 215 (1975).
81. EAGAN, R.T., UTZ, C.D., MYERS, R.P., FURLOW, W.L.: Comparison of adriamycin and the combination of 5-fluorouracil and cyclophosphamide in advanced prostatic cancer. Cancer Chemother. Rep. Part 1, 59, 203 (1975).
82. SANDBERG, A.A., KIRDANI, R.Y., YAMANAKA, H., VARKARAKIS, M.J., MURPHY, G.P.: Potential test systems for drugs against prostatic cancer. Cancer Chemother. Rep. Part 1, 59, 175 (1975).
83. SLOAN, W.R., HESTON, W.D.W., COFFEY, D.S.: New model for studying the effects of cancer chemotherapeutic agents on the growth of the prostate gland. Cancer Chemother. Rep. Part 1, 59, 185 (1975).
84. PEREZ, C.A., ACKERMAN, L.V., SILBER, I., ROYCE, R.K.: Radiation therapy in the treatment of localized carcinoma of the prostate. Cancer 34, 1059 (1974).
85. WASSERMAN, T.H., SLAVIK, M., CARTER, S.K.: Review of CCNU in clinical cancer therapy. Cancer Treat. Rev. 1, 131 (1974).
86. WASSERMAN, T.H., SLAVIK, M., CARTER, S.K.: Methyl-CCNU in clinical cancer therapy. Cancer Treat. Rev. 1, 251 (1974).
87. ALBERTO, P., SENN, H.J.: Hormonal therapy of renal carcinoma alone and in association with cytotoxic drugs. Cancer 33, 1226 (1974).

88. O.E.R.T.C., GROUPE COOPERATEUR DES CANCERS DE L'APPAREIL GENITO-URINAIRE: Essai d'efficacité de la bléomycine dans les cancers de la vessie. Nouv. Presse méd. 3, 601 (1974).
89. JOHNSON, D.E.: Surgery for carcinoma of the urinary bladder. Cancer Treat. Rev. 1, 271 (1974).
90. CARTER, S.K., WASSERMAN, T.H.: The chemotherapy of urologic cancer. Cancer 36, 729 (1975).
91. FLOCKS, R.H., O'DONOGHUE, E.P.N., MILLEMAN, L.A., CULP, D.A.: Surgery of prostatic carcinoma. Cancer 36, 705 (1975).
92. BAGSHAW, M.A., RAY, G.R., PISTENMA, D.A., CASTELLINO, R.A., MEARES, E.M.: External beam radiation therapy of primary carcinoma of the prostate. Cancer 36, 723 (1975).
93. JOHNSON, D.E., CHALBAUD, R.A., HOLOYE, P.Y., SAMUELS, M.L.: Clinical trial of bleomycin (NSC-125066) in the treatment of metastatic renal carcinoma. Cancer Chemother. Rep. Part 1, 59, 433 (1975).
94. SLAVIK, M.: Adriamycin (NSC-123127) activity in genitourinary and gynecologic malignancies. Cancer Chemother. Rep. Part 3, 6, 297 (1975).
95. Van der WERF-MESSING, B.H.P.: Carcinoma of the bladder $T_3N_XM_0$ treated by preoperative irradiation followed by cystectomy. Third report of the Rotterdam Radio-Therapy Institute. Cancer 36, 718 (1975).
96. EAGAN, R.T., HAHN, R.G., MYERS, R.P.: Adriamycin (NSC-123127) versus 5-fluorouracil (NSC-19893) and cyclophosphamide (NSC-26271) in the treatment of metastatic prostate cancer. Cancer Treat. Rep. 60, 115 (1976).
97. JOHNSON, D.E., RODRIGUEZ, L., HOLOYE, P.Y., SAMUELS, M.L.: Combination vincristine (NSC-67574) and hydroxyurea (NSC-32065) for metastatic renal carcinoma. Cancer Chemother. Rep. 59, 1159 (1975).
98. HAHN, R.G., BRODOVSKY, H.: Methyl CCNU, velban, and depo-provera treatment trials in advanced renal cancer. Proc. Amer. Soc. Clin. Oncol. 17, 246 (1976).
99. ISHMAEL, D.R., BOTTOMLEY, R.H., HOGE, A.F.: Treatment of renal cell adenocarcinoma (hypernephroma) with depo-provera and combination chemoimmunotherapy. Proc. Amer. Soc. Clin. Oncol. 17, 265 (1976).
100. YAGODA, A., WATSON, R., GRABSTALD, H., WHITMORE, W.F.: Cis-platinum diammine dichloride (CPDD) in advanced urinary tract cancer. Proc. Amer. Soc. Clin. Oncol. 17, 296 (1976).
101. IZBICKI, R.M., PONTES, E., VAITKEVICIUS, V.K.: Adriamycin bladder instillation. Proc. Amer. Soc. Clin. Oncol. 17, 311 (1976).

Chapter 30
Endocrine Tumors

A. THYROID CARCINOMA

Thyroid carcinomas are relatively rare, accounting for approximately 1% of all cancers. They can occur at any age, but there are two peaks of incidence (at 7-20 and 40-65 years). They are twice as common in females as in males. There does not appear to be any relationship between the development of thyroid carcinoma and preexisting benign thyroid disease. However, irradiation of the neck in children is accepted as a predisposing factor (1, 43).

Several methods have been proposed for the classification of thyroid carcinomas (2, 3). Most take the degree of histologic differentiation and the biologic behavior into account; in this way three different groups of tumors can be distinguished. The majority (70-80%) are differentiated tumors. Four histologic types are included in this group: (1) purely papillary; (2) purely follicular; (3) mixed papillary and follicular; and (4) Hürtle-cell carcinoma. They are characterized by a remarkably benign course. Life expectancy is hardly different from normal. Anaplastic or spindle- and giant-cell carcinomas make up the second group. Their course is rapid, resulting in early death. The medullary (solid) carcinoma of the thyroid falls between the two previous groups in clinical behavior and survival. This tumor is derived from parafollicular cells and has special clinical features, such as a family history, an association with other tumors (pheochromocytoma, parathyroid adenoma, and mucosal neuroma), severe diarrhea, and the production of ectopic hormones (4, 44). Elevated serum levels of calcitonin are a constant feature. Some authors believe that well-differentiated tumors can undergo a transition to a more malignant, anaplastic variety (3).

Papillary carcinomas tend to recur locally after surgery and spread via the lymphatics to regional lymph nodes, while hematogenous dissemination is uncommon. The reverse is true of follicular carcinomas. Lymphatic and hematogenous metastases occur early with anaplastic tumors. The majority of patients have inoperable tumors and metastatic disease when first seen.

1. Chemotherapy

Cytotoxic agents are reserved for cases that are no longer amenable to local measures or ^{131}I (5). After a review of the literature, GOTTLIEB et al. concluded that chemotherapy has produced little subjective or objective improvement in thyroid carcinoma (6, 7), only isolated cases benefiting from 5-FU or cyclophosphamide. They recorded an encouraging response rate of 37% partial remissions with adriamycin in this group (6, 7, 48). Some authors have reported tumor regressions with bleomycir

(8) while others (7) have not been impressed with the drug. The EORTC
recommends further trials with VP-16213 (9). Combination chemotherapy
has not been evaluated in numbers sufficiently large to permit any
conclusions.

2. Hormone Therapy and Radioiodine (^{131}I)

The more differentiated tumors may be hormone (TSH)-dependent (10, 14).
Administration of thyroid, to suppress TSH, results in stabilization
or often even regression of the primary tumors or metastases. CRILE
noted 18 reponders among 32 patients who had either inoperaple tumors or
distant metastases (14). They remained alive and well for 5 to 27 years
(median 13 years), with regression or no progression of their disease. A
beneficial effect was noted only in the papillary variety and the data
indicate that a good response is most likely in female patients under
40 years of age in whom cancer was induced by irradiation in infancy
or childhood. This author also recommends the use of thyroid in inopea-
ble or metastatic cases prior to ^{131}I therapy, since hypothyroidism
and irradiation may stimulate papillary cancers to progress into anaplastic cancers. Medullary carcinoma occasionally responds, which is
surprising in view of its origin (15). Anaplastic carcinomas have shown
no response at all.

3. Strategy

Surgical resection is the treatment of choice and is also indicated
for the papillary variety, because it may transform into an anaplastic
tumor in spite of its usual slow progression (17). Cures can be obtained with subtotal or total thyroidectomy, with or without lymph-node
dissection, depending on the extent of the disease and the histology.
Thyroid therapy should be given systematically after total or partial
thyroidectomy.

For tumors that cannot be completely resected it is recommended that
as much of the tumor as possible be excised, to prevent or alleviate
esophageal and tracheal compression. This is followed by postoperative
irradiation or ^{131}I, depending on the histology.

Inoperable disease can be treated with suppressive therapy with thyroid
if the tumor is of the papillary variety. Radioactive iodine is sometimes effective in papillary and follicular cancers, but not in medullary or anaplastic thyroid cancers (18). Irradiation of the primary
neck tumor is indicated, even if it is inoperable and distant metastases
are present, to reduce or prevent compression phenomena. Chemotherapy
is reserved for patients with refractory recurrent disease, widespread
metastases no longer amenable to surgical or radiotherapeutic approaches,
and all rapidly progressing tumors.

B. ADRENOCORTICAL CARCINOMA

Adrenocortical tumor can present as a large nonfunctioning mass or as
a functioning carcinoma producing a variety of endocrine syndromes.
Depending upon the type of hormone produced, the clinical picture can
be that of Cushing's syndrome, virilization, precocious puberty, feminization, hypertension, or a combination of these. The symptoms are
caused by local invasion of adjacent tissues and distant metastases
(5, 19, 20, 45).

Several compounds that interfere with hormone synthesis have been evaluated (19). Amphenone was abandoned because of its toxicity. Metapyro-
ne has been useful in some cases in the control of Cushing's syndrome.
Aminoglutethimide (Elipten) interferes with corticosteroid synthesis
and produces characteristic histologic changes in the adrenal gland (21).
Palliation of Cushing's syndrome secondary to adrenocortical carcinoma
has been reported.

Investigation of the selective atrophy of the zona fasciculata and zona
reticularis of the adrenal cortex of dog caused by the commercial in-
secticide DDD led to the discovery that a minor component, the ortho-
para derivative (o,p' DDD) was responsible for this effect. Two extensive studies with this derivative have shown objective tumor regression
in 34% and 61% of subjects respectively, and a decrease in steroid excretion in 72% and 85% (22, 23), with a mean duration of 10 months.
Survival is prolonged in responders.

C. MALIGNANT INSULINOMA

Approximately 10-25% of insulinomas are malignant (19, 24, 25). The
clinical course of insulinomas is characterized by recurrent episodes
of lowered blood glucose. Typically plasma immunoreactive insulin is
inappropriately high at a time when blood glucose is low. Metastases
occur most commonly in regional lymph nodes and liver.

The treatment of insulinomas must be directed against both the abnormal
production of hormone and tumor growth.

Antihormonal therapy consists of dietary measures and insulin antagonists. Corticosteroids, human growth hormone, and glucagon have been
effective in individual cases. Diazoxide produces a direct inhibition
of insulin release and its use has been a major advance in the palliation of malignant insulinoma.

Conventional cytotoxic agents have not been extensively investigated in
malignant insulinoma. Some responses have been noted with alkylating
agents and 5-fluorouracil (49).

Several agents have been introduced for clinical use in malignant insulinoma because it was anticipated, on the basis of experimental observations, that they would have selective toxicity against the malignant islet-cell tissue. The most promising drug is streptozotocin (STZ),
a naturally occurring nitrosourea that causes selective destruction of
the pancreatic β-cell (see p. 44) (26-30). The Cancer Therapy Branch
of the National Cancer Institute has information on 52 cases (29). In
their study objective tumor mass regressions occured in 48% of patients
with functioning tumor, 17% attaining complete remission. The median
duration of objective remission has been approximately 1 year. Reponders
had a median survival of 1268 days, compared to 518 for nonresponders.
The activity of STZ in gastrin- or serotonin-secreting islet cell tumors
is not yet known. A weekly schedule of 1-2 g/m^2 is the one that has
been used most frequently. Renal tubular damage is the dose-limiting
criterion of toxicity. It can be avoided by close monitoring of the
urine for protein excretion, and by discontinuation of therapy when
necessary until full reversal to normal renal function has been documented.

Tubercidin, an antibiotic, has undergone limited clinical evaluation.
Although tumor regressions have been recorded, severe toxicity to veins

and local tissues requires special methods of administration and limits its usefulness (30).

D. CARCINOID TUMORS

Carcinoid tumors originate from the argentaffin cells of the intestinal tract and lungs (19, 31, 32). They are found at any point along the gastrointestinal tract, especially the appendix and terminal ileum. Malignant carcinoid tumors secrete biologically active materials which produce different clinical manifestations known as the carcinoid syndrome (33, 36, 46). The main signs and symptoms of the syndrome are chronic diarrhea, cutaneous flush, skin rash, fibrotic right-sided endocardial and valvular lesions, and episodic bronchial asthma. Serotonin (5-hydroxy-tryptamine), 5-hydroxy-tryptophan, kallikrein, histamine, ACTH, insulin, and prostaglandins are among the pharmacologically active products secreted by carcinoid tumors. In some instances the morbidity of these products is greater than that of the actual tumor. Treatment must be directed against both aspects of the disease. Many papers discuss antihormonal rather than cytotoxic therapy (34). Only 4 percent of carcinoid tumors produce vasoactive substances in quantities that produce the debilitating symptom complex that signals its presence (47).

Most efforts to control the carcinoid syndrome have been directed against serotonin, by inhibition of biosynthesis, alteration of the metabolism, or interference with the peripheral effects of serotonin (19, 34). Parachlorophenylalanine and α-methyldopa (Aldomet) inhibit biosynthesis of serotonin (33, 36). Methysergide and cyproheptadine (Periactin) are among the substances that interfere with the peripheral effects of serotonin. Phenothiazines antagonize the peripheral action of kinins and may have a beneficial effect on flushing. Corticosteroids have a similar effect, particularly in cases of bronchial carcinoid, but their mechanism of action is unknown. Alpha-adrenergic blocking agents such as phentolamine and phenoxybenzamine have also been evaluated in the carcinoid syndrome as catecholamines are known to provoke attacks of flushing in some instances.

1. Chemotherapy

Most reports on carcinoid tumors discuss the pharmacological treatment of the carcinoid syndrome; only scattered reports deal with chemotherapy. Cyclophosphamide, thio-TEPA, nitrogen mustard, 5-FU, MTX, actinomycin D, and, more recently, adriamycin, streptozotocin have caused tumor regressions in small numbers of patients (19, 28, 34, 36-42, 50). Some of these agents have also been given by intra-arterial injection into the hepatic artery (37, 38). The combination of 5-FU + STZ appears promising (49).

Since in many patients the course is indolent and the available therapy is suppressive at best, it is recommended that cytotoxic therapy be withheld until the disease is clearly so far advanced as to compromise organ function or cause significant symptoms.

REFERENCES

1. DEGROOT, L., PALOYAN, E.: Thyroid carcinoma and radiation. J. Amer. med. Ass. 225, 487 (1973).
2. WOOLNER, L.B.: Thyroid carcinoma: pathologic classification with data on prognosis. Semin. nucl. Med. 1, 481 (1971).
3. CLARK, R.L., HILL, Jr., C.S.: Thyroid cancer: natural history, diagnosis, and treatment. In: Oncology 1970, Vol. 4, p. 165. Chicago: Year Book Medical Publishers 1970.
4. HILL, jr. C.S.: Medullary carcinoma of the thyroid. Amer.Fam.Physician 7, 99 (1973).
5. DURANT, J.R.: Chemotherapy of endocrine neoplasms. In: Cancer chemotherapy II, p. 167 (eds. I. Brodsky, S.B. Kahn, J.H. Moyer). New York: Grune and Stratton 1972.
6. GOTTLIEB, J.A., HILL, Jr., C.T., IBANEZ, M.L., CLARK, R.L.: Chemotherapy of thyroid cancer. An evaluation of experience with 37 patients. Cancer 30, 848 (1972).
7. GOTTLIEB, J.A., HILL, Jr., C.S.: Chemotherapy of thyroid cancer with adriamycin. New Engl. J. Med. 290, 193 (1974).
8. HARADA, T., NISHIKAWA, Y, SUZUKI, T., ITO, K., BABA, S.: Bleomycin treatment for cancer of the thyroid. Amer. J. Surg. 122, 53 (1971).
9. E.O.R.T.C. Clinical Screening Group: Epipodophyllotoxin VP 16213 in the treatment of acute leukemias, hematosarcomas and solid tumours. Brit. med. J. 3, 199 (1973).
10. BALME, H.W.: Metastatic carcinoma of the thyroid successfully treated with thyroxine. Lancet 1, 812 (1954).
11. CRILE, Jr., G.: The endocrine dependency of certain thyroid cancers and the danger that hypothyroidism may stimulate their growth. Cancer 10, 1119 (1957).
12. CRILE, Jr., G.: Endocrine dependency of papillary carcinomas of the thyroid. J. Amer. med. Ass. 195, 721 (1966).
13. CRILE, Jr., G., HAWK, W.A.: Carcinomas of the thyroid. Cleveland Clinic Quarterly 38, 97 (1971).
14. CRILE, Jr., G.: Thyroid cancer. In: Endocrine therapy in malignant disease, p. 369. London-Philadelphia-Toronto: Saunders 1972.
15. WAHNER, H.W., CUELLO, C., ALJURE, F.: Hormone-induced regression of medullary (solid) thyroid carcinoma. Amer. J. Med. 45, 789 (1968).
16. ESSELSTYN, C.B., CRILE, Jr., G.: Indications for surgical therapy in thyroid disease. Semin. nucl. Med. 1, 474 (1971).
17. SELENKOW, H.A., KARP, P.J.: An approach to diagnosis and therapy of thyroid tumors. Semin. nucl. Med. 1, 461 (1971).
18. POCHIN, E.E.: Radio-iodine therapy of thyroid cancer. Semin. nucl. Med. 1, 503 (1971).
19. SCHEIN, P.S.: Chemotherapeutic management of the hormone-secreting endocrine malignancies. Cancer 30, 1616 (1972).
20. HARRISON, J.H., MAHONEY, E.M., BENNETT, A.H.: Tumors of the adrenal cortex. Cancer 32, 1227 (1973).
21. SCHTEINGART, D.E., CASH, R., CONN, J.W.: Aminoglutethimide and metastatic adrenal cancer. J. Amer. med. Ass. 198, 1007 (1966).
22. HUTTER, A.M., KAYHOE, D.E.: Adrenal cortical carcinoma. Results of treatment with o,p' DDD in 138 patients. Amer. J. Med. 41, 581 (1966).
23. KUBITZ, J.A., FREEMAN, L., OKUN, R.: Mitotane use in inoperable adrenal cortical carcinoma. J. amer. Med. Ass. 223, 1109 (1973).
24. SCHEIN, P.S., DELELLIS, R.A., KAHN, C.R., GORDEN, P., KRAFT, A.R.: Islet cell tumors: current concepts and management. Ann. intern. Med. 79, 239 (1973).
25. BRODER, L.E., CARTER, S.K.: Pancreatic islet cell carcinoma. I. Clinical features of 52 patients. Ann. intern. Med. 79, 101 (1973).
26. CARTER, S.K., BRODER, L., FRIEDMAN, M.: Streptozotocin and metastatic insulinoma. Ann. intern. Med. 74, 445 (1971).
27. DU PRIEST, Jr., R.W., MASSEY, W.H., FLETCHER, W.S.: Search for new cancer drugs: streptozotocin. Amer. Surg. 38, 514 (1972).

28. STOLINSKY, D.C., SADOFF, L., BRAUNWALD, J., BATEMAN, J.R.: Strep-
    tozotocin in the treatment of cancer: phase II study. Cancer 30,
    61 (1972).
29. BRODER, L.E., CARTER, S.K.: II. Results of therapy with streptozo-
    tocin in 52 patients. Ann. intern. Med. 79, 108 (1973).
30. SCHEIN, P., KAHN, R., GORDEN, P., WELLS, S., DEVITA, T.: Streptozo-
    tocin for malignant insulinomas and carcinoid tumor. Arch. intern.
    Med. 132, 555 (1973)
31. SIMPSON, A.J.: Carcinoid syndrome. N. Carolina Med. J. 30, 399,
    and 452 (1969).
32. TEITELBAUM, S.L.: The carcinoid. A collective review. Amer. J.
    Surg. 123, 564 (1972).
33. SATTERLEE, W.G., SERPICK, A., BIANCHINE, J.R.: The carcinoid syn-
    drome: chronic treatment with para-chlorophenylalanine. Ann. intern.
    Med. 72, 919 (1970).
34. HILL, G.J.: Carcinoid tumors: pharmacological therapy. Oncology
    25, 329 (1971).
35. PATCHEFSKY, A.S., SOLIT, R., PHILLIPS, L.D., CRADDOCK, M., HARRER,
    W.V., COHN, H.E., KOWLESSAR, O.D.: Hydroxyindole-producing tumors
    of the pancreas. Carcinoid-islet cell tumor and oat cell carcinoma.
    Ann. intern. Med. 77, 53 (1972).
36. SJOERDSMA, A., LOVENBERG, W., ENGELMAN, K., CARPENTER, W.T., WYATT,
    R.J., GESSA, G.L.: Serotonin now: clinical implications of inhibi-
    ting its synthesis with para-chlorophenylalanine. Ann. intern.
    Med. 73, 607 (1970).
37. ELLIS, F.W.: Carcinoid of the rectum: report of a case of thirteen
    years' survival; treated with intra-arterial nitrogen mustard
    Cancer 10, 138 (1957).
38. REED, M.L., KUIPERS, F.M., VAITKEVICIUS, V.K., CLARK, M.D., DRAKE,
    E.H., EYLER, W.R.: Treatment of disseminated carcinoid tumors in-
    cluding hepatic-artery catheterization. New Engl. J. Med. 269,
    1005 (1963).
39. MENGEL, C.E., KELLY, M.G., CARBONE, P.P., ANLYAN, W.G.: Clinical
    and biochemical effects of cyclophosphamide in patients with malig-
    nant carcinoid. Amer. J. Med. 38, 396 (1965).
40. MENGEL, C.E.: Therapy of the malignant carcinoid syndrome. Ann.
    intern. Med. 62, 587 (1965).
41. MOERTEL, C.G., REITEMEIER, R.J.: Advanced gastrointestinal cancer.
    Clinical management and chemotherapy. New York-Evanston-London:
    Harper and Row 1969.
42. STOLINSKY, D.C., SADOFF, L., BRAUNWALD, J., BATEMAN, J.R.: Strepto-
    zotocin in the treatment of cancer: phase II study. Cancer 30, 61
    (1972).
43. PARKER, L.N., BELSKY, J.L., YAMAMOTO, T., KAWAMOTO, S., KEEHN, R.
    J.: Thyroid carcinoma after exposure to atomic radiation. Ann.
    intern. Med. 80, 600 (1974).
44. CHONG, G.C., BEAHRS, O.H., SIZEMORE, G.W., WOOLNER, L.H.: Medullary
    carcinoma of the thyroid gland. Cancer 35, 695 (1975).
45. HAJJAR, R.A., HICKEY, R.C., SAMAAN, N.A.: Adrenal cortical carci-
    noma. Cancer 35, 549 (1975).
46. URELES, A.L.: Diagnosis and treatment of malignant carcinoid syn-
    drome. J. amer. Med. Ass. 229, 1346 (1974).
47. VAN SICKLE, D.G.: Carcinoid syndrome. Cleve Clin. Q. 39, 79 (1972).
48. GOTTLIEB, J.A., HILL, C.S.: Adriamycin (NSC-123127) therapy in
    thyroid carcinoma. Cancer Chemother. Rep. Part 3, 6, 283 (1975).
49. MOERTEL, C.G.: Clinical management of advanced gastrointestinal
    cancer. Cancer 36, 675 (1975).
50. SOLOMON, A., SONODA, T., PATTERSON, F.K.: Response of metastatic
    malignant carcinoid tumor to adriacycin (NSC-123127). Cancer Treat.
    Rep. 60, 273 (1976).

Chapter 31
Brain Tumors

Brain tumors account for 2% of cancer deaths. They occur at all ages and are the commonest solid tumors before puberty. In this age group cerebellar and brain-stem lesions predominate, while in adults tumors generally arise in the cerebral hemispheres.

Many complex histologic classifications have been proposed. The different tumors can be grouped according to their tissue of origin. We distinguish glial tumors (arising from glial cells, the supporting tissues of the brain), tumors of the membranes (meninges, sheaths of Schwann), embryoplastic tumors (vestigial tumors or metaplastic lesions such as craniopharyngiomas and pinealomas), and mesenchymal tumors (e.g., hemangioblastomas). Glial tumors account for approximately 50% of all brain tumors and range from well-differentiated, low-grade tumors (astrocytomas) to highly anaplastic lesions (glioblastoma multiforme). The brain is often the site of metastatic deposits, especially from cancers of the lung and breast (1).

Brain tumors characteristically spread locally. Because of their growth in a closed space containing vital structures, even histologically benign lesions may prove lethal. Hematogenous dissemination is rare, but some tumors (e.g., medulloblastomas) have a tendency to seed through the cerebrospinal fluid. Peritumoral edema often accentuates symptomatology, and may have the same effect as the expanding mass. Brain tumors are especially problematic for the oncologist, because it is usually not possible to make an adequate assessment of the effects of therapy upon the tumor itself (2, 3). Generally it is necessary to rely on an interpretation of the clinical course and neurologic findings, and on survival data. In addition, they are protected from the action of most cytotoxic agents by the so-called blood-brain barrier. The prognosis of the various types of brain tumors depends on the histology, the location of the tumor and the age of the patient. For glioblastoma multiforme, the mean survival from surgery is 24 weeks (2).

A. CHEMOTHERAPY

1. Single-Agent Chemotherapy

Most of the conventional agents have been ineffective (Table 31-1) (4, 5, 24, 32, 34), but most of them have never been studied (24). Alkylating agents do not appear promising. Vincristine was tried in brain tumors because of its affinity for the nervous tissue. An objective response was noted in 57 percent of subjects; in some patients, especially children with medulloblastoma, the response was of long duration (6). Mithramycin appears to have antitumor activity in glioblastoma

Table 31-1. Effectiveness of single agents and combinations in brain tumors

Drug	Number evaluated	Number of responses	Reference
Methotrexate			
intra-arterial	11	4	LIVINGSTON and CARTER (6)
intrathecal	36	23 (64%)	LIVINGSTON and CARTER (6)
Imidazole carboxamide	7	5	TAYLOR et al. (7)
BCNU	23	11 (48%)	WALKER and HURWITZ (8)
	55	28 (51%)	FEWER et al. (9)
CCNU	115	47 (41%)	WASSERMAN (25)
MeCCNU	25	14 (56%)	LEVINE (11)
Procarbazine	44	12 (27%)	WASSERMAN et al. (26)
Cyclophosphamide	14	0	LIVINGSTON and CARTER (6)
Mithramycin	14	3	RANDSOHOFF et al. (12)
	9	5	KENNEDY et al. (13)
	37	14 (38%)	PITTS (14)
Vincristine	56	32 (57%)	LIVINGSTON and CARTER (6)
VM-26	19	12 (63%)	SKLANSKY et al. (15)
BCNU + VCR	19	6 (31%)	FEWER et al. (9)
DIC + CCNU	5	3	TAYLOR et al. (7)
VM-26 + CCNU (sequentially)	20	5 CR 6 PR 4 stabilisations	POUILLART et al. (23)
MTX, CCNU, VCR	15	6	HILDEBRAND et al. (23)
CCNU, PCZ, VCR	30	12 (+ 6 probable responses)	GUTIN et al. (33)

multiforme (12, 13, 14), but as a result of a controlled study by the Brain Tumor Study Group (BTSG) it was concluded that the toxicity of this agent outweighed its potential benefits (5). The less toxic, alternate-day schedule (16), has not been evaluated. One study suggests that dimethyl-triazeno-imidazole-carboxamide has antitumor activity (7). The data on procarbazine, an agent with prominent CNS toxicity, are insufficient (24). The outlook for brain tumor chemotherapy has appeared considerably brighter since the introduction of two classes of agents which are lipid-soluble and cross the blood-brain barrier. With nitrosoureas (BCNU, CCNU, and MeCCNU) complete and partial remissions occur in one-third to one-half of patients with malignant gliomas and survival is prolonged over no therapy (2, 8-11, 24-28). There have been no comparative trials of these three agents, so that it is not known which, if any, is superior to the others. MeCCNU appears to be inferior (27 percent CR plus PR) to BCNU and CCNU (41 percent CR plus PR) (26). Preliminary results of a controlled study by the BTSG indicate that the combination of chemotherapy (BCNU) plus irradiation yields better survival figures than supportive therapy, BCNU alone, or irradiation alone (2). The EORTC Brain Tumor Cooperative Group is studying the effect of CCNU in patients subjected to surgery and radiation therapy (3).

The second class of agents with promise in brain tumors are the podo-phyllotoxin derivatives. VM-26 resulted in objective neurologic improvement in 5 of 13 patients with progressive neurologic findings at the outset, and 7 asymptomatic patients had a median progression-free interval of 15 months or more (15).

Reviewing the results of chemotherapy in glioblastoma multiforme, GOLDSMITH and CARTER conclude that the lipid-soluble agents, including nitrosoureas, epipodophyllotoxin, procarbazine, and dibromodulcitol should receive highest priority (24).

2. Combination Chemotherapy

One does not expect a multitude of reports on combination chemotherapy as there are few effective agents. Vincristine plus mithramycin had no clinical value (17). FEWER, unexpectedly, found that vincristine decreased the response rate obtained with BCNU (25% for the combination versus 53% for BCNU) (9). TAYLOR et al. treated a small number of patients with DIC combined with CCNU or MeCCNU (7). HILDEBRAND et al. obtained an improvement in 6 of 15 patients treated with a combination of CCNU, VCR, and MTX (40% response rate) (29). POUILLART et al., at our institute, have combined VM-26 and CCNU in a cyclic fashion, obtaining a beneficial effect in 15 out of 17 patients (5 CR, 6 PR, 4 stabilization, 2 F) (see p. 154) (23). The combination of CCNU, PCZ, VCR (33) is slightly more effective than BCNU, VCR (35).

3. Regional Chemotherapy

Because of the problems associated with achieving adequate tissue levels of drugs administered systemically, some investigators have resorted to regional chemotherapy (17). Cytotoxic drugs have been injected into brain tumor cysts, intrathecally, or intra-arterially. Although tumor regressions have been recorded with these approaches, we must continue to stress their experimental nature, as we have done in previous sections.

B. STRATEGY

Surgery is generally necessary to establish the diagnosis. Radical removal of the tumor is the treatment of choice, but is rarely feasible since most brain tumors infiltrate widely into vital areas of the surrounding nervous tissue. Less than 20 percent of glioblastomas are suitable for radical resection. In this event it is generally advisable to remove as much of the tumor as is possible and is deemed safe, and to give radiotherapy postoperatively (18, 24, 25, 34). This approach appears to improve the quality and length of survival but offers no hope of a cure. A surgical intervention is also often necessary to relieve intracranial pressure.

Further studies are necessary to determine how or in what sequence the three treatment modalities (surgery, radiotherapy, and chemotherapy) are best combined for the treatment of primary brain tumors (2, 3, 19, 22). EDLAND et al. could not improve the survival of patients treated with adjuvant 5-FU following surgery and radiotherapy (19). The BTSG, in a preliminary report, indicates that the combination of radiotherapy and BCNU prolongs survival beyond that achieved with either method alone (2). Another preliminary report suggests that radiotherapy plus CCNU prolongs the median time before progression but not the median survival time (21).

A randomized trial failed to show a beneficial effect of adjuvant immunotherapy (autoimmunization with irradiated tumor cells) in patients
with supratentorial glioblastomas treated primarily by radical resection and postoperative irradiation (10).

REFERENCES

1. ZIMMERMAN, H.M.: The ten most common types of brain tumor. Semin.
   Roentgenol. 6, 48 (1971).
2. WALKER, M.D.: Nitrosoureas in central nervous system tumors. Cancer
   Chemother. Rep. Part 3, 4, 21 (1973).
3. HILDEBRAND, J., BRIHAYE, J., GOFFIN, J.C., STAQUET, M.: EORTC protocol for the study of CCNU in the treatment of irradiated, operated malignant glioma of the brain. Europ. J. Cancer 9, 459 (1973).
4. WILSON, C.B., HOSHINO, T.: Current trends in the chemotherapy of
   brain tumors with special reference to gliobastomas. J. Neurosurg.
   31, 589 (1969).
5. KENNEDY, B.J.: Chemotherapy of brain tumors. In: Cancer Chemotherapy,
   Vol. 2, p. 221 (eds. I. Brodsky, S.B. Kahn, J.H. Moyer). Philadelphia: Lea and Febiger 1972.
6. LIVINGSTON, R.B., CARTER, S.K.: Single Agents in Cancer Chemotherapy. New York-Washington-London: IFI/Plenum 1970.
7. TAYLOR, S.G., NELSON, L., BAXTER, D., ROSENBAUM, C., SPONZO, R.W.,
   et al.: Treatment of grade III and IV astrocytoma with dimethyl
   triazeno imidazole carboxamide (DTIC, NSC-45388) alone and in combination with CCNU (NSC-79037) or methyl-CCNU (NSC-95441). Cancer
   36, 1269 (1975).
8. WALKER, M.D., HURWITZ, B.S.: BCNU (1,3 bis(2-chloroethyl)-1-nitro-
   sourea; NSC-409962) in the treatment of malignant brain tumors.
   A preliminary report. Cancer Chemother. Rep. 54, 263 (1970).
9. FEWER, D., WILSON, C.B., BOLDREY, E.B., ENOT, K.J., POWELL, M.R.:
   The chemotherapy of brain tumors. Clinical experience with carmustine (BCNU) and vincristine. J. Amer. med. Ass. 222, 549 (1972).
10. FEWER, D., WILSON, C.B., BOLDREY, E.B., ENOT, J.K.: Phase II study
    of 1-(2-chloroethyl)-3-cyclohexyl-1-nitrosourea (CCNU; NSC-79037)
    in the treatment of brain tumors. Cancer Chemother. Rep. 56, 421
    (1972).
11. LEVINE, M.A., WALKER, M.D., WEISS, H.D.: Intravenous methyl-CCNU
    in the treatment of malignant glioma (Phase II). Proc. Amer. Ass.
    clin. Oncol. 15, 167 (1974).
12. RANSOHOFF, J., MARTIN, B.F., MEDREK, T.J., HARRIS, M.N., GOLOMB,
    F.M., WRIGHT, J.C.: Preliminary clinical study of mithramycin
    (NSC-24559) in primary tumors of the central nervous system. Cancer
    Chemother. Rep. 49, 51 (1965).
13. KENNEDY, B.J., BROWN, J.H., YARBRO, J.W.: Mithramycin (NSC-24559)
    therapy for primary glioblastomas. Cancer Chemother. Rep. 48, 59
    (1965).
14. PITTS, N.: Clinical data accumulated by Pfizer for NDA for mithra-
    mycin. Proceedings of the Chemotherapy Conference, November 5,
    1970. Bethesda: Cancer Therapy Evaluation Branch, National Cancer
    Institute 1970.
15. SKLANSKY, B.D., MANN-KAPLAN, R.S., REYNOLDS, Jr., A.E., ROSENBLUM,
    M.L., WALKER, M.D.: 4'-Demethyl-epipodophyllotoxin-β-D-thenylidene-
    glucoside (PTG) in the treatment of malignant intracranial neo-
    plasms. Cancer 33, 460 (1974).
16. KENNEDY, B.J.: Mithramycin therapy in advanced testicular neoplasms.
    Cancer 26, 755 (1970).

17. MEALEY, Jr., J., CHEN, T.T., PEDLOW, E.: Brain tumor chemotherapy with mithramycin and vincristine. Cancer 26, 360 (1970).
18. SIMPSON, W.J.: The treatment of central nervous system tumours by radiation. Mod. med. Canada 25, 9 (1970).
19. EDLAND, R.W., JAVID, M., ANSFIELD, F.J.: Glioblastoma multiforme. An analysis of the results of postoperative radiotherapy alone versus radiotherapy and concomitant 5-fluorouracil. (A prospective randomized study of 32 cases.) Amer. J. Roentgenol. 3, 337 (1971).
20. WALKER, M.D., GEHAN, E.A.: An evaluation of 1-3-bis(2-chloroethyl)-1-nitrosourea (BCNU) and irradiation alone and in combination for the treatment of malignant glioma. Proc. Amer. Ass. Cancer Res. 13, 67 (1972).
21. BAND, P.R., WEIR, B.K.A., URTASUN, P.C., BLAIN, G., McLEAN, D., WILSON, F., MIELKE, B., GRACE, M.: Radiotherapy and CCNU in grade III and IV astrocytoma. Proc. Amer. Ass. Cancer Res. 15, 161 (1974).
22. ARMENTROUT, S.A., FOLTZ, E., VERMUND, H., OTIS, P.T.: Management of malignant glioma with surgery, irradiation, and BCNU. Proc. Amer. Ass. clin. Oncol. 15, 183 (1974).
23. POUILLART, P., SCHWARZENBERG, L., AMIEL, J.L., MATHE, G., et al.: Chimiothérapies sequentielles. III. Application aux tumeurs primitives du système nerveux central. Nouv. Presse méd. 4, 721 (1975).
24. GOLDSMITH, M.A., CARTER, S.K.: Glioblastoma multiforme - a review of therapy. Cancer Treat. Rev. 1, 153 (1974).
25. WASSERMAN, T.H., SLAVIK, M., CARTER, S.K.: Review of CCNU in clinical cancer therapy. Cancer Treat. Rev. 1, 131 (1974).
26. WASSERMAN, T.H., SLAVIK, M., CARTER, S.K.: Methyl-CCNU in clinical cancer therapy. Cancer Treat. Rev. 1, 251 (1974).
27. HOOGSTRATEN, B., GOTTLIEB, J.A., CAOLI, E., TUCKER, W.G., TALLEY, R.W., HAUT, A.: CCNU in the treatment of cancer. Phase II study. Cancer 32, 38 (1973).
28. YOUNG, R.C., WALKER, M.D., CANELLOS, G.P., SCHEIN, P.S., CHABNER, B.A., DeVITA, V.T.: Initial clinical trials with methyl-CCNU 1-(2-chloroethyl)-3-(4-methyl cyclohexyl)-1-nitrosourea. Cancer 31, 1164 (1973).
29. HILDEBRAND, J., BRIHAYE, J., WAGENKNECHT, L., MICHEL, J., KENIS, Y.: Combination chemotherapy with 1-(2-chloroethyl-3-cyclohexyl-1-nitrosourea) (CCNU), vincristine and methotrexate in primary and metastatic brain tumors. A preliminary report. Europ. J. Cancer 9, 627 (1973).
30. BLOOM, H.J.G.: Combined modality therapy for intracranial tumors. Cancer 35, 111 (1975).
31. VASANTHA KUMAR, A.R., RENAUDIN, J., WILSON, C.B. et al.: Procarbazine didrochloride in the treatment of brain tumors-Phase II study. J. Neurosurg. 40, 365 (1974).
32. SHAPIRO, W.R.: Chemotherapy of primary malignant brain tumors in children. Cancer 32, 965 (1975).
33. GUTIN, P.H., WILSON, C.B., VANSANTHA, A.R., BOLDREY, E.B., LEVIN, V., et al.: Phase II study of procarbazine, CCNU, and vincristine combination chemotherapy in the treatment of malignant brain tumors. Cancer 36, 1398 (1975).
34. WILSON, C.B. (guest editor): Brain tumors. Semin. Oncol. 2, 1-80 (1975).
35. LEVIN, V.A., CRAFTS, D.C., WILSON, C.B., SCHULTZ, M.J., BOLDREY, E.B., et al.: BCNU (NSC-409962) and procarbazine (NSC-77213) treatment for malignant brain tumors. Cancer Treat. Rep. 60, 243 (1976).

Chapter 32
Tumors of Infancy and Childhood

RETINOBLASTOMA

Retinoblastoma is a tumor of the eye found virtually only in children.
The tumor is sometimes present at birth. About 90% of retinoblastomas
become manifest in children under the age of 3. Bilateral involvement
is seen in 25% but the eyes are not necessarily affected simultaneously.
It sometimes occurs as a hereditary form, transmitted as an autosomal
dominant trait, whereby about half the offspring of affected patients
develop the disease. The tumor extends readily within the eye, seeding
itself throughout the interior, even including the iris and anterior
chamber. Direct extension to the brain along the optic nerve is not
uncommon. There are also distant metastases through hematogenous spread
in some cases.

If untreated it is almost invariably fatal. When diagnosed early and
treated properly up to 85% of cases can be cured.

A. Strategy

Biopsy of intraocular tumor is not practical and has led to dangerous
spread and orbital involvement. Enucleation is the treatment of choice
for unilateral disease. As much of the optic nerve as possible is removed along with the eye. If histologic examination of the cut end of
the optic nerve reveals tumor, prophylactic irradiation of the intracranial portion of the optic nerve and chiasma is recommended. Cytologic
examination of the spinal fluid can be used to evaluate spread to the
meningeal spaces.

In the event of bilateral involvement, the more severely affected eye
is enucleated. A combination of radiotherapy and chemotherapy is used
in an attempt to control the disease in the other eye, while preserving
some useful vision. REESE used triethylmelamine (TEM) (1); however, it
has not been demonstrated that this agent is superior to other alkylating agents. HAGGARD reported 5 regressions, of short duration, in 9
patients treated with cyclophosphamide (2). Similar results have been
obtained with vincristine (3).

NEUROBLASTOMA

Neuroblastomas are derived from neural-crest tissue and originate in
the adrenal gland or sympathetic ganglions of the cervical, posterior

mediastinal, retroperitoneal, and abdominal regions (4-8, 40, 41, 42).
The majority are found in the adrenal gland and retroperitoneal area.
They are the second most common solid tumors in children. The peak
incidence occurs within the first three years of life.

Two basic histologic types can be distinguished, neuroblastoma which
is more malignant, and ganglioneuroblastoma, which is more highly differentiated. Many of these tumors synthesize catecholamines. These substances and their metabolites can be found in the urine and help to
establish the diagnosis and monitor the response to therapy (9).

Neuroblastomas tend to break through their capsules and are locally
invasive. Hematogenous dissemination occurs relatively early in the
course of the disease; 70% of children already have metastases,
especially in bones and liver, at the time of diagnosis and are thus
beyond cure by surgery and radiotherapy alone. Several staging systems
have been proposed. The scheme suggested by the Children's Cancer Study
Group A (CCSGA) is reproduced in Table 32-1 (10).

Table 32-1. Staging of neuroblastoma. (From EVANS et al. (10))

Stage	I	Tumor confined to the organ or structure of origin
Stage	II	Tumors extending in continuity beyond the organ or structure of origin but not crossing the midline. Regional lymph nodes on the homolateral side may be involved
Stage	III	Tumors extending in continuity beyond the midline. Regional lymph nodes may be involved bilaterally
Stage	IV	Remote disease involving skeleton, organs, soft tissues, or distant lymph node groups, etc. (See IV-S.)
Stage	IV-S	Patients who would otherwise be Stage I or II, but who have remote disease confined to one or more of the following sites: liver, skin, or bone marrow (without radiographic evidence of bone metastases on complete skeletal survey)

It has been recognized that neuroblastoma can have an unpredictable
course, including spontaneous regressions or maturation to a ganglio-
neuroma.

A number of variables influence the outcome (40, 42, 43). Patients
under 2 years of age have a more favorable prognosis than older children and girls have a better survival than boys (43). The site of the
origin has an effect on survival, the best results having been reported
for mediastinal tumors. As with almost all tumors, the degree of differentiation and the extent of the disease are the most important features of prognosis. However, there is one group of children with disseminated neuroblastoma in whom prognosis is surprisingly good (Stage IV-S,
Table 32-1) (11). Finally, the outcome is more favorable when there is
evidence of immune reactivity.

A. CHEMOTHERAPY

Alkylating agents are the substances that have been used most frequently, especially cyclophosphamide (CPM), with approximately one- to two-thirds of patients responding (12, 44). About one-third patients respond to vincristine (VCR). Antimetabolites, actinomycin D (ACD), and cortico-steroids have been of no value (8, 44).

Inconsistent results have been reported for daunorubicin (DRB) (Table 32-2) (13-15). Adriamycin (ADM) is also effective (16, 45). Thus far we have no data on nitrosoureas. Most combination studies so far have combined the two active single agents, CPM and VCR, with an overall response rate of 50 percent (Table 32-3) (17-20, 44). The addition of daunorubicin to this combination did not improve cure rates but did increase survival time (21). A four-drug sequential combination (CPM, ACD, ADM, VCR) was not superior to the three-drug regimen (46). Res-ponders (59 percent) to a combination of CPM, ADM, and VCR enjoyed a significantly increased survival rate (17.5 months) compared with that of non-responders (5 months) (47). The SWCCG is comparing a combination of prednisone, ACD, CPM, VCR, and DRB with the dual combination of CPM and VCR. They reported 7 responses in 16 patients treated with a combi-nation of ADM plus DIC (48). The CCSGA is studying the combination of CPM and VCR with and without cytosine arabinoside. The same group has

Table 32-2. Effectiveness of single agents in neuroblastoma

Drug	Number evaluated	Responses	Reference
Procarbazine	3	1/ 3	LIVINGSTON and CARTER (12)
Chlorambucil	10	2/10	LIVINGSTON and CARTER (12)
Cyclophosphamide	78	67%	LIVINGSTON AND CARTER (12)
Daunorubicin	15	40%	TAN et al. (13)
	29	10%	SUTOW et al. (14)
	43	7%	SAMUELS et al. (15)
Adriamycin	71	30%	BLUM (16)
Vincristine	71	40%	LIVINGSTON and CARTER (12)

Table 32-3. Response rates to combinations in neuroblastoma

Combination	Number evaluated	Number of responses	Reference
CPM, VCR	14	11	PRATT et al., 1968 (18)
	28	9	EVANS et al., 1969 (19)
	48	26	SAWITSKY et al., 1970 (20)
	11	5	STARLING et al., 1974 (44)
CPM, ADM	28	23 (86%)	GREEN et al., 1976 (17)
DIC, ADM	16	7	CANGIR et al., 1975 (48)
	18	2 (PR)	LEIKIN et al., 1975 (54)
CPM, DRB, VCR	20	60%	HELSON et al., 1972 (21)
CPM, ADM, VCR	19	59%	GASPARINI et al., 1974 (47)
DIC, CPM, VCR	26	73%	FINKLESTEIN et al., 1974 (22)
CPM, ACD, ADM, VCR	10	5	HELSON 1974 (21)

reported a 73 percent total response rate with a combination of CPM, VCR, and imidazole carboxamide (22). GREEN et al. (17) obtained 86% regressions with CPM, ADM.

B. STRATEGY

1. Localized Neuroblastoma

Surgical removal of the entire tumor offers the best hope of a cure (40, 41). However, it appears that for tumors that cannot be completely resected it is still advisable to remove as much of the lesion as is technically feasible, irrespective of local invasion. Incomplete resection of the bulk of the tumor has been shown to be more beneficial than mere biopsy.

Neuroblastomas are very radiosensitive, and postoperative radiotherapy applied to the tumor bed and regional lymph nodes or residual tumor is recommended. Some authors are of the opinion that postoperative radiotherapy is not necessary if the surgeon is certain that the primary tumor has been completely removed (5, 41), especially in children under the age of one year. Preoperative radiotherapy is indicated if the tumor is massive, and is followed by surgical excision of the remaining tumor tissue.

Because of the high incidence of hematogenous dissemination, many authorities recommend adjuvant chemotherapy. Its value is under study by the CCSGA. Following curative local measures, patients with localized or regional disease (Stage I, II and III) are selected by random choice to receive either no further therapy or cyclophosphamide maintenance (10 mg/kg p.o., 10-day courses every month for 12 months) (5).

The value of immunotherapy is also being investigated (23). In-vitro studies have shown that there are cellular and humoral immune responses to neuroblastoma. It is possible that spontaneous regressions of neuroblastoma are the result of this type of reaction and that immunity can be increased by immunotherapy applied after the number of cells has been reduced by other forms of treatment.

2. Disseminated Neuroblastoma

Patients who present with disseminated disease are treated with chemotherapy, with or without irradiation of local tumor masses (5 - 8, 42). Surgical resection can be considered at a later date if only local residual tumor persists following chemoradiotherapy.

WILMS' TUMOR

Wilms' tumor (embryonal sarcoma of the kidney) is a common tumor of infancy and childhood, with a peak incidence at age 3-4 years (5-7, 24-28, 49, 50). It is usually diagnosed before the age of 5 and is sometimes present at birth. Patients with congenital anomalies such as hemihypertrophy, aniridia, hypospadias, cryptorchidism, and pigmented nevi seem to be at higher risk, as are their siblings and identical twins (24). The tumor affects both kidneys in 3-10%, in two-thirds of cases simultaneously, while in the remaining one-third the contralateral kidney becomes involved within 3-10 years (29). It is not known whether bilateral involvement is the result of a multifocal origin or rather of a metastatic process.

The term "Wilms' tumor" refers to a spectrum of renal embryomas of the adenosarcomatous type. The varied histologic picture is in keeping with the concept that it arises from embryonic tissue not definitely committed to any one mode of differentiation. The "mesoblastic nephroma of infancy" has been segregated from this heterogenous group as a histologically distinct tumor with a characteristic clinical course. Although this tumor can attain a huge size and extend locally, it does not tend to metastasize and can be cured by surgery alone.

Table 32-4. Staging of Wilms' tumor (National Wilms' Tumor Study (24))

Stage	I	Tumor limited to kidney and completely resected
Stage	II	Tumor extends beyond kidney but is completely resected (includes penetration beyond pseudocapsule, periaortic lymph node involvement and infiltration of renal vessels or tumor thrombi in vessels when there is no residual beyond margin of resection)
Stage	III	Residual nonhematogenous tumor confined to abdomen, inclu-including:
		1. Tumor biopsy; tumor rupture before or during surgery
		2. Peritoneal implants
		3. Lymph node involvement beyond the periaortic chain
		4. Incomplete resection due to local infiltration of vital structures
Stage	IV	Hematogenous metastases (lung, liver, bone, brain)
Stage	V	Bilateral involvement either initially or subsequently

Locally, Wilms' tumor invades the adjacent tissues and it has a marked tendency to venous invasion, which explains the frequency of pulmonary metastases (27). Approximately 20% of patients have evidence of distant metastases at the time of diagnosis.

The National Wilms' Tumor Study (NWST) has proposed a staging system based on clinical, surgical and histologic findings (Table 32-4) (24).

The extent of the disease (stage) is the major determinant of the outcome. Invasion of the renal capsule, the renal vein, or regional lymph nodes and distant metastases all have an adverse effect on prognosis (26). The influence of age is less definite, some authors, but not all, reporting better results in younger patients (under 2 years) (26-28). It is generally accepted that if a child remains free of evidence of disease for two years after therapy, he is very probably cured.

A. CHEMOTHERAPY

Several classes of agents are effective in disseminated Wilms' tumor. In 1955 FARBER (30) pioneered in the use of actinomycin D (ACD), and its effectiveness has since been amply demonstrated, both in disseminated disease and as an adjuvant (Table 32-5) (31-33). Impressive results have been obtained with vincristine (VCR) (12, 34). A comparison of these two drugs and combinations of both is now in progress (23, 34). Cyclophosphamide appears to be less active (12, 35). Among the newer agents adriamycin (ADM) holds promise (16, 45) and can be used in patients who have become refractory to ACD and VCR. TAN et al. are evaluating a combination of ACD, ADM, and CPM (multidisciplinary protocol T 2) in a variety of solid tumors in children, including Wilms' tumor (51).

B. STRATEGY

For no other solid tumor have surgery, radiotherapy, and chemotherapy been more integrated in an attempt to destroy the total tumor-cell population (24-28, 49, 50, 52). This combined approach has considerably improved the cure rate and this justifies the pursuit of vigorous treatment.

1. Localized Wilms' Tumor

The primary treatment consists of surgery to establish the diagnosis, to stage the disease, and to remove the tumor. Because of the risk of tumor emboli, manipulation of the tumor is avoided until after ligation of the renal vein. The opposite kidney is carefully inspected as well as the liver, spleen, lymph nodes, and other abdominal organs. When possible all tumor is removed. This may involve the resection of contiguous organs. Great care should be exercised to avoid tumor spillage at surgery. Clips are placed at appropriate points to outline the tumor bed or residual tumor.

Postoperative radiotherapy applied to the entire renal bed or a larger field, depending on the operative findings, is usually initiated within 24 hours of laparotomy. It has been recommended that the entire abdomen be treated if tumor spill has occurred before or during surgery (27, 28). Some authors question the need for routine postoperative radiotherapy for patients with well-encapsulated, localized lesions (Stage I) which have been completely excised. This problem is under study in a prospective trial by the NWTS (25). A preliminary report shows in fact that the 2-year disease-free rate is equally good (80%) in Stage-I patients (tumor confined to kidney) irrespective of whether or not they have received postoperative flank radiotherapy (36). Both groups received ACD for 15 months.

Chemotherapy is also initiated at the time of laparotomy. Actinomycin D is given daily for 5-7 days (10-15 µg/kg). A co-operative study has shown that intermittent maintenance with ACD is more effective than a single course given in addition to surgery and radiotherapy (37). Eighty-six percent of patients who received maintenance therapy had no recurrence, as against 48% in the group without maintenance ACD. In this study ACD was given for five consecutive days (15 µg/kg); patients on maintenance were given the same course at six weeks and three months after the operation and every three months thereafter for the first 15 months of the postoperative period. A more recent analysis of these same patients indicated that the beneficial effect of maintenance therapy with ACD is not sustained as far as survival is concerned but the disease-free remission is prolonged (53). However, the occurrence of fewer relapses in the patients given maintenance therapy (ACD), requiring less control measures (additional surgery, radiotherapy, or chemotherapy) for recurrent tumor allowed a lower morbidity from the disease and its treatment. Vincristine appears be equally effective as an ad-

Table 32-5. Effectiveness of single agents in Wilms' tumor

Drug	Number evaluated	Responses (%)	Reference
Cyclophosphamide	45	27	LIVINGSTON and CARTER (12)
Actinomycin D	26	39	LIVINGSTON and CARTER (12)
Adriamycin	40	65	BLUM (16)
Vincristine	31	74	LIVINGSTON and CARTER (12)

juvant (38, 39). The NWTS is now comparing the value of ACD, VCR, and the combination of ACD and VCR as adjuvant to surgery and radiotherapy in Stages II and III of the disease (25). A similar study is in progress in Great Britain (23). Early results obtained in the NTWS study suggest that the 2-year disease-free rate is better for the combination (79%) than for ACD (50%) or VCR (44%) alone (36).

Preoperative radiotherapy, chemotherapy, and combinations of the two have been used for very large tumors. Several authors have stressed the need to establish the diagnosis first (25, 26). Vincristine is recommended in preference to ACD for preoperative use, because of its lack of myelotoxicity (25, 36).

2. Disseminated Wilms' Tumor

A vigorous attack with a combination of treatment modalities is indicated even when the disease appears to be hopelessly disseminated. Cures can still be achieved (up to 50%) (25), and this must be the objective of therapy. Treatment should be individually selected in each case. All patients are given chemotherapy. Radiotherapy is sometimes prescribed in addition, in an attempt to cure metastatic disease. Lungs, liver and other metastatic foci have been irradiated (26-28). Hemihepatectomy, thoracotomy, etc. can also be carried out for surgical excision of localized and accessible metastatic foci.

Several studies have shown that the results are distinctly better when the combined treatment is carried out mainly in a specialized cancer center, where this multidisciplinary approach is most feasible (27, 28, 30). Eighty percent of children can be expected to survive when modern techniques of surgery, radiotherapy, and chemotherapy are employed by well-coordinated, experienced groups of clinicians.

REFERENCES

1. REESE, A.B., HYMAN, G.A., TAPLEY, N. du V., FORREST, A.W.: The treatment of retinoblastoma by X-ray and triethylene melamine. Arch. Ophthal. 60, 897 (1958).
2. HAGGARD, M.W.: Cyclophosphamide (NSC-26271) in the treatment of children with malignant neoplasms. Cancer Chemother. Rep. 51, 403 (1967).
3. SELAWRY, O.S., HOLLAND, J.F., WOLMAN, I.J.: Effect of vincristine (NSC-67574) on malignant solid tumors in children. Cancer Chemother. Rep. 52, 497 (1968).

4. EVERETT KOOP, C.: Solid tumors of children - neuroblastoma. In: Oncology 1970, Vol. 4, p. 377 (eds. R.L. Clark, R.W. cumley, J.E. McCay, M.M. Copeland). Chicago: Year Book Medical Publisher 1971.
5. EVANS, A.E.: Refinements in the treatment of children with solid tumors. In: Cancer Chemotherapy, Vol. 2, p. 181 (eds. I. Brodsky, S.B. Kahn, J.H. Moyer) New York: Grune & Stratton 1972.
6. LAWHORN, T.I., STONE, H.H., MARTIN, Jr., J.D.: Chemotherapy in solid tumors of childhood. Oncology 26, 250 (1972).
7. SUTOW, W.W.: Considerations in the management of solid tumors in children. Cancer Bull. 24, 17 (1972).
8. EVANS, A.E.: Treatment of neuroblastoma. Cancer 30, 1595 (1972).
9. LIEBNER, E.J., ROSENTHAL, I.M.: Serial catecholamines in the radiation management of children with neuroblastoma. Cancer 32, 632 (1973).
10. EVANS, A.E., D'ANGIO, G.J., RANDOLPH, J.: A proposed staging for children with neuroblastoma. Children's cancer study group A. Cancer 27, 374 (1971).
11. D'ANGIO, G.J., EVANS, A.E., KOOP, C.E.: Special pattern of widespread neuroblastoma with a favorable prognosis. Lancet 1, 1046 (1971).
12. LIVINGSTON, R.B., CARTER, S.K.: Single Agents in Cancer Chemotherapy. New York-Washington-London: IFI/Plenum 1970.
13. TAN, C., TASAKA, H., YU, K.P., MURPHY, L.M., KARNOFSKY, D.A.: Daunomycin, an antitumor antibiotic, in the treatment of neoplastic disease. Clinical evaluation with special reference to childhood leukemia. Cancer 20, 333 (1967).
14. SUTOW, W.W., FERNBACH, D.J., THURMAN, W.G., HOLTON, C.P., WATKINS, W.L.: Daunomycin (NSC-92151) in the treatment of metastatic neuroblastoma. Cancer Chemother. Rep. 54, 283 (1970).
15. SAMUELS, L.D., NEWTON, Jr., W.A., HEYN, R.: Daunorubicin therapy in advanced neuroblastoma. Cancer 27, 831 (1971).
16. BLUM, R.H.: An overview of studies with adriamycin (NSC-123127) in the United States. Cancer Chemother. Rep. Part 3, 6, 247 (1975).
17. GREEN, A.A., HUSTU, H.O., KUMAR, M.: The response of neuroblastoma to sequential low-dose cyclophosphamide and adriamycin therapy. Proc. Amer. Ass. Cancer Res. 17, 120 (1976).
18. PRATT, C.B., JAMES, Jr., D.H., HOLTON, C.P., PINKEL, D.: Combination chemotherapy including vincristine in the management of childhood malignant solid tumors. Cancer Chemother. Rep. 52, 489 (1968).
19. EVANS, A.E., HEYN, R.M., NEWTON, Jr., W.A., LEIKIN, S.L.: Vincristine sulfate and cyclophosphamide for children with metastatic neuroblastoma. J. Amer. med. Ass. 207, 1325 (1969).
20. SAWITSKY, A., DESPOSITO, F., et al.: Vincristine and cyclophosphamide therapy in generalized neuroblastoma; a collaborative study. Amer. J. Dis. Childh. 119, 308 (1970).
21. HELSON, L., VANICHAYANGKUL, P., TAN, C.C., WOLLNER, N., MURPHY, M.L.: Combination intermittent chemotherapy for patients with disseminated neuroblastoma. Cancer Chemother. Rep. 56, 499 (1972).
22. FINKLESTEIN, J.Z., LEIKIN, S., EVANS, A., KLEMPERER, M., BERNSTEIN, I., HITTLE, R., HAMMOND, G.D.: Combination chemotherapy for metastatic neuroblastoma. Proc. Amer. Ass. Cancer Res. 15, 44 (1974).
23. EDITORIAL: Nephroblastoma and neuroblastoma in children. Brit. med. J. 1, 304 (1971).
24. SULLIVAN, M.P.: Wilms' tumor. Oncology 1970, Vol. 4, p. 370. Chicago: Year Book Medical Publishers 1970.
25. D'ANGIO, G.T.: Management of children with Wilms' tumor. Cancer 30, 1528 (1972).
26. PEREZ, C.A., KAIMAN, H.A., KEITH, J., MILL, W.B., VIETTI, T.J., POWERS, W.E.: Treatment of Wilms' tumor and factors affecting prognosis. Cancer 32, 609 (1973).

27. CASSADY, J.R., TEFFT, M., FILLER, R.M., JAFFE, N., PAED, D., HELL-MAN, S.: Considerations in the radiation therapy of Wilms' tumor. Cancer 32, 598 (1973).
28. MARGOLIS, L.W., SMITH, W.B., WARA, W.M., KUSHNER, J.H., DeLORIMIER, A.A.: Wilms' tumor - an interdisciplinary treatment program with and without dactinomycin. Cancer 32, 618 (1973).
29. RAGAB, A.H., VIETTI, T.J., CRIST, W., PEREZ, C., McALLISTER, W.: Bilateral Wilms' tumor. Cancer 30, 983 (1972).
30. FARBER, S.: Chemotherapy in the treatment of leukemia and Wilms' tumor. J. Amer. med. Ass. 198, 826 (1966).
31. HOWARD, R.: Actinomycin D in Wilms' tumor treatment of lung metastases. Arch. Dis. Childh. 40, 200 (1965).
32. FERNBACH, D.J., MARTYN, D.T.: Role of dactinomycin in the improved survival of children with Wilms' tumor. J. Amer. med. Ass. 195, 1005 (1966).
33. BURGERT, Jr., E.O., GLIDEWELL, O.: Dactinomycin in Wilms' tumor. J. Amer. med. Ass. 199, 464 (1967).
34. SULLIVAN, M.P.: Vincristine (NSC-67574) therapy for Wilms' tumor. Cancer Chemother. Rep. 52, 481 (1968).
35. SUTOW, W.W.: Cyclophosphamide (NSC-26271) in Wilms' tumor and rhabdomyosarcoma. Cancer Chemother. Rep. 51, 407 (1967).
36. D'ANGIO, G., BECKWITH, J.B., BISHOP, H., BRESLOW, N., FEIGL, P., EVANS, A., GOODWIN, W., PICKETT, L., SINKS, L., SUTOW, W., TEFFT, M., WOLFF, J.: The national Wilms' tumor study (NWST): preliminary results. Proc. Amer. Ass. Cancer Res. 15, 68 (1974).
37. WOLFF, J.A., KRIVIT, W., NEWTON, Jr., W.A., D'ANGIO, G.J.: Single versus multiple dose dactinomycin therapy of Wilms' tumor. New Engl. J. Med. 279, 290 (1968).
38. VIETTI, T.J., SULLIVAN, M.P., HAGGARD, M.E., HOLCOMB, T.M., BERRY, D.H.: Vincristine sulfate and radiation therapy in metastatic Wilms' tumor. Cancer 25, 12, (1970).
39. SCHWEISGUTH, O., TARIS, N., LEMERLE, J., TCHERNIA, G.: Action de la vincristine dans les néphroblastomes. Bull. Cancer 57, 93 (1970).
40. GERSON, J.M., KOOP, C.E.: Neuroblastoma. Semin. Oncol. 1, 35 (1974).
41. KOOP, C.E., SCHAUFNER, L.: The management of abdominal neuroblastoma. Cancer 35, 905 (1975).
42. JAFFE, N.: Neuroblastoma: Review of the literature and an examination of factors contributing to its enigmatic character. Cancer Treat. Rev. 3, 61 (1976).
43. KINNIER WILSON, L.M., DRAPER, G.J.: Neuroblastoma, its natural history and prognosis: a study of 487 cases. Brit. med. J. 3, 301 (1974).
44. STARLING, K.A., SUTOW, W.W., DONALDSON, M.H., LAND, V.J., LANE, D.M.: Drug trials in neuroblastoma: cyclophosphamide alone; vincristine plus cyclophosphamide; 6-mercaptopurine plus 6-methylmercaptopurine riboside; and cytosine arabinoside alone. Cancer Chemother. Rep. Part 1, 58, 683 (1974).
45. RAGAB, A.H., SUTOW, W.W., KOMP, D.M., STARLING, K.A., LYON, G.M.: Adriamycin in the treatment of childhood acute leukemia and solid tumors. Proc. Am. Soc. Clin. Oncol. 16, 228 (1975).
46. HELSON, L., DENOIX, L.: Four drug sequential chemotherapy for metastatic neuroblastoma. Europ. J. Cancer 9, 883 (1973).
47. GASPARANI, M., BELLANI, F.F., MUSUMECI, R., BONADONNA, G.: Response and survival of patients with metastatic neuroblastoma after combination chemotherapy with adriamycin, cyclophosphamide, and vincristine. Cancer Chemother. Rep. Part 1, 58, 365 (1974).
48. CANGIR, A., LAND, V., STARLING, K.A., NITSCHKE, R., HOWE, C.D.: Combination chemotherapy with dimethyl triazeno imidazole carboxamide and adriamycin in children with metastatic solid tumors. Proc. Am. Soc. Clin. Oncol. 16, 240 (1975).
49. ROSENSTOCK, J.G., BISHOP, H.C.: Wilms' tumor and its treatment. Semin. Oncol. 1, 27 (1974).

50. WOLFF, J.A: Advances in the treatment of Wilms' tumor. Cancer <u>35</u>, 901 (1975).
51. TAN, C., GILLADOGA, A., GHAVIMI, F., HAGHBIN, M., WOLLNER, N., HELSON, L., MURPHY, M.L.: Adriamycin alone and in combination in the treatment of childhood neoplastic diseases. In: Adriamycin Review, EORTC international symposium, p. 175 (eds. M. Staquet, H, Tagnon, Y. Kenis et al.) Ghent: European Press Medikon 1975
52. BENJAMIN, J.T., JOHNSON, W.D., McMILLAN, C.W.: The management of Wilms' tumor: a comparison of two regimens. Cancer <u>34</u>, 1233 (1974).
53. WOLFF, J.A., D'ANGIO, G.J., HARTMANN, J., KRIVIT, W., NEWTON, Jr., W.A.: Long-term evaluation of single versus multiple courses of actinomycin-D therapy of Wilms' tumor. New Engl. J. Med. <u>290</u>, 84 (1974).
54. LEIKIN, S., et al.: Use of combination adriamycin (NSC-123127) and DTIC (NSC-45388) in children with advanced stage IV neuroblastoma. Cancer Chemother. Rep. Part 1, <u>59</u>, 1015 (1975).

Chapter 33
Osteogenic Sarcoma, Ewing's Sarcoma, Soft-Tissue Sarcoma

A. OSTEOGENIC SARCOMA

Osteosarcomas are the commonest of the bone tumors; males are more frequently affected than females and the peak incidence is in the second
decade. The metaphyseal region of the long bones is the commonest site,
the distal end of the femur and the proximal end of the humerus being
most affected. The histologic picture shows dense connective and osteoid
tissue. It used to be generally thought that these tumors spread far
into the marrow cavity, a feature to be reckoned with during therapy.
LEWIS et al., however, failed on pathologic examination of 20 amputation specimens to find any unappreciated tumor extension or skip areas
in the marrow cavity (1). Dissemination is mainly hematogenous, with
predominant involvement of the lungs and other bones. It occurs early,
most often by the time of diagnosis or within 6 months. The majority
of patients die within 2 years of diagnosis of pulmonary metastatic
disease. The best obtainable 5-year survival rates are about 20%.

1. Chemotherapy

Osteosarcoma has proved resistant to most cytotoxic agents (Table 33-1).
Response rates for agents that have been tried in at least 10 patients
are approximately 15% for cyclophosphamide (CPM) or melphalan, and 23%
for mitomycin C (MTC). No regressions were registered for vincristine
or uracil mustard. For only two drugs have regressions been noted in
more than one-quarter of patients: adriamycin (ADM) (27.5%) (3, 62) and
high-dose MTX with folinic acid rescue (4/10, i.e., 40%) (2, 63).

GOTTLIEB et al. (3) obtained 44% responses with the combination of ADM
and imidazole carboxamide (DIC) (Table 33-2)) and the duration of response was considerably longer than with ADM alone. ROSEN et al. used
adriamycin and high-dose MTX-FA in sequence in repeated cycles and obtained 7 objective tumor regressions in 13 patients (7). More recently,
ROSEN et al. (9) and WILBUR et al. (10) have combined MTX-FA, CPM, ADM,
and VCR.

2. Strategy

The management of both localized and disseminated disease has been unsatisfactory. Recent advances in chemotherapy promise significant
improvement in the overall management of the disease.

The treatment of choice for apparently localized disease has not been
defined. Some workers advocate immediate amputation or radical local
excision for tumors not in the extremities, while others propose radio-

Table 33-1. Effectiveness of single agents in osteogenic sarcoma

Drug	Number evaluated	Number of responses	Reference
Methotrexate and FA rescue	10	4	JAFFE (2)
Imidazole carboxamide (DIC)	6[a]	1	GOTTLIEB et al. (3)
5-Fluorouracil	2	1	GROESBECK and CUDMORE (72)
Hydroxyurea	5	O	SUTOW et al. (4)
Cyclophosphamide	28[a]	4 (14%)	JAFFE (2)
Melphalan	32[a]	5 (15.5%)	JAFFE (2)
Uracil mustard	10	O	SUTOW et al. (4)
Mitomycin C	22[a]	6 (28%)	LIVINGSTON and CARTER (5)
Daunorubicin	2	O	SUTOW et al. (4)
Adriamycin	35[a]	10 (27.5%)	GOTTLIEB et al. (3)
Vincristine	7	O	SUTOW et al. (4)
	4	O	SELAWRY et al. (6)

[a] Results of several studies combined.

Table 33-2. Response to combinations in osteogenic sarcoma

Combination	Number evaluated	Number of responses	Reference
DIC, ADM	18	8	GOTTLIEB et al. (3) 1972
	31	13	GOTTLIEB (70) 1974
MTX-FA, ADM	13	7	ROSEN et al. (7) 1974
DIC, ADM, VCR	5	1	GOTTLIEB et al. (70) 1974
MPH, MTC, VCR	10	1	JAFFE et al. (8) 1971
MTX-FA, CPM, ADM, VCR	9	7	ROSEN et al. (9) 1975
MTX-FA, CPM, ADM, VCR	8	3	WILBUR et al. (10) 1974

therapy followed by a waiting period of several months and delayed surgery in patients who have not developed metastases during the period
of observation. Both approaches have their advocates (11-14, 64, 66,
76, 77). It appears that radical radiotherapy cannot offer long-term
control of the primary tumor (as in Ewing's sarcoma) (14). The majority
of patients develop local recurrences within 3-4 months, with considerable morbidity (14). Immediate surgery is therefore generally recommended nowadays.

Mutilating surgery is necessary in most patients for control of the
local disease, and even more frustrating is the fact that the majority
of patients subjected to these operations develop metastases while they
are still trying to adapt to their amputation. Obviously survival rates
will not improve until effective adjuvant therapy (chemotherapy or immunotherapy) becomes available to prevent subsequent clinical metas-

tases (78). Preliminary reports with adjuvant chemotherapy are encouraging. It appears to be able to modify the natural course of the malignant tumor by eradicating microfoci of metastatic disease. CORTES et al. use adriamycin (15, 68), JAFFE et al. use MTX-FA (16), PRATT et al. use MTX-FA, CPM, and DRB (17), ROSEN et al. (9) and WILBUR et al. (10) give MTX-FA, CPM, ADM, and VCR, while SUTOW et al. have been investigating 4- and 5-drug combinations: CPM, VCR, MPH, ADM, +/- MTX-FA (18).

Chemotherapy has been disappointing in disseminated disease until recently. Recent reports with the combination of ADM and DIC and high-dose MTX-FA +/- ADM and three- and four-drug combinations are promising (2, 3, 7, 9, 64). A surgical attack on pulmonary metastases has been advocated in selected cases (19, 65, 68, 70, 71). It is obvious that for both localized and disseminated osteogenic sarcoma a multidisciplinary approach is necessary.

B. EWING'S SARCOMA

Ewing's sarcoma is a highly malignant primary tumor of the bone. Ninety-five percent are seen in people aged 4-25 years. Males are affected twice as often as females. The majority of tumors (75%) occur in the pelvic girdle and long tubular bones of the extremities, but almost any bone can be involved.

The histogenesis of the tumor remains an enigma, but it is generally thought of as a specific disease entity (20). The endothelial origin, suggested by Ewing, is a matter of controversy. The tumor is composed of highly anaplastic, small, round cells. It originates in the medulla and spreads locally in the marrow cavity, bone, and soft tissues. The bone is involved much more extensively than can be suspected on the grounds of clinical or radiologic evaluation. Hematogenous spread takes place early in the course. Some 20% of patients already have evident metastases at the time of diagnosis, while 70% of those presenting with apparently localized disease develop dissemination within 12 months. Metastases occur predominantly in lungs and other bones. Lymphangitic spread is less common (20%).

The 5-year survival taken from several series is about 10%. Eighty-five percent of patients die within two years (21). Survival is better in patients presenting with localized disease, with involvement of long bones (extremities), with increasing age at diagnosis and absence of systemic symptoms (22, 73).

1. Chemotherapy

Several agents are useful in disseminated disease. Tumor regressions have been reported most frequently with cyclophosphamide (CPM) (4, 24), actinomycin D (ACD) (25) and vincristine (VCR) (4, 6) of the conventional agents (Table 33-3). Among the newer agents, BCNU (4, 23), daunorubicin (DRB) (4, 27) and, especially, adriamycin (ADM) (3, 28) deserve further trials.

Cyclophosphamide and vincristine with or without actinomycin D have been used in various schedules to treat disseminated disease or as long-term adjuvant therapy for localized Ewing's sarcoma (29 – 33, 67).

Most reports involve small numbers of patients since Ewing's sarcoma is a relatively uncommon tumor.

Table 33-3. Effectiveness of single agents in Ewing's sarcoma

Drugs	Number evaluated	Number of responses	References
Imidazole carboxamide (DIC)	2	0	GOTTLIEB et al. (3)
5-Fluorouracil	5[a]	3	LIVINGSTON and CARTER (5)
BCNU	5	0	SUTOW et al. (4)
	12	5	PALMA et al. (23)
Cyclophosphamide	21[a]	13 (61%)	LIVINGSTON and CARTER (5)
Melphalan	3	0	SUTOW et al. (4)
	5	0	SAMUELS and HOWE (24)
Uracil mustard	12	1	SUTOW et al. (4)
Actinomycin D	9	3	SENYSZYN et al. (25)
Mithramycin	5	2	KOFMAN et al. (26)
Daunorubicin	9	4	SUTOW et al. (4)
	3	0	TAN et al. (27)
Adriamycin	11	6	OLDHAM and POMEROY (28)
	20[a]	12 (60%)	GOTTLIEB et al. (3)
Vincristine	8[a]	4	LIVINGSTON and CARTER (5)

[a] Results of several studies combined.

2. Strategy

(i) Localized Ewing's Sarcoma

Since the primary lesion can be controlled as well by radiotherapy as by amputation or en-bloc resection, most workers currently prefer to recommend irradiation (22, 34, 35, 66, 73, 74, 76). Mutilating operations do not seem justified in patients who have such a short anticipated survival, and are an unnecessary strain on the patient. The entire bone and surrounding soft tissues should be irradiated. Ewing's sarcoma is radiosensitive, but substantial doses are required to avoid local recurrences.

Since patients presenting with localized disease die not of their primary tumor but of subsequent disseminated disease, a great deal of effort is now devoted to the prevention of this course of events. It is assumed that the disease is already disseminated at diagnosis, if not clinically, at least microscopically. Clinical trials are now in progress to examine the possibility of eradicating these subclinical metastases by adjuvant chemotherapy (22, 39, 31-33, 36, 73, 74), total-body irradiation (35, 37), or prophylactic irradiation of both lung fields (36) at the time of diagnosis. Preliminary reports have already indicated a beneficial effect of adjuvant chemotherapy on survival and quality of life (29, 31-33, 73, 74). One author also recommends prophylactic irradiation of the brain to prevent recurrences in the CNS (29, 30, 73).

(ii) Disseminated Ewing's Sarcoma

As more effective cytotoxic agents become available it is anticipated that the management of Ewing's sarcoma will become more aggressive, using combination chemotherapy and radiotherapy (32, 38, 66, 76) and aiming at long-term control of the disease rather than palliation only.

C. SOFT-TISSUE SARCOMAS

Soft-tissue sarcomas are tumors of supporting tissue other than the skeleton. They make up less than 1% of all malignant tumors, occur at all ages and can involve almost any part of the body (39, 40).

They are classified histologically according to the tissue they most resemble. There are about 20 varieties, originating from nonepithelial, nonosseous and nonlymphoid tissues of mesenchymal and nervous origin, each with its own histology and biological behavior, with varying tendencies to local, lymphatic and hematogenous spread. Generally they tend to infiltrate locally beyond the obvious zone of disease and disseminate through the blood stream rather than lymphatics. Approximately 10% of patients already have clinical metastases at the time of diagnosis. Survival rates for most of these tumors are poor (39).

1. Chemotherapy

The treatment of soft-tissue sarcomas with cytotoxic agents has been reviewed by several authors in recent years (3, 5, 40, 41, 81). It is a difficult subject because of the many different histological types and the rarity of these tumors, in addition to the usual problems associated with any review of chemotherapeutic reports. The following agents seem to have some activity: cyclophosphamide (CPM) (44-47), vincristine (VCR) (6, 43), methotrexate (MTX) (48), actinomycin D (ACD), adriamycin (ADM) (3), daunorubicin (DRB) (27, 42), mitomycin C (MTC), and imidazole carboxamide (DIC) (3). The response rates obtained with these agents in rhabdomyosarcoma are given as an example of their effectiveness in soft-tissue sarcomas (Table 33-4). Over half of the patients respond to cyclophosphamide, one-third to VCR, ACD, or MTC, one-quarter to DRB, and one in eight to ADM or DIC. The results with various combinations of these agents in rhabdomyosarcoma are listed in Table 33-5, from which it can be seen that two-thirds of patients respond (77). The most popular combinations for soft-tissue sarcomas contain the most active single agents, namely CPM, VCR, and ACD, in various schedules. In one study, the new combination of ADM and DIC gave a 41% response rate in a variety of metastatic soft-tissue sarcomas (3, 70). A three-drug combination (DIC, ADM, VCR) yielded an overall response rate of 48.5% (70). The addition of cyclophosphamide to DIC, ADM, VCR has further improved the response rate (60% in 82 evaluable patients) (53). No great difference was noted in the response rates between the major histologic variants studied, except for a lesser response in chondrosarcomas and liposarcomas (70).

One sarcoma that deserves special mention because of its unusual sensitivity to chemotherapy is Kaposi's sarcoma. This tumor, although rare in Europe and the United States, is common in many parts of Africa. High response rates have been obtained with actinomycin D alone or in combination with vincristine (54), and with DIC (55), BCNU (56), and bleomycin (56) (Table 33-6). Complete remissions were obtained in 10 out of 14 patients with the combination of ACD and VCR (92).

Table 33-4. Effectiveness of single agents in rhabdomyosarcoma

Drugs	Number evaluated	Number of responses	References
Imidazole carboxamide (DIC)	13[a]	2	GOTTLIEB et al. (3)
Cyclophosphamide,			
intermittent	29[a]	24 (83%)	LIVINGSTON and CARTER (5)
daily	27[a]	9 (33%)	LIVINGSTON and CARTER (5)
total	56[a]	33 (59%)	LIVINGSTON and CARTER (5)
Mitomycin C	11[a]	4	LIVINGSTON and CARTER (5)
Actinomycin D	21[a]	6 (29%)	LIVINGSTON and CARTER (5)
Daunorubicin	10	3	TAN et al. (27)
	13	2	SUTOW et al. (42)
	23	22%	
Adriamycin	16[a]	2 (12,5%)	GOTTLIEB et al. (3)
Vincristine	7	3	SUTOW et al. (43)
	11	3	SELAWRY et al. (6)
	18	6	

[a] Results of several studies combined

2. Strategy

(i) Localized Soft-Tissue Sarcomas

Therapy must be adequate and aggressive when first started since the survival rate is considerably lower if local recurrences are permitted to occur.

Table 33-5. Response rates to combinations in rhabdomyosarcoma

Combination	Number evaluated	Number of responses	Reference
5-FU, VCR	2	1	ENZINGER and SHIRAKI (49)
DIC, ADM	5	3	GOTTLIEB et al. (3)
MPH, ACD	2	1	LINDBERG (50)
ACD, VCR	6	6	JAMES et al. (51)
ACD, VCR	1	0	PRATT et al. (52)
	26	7	HEYN et al. (75)
MTX, CLB, ACD	11	4	GOLBEY (cited in 41)
CPM, ACD, VCR	7	7 (6PR, 1CR)	PRATT et al. (52)
CPM, ACD, VCR	4	3	JACOBS (41)
CPM, ACD, VCR, MTM	1	1	JACOBS (41)
DIC, CPM, ADM, VCR	12	8 (3CR, 5PR)	GOTTLIEB et al. (53)
	51	34 (66%)	

543

Table 33-6. Response rates to chemotherapy in Kaposi's sarcoma

Drugs	Number evaluated	Complete remission	Partial remission	Total response (%)	References
Imidazole carb-oxamide (DIC)	10	3	2	50	VOGEL et al. (55)
BCNU	21	4	5	43	VOGEL et al. (56)
Cyclophosphamide					VOGEL et al. (57)
Actinomycin D	10	4	5	90	VOGEL et al. (54)
Daunorubicin	3	0	0	-	VOGEL et al. (54)
Bleomycin	10	0	6	60	VOGEL et al. (56)
ACD, VCR	14	10	3	92	VOGEL et al. (54)
MOPP (HN2, VCR, PCZ, PDN)	5	0	0		VOGEL et al. (54)

The treatment of soft-tissue sarcomas is primarily by wide local excision; frozen section is used to ensure total removal (79-81). The surgeon must realize that these tumors do not have a true capsule and spread by local extension along tissue planes, often far from any palpable tumor. Amputation may be necessary if the mass cannot be encompassed by wide excision or if the operation would leave a useless extremity without an adequate vascular or neurologic supply. Lymph-node dissection is generally not necessary unless the nodes are involved.

Control of the disease at the primary site remains a serious problem. Local recurrences occur in 60% of cases, and even experienced cancer surgeons have not been able to reduce this figure below 30% (58).

The radiosensitivity of soft-tissue sarcomas varies according to histologic group, and also within each histological type (59, 60, 80). Radiotherapy may have an adjunctive role in the treatment of the primary tumor, but randomized studies are needed to prove that preoperative radiotherapy is genuinely better than surgery alone. Postoperative irradiation is indicated if residual microscopic disease is left behind. Radical radiotherapy may be indicated if surgery is refused by the patient or medically contraindicated.

The high recurrence rates after primary therapy indicate the need for adjuvant chemotherapy and/or immunotherapy studies (82).

As mentioned earlier, local recurrences are common, occurring in 30-60% of cases. Approximately 55% are noted within one year, 85% within two years of primary treatment. Locally recurrent sarcoma behaves more aggressively than the primary tumor and the prognosis is less favorable. At least 65% of patients with local recurrences develop distant metastases. Local recurrences are treated with further surgery and/or radiotherapy.

The CCSGA has already proven the value of adjuvant combination chemotherapy (ACD + VCR) for 1 year in preventing growth of metastatic or recurrent disease when children with rhabdomyosarcoma are made grossly tumor-free by surgery and radiotherapy (75).

(ii) Advanced and Disseminated Soft-Tissue Sarcomas

Surgery, for example amputation, may still be indicated, because of bleeding, pain, or odor, for a local tumor that cannot be palliated by drug therapy. A surgical approach is sometimes justified for solitary metastases, for instance in the lungs.

Radiotherapy offers worthwhile palliation (59). Combination chemotherapy with CPM, VCR, ACD, or ADM + DIC is recommended for widely disseminated disease (53, 61, 69, 81).

REFERENCES

1. LEWIS, R.J., LOTZ, M.J.: Medullary extension of osteosarcoma. Implications for rational therapy. Cancer 33, 371 (1974).
2. JAFFE, N.: Recent advances in the chemotherapy of metastatic osteogenic sarcoma. Cancer 30, 1627 (1972).
3. GOTTLIEB, J.A., BAKER, L.H., QUAGLIANA, J.M., LUCE, J.K., WHITECAR, J.P., SINKOVICS, J.G., RIVKIN, S.E., BROWNLEE, R., FREI, E.III: Chemotherapy of sarcomas with a combination of adriamycin and dimethyl triazeno imidazole carboxamide. Cancer 30, 1632 (1972).
4. SUTOW, W.W., VIETTI, T.J., FERNBACH, D.J., LANE, D.M., DONALDSON, M.H., LONSDALE, D.: Evaluation of chemotherapy in children with metastatic Ewing's sarcoma and osteogenic sarcoma. Cancer Chemother. Rep. 55, 67 (1971).
5. LIVINGSTON, R.B., CARTER, S.K.: Single Agents in Cancer Chemotherapy. New York: IFI/Plenum 1970.
6. SELAWRY, O.S., HOLLAND, J.F., WOLMAN, I.J.: Effect of vincristine (NSC-67574) on malignant solid tumors in children. Cancer Chemother. Rep. 52, 497 (1968).
7. ROSEN, G., SUWANSIRIKUL, S., KWON, C., TAN, C., WU, S.U., BEATTIE, E.J., MURPHY, M.L.: High-dose methotrexate with citrovorum factor rescue and adriamycin in childhood osteogenic sarcoma. Cancer 33, 1151 (1974).
8. JAFFE, N., TRAGGIS, D., ENRIQUEZ, C.: Evaluation of a combination of mitomycin C (NSC-26980), phenylalanine mustard (NSC-14210), and vincristine (NSC-67574) in the treatment of osteogenic sarcoma. Cancer Chemother. Rep. 55, 189 (1971).
9. ROSEN, G., TAN, C., SANMANEECHAI, A., BEATTIE, E.J., MARCOVE, R., MURPHY, M.L.: The rationale for multiple drug chemotherapy in the treatment of osteogenic sarcoma. Cancer 35, 936 (1975).
10. WILBUR, J.R., ETCUBANAS, E., LONG, T., GLATSTEIN, E., LEAVITT, T.: Drug therapy and irradiation in primary and metastatic osteogenic sarcoma. Proc. Amer. Ass. Cancer Res. 15, 188 (1974).
11. SWEETNAM, R., KNOWELDEN, J., SEDDON, H.: Bone sarcoma: Treatment by irradiation, amputation, or a combination of the two. Brit. med. J. 2, 363 (1971).
12. CACERES, E., ZAHARIA, M.: Massive preoperative radiation therapy in the treatment of osteogenic sarcoma. Cancer 30, 634 (1972).
13. ALLEN, C.V., STEVENS, K.R.: Preoperative irradiation for osteogenic sarcoma. Cancer 31, 1364 (1973).

14. JENKIN, R.D.T., ALLT, W.E.C., FITZPATRICK, P.J.: Osteosarcoma. An assessment of management with particular reference to primary irradiation and selective delayed amputation. Cancer 30, 393 (1972)
15. CORTES, E.P., HOLLAND, J.F., WANG, J.J., SINKS, L.F., BLOM, J., SENN, H., BANK, A., GLIDEWELL, O.: Amputation and adriamycin in primary osteosarcoma. New Engl. J. Med. 291, 998 (1974).
16. JAFFE, N., FREI, E.III, TRAGGIS, D., BISHOP, Y.: Adjuvant methotrexate and citrovorum factor treatment of osteogenic sarcoma. New Engl. J. Med. 291, 994 (1974).
17. PRATT, C.B., HUTSU, H.O., SHANKS, E.: Cyclic multiple drug adjuvant chemotherapy for osteosarcoma. Proc. Amer. Ass. Cancer Res. 15, 19 (1974).
18. SUTOW, W.W., SULLIVAN, M.P., FERNBACH, D.J., CANGIR, A., GEORGE, S.L.: Adjuvant chemotherapy in primary treatment of osteogenic sarcoma. Cancer 36, 1598 (1975).
19. MARTINI, N., HUVOS, A.G., MIKE, V., MARCOVE, R.C., BEATTIE, E.J.: Multiple pulmonary resections in the treatment of osteogenic sarcoma. Ann. Thoracic Surg. 12, 271 (1971).
20. KADIN, M.E., BENSCH, K.G.: On the origin of Ewing's tumor. Cancer 27, 257 (1971).
21. FALK, S., ALPERT, M.: Five year survival of patients with Ewing's sarcoma. Surg. Gynec. Obstet. 124, 319 (1967).
22. PHILIPS, R.F., HIGINBOTHAM, N.L.: The curability of Ewing's endothelioma of bone in children. J. Pediat. 70, 391 (1967).
23. PALMA, J., GAILANI, S., FREEMAN, A., SINKS, L., HOLLAND, J.F.: Treatment of metastatic Ewing's sarcoma with BCNU. Cancer 30, 909 (1972).
24. SAMUELS, M.L., HOWE, C.D.: Cyclophosphamide in the management of Ewing's sarcoma. Cancer 20, 961 (1967).
25. SENYSZYN, J.J., JOHNSON, R.E., CURRAN, R.E.: Treatment of metastatic Ewing's sarcoma with actinomycin D (NSC-3053). Cancer Chemother. Rep. 54, 103 (1970).
26. KOFMAN, S., PERLIA, C.P., ECONOMOU, S.G.: Mithramycin in the treatment of metastatic Ewing's sarcoma. Cancer 31, 889 (1973).
27. TAN, C., TASAKA, H., YU, K.P., MURPHY, L.M., KARNOFSKY, D.A.: Daunomycin, an antitumor antibiotic, in the treatment of neoplastic disease. Clinical evaluation with special reference to childhood leukemia. Cancer 20, 333 (1967).
28. OLDHAM, R.K., POMEROY, T.C.: Treatment of Ewing's sarcoma with adriamycin (NSC-123127). Cancer Chemother. Rep. 56, 635 (1972).
29. JOHNSON, R.E., POMEROY, T.C.: Integrated therapy for Ewing's sarcoma. Amer. J. Roentgenol. 114, 532 (1972).
30. MARSA, G.W., JOHNSON, R.E.: Altered pattern of metastasis following treatment of Ewing's sarcoma with radiotherapy and adjuvant chemotherapy. Cancer 27, 1051 (1971).
31. HUSTU, H.O., PINKEL, D., PRATT, C.B.: Treatment of clinically localized Ewing's sarcoma with radiotherapy and combination chemotherapy. Cancer 30, 1522 (1972).
32. JAFFE, N., SALLAN, S., TRAGGIS, D., CASSADY, R., WAWTER, G.: Improved outlook for Ewing's sarcoma with combination chemotherapy and radiotherapy. Proc. Amer. Ass. Cancer Res. 15, 184 (1974).
33. ROSEN, G., WOLLNER, N., TAN, C., WU, S.J., HAJDOU, S.I., CHAM, W., D'ANGIO, G.J., MURPHY, M.L.: Disease-free survival in children with Ewing's sarcoma treated with radiation therapy and adjuvant four-drug sequential chemotherapy. Cancer 33, 384 (1974).
34. BOYER, C.W., BRICKNER, T.J., PERRY, R.H.: Ewing's sarcoma. Case against surgery. Cancer 20, 1602 (1967).
35. MILLBURN, L.F., O'GRADY, L., HENDRICKSON, F.R.: Radical radiation therapy and total body irradiation in the treatment of Ewing's sarcoma. Cancer 22, 919 (1968).

36. National Ewing's Sarcoma Study: unpublished data.
37. JENKIN, R.D.T., RIDER, W.D., SONLEY, M.J.: Ewing's sarcoma. Radiology 96, 151 (1970).
38. MARGOLIS, L.W., PHILLIPS, T.L.: Whole-lung irradiation for metastatic tumor. Radiology 93, 1173 (1969).
39. FERRELL, H.W., FRABLE, W.J.: Soft part sarcomas revisited. Review and comparison of a second series. Cancer 30, 475 (1972).
40. SHNIDER, B.I.: Soft-tissue sarcomas. In: Cancer Chemotherapy, Vol. 2, p. 209 (eds. I. Brodsky, S.B. Kahn, J.H. Mayer). New York: Grune and Stratton 1972.
41. JACOBS, E.M.: Combination chemotherapy of metastatic testicular germinal cell tumors and soft part sarcomas. Cancer 25, 324 (1970).
42. SUTOW, W.W., VIETTI, T.J., LONSDALE, D., TALLEY, R.W.: Daunomycin in the treatment of metastatic soft tissue sarcoma in children. Cancer 29, 1291 (1972).
43. SUTOW, W.W., BERRY, D.H., HADDY, T.B., SULLIVAN, M.P., WATKINS, W.L., WINDMILLER, J.: Vincristine sulfate therapy in children with metastatic soft tissue sarcoma. Pediatrics 38, 465 (1966).
44. BERGSAGEL, D., LEVIN, W.: A prelusive clinical trial of cyclophosphamide. Cancer Chemother. Rep. 8, 120 (1960).
45. STEINBERG, J., HADDY, T., PORTER, F., THURMAN, W.G.: Clinical trials with cyclophosphamide in children with soft tissue sarcoma. Cancer Chemother. Rep. 28, 39 (1963).
46. SUTOW, W.W.: Cyclophosphamide (NSC-26271) in Wilms' tumor and rhabdomyosarcoma. Cancer Chemother. Rep. 51, 407 (1967).
47. FINKELSTEIN, J.Z., HITTLE, R.E., HAMMOND, G.D.: Evaluation of a high dose cyclophosphamide regimen in childhood tumors. Cancer 23, 1239 (1969).
48. WILTSHAW, E.: Methotrexate in treatment of sarcomata. Brit. med. J. 2, 142 (1967).
49. ENZINGER, F.M., SHIRAKI, M.: Alveolar rhabdomyosarcoma. An analysis of 110 cases. Cancer 24, 18 (1969).
50. LINDBERG, R.D.: Rhabdomyosarcoma in children: treatment and results. In: Neoplasia in Childhood, p. 209. Chicago: Year Book Publishers 1969.
51. JAMES, Jr., D.H., HUSTU, O., WRENN, E.: Combination actinomycin D-vincristine sulfate chemotherapy of childhood malignant tumors. Proc. Amer. Ass. Cancer Res. 7, 34 (1966).
52. PRATT, C.B., JAMES, Jr., D.H., HOLTON, C.P., PINKEL, D.: Combination therapy including vincristine (NSC-67547) for malignant solid tumors in children. Cancer Chemother. Rep. 52, 489 (1968).
53. GOTTLIEB, J.A., BODEY, G.P., SINKOVICS, J.G., RODRIGUEZ, V., BURGESS, M.A.: An effective new 4-drug combination regimen (CY-VA-DIC) for metastatic sarcomas. Proc. Amer. Ass Cancer Res. 15, 162 (1974).
54. VOGEL, C.L., PRIMACK, A., DHRU, D, et al.: Treatment of Kaposi's sarcoma with a combination of actinomycin D and vincristine: results of a randomized clinical trial. Cancer 31, 1382 (1973).
55. VOGEL, C.L., PRIMACK, A., OWER, R., KYALWAZI, S.K.: Effective treatment of Kaposi's sarcoma with 5-(3,3-dimethyl-1-triazeno)imidazole-4-carboxamide (NSC-45388). Cancer Chemother. Rep. 57, 65 (1973).
56. VOGEL, C.L., CLEMENTS, D., WANUME, A.K., TOYA, T., PRIMACK, A., KYALWAZI, S.: Phase II clinical trials of BCNU (NSC-409962) and bleomycin (NSC-125066) in the treatment of Kaposi's sarcoma. Cancer Chemother. Rep. 57, 325 (1973).
57. VOGEL, C.L., TEMPLETON, C.J., TEMPLETON, A.C. et al. Treatment of Kaposi's sarcoma with actinomycin D and cyclophosphamide: results of a randomized clinical trial. Int. J. Cancer 8, 136 (1971).
58. CANTIN, J., McNEER, G.P., CHU, F.C., BOOHER, R.J.: The problem of local recurrence after treatment of soft tissue sarcoma. Ann. Surg. 168, 47 (1968)
59. PERRY, H., CHU, F.C.H.: Radiation therapy in the palliative management of soft tissue sarcoma. Cancer 15, 179 (1962).

60. McNERR, G.P., CANTIN, J., CHU, F., NICKSON, J.J.: Effectiveness of radiation therapy in the management of sarcoma of the soft somatic tissue. Cancer 22, 391 (1968).
61. MOLANDER, D.W.: Palliative treatment of metastatic tumors of the soft somatic tissues with irradiation and chemotherapy. Amer. J. Roentgenol. 96, 150 (1966).
62. CORTES, E.P., HOLLAND, J.F., WANG, J.J., SINKS, L.F.: Doxorubicin in disseminated osteosarcoma. J. Amer. Med. Ass. 221, 1132 (1972).
63. JAFFE, N., TRAGGIS, D.: Toxicity of high-dose methotrexate (NSC-740) and citrovorum factor (NSC-3590) in osteogenic sarcoma. Cancer Chemother. Rep. Part 3, 6, 31 (1975).
64. ROSEN, G., TEFFT, M., MARTINEZ, A., CHAM, W., MURPHY, M.L.: Combination chemotherapy and radiation in the treatment of metastatic osteogenic sarcoma. Cancer 35, 622 (1975).
65. BEATTIE, E.J., MARTINI, N., ROSEN, G.: The management of pulmonary metastases in children with osteogenic sarcoma with surgical resection combined with chemotherapy. Cancer 35, 618 (1975).
66. KINNEY, T.R., CHUNG, S.M.K.: Advances in the treatment of tumors arising in bone. Semin. Oncol. 1, 47 (1975).
67. GUTIERREZ, M., MARCOVE, M., ROSEN, G.: Four-drug chemotherapy in Ewing's sarcoma: follow-up of prolonged disease-free survival. Proc. Amer. Soc. Clin. Oncol. 17, 268 (1976).
68. CORTES, E.P., HOLLAND, J.F., WANG, J.J., GLIDEWELL, O.: Adriamycin (NSC-123127) in 87 patients with osteosarcoma. Cancer Chemother. Rep. Part 3, 6, 305 (1975).
69. BENJAMIN, R.S., GOTTLIEB, J.A., BAKER, L.O., SINKOVICS, J.G.: CYVADIC vs CYVADACT - a randomized trial of cyclophosphamide, vincristine, and adriamycin, plus dacarbazine, or actinomycin-D in metastatic sarcomas. Proc. Amer. Soc. Clin. Oncol. 17, 256 (1976).
70. GOTTLIEB, J.A.: Combination chemotherapy for metastatic sarcoma. Cancer Chemother. Rep. Part 1, 58, 265 (1974).
71. SUTOW, W.W., FERNANDEZ, C.H., MOUNTAIN, C.F., KING, O.Y., RIVERA, R.L., MUMFORD, D.M.: Multimodal treatment of pulmonary metastases in osteogenic sarcoma. Proc. Am. Ass. Cancer Res. 16, 39 (1975).
72. GROESBECK, H., CUDMORE, J.: Evaluation of 5-fluorouracil in surgical practice. Am. Surg. 29, 683 (1968).
73. POMEROY, T.C., JOHNSON, R.E.: Combined modality therapy of Ewing's sarcoma. Cancer 35, 36 (1975).
74. FERNANDEZ, C.H., LINDBERG, R.D., SUTOW, W.W., SAMUELS, M.L.: Localized Ewing's sarcoma. Treatment and results. Cancer 34, 143 (1974).
75. HEYN, R.M., HOLLAND, R., NEWTON, W.A., TEFFT, M., BRESLOW, N., HARTMANN, J.R.: The role of combined chemotherapy in the treatment of rhabdomyosarcoma in children. Cancer 34, 2128 (1974).
76. JAFFE, N.: The potential of combined modality approaches for the treatment of malignant bone tumors in children. Cancer Treatment Rev. 2, 33 (1975).
77. MAURER, H.M.: Intergroup rhabdomyosarcoma study: progress report. Proc. Amer. Soc. Clin. Oncol. 17, 242 (1976).
78. HANDELSMAN, H., CARTER, S.K.: Current therapies in osteosarcoma. Cancer Treat. Rev. 2, 77 (1975).
79. RANEY, R.B., SCHNAUFER, L., DONALDSON, M.H.: Soft-tissue sarcoma in childhood. Semin. Oncol. 1, 57 (1974).
80. SUIT, H.D., RUSSELL, W.O.: Radiation therapy of soft tissue sarcomas. Cancer 36, 759 (1975).
81. WILBUR, J.R., SUTOW, W.W., SULLIVAN, M.P., GOTTLIEB, J.A.: Chemotherapy of sarcomas. Cancer 36, 765 (1975).
82. TOWNSEND, C.M., EILBER, F.R., MORTON, D.L.: Skeletal and soft tissue sarcomas: results of surgical adjuvant chemotherapy. Proc. Amer. Soc. Clin. Oncol. 17, 265 (1976).

Appendix

MNM	mannomustine
6-MP	6-mercaptopurine, <u>Purinethol</u>
6-MMPR	6-methylmercaptopurine ribonucleotide
MCM	mitoclomine
MPH	melphalan, L-phenylalanine mustard, <u>Alkeran</u>
MTC	mitomycin C, <u>Mutamycin</u>
MTM	mithramycin, <u>Mithracin</u>
MTX	methotrexate, amethopterin, <u>Methotrexate</u>
O,p'DDD	ortho para DDD, <u>Mitotane</u>
Poly-IC	polyinosinic polycytidylic acid
PCZ	N-methylhydrazine, procarbazine, <u>Matulane</u>
PDL	prednisolone
PDN	prednisone
PPB	pipobroman, <u>Vercyte</u>
PDD	cis-platinum diamminodichloride
PPS	piposulfan, <u>Ancyte</u>
PRM	puromycin
QNC	quinacrine, <u>Atabrine</u>
RFC	rufochromomycin
STN	streptonigrin
STZ	streptozotocin
TACE	chlorotrianisene
TEM	triethylene melamine
6-TG	6-thioguanine, <u>Thioguanine</u>
ThioTEPA	triethylene thiophosphoramide, <u>Thiotepa</u>
TIC-mustard	5-(3,3-bis(2-chloroethyl)-1-triazeno)imidazole-4-carboxamide
TMCA	trimethylcolchicinic acid
VCR	vincristine, <u>Oncovin</u>
VLB	vinblastine, <u>Velban</u>
VM-26	EPT, 4'demethyl-epipodophyllotoxin-β-D-thenylidene glucoside
VP-16-203	EPE, 4'demethyl-epipodophyllotoxine-β-D-ethylidene glucoside

Achronyms of Combinations

ABVD	adriamycin, bleomycin, vinblastine, imidazole carboxamide
A-OAP	adriamycin, vincristine, cytosine arabinoside, prednisone
AVmCP	adriamycin, VM 26, cyclophosphamide, prednisone
C.A.F.	cyclophosphamide, adriamycin, fluorouracil
CAVe	CCNU, adriamycin, vinblastine
CHOP	cyclophosphamide, adriamycin, vincristine, prednisone
C.M.F.	cyclophosphamide, methotrexate, fluorouracil
COMB	cyclophosphamide, vincristine, MeCCNU, bleomycin

COMF	cyclophosphamide, vincristine, methotrexate, 5-fluorouracil
COP	cyclophosphamide, vincristine, prednisone
CVP	cyclophosphamide, vincristine, prednisone
CY-VA-DIC	cyclophosphamide, vincristine, adriamycin, imidazole carboxamide
HOP	adriamycin, vincristine, prednisone
MOPP	nitrogen mustard, vincristine, procarbazine, prednisone
POMP	6-mercaptopurine, vincristine, methotrexate, prednisone
V.A.C.	vincristine, actinomycin D, cyclophosphamide
VAMP	vincristine, methotrexate, 6-mercaptopurine, prednisone

ABBREVIATIONS FOR COOPERATIVE GROUPS

ALGB	Acute Leukemia Group B
BTSG	Brain Tumor Study Group
CBCG	Cooperative Breast Cancer Group
CCSGA	Chidren's Cancer Study Group A
COG	Central Oncology Group
ECOG	Eastern Cooperative Oncology Group
EORTC	European Organization for Research on the Treatment of Cancer
NSABP	National Surgical Adjuvant Breast Project
NWTSG	National Wilms' Tumor Study Group
SECSG	Southeastern Cancer Study Group
SWCCG	Southwestern Cancer Chemotherapy Group
VACURG	Veterans Administration Cooperative Urological Research Group

OTHER ABBREVIATIONS USED IN THIS TEXT

Malignant Diseases

ALL	acute lymphoid leukemia
AML	acute myeloid leukemia
AMMoL	acute myelomonocytoid leukemia
AMol	acute monocytoid leukemia
HD	Hodgkin's disease
H + N	head and neck cancers
LS	lymphosarcoma
mLbAL	microlymphoblastic ALL
MLbAL	macrolymphoblastic ALL

PLbAL	prolymphoblastic ALL
PLcAL	prolymphocytic ALL
RS	reticulosarcoma, reticulum cell sarcoma

Others

ACR	apparent complete remission
CNS	central nervous system
CR	complete response, unspecified whether complete remission or complete regression
CRg	complete regression
CRm	complete remission
CRX	chemotherapy
DT	doubling time
F	failure
GF	growth fraction
ICIG	Institut de cancérologie et d'immunogénétique, Villejuif, France
IRX	immunotherapy
IT	intrathecal
NCI	National Cancer Institute
PR	partial response
RR	response rate
TNR	total nodal radiation
XRT	radiotherapy

Subject Index

Recent Results in Cancer Research

Sponsored by the Swiss League against Cancer. Editor in Chief: P. Rentchnick, Genève

Further publications by Georges Mathé

L'aplasie myélo-lymphoide de l'irradiation totale (with J. L. AMIEL). 1 Vol. Paris: Gauthier-Villars 1965.

Bone marrow transplantation and white cell transfusions (with J. L. AMIEL and L. SCHWARZENBERG). 1 Vol. Springfield: Ch. C. Thomas 1971.

Histocytological typing of the neoplastic diseases of the hematopoietic and lymphoid tissues (with H. RAPPAPORT). 1 Vol. Geneva: World Health Organisation, in press 1975.

Cancer Active Immunotherapy, Immunoprophylaxis and Immunorestoration. Recent Results in Cancer Research Vol. 55. Berlin-Heidelberg-New York: Springer Verlag 1976.

Cancerologie (with A. CATTAN) 1 Vol. Paris: Expansion Scientifique, in press.